Pharmacology

made Incredibly Easy!

Fifth Edition

Pharmacology

made Incredibly Easy!

Fifth Edition

Clinical Editors

Cherie R. Rebar, PhD, MBA, RN, CNE, CNEcl, COI, FAADN
Professor of Nursing
Wittenberg University
Springfield, Ohio

Nicole M. Heimgartner, DNP, RN, CNE, CNEcl, COI
Nursing Faculty
Galen College of Nursing
Louisville, Kentucky

Carolyn J. Gersch, PhD, MSN, RN, CNE
Professor of Practice
Wittenberg University
Springfield, Ohio

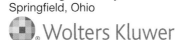

Philadelphia • Baltimore • New York • London
Buenos Aires • Hong Kong • Sydney • Tokyo

Not authorised for sale in United States, Canada, Australia, New Zealand, Puerto Rico, and U.S. Virgin Islands.

Acquisitions Editor: Jamie Blum
Development Editor: Maria M. McAvey
Editorial Coordinator: Christopher Rodgers
Production Project Manager: Bridgett Dougherty
Design Coordinator: Stephen Druding
Manufacturing Coordinator: Kathleen Brown
Marketing Manager: Linda Wetmore
Prepress Vendor: Straive

Fifth edition

9 8 7 6 5 4 3 2 1

Printed in Singapore

Cataloging-in-Publication Data available on request from the Publisher
ISBN: 978-1-9751-7755-3

shop.lww.com

Dedication

For the nurses, nursing students, and other health care heroes on the front lines of COVID-19, thank you for your unwavering commitment to the promises you made to care for others.

For my husband, children, and grandchildren—thank you for your love and support!

Carolyn

For Jeremy, Alayna, and Addison—my sunshine and inspiration.

Nicole

For Michael and Gillian and Flash—I could not possibly love you any more than I do.

Cherie

Contributors

Marie Bashaw, DNP, RN, NEA-BC
Director of Nursing
Wittenberg University
Springfield, Ohio

Gretchen Carolan, MSN, APRN, FNP-BC
Nurse Practitioner
University of Louisville
Louisville, Kentucky

Lorraine Chiappetta, MSN, RN, CNE
Emeritus Professional Faculty
Washtenaw Community College
Ann Arbor, Michigan

Beverly Cobb, PhD, MSN, RN, PMHNP-BC
Psychiatric-Mental Health Nurse
  Practitioner
Kettering Behavioral Medical Center
Kettering, Ohio

Jared Collins, MS, APRN-CNP, ACNPC-AG, CCRN
Critical Care Nurse Practitioner
Mount Carmel Health System
Columbus, Ohio

Keelin Cromar, MSN, RN
Nursing Consultant
Wichita County Public Health District
Wichita Falls, Texas

Carolyn J. Gersch, PhD, MSN, RN, CNE
Professor of Practice
Nursing Program
Wittenberg University
Springfield, Ohio
Educational Strategist
Connect: RN2ED
Beavercreek, Ohio

Stacy Gilson, MSN, RN, CEN, NE-BC
Assistant Professor of Practice
Nursing Resource Center and Simulation
  Lab Coordinator
Wittenberg University
Springfield, Ohio

Charity L. Hacker, MSN-Ed, RN
Assistant Professor
Department of Nursing
Ivy Tech Community College
Madison, Indiana
Adjunct Faculty
Department of Nursing
Indiana University–Purdue University
  Columbus
Columbus, Indiana

Nicole M. Heimgartner, DNP, RN, CNE, CNEcl, COI
Nursing Faculty
Galen College of Nursing
Louisville, Kentucky
Educational Strategist
Connect: RN2ED
Beavercreek, Ohio

Katherine Marie Hendricks, MSN, APRN,
FNP-C, AGACNP-BC
Trauma/Acute Surgery Nurse Practitione
Critical Care Medicine
Wake Forest Baptist Medical Center
Winston Salem, North Carolina

Hannah Lopez, MSN, RN, OCN, CBCN
Clinical Nurse Manager
Hematology/Oncology & Supportive
  Palliative Care
Baylor Scott & White Health
Round Rock, Texas

Melanie DeGonzague Luttrell, DNP, MSN,
APRN, AGPCNP-BC
Certified Nurse Practitioner
Internal Medicine
The Christ Hospital Medical Associates
Cincinnati, Ohio

Abby Pippin, MSN, RN, CNP
Family Nurse Practitioner
Matrix Medical
Washington Courthouse, Ohio

Cherie R. Rebar, PhD, MBA, RN, CNE, CNEcl, COI, FAADN
Professor of Nursing
Wittenberg University
Springfield, Ohio
Educational Strategist
Connect: RN2ED
Beavercreek, Ohio

Jeffrey W. Schultz, MS, APRN, ACNP-BC, CCNS, CV-BC, CCRN-CSC, CEN, NE-BC, NR-P
Senior APP-CVICU
Cardiothoracic Surgery
North Florida Regional Medical Center
Flight Nurse
University of Florida Health
ShandsCair Critical Care Transport Program
Gainesville, Florida

Russell N. Ludwig Worthen, MSN, AGACNP-BC, FNP-C
Critical Care Nurse Practitioner
Critical Care Medicine
Wake Forest Baptist Medical Center
Winston Salem, North Carolina

Michelle Yeager, MSN, APRN, NP-C
Assistant Professor of Practice
Wittenberg University
Springfield, Ohio
Nurse Practitioner
Community Emergency Medicine Partners
Washington Courthouse, Ohio

Previous Edition Contributors

Adair Lattimer, DNP, RN

Amy Beckmann, CMN

Charity L. Hacker, MSN-Ed, RN

Emily Sheff, MSN, CMSRN, FNP-BC

Katrin Moskowitz, DNP, APRN

Margaret M. Gingrich, CRNP

Sarah Clark, RN, BA

Sharon Wing, PhDc, RN, CNL

Tracy Taylor, MSN, RN

Victoria Wilson, RN

Foreword

Let's cut right to the chase about why this book is so useful:

1. It emphasizes the important things you need to know about nursing pharmacology.
2. It helps you remember what you've learned.
3. It builds your confidence while enhancing your knowledge, skills, and clinical judgment.

Special logos highlight important points:

Prototype pro—details actions, indications, and nursing considerations for common prototype drugs.

Pharm function—explains and illustrates the way drugs act in the body.

Before you give that drug—alerts you to important drug warnings that should be considered before administration.

Education edge—provides important information you should share with your patient.

Look for Nurse Joy, Nurse Jake, and the other individuals or characters in the margins throughout this book. They will be there to explain key concepts, provide important care reminders, offer reassurance, and teach in a way that no other resource can. Also, take note of three *new* special features: 🅱️ *Black Box Warning* boxes draw attention to life-threatening concerns. 🔧 *Pharm Fact Alert* boxes feature key information about a specific drug or class of drugs that the nurse should remember. 💡 *Lifespan Lightbulb* boxes highlight information about how a drug or drug class may affect patients of different ages.

- A three-step process is provided throughout the chapters to help you care for individuals taking commonly prescribed medications.
- Preparing for Practice boxes emphasize special concerns about medications that may cause harm to patients
- In addition to the end-of-chapter questions, Practice Makes Perfect helps you practice NCLEX style questions.

We hope you find this book helpful, and we wish you the very best as you continue providing safe, effective, compassionate nursing care.

Cherie R. Rebar, PhD, MBA, RN, CNE, CNEcl, COI, FAADN
Nicole M. Heimgartner, DNP, RN, CNE, CNEcl, COI
Carolyn J. Gersch, PhD, MSN, RN, CNE

Contents

Chapter 1

Fundamentals of nursing pharmacology

Just the facts

In this chapter, you'll learn:

♦ pharmacology basics

♦ key concepts of pharmacokinetics, pharmacodynamics, and pharmacotherapeutics

♦ key types of drug interactions and adverse reactions

♦ priority patient needs.

Pharmacology basics

Pharmacology is the scientific study of the origin, nature, chemistry, effects, and uses of drugs. Drugs are chemicals that are used to cause an effect on the body (Karch, 2020). Knowledge about drugs and how they affect the body is essential to providing safe medication administration to your patients.

The big three

This chapter reviews the three basic concepts of pharmacology:
1. pharmacokinetics—the movement of drugs through the body: absorption, distribution, metabolism, and excretion
2. pharmacodynamics—the biochemical and physical effects of drugs and the mechanisms of drug actions on the body
3. pharmacotherapeutics—the use of drugs to prevent and treat diseases.

In addition, it discusses other important aspects of pharmacology, including:
- how drugs are named and classified
- how drugs are derived
- how drugs are administered
- how new drugs are developed.

Naming and classifying drugs

Drugs have a specific kind of nomenclature—that is, a drug can go by three different names:
- The *chemical name* is a scientific name that describes the drug's atomic and molecular structure.
- The *generic*, or *nonproprietary*, *name* is an abbreviation of the chemical name.
- The *trade name* (also known as the *brand name* or *proprietary name*) is selected by the drug company selling the product. Trade names are protected by copyright. The symbol® after a trade name indicates that the name is registered by and restricted to the drug manufacturer.
To avoid confusion, it's best to use a drug's generic name because any one drug can have a number of trade names.

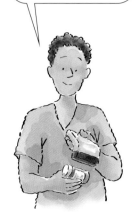

Drugs may have many different trade names. To avoid confusion, refer to a drug by its generic name.

Making it official

In 1962, the federal government mandated the use of official names so that only one official name would represent each drug. The official names are listed in the *United States Pharmacopeia* and *National Formulary (USP-NF) (2020)*.

Classifications

Drugs that share similar characteristics are grouped together as a *pharmacologic class* (or family). Beta-adrenergic blockers are an example of a pharmacologic class, because all drugs in that class perform in the same way.

A second type of drug grouping is the *therapeutic class*, which categorizes drugs by therapeutic use. Antihypertensives are an example of a therapeutic class, because all drugs in that class are used to treat hypertension.

A pharmacologic class groups drugs by their shared characteristics. A therapeutic class groups drugs by their therapeutic use.

Where drugs come from

Traditionally, drugs were derived from *natural* sources, such as plants, animals, or minerals. In addition to natural sources, laboratory researchers use traditional knowledge and chemical science to develop *synthetic* drug sources. Synthetic drugs are free from the impurities found in natural substances. Researchers and drug developers can manipulate the molecular structure of substances so that a slight change in the chemical structure makes the drug effective against different organisms.

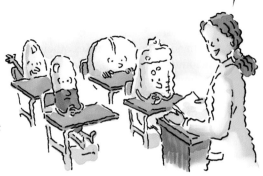

For example, cephalosporins have been manipulated at different times to be more effective and are now known as first-, second-, third-, fourth-, or fifth-generation cephalosporins.

Sowing the seeds of drugs

The earliest drug concoctions from plants used everything: the leaves, roots, bulb, stem, seeds, buds, and blossoms. As a result, harmful substances often found their way into the mixture.

Reaping the rewards of research

As the understanding of plants as drug sources became more sophisticated, researchers sought to isolate and intensify *active components* while avoiding harmful ones. The active components of plants vary in character and effect:

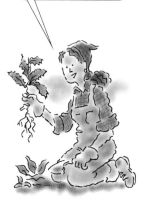

Active components of plant sources include alkaloids, glycosides, gums, resins, and oils.

- *Alkaloids*, the most active component in plants, react with acids to form a salt that's able to dissolve more readily in body fluids. The names of alkaloids and their salts usually end in "-ine"; examples include atropine, caffeine, and nicotine.
- *Glycosides* are naturally occurring active components that are found in plants and have both beneficial and toxic effects. They usually have names that end in "-in," such as digoxin.
- *Gums* give products the ability to attract and hold water. Examples include seaweed extractions and seeds with starch.
- *Resins*, of which the chief source is pine tree sap, commonly act as local irritants or as laxatives and caustic agents.
- *Oils*, thick and sometimes greasy liquids, are classified as volatile or fixed. Examples of volatile oils, which readily evaporate, include peppermint, spearmint, and juniper. Fixed oils, which aren't easily evaporated, include castor oil and olive oil.

Aid from animals

The body fluids or glands of animals are also natural drug sources. The drugs obtained from animal sources include:

- *hormones*, such as insulin
- *oils* and *fats* (usually fixed), such as cod liver oil
- *enzymes*, which are produced by living cells and act as catalysts, such as pancreatin and pepsin
- *vaccines*, which are suspensions of killed, modified, or attenuated microorganisms; certain vaccines require the use of chicken eggs for creation.

Minerals

Metallic and nonmetallic minerals provide various inorganic materials not available from plants or animals. Mineral sources are used as they occur in nature or they're combined with other ingredients. Examples of drugs that contain minerals are iron, iodine, and Epsom salts.

Lab production

Today, most drugs are produced in laboratories. Examples of such drugs include thyroid hormone (from natural sources) and cimetidine (from synthetic sources).

DNA paving the way

Recombinant deoxyribonucleic acid (DNA) research has led to another chemical source of organic compounds. For example, the reordering of genetic information enables scientists to develop bacteria that produce insulin for humans.

How drugs are administered

A drug's administration route influences the quantity given and the rate at which the drug is absorbed and distributed. These variables affect the drug's action and the patient's response.

Buccal, sublingual, and translingual

Certain drugs are given buccally (in the pouch between the cheek and teeth), sublingually (under the tongue), or translingually (on the tongue) to prevent their destruction or transformation in the stomach or small intestine.

Gastric

The gastric route allows direct administration of a drug into the GI system. This route is used when patients can't ingest the drug orally. This route is accessed through a tube placed directly into the GI system, such as a "G-tube."

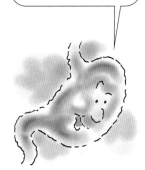

Looks like I need to get involved here. The gastric route is used when a patient can't ingest a drug orally.

Intradermal

In intradermal administration, drugs are injected into the skin. A needle is inserted at a 10- to 15-degree angle so that it punctures only the skin's surface. This form of administration is used mainly for diagnostic purposes, such as testing for allergies or tuberculosis.

Intramuscular

The IM route allows drugs to be injected directly into various muscle groups. This form of administration provides rapid systemic action and allows for absorption of relatively large doses (up to 3 mL). Aqueous suspensions, solutions in oil, and drugs that aren't available in oral forms are given IM.

Intravenous

The IV route allows injection of drugs and other substances directly into the bloodstream through a vein. Appropriate substances to administer IV include drugs, fluids, blood or blood products, and diagnostic contrast agents. Administration can range from a single dose to an ongoing infusion.

Oral

Oral administration is usually the safest, most convenient, and least expensive route. Oral drugs are administered to patients who are conscious and able to swallow.

Rectal and vaginal

Suppositories, ointments, creams, or gels may be instilled into the rectum or vagina to treat local irritation or infection. Some drugs applied to the mucosa of the rectum or vagina can also be absorbed systemically.

Respiratory

Drugs that are available as gases can be administered into the respiratory system through inhalation. These drugs are rapidly absorbed. In addition, some of these drugs can be self-administered by devices such as the metered-dose inhaler. The respiratory route is also used in emergencies, such as to administer drugs directly into the lungs via an endotracheal tube.

Subcutaneous

In subcutaneous administration, small amounts of a drug are injected beneath the dermis and into the subcutaneous tissue, usually in the patient's upper arm, thigh, or abdomen. This allows the drug to move into the bloodstream more rapidly than if given by mouth. Drugs given by the subcutaneous route include nonirritating aqueous solutions and suspensions contained in up to 1 mL of fluid, such as heparin and insulin.

Topical

The topical route is used to deliver a drug via the skin or a mucous membrane. This route is used for most dermatologic, ophthalmic, otic, and nasal preparations.

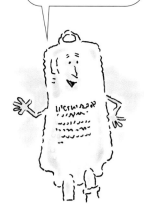

Talk about going with the flow! IV administration puts substances right into the bloodstream.

Specialized infusions

Drugs may also be given as specialized infusions. These are given directly to a specific site in the patient's body. Specific types of infusions include:

- epidural—into the epidural space
- intrapleural—into the pleural cavity
- intraperitoneal—into the peritoneal cavity
- intraosseous—into the rich vascular network of a long bone
- intra-articular—into a joint
- intrathecal—into the spinal canal.

New drug development

Newly identified chemical compounds (a new drug) must undergo a rigorous process involving systematic scientific research controlled by the U.S. Food and Drug Administration (FDA) (FDA, 2020). (See *Phases of new drug development.*)

> Drugs are primarily developed by systematic scientific research conducted under FDA guidelines.

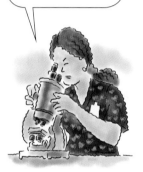

Phases of new drug development

Once a drug has been identified, it will be tested in the lab (preclinical trials); then, it will go through four phases.

Preclinical trials
The drug continues to be tested in the laboratory and on living animals.

Phase I
In phase I, the drug is tested on healthy volunteers to make sure that the drug can be given safely to people.

Phase II
Phase II involves trials with human subjects who have the disease for which the drug is thought to be effective.

Phase III
Large numbers of patients in medical research centers receive the drug in phase III. This larger sampling provides information about infrequent or rare adverse effects. The FDA approves a new drug application if phase III studies are satisfactory.

Phase IV
Phase IV is voluntary and involves postmarket surveillance of the drug's therapeutic effects at the completion of phase III. The pharmaceutical company receives obligatory reports from prescribers and other health care professionals about the therapeutic results and adverse effects of the drug. Some drugs, for example, have been found to be toxic and have been removed from the market after their initial release.

On the FDA fast track

Although most new drugs undergo all four phases of clinical evaluation mandated by the FDA, some can receive expedited approval. Because of the public health threat posed by severe acute respiratory syndrome coronavirus 2 (SARS-CoV-2, known as COVID-19), the FDA has shortened the approval process for certain drugs and provided Emergency Use Authorization (EUA) for others. The FDA also determines the safety and efficacy of drugs that can be purchased without a prescription. (See *Cheaper and easier.*)

Pharmacokinetics

The term *kinetics* refers to movement. Pharmacokinetics describes a drug's actions as it moves through the body and what the body does to the drug. Therefore, pharmacokinetics discusses how a drug is:

- absorbed (taken into the body)
- distributed (moved into various tissues)
- metabolized (changed into a form that can be excreted)
- excreted (removed from the body).

This branch of pharmacology is also concerned with a drug's onset of action, peak concentration level, and duration of action.

Absorption

Drug absorption covers the progress of a drug from the time it's administered, through the time it passes to the tissues, until it becomes available for use by the body.

How drugs are absorbed

On a cellular level, drugs are absorbed by several means—primarily through active or passive transport.

Passive transport

Passive transport requires no cellular energy because the drug moves from an area of higher concentration to one of lower concentration (diffusion). It occurs when small molecules diffuse across membranes. Diffusion stops when the drug concentrations on both sides of the membrane are equal. Oral drugs use passive transport; they move from higher concentrations in the GI tract to lower concentrations in the bloodstream.

Cheaper and easier

The phrases "over the counter" and "nonprescription medicine" refer to drugs that can be purchased without a prescription. The FDA determines safety and efficacy of these drugs and provides approval for over-the-counter use, increasing accessibility while decreasing cost to consumers. These drugs are acknowledged to be safe and effective when used as directed on the label (Food and Drug Administration, 2018). Examples include GI medications (such as cimetidine), antihistamines (such as loratadine), analgesics (like acetaminophen), and topical antibiotics (like triple-antibiotics for skin abrasions).

Active transport

Active transport requires cellular energy to move the drug from an area of lower concentration to one of higher concentration. Active transport is used to absorb electrolytes, such as sodium and potassium, as well as some drugs, such as levodopa.

Pinocytosis

Pinocytosis is a unique form of active transport that occurs when a cell engulfs a drug particle. Pinocytosis is commonly employed to transport the fat-soluble vitamins (A, D, E, and K).

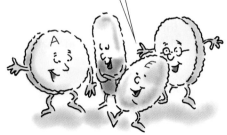

We're fat-soluble, which means we're absorbed through pinocytosis.

Factors affecting absorption

Various factors—such as the route of administration, the amount of blood flow, and the form of the drug— can affect the rate of a drug's absorption.

Cellular layers

If only a few cells separate the active drug from systemic circulation, absorption occurs rapidly and the drug quickly reaches therapeutic levels in the body. Typically, drug absorption occurs within seconds or minutes when administered sublingually, IV, or by inhalation.

Slow but steady

Absorption occurs at slower rates when drugs are administered by the oral, IM, or subcutaneous routes because the complex membrane systems of GI mucosal layers, muscle, and skin delay drug passage.

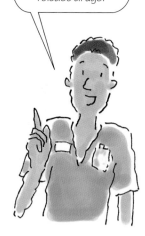

Sublingual, IV, or inhaled drugs are usually absorbed much faster than rectally adminis-tered or sustained-release drugs.

Slow absorption

At the slowest absorption rates, drugs can take several hours or days to reach peak concentration levels. A slow rate usually occurs with rectally administered or sustained-release drugs.

Intestinal interference

Several other factors can affect absorption of a drug. For example, most absorption of oral drugs occurs in the small intestine. If a patient has had large sections of the small intestine surgically removed, drug absorption decreases because of the reduced surface area and the reduced time the drug is in the intestine.

Liver-lowered levels

Drugs absorbed by the small intestine are transported to the liver before being circulated to the rest of the body. The liver may metabolize much of the drug before it enters circulation. This mechanism is referred to as the *first-pass effect*. Liver metabolism may inactivate the drug; if so, the first-pass effect lowers the amount of active drug released into the systemic circulation. Therefore, higher drug dosages must be administered to achieve the desired effect.

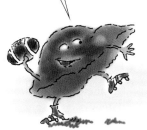

Watch out for my first-pass effect! It lowers the amount of active drug released into the systemic circulation.

More blood, more absorption

Increased blood flow to an absorption site improves drug absorption, whereas reduced blood flow decreases absorption. More rapid absorption leads to a quicker onset of drug action.

For example, the muscle area selected for IM administration can make a difference in the drug absorption rate. Blood flows faster through the deltoid muscle (in the upper arm) than through the gluteal muscle (in the buttocks). The gluteal muscle, however, can accommodate a larger volume of drug than the deltoid muscle.

More pain, more stress, less drug

Pain and stress can also decrease the amount of drug absorbed. This may be due to a change in blood flow, reduced movement through the GI tract, or gastric retention triggered by the autonomic nervous system's response to pain.

Does eating matter?

High-fat meals and solid foods slow the rate at which contents leave the stomach and enter the intestines, delaying intestinal absorption of a drug.

Form factors

Drug formulation (such as tablets, capsules, liquids, sustained-release formulas, inactive ingredients, and coatings) affects the drug absorption rate and the time needed to reach peak blood concentration levels. For example, enteric coated drugs are specifically formulated so that they don't dissolve immediately in the stomach. Rather, they release in the small intestine. Liquid forms, however, are readily absorbed in the stomach and at the beginning of the small intestine.

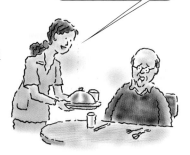

Watch what your patient eats. High-fat meals and solid food can delay intestinal absorption of a drug.

Combo considerations

Combining one drug with another drug or with food can cause interactions that increase or decrease drug absorption, depending on the substances involved.

Distribution

Drug distribution is the process by which the drug is delivered to the tissues and fluids of the body. Distribution of an absorbed drug within the body depends on several factors, including:
- blood flow
- solubility
- protein binding.

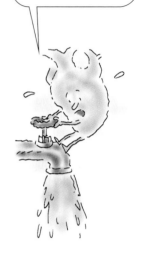

Having a large blood supply, like I do, means drugs flow quickly toward me. Let's keep that flow going!

Blood flow

After a drug has reached the bloodstream, its distribution in the body depends on blood flow. The drug is distributed quickly to those organs with a large supply of blood, including the heart, liver, and kidneys. Distribution to other internal organs, skin, fat, and muscle is slower.

Breaching the barrier

The ability of a drug to cross a cell membrane depends on whether the drug is water or lipid (fat) soluble. Lipid-soluble drugs easily cross through cell membranes, whereas water-soluble drugs can't. Lipid-soluble drugs can also cross the blood-brain barrier and enter the brain.

Protein binding

As a drug travels through the body, it comes in contact with proteins, such as the plasma protein albumin. The drug can remain free or bind to the protein. The portion of a drug that's bound to a protein is inactive and can't exert a therapeutic effect. Only the free, or unbound, portion remains active. A drug is said to be *highly protein-bound* if more than 80% of it binds to protein.

Metabolism

Drug metabolism, or *biotransformation*, refers to the body's ability to change a drug from its dosage form to a more water-soluble form that can then be excreted. Drugs can be metabolized in several ways:
- Most commonly, a drug is metabolized into inactive metabolites (products of metabolism), which are then excreted.
- Some drugs can be converted to active metabolites, meaning they're capable of exerting their own pharmacologic action. These metabolites may undergo further metabolism or may be excreted from the body unchanged.
- Other drugs can be administered as inactive drugs, called *prodrugs*, and don't become active until they're metabolized.

Where the magic happens

Most drugs are metabolized by enzymes in the liver; however, metabolism can also occur in the plasma, kidneys, and membranes of the intestines. Some drugs inhibit or compete for enzyme metabolism, which can cause the accumulation of drugs when they're given together. This accumulation increases the potential for an adverse reaction or drug toxicity.

Metabolism busters

Certain diseases can reduce metabolism. These include liver disease, such as cirrhosis, and heart failure, which reduces circulation to the liver.

In the genes

Genetics allow some people to be able to metabolize drugs rapidly, whereas others metabolize them more slowly.

Environmental effects

The environment can alter drug metabolism. For example, if a person is surrounded by cigarette smoke, the rate of metabolism of some drugs may be affected. A stressful environment, such as one involving prolonged illness or surgery, can also change how a person metabolizes drugs.

Age alterations

Developmental changes can also affect drug metabolism. For example, infants have immature livers that reduce the rate of metabolism, and older adults experience a decline in liver size, blood flow, and enzyme production that also slows metabolism.

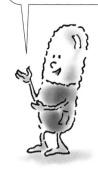

Although most drugs are metabolized in the liver, metabolism can also occur in the plasma, kidneys, and intestines.

Excretion

Drug excretion refers to the elimination of drugs from the body. Most drugs are excreted by the kidneys and leave the body through urine. Drugs can also be excreted through the lungs, exocrine glands (sweat, salivary, or mammary glands), skin, and intestinal tract.

Half in and half out

The half-life of a drug is the time it takes for the plasma concentration of a drug to fall to half its original value—in other words, the time it takes for one half of the drug to be eliminated by the body. Factors that affect a drug's half-life include its rates of absorption, metabolism, and excretion. Knowing how long a drug remains in the body helps determine how frequently a drug should be taken.

A drug that's given only once is eliminated from the body almost completely after four or five half-lives. A drug that's administered at regular intervals, however, reaches a steady concentration (or *steady state*) after about four or five half-lives. Steady state occurs when the rate of drug administration equals the rate of drug excretion.

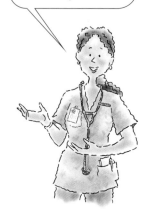

A drug's half-life is the time it takes for its plasma concentration to drop to its original value.

Onset, peak, and duration

In addition to absorption, distribution, metabolism, and excretion, three other factors play important roles in a drug's pharmacokinetics:
- onset of action
- peak concentration
- duration of action.

Action!

Onset of action refers to the time interval that starts when the drug is administered and ends when the therapeutic effect actually begins. Rate of onset varies depending on the route of administration and other pharmacokinetic properties.

Peak performance!

As the body absorbs more drugs, blood concentration levels rise. The peak concentration level is reached when the absorption rate equals the elimination rate. However, the time of peak concentration isn't always the time of peak response.

How long will it last?

The duration of action is the length of time the drug produces its therapeutic effect.

Pharmacodynamics

Pharmacodynamics is the study of the drug and body mechanisms that produce biochemical or physiologic changes in the body. The interaction at the cellular level between a drug and cellular components, such as the complex proteins that make up the cell membrane, enzymes, or target receptors, represents *drug action*. The response resulting from this drug action is called the *drug effect*.

Fooling with function

A drug can modify cell function or the rate of function, but a drug can't impart a new function to a cell or target tissue. Therefore, the drug effect depends on what the cell is capable of accomplishing.

A drug can alter the target cell's function by:

- modifying the cell's physical or chemical environment
- interacting with a receptor (a specialized location on a cell membrane or inside a cell).

> A drug's action refers to the interaction between the drug and the body's cellular components. Pleased to meet you!

Agonist: Stimulating response

An *agonist* is an example of a drug that interacts with receptors. An agonist drug has an attraction, or affinity, for a receptor and stimulates it. The drug then binds with the receptor to produce its effect. The drug's ability to initiate a response after binding with the receptor is referred to as *intrinsic activity*.

Antagonist: Preventing response

If a drug has an affinity for a receptor but displays little or no intrinsic activity, it's called an *antagonist*. The antagonist prevents a response from occurring.

Antagonists can be competitive or noncompetitive:

- A *competitive antagonist* competes with the agonist for receptor sites. Because this type of drug binds reversibly to the receptor site, administering large doses of an agonist can overcome the antagonist's effects.
- A *noncompetitive antagonist* binds to receptor sites and blocks the effects of the agonist. Administering large doses of the agonist can't reverse its action.

Not so choosy

If a drug acts on a variety of receptors, it's said to be *nonselective* and can cause multiple and widespread effects.

Potency

Drug potency refers to the relative amount of a drug required to produce a desired response. Drug potency is also used to compare two drugs. If drug X produces the same response as drug Y but at a lower dose, then drug X is more potent than drug Y.

Dose–response curve

As its name implies, a dose-response curve is used to graphically represent the relationship between the dose of a drug and the response it produces. (See *Dose-response curve*, page 14.)

On the dose-response curve, a low dose usually corresponds with a low response. At a low dose, an increase in dose produces only a slight increase in response. With further increases in dose, there's a marked rise in drug response. After a certain point, an increase in dose yields little or no increase in response. At this point, the drug is said to have reached *maximum effectiveness*.

Dose-response curve

This graph shows the dose-response curve for two different drugs. As you can see, at low doses of each drug, a dosage increase results in only a small increase in drug response (for example, from point A to point B). At higher doses, an increase in dosage produces a much greater response (from point B to point C). As the dosage continues to climb, an increase in dose produces very little increase in response (from point C to point D).

This graph also shows that drug X is more potent than drug Y because it results in the same response, but at a lower dose (compare point A to point E).

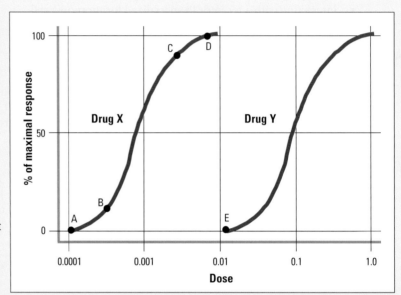

From desired effect to dangerous dose

Most drugs produce multiple effects. The relationship between a drug's desired therapeutic effects and its adverse (toxic) effects is called the drug's *therapeutic index* (U.S. National Library of Medicine, n.d.).

The therapeutic index usually measures the difference between:
- an effective dose for 50% of the patients treated
- the minimal dose at which adverse (toxic) reactions occur.

A drug's *margin of safety* is the ratio of the toxic dose to 1% of the population to the dose that is an effective dose to 99% of the population.

The lowdown on a low index

A drug with a low or narrow therapeutic index has a narrow range of safety between an effective dose and a lethal one. On the other hand, a drug with a high therapeutic index has a wide range of safety and less risk of toxic effects.

Pharmacotherapeutics

Pharmacotherapeutics is the use of drugs to treat disease or symptoms. When choosing a drug to treat a particular condition, health care providers consider the drug's effectiveness, cost, and availability in relation to the patient's condition.

Drug therapy

The type of therapy prescribed depends on the severity, urgency, and prognosis of the patient's condition. Therapy types include:
- *acute therapy*, if the patient is critically ill and requires acute intensive therapy
- *empiric therapy*, based on practical experience rather than on pure scientific data
- *maintenance therapy*, for patients with chronic conditions that don't resolve
- *supplemental* or *replacement therapy*, which replenishes or substitutes missing substances in the body
- *supportive therapy*, which doesn't treat the cause of the disease but maintains other threatened body systems until the patient's condition resolves
- *palliative therapy*, therapies used to improve the patient's and their family's quality of life when the patient is faced with life-threatening conditions (World Health Organization, 2020).

It's all personal

A patient's overall health as well as other individual factors can alter the drug response. Coinciding medical conditions and personal lifestyle characteristics must also be considered when selecting drug therapy. (See *Factors affecting patient response to a drug.*)

Decreased response...

Certain drugs have a tendency to create drug tolerance and drug dependence in patients. *Drug tolerance* occurs when a patient has a decreased response to a drug over time. The patient then requires larger doses to produce the same response.

... and increased desire

Tolerance differs from *drug dependence*, in which a patient displays a physical or psychological need for the drug. Physical dependence produces withdrawal symptoms when the drug is stopped, whereas psychological dependence is based on a desire to continue taking the drug to relieve tension and avoid discomfort.

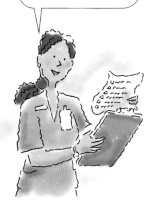

When reviewing patient's ordered medication, also be sure to review coinciding medical conditions and lifestyle.

Drug interactions

Drug interactions can occur between drugs or between drugs and foods. They can interfere with the results of a laboratory test or produce physical or chemical incompatibilities. The more drugs a patient receives, the greater the chances are that a drug interaction will occur.

Potential drug interactions include:

- additive effects
- potentiation
- antagonistic effects
- decreased or increased absorption
- decreased or increased metabolism and excretion.

Additive effect

An *additive* effect can occur when two drugs with similar actions are administered to a patient. The effects are equivalent to the sum of the effects of either drug administered alone in higher doses. Giving two drugs together, such as two analgesics (pain relievers), has these potential advantages:

- Lower doses of each drug can be administered, which can decrease the probability of adverse reactions because higher doses increase the risk of adverse reactions.
- Greater pain control than can be achieved from administration of one drug alone (most likely because of different mechanisms of action).

Potentiation

A synergistic effect, also called *potentiation*, occurs when two drugs that produce the same effect are given together and one drug potentiates (enhances the effect) of the other drug. This produces greater effects than either drug taken alone.

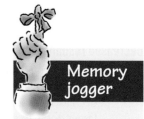

Memory jogger

When a drug is said to be **potentiated** by another drug, the results are more **potent**—the drug goes beyond its original potential.

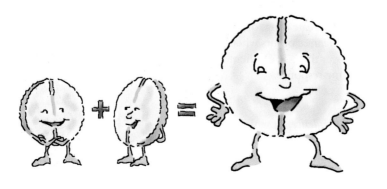

Antagonistic drug interactions

An *antagonistic* drug interaction occurs when the combined response of two drugs is less than the response produced by either drug alone.

Altering absorption

Two drugs given together can change the absorption of one or both of the drugs. For example, drugs that change the acidity of the stomach can affect the ability of another drug to dissolve in the stomach. Other drugs can interact and form an insoluble compound that can't be absorbed. Sometimes, an absorption interaction can be avoided by separating drug administration by at least 2 hours.

Binding battles

After a drug is absorbed, blood distributes it throughout the body as a free drug or one that's bound to plasma protein. When two drugs are given together, they can compete for protein-binding sites, leading to an increase in the effects of one drug as that drug is displaced from the protein and becomes a free, unbound drug.

Turning toxic

Toxic drug levels can occur when a drug's metabolism and excretion are inhibited by another drug. Some drug interactions affect excretion only.

Tampering with tests

Drug interactions can also alter laboratory tests and can produce changes seen on a patient's electrocardiogram.

Factor in food

Food can alter the therapeutic effects of a drug as well as the rate and amount of drug absorbed from the GI tract, affecting *bioavailability* (the amount of a drug dose available to the systemic circulation). Dangerous interactions can also occur. For example, when food that contains tyramine (such as aged cheddar cheese) is eaten by a person taking a monoamine oxidase inhibitor, hypertensive crisis can occur. Also, grapefruit can inhibit the metabolism of certain drugs and result in toxic blood levels such as some of the statin drugs (for example, simvastatin).

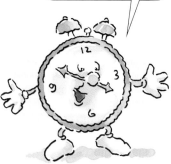

For some drugs, you can avoid absorption interactions by separating their administration times by at least 2 hours.

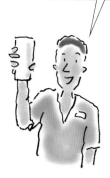

Patients may need to avoid certain foods when taking drugs. For example, grapefruit can inhibit the metabolism of certain drugs and result in toxic blood levels. Here, have some orange juice instead!

Elevating enzymes

Some drugs stimulate enzyme production, increasing metabolic rates and the demand for vitamins that are enzyme cofactors (which must unite with the enzyme in order for the enzyme to function). Drugs can also impair vitamin and mineral absorption.

Side effects and adverse drug reactions

A drug's desired effect is called the *expected therapeutic response*. A *side effect* is an expected response, either therapeutic or nontherapeutic, as a result of taking the drug. A side effect does not impact the therapeutic response of the drug; however, it may cause unwanted mild effects such as headache or nausea. An *adverse drug reaction (ADR)* is a harmful, undesirable response that can have a negative impact on the treatment and can cause harm to the patient. Adverse drug reactions can range from mild reactions that disappear when the drug is stopped to debilitating diseases that become chronic, to death.

Iatrogenic effects

Some adverse drug reactions, known as *iatrogenic effects*, can mimic pathologic disorders. For example, such drugs as antineoplastics, aspirin, corticosteroids, and indomethacin commonly cause GI irritation and bleeding. Other examples of iatrogenic effects include induced asthma with propranolol and induced deafness with gentamicin.

Adverse drug reactions: Type A or B?

Adverse drug reactions (ADRs) can be classified as type A or type B reactions.

Type A adverse drug reactions

Type A reactions are related to known pharmacologic effects of a drug and are typically dose related. These types of reactions are predictable. Type A reactions include:
- side effects (see *Side effects and adverse drug reactions*)
- drug interactions (see *Drug interactions*)
- overdose or toxic drug reaction.

Toxic drug reaction

A *toxic drug reaction or overdose* can occur when an excessive dose is taken, either intentionally or accidentally. The result is an exaggerated response to the drug that can lead to transient changes or more serious reactions, such as respiratory depression, cardiovascular collapse, and even death. To avoid toxic reactions, chronically ill or older adults may be prescribed lower drug doses.

Type B adverse drug reactions

Type B ADRs are typically unpredictable and are patient related (not dose related). Type B reactions include:
- idiosyncratic reactions
- immunological reactions (allergy).

Idiosyncratic reactions

An *idiosyncratic reaction* is an uncommon response due to an individual's genetic predisposition.

Immunological reactions

An immunological reaction results when a drug or its metabolites interact with a protein resulting in immunogenicity also known as a drug allergy. A *drug allergy* occurs when a patient's immune system identifies a drug, a drug metabolite, or a drug contaminant as a dangerous foreign substance that must be neutralized or destroyed. Previous exposure to the drug or to one with similar chemical characteristics sensitizes the patient's immune system, and subsequent exposure causes an allergic reaction (hypersensitivity). Hypersensitivity reactions can be classified as type I (IgE mediated—mild local reaction to anaphylaxis), II (cytotoxic reactions), III (serum sickness), or IV (delayed allergic response).

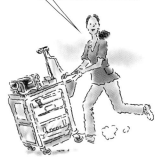

Allergic reactions to drugs can range from a mild rash to life-threatening anaphylaxis. Get some help! Stat!

The three-step approach—Safe medication administration

Several approaches or frameworks can be used to ensure safe medication administration such as the Nursing Process, Tanner's Model, or the Clinical Judgment Measurement Model. (See *Education edge*.) The important thing to remember is to use the approach or framework consistently every time medications are administered.

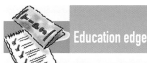

Education edge

The nursing process and CJMM are closely related.

	Nursing process	Clinical judgment measurement model
Preadministration	Assessment Diagnosis Planning	Recognize cues Analyze cues Prioritize hypotheses Generate solutions
Medication administration	Implementation	Take action
Postadministration	Evaluation	Evaluate outcomes

For this text, the three-step approach is used based on the timing of medication administration. These are congruent with the National Council of State Boards of Nursing's (NCSBN) Clinical Judgment Measurement Model (CJMM) (2020):

- Preadministration
- Medication administration
- Postadministration

Preadministration

The first step, preadministration, is what occurs before medications are administered. Recognizing and analyzing cues involves collecting data that are used to make hypotheses. Cues are obtained by taking a health history, performing a physical examination, and reviewing relevant laboratory and diagnostic information. The health history includes documenting drugs and supplements (including vitamins and herbal preparations) that the patient is taking, as well as recording any allergies. During the assessment, the nurse determines which cues are relevant or irrelevant and which are the most important to make hypotheses.

Once hypotheses are made and prioritized according to the patient's situation, planning begins by generating solutions including expected outcomes and actions. *Expected outcomes* are the desired results from the administration of the medication(s). Expected outcomes and actions are based on the patient's situation and the use of the medication rights (right patient, time, drug, dose, route, reason, response, and documentation). (See Chapter 2.)

Medication administration

The second step, medication administration, is the act (taking action) of administering medications to the patient to achieve the planned expected outcomes. The nurse collaborates with the patient, the patient's family, caregivers, and health care team members as needed for safe medication administration. Communication (documentation) of medication administration is an essential aspect of safe patient care.

Postadministration

The third step, postadministration, involves evaluating outcomes. During evaluation, the nurse must determine if the actions taken have enabled the patient to achieve the desired outcomes. If the outcome is stated in measurable terms, then the nurse can easily evaluate the extent to which the outcomes were met. This includes evaluating the effectiveness of drug interventions, such as achievement of all or a degree of pain relief after the patient received an analgesic. Evaluation is an ongoing process and assists the nurse with determining if the treatment is effective, ineffective, or did not make any differences.

Quick quiz

1. Which factor plays a role in drug absorption? **Select all that apply.**
    A. Route of administration
    B. Blood flow
    C. Form of drug
    D. High-fat diet
    E. Renal function

Answer: A, B, C, D. Several factors impact drug absorption including route, form of drug, amount of blood flow, high-fat diet, pain, and stress. Renal function plays a role in excretion of the drug.

2. A nurse is administering a drug that is considered an agonist. Which action does the nurse understand about the drug?
    A. Stimulates the receptor
    B. Increases the duration time
    C. Blocks the receptor from responding
    D. Changes what the receptor produces

Answer: A. An agonist interacts with the receptor and stimulates it to produce the desired effect. It does not increase the duration time, block the receptor response, or change what the receptor produces.

3. A nurse is reviewing dose-related and adverse reactions with a group of new nurses. Which statement would the nurse include in the review?
    A. Iatrogenic effects occur when the patient overdoses on a medication.
    B. A drug allergy occurs when the patient is exposed to a drug for the first time.
    C. A toxic drug reaction can occur when the patient takes an excessive dose or doses.
    D. Idiosyncratic effects are reactions that are harmful to patients when taking the drug for the second time.

Answer: C. A toxic drug reaction can occur when an excessive dose (or doses) is taken, either intentionally or accidentally. Iatrogenic effects mimic pathologic disorders. Drug allergy occurs when a previous exposure to the drug or to one with similar chemical characteristics sensitizes the patient's immune system causing an allergic reaction. An idiosyncratic effect is an uncommon response due to an individual's genetic predisposition.

4. Which term refers to the mechanism of drug action?
    A. Pharmacokinetics
    B. Classifications
    C. Transport
    D. Pharmacodynamics

Answer: D. Pharmacodynamics is the biochemical and physical effects of drugs and the mechanisms of drug actions. Pharmacokinetics is the movement of drugs through the body and includes absorption, distribution, metabolism, and excretion. Drug classifications are groups of drugs with similar characteristics. Transport is how drugs are absorbed through passive or active energy mechanisms.

5. Which factor must be in place for outcomes of medication administration to be evaluated?
- A. Only one or two outcomes can be stated.
- B. Another nurse must be able to state the outcome criteria.
- C. Outcome criteria must be stated in measurable terms.
- D. The patient must design the outcomes.

Answer: C. Expected outcomes are realistic, measurable goals for the patient. More than two outcomes can be stated, and outcomes must be documented for all health care team members to evaluate. The patient should be included in the development of outcomes.

Scoring

☆☆☆   If you answered all five questions correctly, fantastic! You obviously know your fundamental pharm facts.

☆☆   If you answered three-four questions correctly, terrific! You can clearly interact well with this material.

☆   If you answered two or fewer questions correctly, you can improve your absorption of this chapter with a quick review.

Suggested References

Center for Disease Control and Prevention. (2020). *How influenza (flu) vaccines are made*. Retrieved from https://www.cdc.gov/flu/prevent/how-fluvaccine-made.htm

Hess, D., & Dhand, R. (2020). Delivery of inhaled medication in adults. In B. Bochner, & H. Hollingsworth (Eds.), *UpToDate*. Waltham, MA: UpToDate.

Karch, A. (2020). *Focus on nursing pharmacology* (8th ed.). Philadelphia, PA: Wolters Kluwer.

National Council of State Boards of Nursing. (2020). *NCSBN clinical judgment measurement model*. Retrieved from https://www.ncsbn.org/14798.htm

Oliveira, P., Ribeiro, J., Donato, H., et al. (2017). Smoking and antidepressants pharmacokinetics: A systematic review. *Annals of General Psychiatry, 16*, 17. https://doi.org/10.1186/s1299-017-0140-8

O'Toole, M. (Ed.). (2021). *Mosby's dictionary of medicine, nursing & health professions* (11th ed.). St. Louis, MO: Elsevier/Mosby.

Pichler, W. (2020). Drug hypersensitivity: Classification and clinical features. In D. Adkinson, & A. Feldwag (Eds.), *UpToDate*. Waltham, MA: UpToDate Inc.

Schull, P. (2013). *McGraw-Hill nurse's drug handbook* (7th ed.). New York, NY: McGraw-Hill.

The Food and Drug Administration. (2018). *Understanding over-the-counter medicines*. Retrieved from https://www.fda.gov/drugs/buying-using-medicine-safely/understanding-over-counter-medicines

The Food and Drug Administration. (2020). *The drug development process*. Retrieved from https://www.fda.gov/patients/learn-about-drug-and-device-approvals/drug-development-process

United States Pharmacopeia and National Formulary. (2020). Pharmacopeia forum table of contents. Retrieved from https://www.uspnf.com/

U.S. National Library of Medicine. (n.d.). *Determining the safety of a drug*. Retrieved from https://toxtutor.nlm.nih.gov/02-005.html#One

World Health Organization. (2020). *Palliative care*. Retrieved from https://www.who.int/news-room/fact-sheets/detail/palliative-care

Chapter 2

Principles of safe medication administration

Just the facts

In this chapter, you'll learn:

◆ the "rights" of drug administration

◆ the medication administration process

◆ elements that contribute to drug administration safety

◆ strategies to reduce drug error rates

Getting started...

Understanding basic pharmacology is essential to providing safe and accurate medication administration to your patients, especially because drug therapy is the primary intervention used to address many illnesses and to facilitate healing of injuries. Proper administration of drug therapy benefits many patients, yet is also a leading cause of patient harm from unintended consequences of therapy (*drug side effects* or *adverse reactions*), or medication-related errors (adverse *events*).

The National Coordinating Council for Medication Error Reporting and Prevention (NCCMERP) (https://www.nccmerp.org/about-medication-errors) defines a *medication error* as "any preventable event that may cause or lead to inappropriate medication use or patient harm while the medication is in the control of the health care professional, patient, or consumer. Such events may be related to professional practice, health care products, procedures, and systems, including prescribing, order communication, product labeling, packaging, and nomenclature, compounding dispensing, distribution, administration, education, monitoring, and use" (NCCMERP, 2021).

Understanding evidence about drug administration and outcomes is important, as this serves as a reminder of why nurses must always be cautious when preparing and giving medications.

Toward safer practice

The Institute for Safe Medication Practices (ISMP) is a nonprofit organization entirely dedicated to preventing medication errors and using medications safely. In addition, The Joint Commission has established National Patient Safety Goals to improve the safe use of medications in its accredited facilities.

Historically, teaching nurses to safely administer drugs focused on the individual nurse's practice and the application of "rights" of safe medication administration. (See *The "rights" of medication administration.*) These "rights" provide a framework for the nurse to use when preparing to administer medication. It is important to recognize that these rights are *goals* or *desired outcomes* of safe medication delivery; they are not a procedural guideline for how to achieve those outcomes (Federico, 2021). The rights do not focus on individual performance nor on human factors or problems that are inherent within a system that may contribute to errors (Federico, 2021). To that end, nurses must be aware of the rights, yet base their practice in procedural rules set forth by the agency in order to achieve the best outcomes (See *Agency Policy*, Page 26.) (Federico, 2021). This practice mitigates risk by following a uniform and consistent process in the delivery of medication, as noted in Chapter 1.

"Rights" of medication administration

Historically, nurses have been taught the "five rights" of medication administration (Institute for Healthcare Improvement, 2020). These are broadly stated goals or desired outcomes of safe medication delivery.

- The *right drug*: Check the drug label and verify that the drug and form to be given is the drug that was prescribed.
- The *right patient*: Confirm the patient's identity by checking at least two patient identifiers.
- The *right dose*: Verify that the dose and form to be given are appropriate for the patient and check the drug label with the prescriber's order.
- The *right time*: Ensure that the drug is administered at the correct time and frequency.
- The *right route*: Verify that the route by which the drug is to be given is specified by the prescriber and is appropriate for the patient.

Besides the traditional "five rights" of individual practice, best practice researchers added three more "rights":

- The *right reason*: Verify that the drug prescribed is appropriate to treat the patient's condition.
- The *right response*: Monitor the patient's response to the drug administered.
- The *right documentation*: Completely and accurately document in the electronic health record the drug administered, monitoring performed, and any other accompanying nursing interventions.

Agency Policy

Each agency must have tools and policies in place for the documentation of medication administration. For example: Each prescribed medication order must be fully documented in the electronic health record, or clearly written. Verbal orders should be avoided; however, when given, these must be documented appropriately according to agency policy as soon as possible after conveying them. Each verbal order should be read back and verified with the prescriber before the drug is administered. The patient's condition must be monitored after each medication is given, and the patient's response and any associated nursing interventions must be documented appropriately.

Although individual nursing practice is still an extremely important part of safe drug administration, the responsibility for safe practice extends to many individuals and to systems within health agencies. Organizational processes, management decisions, inadequate medication administration protocols, staffing shortages, environmental conditions, poor communication, inadequate drug knowledge and resources, and individual mistakes or protocol violations may all contribute to errors. Medication errors are complex events with multiple factors and are often caused by failures within systems. As a result of these findings, research focuses now on preventing medication errors by identifying the root cause, and developing and validating evidence-based strategies to decrease risk.

The medication administration process

Medication errors can occur from administration process problems within any one or within more than one of the "rights" and at any stage within the delivery of care. Here are some of the types of errors that have been reported by stage.

Preadministration
- Prescriber's orders are incomplete or illegible.
- Contraindicated drugs (such as drugs to which the patient is allergic) are prescribed.
- The prescriber specifies the wrong drug, dose, route, or frequency.
- Drugs are prescribed using inappropriate or inadequate verbal orders.
- An incorrect drug, dose, route, time, or frequency is transcribed into the medication administration record (MAR) by the pharmacist or nurse.

- Drug verification and documentation in the MAR by the pharmacist or nurse are inadequate.
- The prescribed drug is filled incorrectly by the pharmacy.
- Failure to deliver the right drug to the right place (where the right patient is located) occurs.

Administration

- The wrong drug is given to the wrong patient.
- The wrong dose is calculated and given or infused.
- The right drug is incorrectly prepared (such as crushing a drug that shouldn't be crushed).
- The right drug is administered by the wrong route (such as an oral drug that is injected intramuscularly (IM)).
- The right drug is given at the wrong time or at the wrong frequency.

Postadministration

- The patient is not adequately monitored after the medication is given.
- Documentation of the patient's condition after medication administration lacks detail and does not fully represent the patient's response to drug therapy.
- Hand-off communication between licensed health care professionals is incomplete.
- There is inadequate reporting of medication errors.

Dosage calculation

Specific methods of dosage calculation can be obtained in resources that are developed specifically for this purpose. Three methods of dosage calculation include Dimensional Analysis, Ratio Proportion, and Formula (or Desired Over Have Method) (Toney-Butler & Wilcox, 2021). Nursing students should study the calculation method taught during their curriculum and use credible online tools to check and double-check dosage calculations.

Elements contributing to safer drug administration

Ensuring the safe delivery of medication involves a system-wide approach, and research has shown that improvements in communication and education can facilitate the safer delivery of medication.

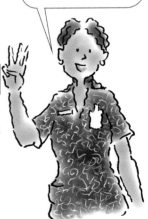

Three methods of dosage calculation include Dimensional Analysis, Ratio Proportion, and Formula.

Communication improvements

Communication issues are responsible for numerous reported medication errors. This communication may be between the providers of care (for example, health care provider and nurse), or communication may be lacking from the patient. For example, a provider may prescribe correctly, and the nurse may exactly follow the right of medication administration. However, an allergic reaction may occur if the patient has not communicated this allergy information to the health care team. Therefore, all avenues of communication must be clear as possible in an effort to prevent errors from occurring.

Many health care facilities have instituted measures to help standardize and organize appropriate communication. One tool commonly used is SBAR (Situation, Background, Assessment, and Recommendation); its purpose is to logically organize information to optimize proper communication among health care providers. TeamStepps® is an evidence-based program created to optimize health care performance through communication. They offer curriculum for generalized team care, office-based care, long-term care, dental care, and rapid response care (Agency for Healthcare Research and Quality, 2019).

The Joint Commission (TJC) has developed goals and standards regarding *medication reconciliation*—the process of comparing a patient's medication regimen at every transition in care (for example, on admission, on discharge, and between care settings and levels). Medication reconciliation helps ensure that essential information about the patient's medication regimen is communicated to the health care team. This process also helps prevent the inadvertent omission of needed medications, prevents medication duplication, and helps identify medications with potentially harmful interactions.

Education improvements

Improving education about medications is essential to safe administration. All health care team members involved in the process of medication administration, including the prescriber, pharmacist, and nurse, must have access to accurate information about each drug's indications, appropriate dosing regimen, appropriate route, frequency, possible drug interactions, appropriate monitoring, any cautions, and possible adverse effects. Each agency should have processes in place to educate staff and communicate important drug information.

Governmental and nongovernmental agencies are doing their part toward educating facilities, prescribers, and nurses. The U.S. Food and Drug Administration's (FDA) black box warning system alerts prescribers to drugs with increased risks to patients. These boxed warnings are the strongest labeling requirements for drugs that can have serious reactions. The Joint Commission provides an official "do not use" list that must be followed and requires accredited health care facilities to develop their own list of abbreviations to avoid in all medication communications. The Institute for Safe Medication Practices (ISMP) maintains a list of high-alert medications that may cause significant patient harm. Each agency should have protocols in place for administering these high-alert medications with safeguards built into the process. The FDA and ISMP publish a list of drugs with similar names that can be easily confused. Dissimilarities in each drug's name are highlighted with "Tall man" letters (a mix of capitals and lowercase letters, See a sample of this type of list below in the "Drug Name/Confused Drug Name" figure.) making each drug less prone to mix-ups.

Drug name	Confused drug name
Abelcet	*amphotericin B*
Accupril	Aciphex
acetaminophen	*aceta**ZOLAMIDE***
*aceta**ZOLAMIDE***	*acetaminophen*
*aceta**ZOLAMIDE***	*aceto**HEXAMIDE***

Institute for Safe Medication Practices. (2019). *List of confused drug names*. Retrieved from https://www.ismp.org/recommendations/confused-drug-names-list

Black box warning

A black box warning (BBW) is the Food and Drug Administration's strongest warning about drugs and medical devices. This specific marking serves as an alert about known health risks associated with use of a specific medication. Often these risks are associated with suicidality, older adult mortality, risk for dependence or abuse, or life-threatening hepatic failure (Leahy, 2017). Safer administration can take place when nurses recognize the implications of specific BBWs and adhere to that knowledge throughout the administration and teaching processes (Leahy, 2017).

Abbreviation and symbol avoidance

In 2001, The Joint Commission (TJC) created an official "Do Not Use" list of abbreviations, which continues to be used in practice (TJC, 2019). Agencies are encouraged to avoid all abbreviations and symbols in addition to this absolute list. (See *Official "Do Not Use" List*, page 30.)

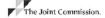 The Joint Commission.

Official "Do Not Use" List

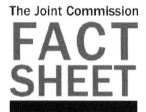

The Joint Commission

FACT SHEET

- This list is part of the Information Management standards
- Does not apply to preprogrammed health information technology systems (i.e. electronic medical records or CPOE systems), but remains under consideration for the future

Organizations contemplating introduction or upgrade of such systems should strive to eliminate the use of dangerous abbreviations, acronyms, symbols and dose designations from the software.

For more information

- Contact the Standards Interpretation Group at 630-792-5900.
- Complete the Standards Online Question Submission Form.

Official "Do Not Use" List

Do Not Use	Potential Problem	Use Instead
U, u (unit)	Mistaken for "0" (zero), the number "4" (four) or "cc"	Write "unit"
IU (International Unit)	Mistaken for IV (intravenous) or the number 10 (ten)	Write "International Unit"
Q.D., QD, q.d., qd (daily)	Mistaken for each other	Write "daily"
Q.O.D., QOD, q.o.d, qod (every other day)	Period after the Q mistaken for "I" and the "O" mistaken for "I	Write "every other day"
Trailing zero (X.0 mg)* Lack of leading zero (.X mg)	Decimal point is missed	Write X mg Write 0.X mg
MS	Can mean morphine sulfate or magnesium sulfate	Write "morphine sulfate" Write "magnesium sulfate"
MSO₄ and MgSO₄	Confused for one another	

¹ Applies to all orders and all medication-related documentation that is handwritten (including free-text computer entry) or on pre-printed forms.

Exception: A "trailing zero" may be used only where required to demonstrate the level of precision of the value being reported, such as for laboratory results, imaging studies that report size of lesions, or catheter/tube sizes. It may not be used in medication orders or other medication-related documentation.

Development of the "Do Not Use" List
In 2001, The Joint Commission issued a *Sentinel Event Alert* on the subject of medical abbreviations. A year later, its Board of Commissioners approved a National Patient Safety Goal requiring accredited organizations to develop and implement a list of abbreviations not to use. In 2004, The Joint Commission created its "Do Not Use" List to meet that goal. In 2010, NPSG.02.02.01 was integrated into the Information Management standards as elements of performance 2 and 3 under IM.02.02.01.

6/19

Further strategies for reducing error rates

In addition to improvements in communication and education, other strategies that have helped reduce medication administration error rates include the following:

Encouraging safer prescribing

- switching from intravenous (IV) to oral or subcutaneous forms of drug therapy as soon as possible based on the prescriber's order
- avoiding unapproved abbreviations (see *"Official Do Not Use List"*, page 30)
- requiring that medication orders be prescribed by metric weight, not by volume (for example, in mg/kg instead of mL)
- establishing protocols and checklists to double-check and document unusual drugs, dosages, or regimens
- recalculating doses before giving drugs to children or neonates, making sure that the dose formula is included for calculating the dose
- having a second clinician (preferably a pharmacist) double-check the calculations for drugs given to children or neonates.

Enhancing staffing

- providing adequate nurse-to-patient staffing ratios so that each patient is monitored appropriately before, during, and after drug administration.

Improving areas for preparing medications

- designating specific areas as safety zones where others do not disturb the nurse who is preparing medication
- improving the medication administration environment (noise not greater than 50 dB, improved lighting, nonglare computer screens)
- ensuring emergency equipment is always available in areas where high-alert medications are given.

Improving drug delivery

- dispensing medications in unit-dose or unit-of-use packaging
- dispensing IV and epidural infusions only from the pharmacy
- restricting high-alert drugs and administration routes (limiting their number, variety, and concentration in patient care areas). For example: Remove all neuromuscular blockers from units in which patients aren't normally intubated.
- labeling all medications on and off the sterile field
- using infusion rate and dosing charts in patient care areas
- having appropriate monitoring equipment (cardiac monitors, capnography, pulse oximetry) available as needed.

Using technology to promote safety

Technology continues to be a critical component providing safer drug administration. The goal of medication administration technology is to enhance individual practice and help build safeguards into the medication administration process.

Computerized order entry

In computerized provider order entry (CPOE), the prescriber enters the medication orders into a computerized record, thus eliminating errors due to illegible handwriting or missed pages within a paper record. Safeguards such as immediate order checking for errors (for example, incorrect dosing or routes of administration) and drug interactions, allergy checks, and administration protocols can be built into the system. Orders can be immediately transmitted to the appropriate department and be linked to drug information databases.

Bar codes

Bar code technology is used for safer drug administration, dispensing, inventory control, and drug storage and preparation. This method has been endorsed by the Institute of Medicine (IOM), The Joint Commission, Agency for Healthcare Research and Quality, and ISMP. With this technology, the patient wears a bar code identifier on a wristband; the medication also has a bar code that uses the medication's own unique National Drug Code to identify the name, dose, manufacturer, and type of packaging. The nurse scans the bar code using an optical scanner, verifying the patient's identity and medication. The system supports but does not replace the traditional "rights" of safe medication administration; however, it does greatly enhance that process.

Bar code systems have been shown to reduce medication errors, but they aren't without occasional complications. They require time to perform the scanning process. There are inherent technology problems that may arise, such as wristbands that become unreadable over time, or a scanner that malfunctions. It is important that the nurse has received full training and education regarding what to do to troubleshoot these problems.

Automated dispensing cabinets

Automated dispensing cabinets (ADCs) are computer-controlled medication distribution systems in the patient care unit that are used to store, track, and dispense medications. ADCs can provide nurses with near-total access to medications needed in their patient care area and promote the control and security

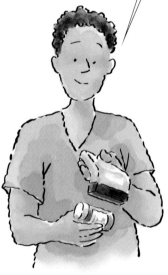

Remember to scan the bar code verifying the patient's identity and medication.

of medications. They electronically track the use of such drugs as controlled substances. They may have bar code capabilities for restocking and correct medication selection and can be programmed to provide such safeguards as drug safety alerts. ADCs can be linked with external databases and billing systems to increase the efficiency of drug dispensing and billing.

"Smart" pumps

Initiatives have been implemented to improve infusion systems and technology. "Smart" IV pumps, which are often wireless, have features such as programmable drug libraries and dosage limits. They can perform automatic calculations and be programmed to signal dosage alerts. They can be integrated with bar code and CPOE technologies. Smart pumps can alert nurses when incorrect dosages have been selected or indicate dosages that may exceed recommended levels. Although very efficient and helpful, smart pumps can't detect all problems with IV drug infusions. For example, an incorrect drug can be selected from the library database, and some pumps will allow the nurse to override safety alerts.

Other infusion pump problems include software defects and failure of built-in safety alarms. Some pumps have ambiguous on-screen directions that can lead to dosing errors. The FDA recommends reporting all infusion-related adverse events, planning ahead in case a pump fails, labeling the channels and tubing to prevent errors, checking all settings, and monitoring patients for signs and symptoms of infusion problems. Nurses should perform independent calculation of all doses and infusion rates and not rely solely on the pump. It is essential to double-check each dose calculation. Nurses must not bypass pump alarms and must verify that the pump is functioning properly before beginning an infusion.

Other technologies

Using only oral syringes that don't have Luer locks to administer oral or enteral medications helps prevent oral or enteral medications from being administered via the wrong route. (The ISMP has reported cases in which oral medications were drawn into parenteral syringes and inadvertently injected into IV lines, resulting in patient deaths.) Utilizing special tubing for epidural medication administration that doesn't have side ports prevents inadvertent injection of an additional drug into the epidural catheter.

Reporting medication errors

Sharing and analyzing data, and performing more research about medication errors, can lead to evidence-based quality improvement processes. Select agencies and organizations provide voluntary reporting systems to study the causes and prevalence of medication errors. The U.S. Food and Drug Administration (FDA) has the Adverse Event Reporting System (FAERS). The Institute for Safe Medication Practices (ISMP) maintains a voluntary medication error reporting program (2021). The reports are analyzed by these agencies, and information is published about their findings. Nurses should be encouraged to report medication errors and "near misses" and to help identify problems within systems.

Quick quiz

1. Which "right" is included in the traditional five rights of medication administration? **Select all that apply.**
   A. Drug
   B. Time
   C. Dose
   D. Route
   E. Patient

Answer: A, B, C, D, E. The traditional five rights of medication administration include the right drug, the right patient, the right dose, the right time, and the right route.

2. Which process will the nurse use to provide information to other members of the interprofessional health care team?
   A. FMLA
   B. OSHA
   C. PDCA
   D. SBAR

Answer: D. The SBAR method of handoff communication is used between members of the interprofessional health care team. This stands for Situation, Background, Assessment, Recommendation. FMLA is the Family Medical Leave Act. OSHA is the Occupational Safety and Health Act. PDCA is the Plan Do Check Act process. FMLA, OSHA, and PCDA are not handoff tools.

3. The nurse receives a written medication order for MS. Which nursing action is appropriate?
   A. Contact the pharmacy for clarity.
   B. Gather dose of magnesium sulfate.
   C. Ask the provider to rewrite the order.
   D. Prepare to administer morphine sulfate.

Answer: C. Using MS in an abbreviation is part of The Joint Commission's (TJC) Do Not Use List. The nurse should not assume anything about the order, and instead contact the provider (not the pharmacy) to rewrite the order for clarity.

Scoring

☆☆☆ If you answered all three questions correctly, fantastic! You know basic safe medication administration facts.

☆☆ If you answered two questions correctly, terrific! You have a beginning grasp of medication safety.

☆ If you answered one question correctly, just go back and read the chapter again.

Suggested References

Agency for Healthcare Research and Quality. (2019). *Curriculum materials*. Retrieved from https://www.ahrq.gov/teamstepps/curriculum-materials.html

Federico, F. (2021). *The five rights of medication administration*. Institute for Healthcare Improvement. Retrieved from http://www.ihi.org/resources/Pages/ ImprovementStories/FiveRightsofMedicationAdministration.aspx

Institute for Healthcare Improvement (IHI). (2021). *The five rights of medication administration*. Retrieved from http://www.ihi.org/resources/Pages/ ImprovementStories/FiveRightsofMedicationAdministration.aspx

Institute for Safe Medication Practices (ISMP). (2019). *List of confused drug names*. Retrieved from https://www.ismp.org/recommendations/confused-drug-names-list

Institute for Safe Medication Practices (ISMP). (2021). *Report an error*. Retrieved from https://www.ismp.org/report-medication-error

Leahy, L. (2017). Medication safety: What nurses should know about black box warnings. *Journal of Psychosocial Nursing and Mental Health Services, 55*(6), 11–15.

National Coordinating Council for Medication Error Reporting and Prevention. (2021). *About medication errors: What is a medication error?* Retrieved from http://www. nccmerp.org/about-medication-errors

The Joint Commission. (2019). *Official "Do Not Use" List*. Retrieved from https://www. jointcommission.org/-/media/tjc/documents/resources/patient-safety-topics/ do_not_use_list_6_28_19.pdf

Toney-Butler, T., & Wilcox, L. (2021). Dose calculation desired over have formula method. In *StatPearls [Internet]*. Treasure Island, FL: StatPearls Publishing; 2020. Retrieved from https://www.ncbi.nlm.nih.gov/books/NBK493162/

Chapter 3

Patient education and medication safety

Just the facts

In this chapter, you'll learn:

- ◆ the importance of patient education in medication administration
- ◆ the patient education process for medication safety
- ◆ general patient education common to all medications.

Patient education

Part of providing safe and effective nursing care is the provision of patient education. This is especially important in teaching patients about medications. A patient's safety is often directly connected to their understanding of prescribed medications. Further, understanding the purpose of medications and what to expect with prescribed medication can improve adherence to a medication regimen.

Active participation

Part of being an active participant in care is understanding the purpose of newly prescribed medications. This active participation in the plan of care is important for the patient as well as family members of the patient. The patient and family need to be taught what to watch for, how the patient's condition will be monitored, what signs and symptoms to report, and to report anything that doesn't seem right. Before administering a medication, the nurse needs to verify with the patient medication allergies or unusual past reactions to medications.

The teaching process

There is no standard approach to patient education for drug therapy (Bowen et al., 2017). Most facilities have a standard process for discharge education that includes medication teaching. The following process provides a simple structure for the nurse to use when providing patient education about medication. This process will help ensure that the patient receives the maximum therapeutic benefit from the medication regimen and help to avoid adverse reactions, accidental overdose, and harmful changes in effectiveness. This process should be used anytime the nurse is discussing and administering medications, as discharge education starts with the patient's admission.

- Begin by introducing the drug. Explain that drugs have two names, generic and trade, and provide both names of the drug to the patient.
- Explain in clear terms what the drug is used for. For example, if the patient is prescribed furosemide, the nurse will explain that this drug is a diuretic that will help remove fluid from the body by increasing urination. Depending on the patient's educational level, the nurse can tailor the instruction appropriately. The nurse may need to be even more specific by saying, "This medication works by making you go to the bathroom more than you normally do."
- Provide the patient with concise directions on how to take the medication. This should include the route of the medication, dose, frequency, and timing of administration. Providing this through verbal and written instruction is important for adherence to therapy.
- Next, provide details on how to take the medication. This includes what the medication should and should not be taken with. For example, some medications must be taken on an empty stomach to increase absorption.
- Discuss potential interactions with the patient. This will require the nurse to be prepared by reviewing the medications that the patient is currently taking. Remember to include any potential food interactions, such as the avoidance of grapefruit juice with simvastatin (Food and Drug Administration, 2021).
- Spend time discussing side effects with the patient. Remember, side effects are associated with the drug. For example, a side effect of furosemide is orthostatic hypotension. As such, it is important to teach the patient that this can occur and how to avoid by changing positions slowly.
- Next, discuss adverse effects of the medication. Remember, adverse effects need to be reported to the health care provider. Adverse effects of furosemide include dehydration and significant loss

Education edge

Teaching template....

1. Drug Name
2. Used for?
3. How to (Route, dose, timing) take?
4. How to specifics!

5. Interactions
6. Side Effects
7. Adverse Effects (Call the Provider!)
8. Tips for Success!!

of potassium. Signs that this is occurring include muscle cramps and weakness, as well as fast or irregular heartbeat. Be sure to differentiate between side effects and adverse effects, by ensuring the patient understands when to call the provider.

- Be sure to conclude with specific tips to ensure drug safety such as the importance of adherence to therapy. For example, if the patient is prescribed antibiotics, specific teaching tips include explaining the need to take the full prescription even if the symptoms improve.

The teach-back approach

The teach-back approach is a common teaching method used to ensure that patients and their family members understand medical information that has been presented to them. Evidence does demonstrate that this strategy increases patient adherence and improves patient outcomes (Agency for Healthcare Research and Quality, 2017). Using this approach, after teaching the nurse will ask the patient to use their own words to "teach-back" what they learned. The goal is not repeating what has been said, but rather showing clear understanding of the critical elements of teaching. This process provides the nurse with immediate feedback regarding the clarity of teaching as well as the overall understanding of the patient and family.

Common teaching points

While every drug is unique, there are elements of medication teaching that are common for all medications. The following list provides common teaching points to include with all medication instruction:

- Instruct the patient to learn the names and dosages of all prescribed drugs and supplements (such as herbs and vitamins).
- Tell the patient to notify the pharmacist and health care provider about all medications, including prescription drugs, over-the-counter drugs, herbal or other supplements, and about any drug allergies.
- Advise the patient to always read the label before taking a drug, to take it exactly as prescribed, and never to share prescription drugs.
- Tell the patient to check the expiration date before taking a drug.
- Caution the patient to keep all drugs safely out of the reach of children and pets.
- Advise the patient to store drugs in their original container, at the proper temperature, and in areas where they won't be exposed to sunlight or excessive heat or humidity. Sunlight, heat, and humidity can cause drug deterioration and reduce a drug's effectiveness.
- Suggest that the patient have all prescriptions filled at the same pharmacy so that the pharmacist can warn against potentially harmful drug interactions.
- Instruct the patient to call the health care provider, poison control center, or pharmacist immediately and to seek immediate medical attention if an overdose is suspected. The National Poison Control Center phone number is 1-800-222-1222. Tell the patient to keep this and other emergency numbers handy at all times.
- Advise the patient to make sure there is a sufficient supply of drugs when traveling. Also, carry the medications in their original containers and do not pack them in luggage.

Are you on "High-Alert"?

While it is important to teach patients about every medication, some medications have higher-risk profiles than others. The Institute for Safe Medication Practices (ISMP) has designated certain medications as "high-alert" drugs. This means that while the drug has been proven to be safe and effective, serious harm can occur if the medication is not taken exactly as prescribed. Learning guides for these medications can be found online at consumermedsafety.org

Selected examples of high-alert medications and categories include: heparin, warfarin, metformin, digoxin, anticoagulants, opioids, and insulins.

Quick quiz

1. Which effect is considered an adverse effect of a medication? Select all that apply.
   A.   Dry cough
   B.   Headache
   C.   Angioedema
   D.   Chest pain
   E.   Rapid heart rate

Answer: C, D, E. Adverse effects are effects of a drug that require notification of the health care provider and prompt treatment. Adverse effects can be life-threatening if untreated. Angioedema, chest pain, and rapid heart rate are considered adverse effects that require urgent treatment.

2. Which nursing statement reflects the teach-back process of patient education?
   A.   "Repeat after me as I state the name of the drug."
   B.   "Using your own words, tell me about the drug we just talked about."
   C.   "Let me show you how to use a pill-organizer."
   D.   "I am leaving a pamphlet that covers what we discussed today."

Answer: B. The teach-back approach is a common teaching method used to ensure that patients and their family members understand medical information that has been presented to them. Using this approach, after teaching the nurse will ask the patient to use their own words to "teach-back" what they learned.

3. Which general teaching will the nurse include with drug education? Select all that apply.
   A.   Since you are taking multiple drugs, you may need to use multiple pharmacies to get the best prices.
   B.   Be sure to review the discharge instructions not the labels on your medication.
   C.   Make sure to leave your medications in the bottles when you travel.
   D.   Be sure that you know the name and dose of your medication.
   E.   Do not share medications or take medications from someone else.

Answer: C, D, E. Patients should be advised to use one pharmacy, not multiple as this allows the pharmacist to monitor for potential drug interactions. The patient should be advised to read and follow the labels on the medication bottle. Medications should remain in the bottle while traveling. Medications should not be shared, and it is critical for patients to be aware of prescribed medication name and dose.

Scoring

☆☆☆ If you answered all three questions correctly, fantastic! You know basic patient education and medication safety facts.

☆☆ If you answered two questions correctly, terrific! You have a beginning grasp of patient education and medication safety.

☆ If you answered one question correctly, just go back and read the chapter again.

Suggested References

Agency for Healthcare Research and Quality. (2017). *Implementation quick-start guide teach back.* Retrieved from https://www.ahrq.gov/sites/default/files/wysiwyg/professionals/quality-patient-safety/patient-family-engagement/pfeprimarycare/teach-back_quickstart_full.pdf

Bowen, J. F., Rotz, M. E., Patterson, B. J., & Sen, S. (2017). Nurses' attitudes and behaviors on patient medication education. *Pharmacy practice, 15*(2), 930. https://doi.org/10.18549/PharmPract.2017.02.930

Institute for Safe Medication Practices. (2018). *High-alert medication guides for consumers.* Retrieved from https://www.ismp.org/resources/high-alert-medication-learning-guides-consumers

Institute for Safe Medication Practices. (2020). *ISMP high-alert medications.* Retrieved from https://forms.ismp.org/Tools/highAlertMedicationLists.asp

National Capital Poison Center. (2020). *Get poison control help.* Retrieved from https://www.poison.org

U.S. Food and Drug Administration. (2021). *Grapefruit juice and some drugs don't mix.* Retrieved from https://www.fda.gov/consumers/consumer-updates/grapefruit-juice-and-some-drugs-dont-mix

Chapter 4

Dermatologic drugs

Just the facts

In this chapter, you'll learn:

◆ classes of drugs used to treat dermatologic disorders

◆ uses and varying actions of these drugs

◆ absorption, distribution, metabolization, and excretion of these drugs

◆ drug interactions and adverse reactions to these drugs.

Drugs and the integumentary system

The integumentary system, also known as the dermatologic system, is comprised of skin, hair, nails, glands, and receptors, which help protect the body. Types of drugs used to treat disorders of the integumentary system include:

- anti-infective drugs
- anti-inflammatory drugs
- hair growth stimulant drug
- antiacne drugs
- antiparasitic drugs.

Note: antihistamine drugs are covered in Chapter 17.

This chapter may look a little different than other chapters in this book. Rest assured, that is purposeful. The method in which information is presented for dermatologic drugs will help you organize your thoughts in the best way possible to provide safe administration of the medications included.

Drug formulations and information

This chapter focuses on *topical* dermatologic drugs, with limited coverage of drugs that may be used *systemically* for dermatologic issues. Drug formulations used as topical therapies come in the forms of solids (for example, dry powder), semisolids (for example, creams, ointment, gels, and pastes), and liquids.

Note that not all trade names are included for each drug, as there are multiple manufacturers for many of these products. For drugs that are referred to only by the generic name, no trade name was available at time of publication. Within this chapter, narrative information may only include the generic name for drugs.

Anti-infective drugs

Anti-infective drugs treat infections caused by bacteria, fungi, or viruses. They do so by killing or slowing the growth of the targeted microbe. This section discusses anti-infective drugs—antibacterial, antifungals, and antivirals—used to treat or prevent different types of infections.

Topical antibacterials

Antibacterial drugs are used to treat different types of bacterial infections. Antibacterial drugs can be administered using different routes depending on location and type of bacterial infection. This section focuses on topical antibacterial drugs.

Select examples of antibacterial drugs include:

Topical antibacterial drugs	Common indications
Azelaic acid (Azelex, Finacea)	Acne, rosacea
Bacitracin *usually mixed with one or more other topical agents, such as polymyxin B sulfate, neomycin, and/or hydrocortisone acetate*	Bacterial eye infections, prevention, or treatment of superficial bacterial skin infections
Clindamycin (Cleocin, Cleocin T, Clindagel, Clindets, Clinda-Derm, Clindesse, Evoclin)	Acne, bacterial vaginosis
Erythromycin (Erygel)	Conjunctivitis, blepharitis, perioral dermatitis, *Chlamydia trachomatis* of conjunctiva or nasopharynx
Gentamicin	Prevention of peritoneal catheter site infection/peritonitis
Metronidazole (MetroCream, Metrogel, Metrogel-Vaginal, MetroLotion, Noritate, Nuvessa, Vandazole)	Rosacea, perioral dermatitis, bacterial vaginosis, trichomoniasis
Mupirocin (Centany)	Superficial bacterial skin infections, secondary bacterial skin infections, prevention of peritoneal catheter exit-site and tunnel infection (off-label), *Staphylococcus aureus* decolonization (including methicillin resistant)

Topical antibacterial drugs	Common indications
Neomycin •*always mixed with one or more other topical agents, such as polymyxin B sulfate, hydrocortisone, gramicidin, colistin, thonzonium bromide, fluocinolone, dexamethasone, and/or bacitracin. For exam, Neosporin is neomycin, polymyxin B sulfate, and gramicidin*	Prevention or treatment of superficial bacterial skin infections
Polymyxin B *always mixed with one or more other topical agents, such as bacitracin, neomycin, dexamethasone, trimethoprim, and/or hydrocortisone. For exam, Neosporin is neomycin, polymyxin B sulfate, and gramicidin*	Bacterial infection of eye, prevention or treatment of superficial bacterial skin infections
Silver sulfadiazine (Silvadene, SSD, Thermazene)	Burn treatment
Sulfacetamide (Klaron, Bleph-10, Blephamide, Blephamide S.O.P.)	Acne, rosacea, bacterial skin infections, scaling dermatoses, seborrheic dermatitis, superficial ocular infections, *Chlamydia trachomatis* infection of the eye

*Topical antibiotics are often mixed with other active ingredients, such as with another topical antibiotic, topical corticosteroid, and/or topical keratolytic.
*Not all trade names are included for each drug, as there are multiple manufacturers for many of these products.

Pharmacokinetics

The general pharmacokinetics of topical drugs used for dermatology conditions are similar. Many are applied directly to the skin, whereas ophthalmic drugs are applied to the eyes. Be certain to pay close attention to the prescribed route in order to provide safe administration.

When a topical antibacterial drug is applied to an affected area, most of the drug remains localized. Only a small amount penetrates the skin, so higher concentrations of the drug may be applied to the targeted site with low risk for systemic side effects or toxicity. Medications administered through the eyes have a higher potential for systemic absorption; be certain to understand systematic (as well as local) side effects or interactions prior to administration.

Pharmacodynamics

Antibacterial drugs kill or slow the growth of bacteria.

Pharmacotherapeutics

Topical antibacterial drugs are used to prevent or treat infections of the skin, eye, ear, nasal cavity, oral cavity, vulva/vagina, or respiratory tract. Some topical antibacterial drugs can also be used to treat seborrheic dermatitis (for example, sulfacetamide), burns (for example, mafenide, silver sulfadiazine, sulfacetamide), rosacea (for example, azelaic acid, clindamycin, metronidazole, sulfacetamide), bacterial vaginosis (for example, metronidazole, clindamycin), and trichomoniasis (for example, metronidazole). Others may be used as an adjunctive therapy for acne (azelaic acid, erythromycin, clindamycin, sulfacetamide) or rosacea (for example, erythromycin, metronidazole). Mupirocin can be used for impetigo, methicillin-resistant *Staphylococcus aureus* (MRSA) decolonization, peritoneal dialysis catheter tunnel site prophylaxis, folliculitis (off-label), and nasal vestibulitis (off-label).

Drug interactions

While topical antibacterials are generally perceived as very safe, there are potential drug interactions. This is a very abbreviated list:
- Erythromycin (systemic or topical) in combination with clindamycin (systemic or topical) may reduce the therapeutic effect of each other.
- Clindamycin may increase effect of neuromuscular-blocking agents.
- Isotretinoin (topical) may increase adverse/toxic effects of erythromycin.
- Mafenide may reduce the therapeutic effects of BCG (Bacille Calmette-Guérin vaccine), cholera vaccine, typhoid vaccine, lactobacillus, estriol, and sodium picosulfate.
- Metronidazole may increase adverse/toxic effects of alcohol, disulfiram, lopinavir, and tipranavir.
- Topical antibiotics used in combination with a corticosteroid may mask signs of infection or allergic reaction or increase the risk for a superimposed infection.
- Caution should be used when consuming alcohol while using topical antibacterial drugs. Alcohol may reduce efficacy of the drug or increase the effect resulting in toxicity or an adverse drug reaction. For example, concurrent use of topical metronidazole and alcohol can cause headache, nausea, vomiting, chest or abdominal discomfort, dizziness face flushing, weakness, blurred vision, altered mental status, or low blood pressure.

Adverse reactions

The most common adverse reactions to topical skin applications include contact dermatitis (commonly seen with neomycin and bacitracin), acne, skin burning, itching, stinging, redness, or dryness, headache, nausea, and hypopigmentation. Other specific concerns include:
- Asthma exacerbation, which can occur with azelaic acid
- Avoidance of any antibacterial drugs that contain benzyl alcohol or propylene glycol in neonates, which can lead to fatal toxicity
- Rare side effects can occur, such as hearing loss (usually with aminoglycosides), metabolic acidosis (specifically with mafenide), and severe allergic reaction (swelling and itching of face, tongue, or throat, generalized rash, hives, dizziness, trouble breathing)

Cautions

Topical antibacterial drugs such as mafenide, sulfacetamide, and silver sulfadiazine are used with caution in with sulfonamide allergy as there are chemical similarities between sulfonamides, sulfonylureas, carbonic anhydrase inhibitors, thiazides, and loop diuretics.

It is important to avoid occlusive dressings when using topical antibacterial drugs, unless prescribed otherwise. Dressings can increase drug absorption, leading to unwanted side effects.

Teaching

In addition to following basic teaching information as contained in Chapter 3, teach patients how to properly use topical preparations based on the box *Teaching about use of topical drugs*. This same information will be used when teaching about any topical drug contained within this chapter.

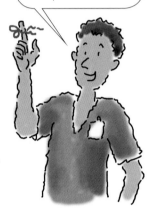

Remember to avoid occlusive dressing placement over topical antibacterial drugs, unless otherwise prescribed.

Topical Antifungals

Antifungal drugs are used to treat different types of fungal infections. These drugs can be used in combination with a topical steroid. Some are available over-the-counter, such as Lotrimin AF and select Monistat products. It is important to note that some drugs are available as foam preparations. These should be used with extreme

---

Teaching about use of topical drugs

If topical drugs are prescribed, review these points with the patient/caregivers:

- Wash your hands before and after applying medication.
- Apply the drug as prescribed.
- Unless instructed otherwise, wash the affected area with mild soap and water and then pat dry before applying the topical drug.
- Don't stop application of the drug until directed by health care professional.
- Do not place the drug into deep wounds, puncture wounds, animal bites, onto serious burns, or on large wounds. This minimizes systemic absorption.
- If site of infection does not improve within 5 to 7 days or if it worsens, contact your health care provider.

- Don't take over-the-counter preparations, other drugs, or herbal remedies without first talking to your health care provider.
- Refrain from drinking alcohol while using topical drugs, as these may reduce efficacy or result in toxicity or adverse drug reaction.
- If you develop any signs of an allergic reaction, such as hives, difficulty breathing, swelling of face, lips, tongue, or throat, seek emergency medical help.
- Report planned or known pregnancy right away, as certain topical medications are known teratogens.

caution and should never be used around fire or flame. Patients should be taught to avoid smoking after application due to risk of flammability.

Examples of topical antifungal drugs include:

Azoles
- Clotrimazole (Lotrimin AF, Trivagizole 3)
- Econazole (Ecoza, Spectazole)
- Ketoconazole (Nizoral, Nizoral A-D)
- Miconazole (Miconazole 3, Monistat 1 combination pack, Monistat 3, Monistat 7)
- Oxiconazole (Oxistat)
- Sulconazole (Exelderm)

Allylamines
- Butenafine (Lotrimin Ultra, Mentax)
- Naftifine (Naftin)
- Terbinafine (Lamisil, Lamisil AT)

Hydroxypyridone
- Ciclopirox (Loprox, Penlac)

Polyenes
- Nystatin (Nystop)

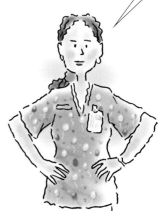

Cream is preferred over ointment when applied to skin folds and a powder formulation is preferred for very moist areas.

Pharmacokinetics

Similar to antibacterials, topical antifungal drugs are poorly absorbed.

Pharmacodynamics

Antifungal drugs kill or slow down growth of fungi.

Pharmacotherapeutics

Antifungal drugs are used to treat or prevent fungal infections, which are caused by dermatophytes, yeasts, or molds. Topical antifungals are specifically used for fungal infections of the skin, scalp hair, beard hair, eye, ear, nasal cavity, oral cavity, or vulva/vagina, as well as seborrheic dermatitis. Topical antifungals are usually used before systemic ones. The type of antifungal chosen by the health care provider (for example, cream, powder, ointment, etc.) depends mainly on the area of infection.

Drug interactions

While topical antifungals are generally considered safe, there are some potential drug interactions.
- Antifungal drugs may reduce the therapeutic effect of progesterone.
- Clotrimazole may increase the serum concentration of sirolimus or tacrolimus.
- Econazole and miconazole may increase the serum concentration of vitamin K antagonists (for example, warfarin).

- Topical antifungals used in combination with a corticosteroid may mask signs of infection or allergic reaction in addition to increase risk for fungal infections.

Adverse reactions

- The most common adverse reaction to topical antifungal drugs is a localized site reaction at the point of application (for example, burning, itching, stinging, redness, or dryness).
- Rare side effects include other types of skin infections, foul smelling vaginal discharge, contact dermatitis, hair loss, hair discoloration, change in hair texture, nail discoloration/disease, headache, dizziness, acne, abdominal cramps, fast/abnormal heartbeat, severe allergic reaction (swelling and itching of face, tongue, or throat, generalized rash, hives, dizziness, trouble breathing), and Stevens-Johnson syndrome.

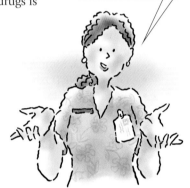

Rare side effects may include hair loss or discoloration, or change in hair texture.

Cautions

- As there are not enough studies on use of antifungal drugs in the pediatric, pregnant/lactating women, or the older adult populations, use with caution.
- Topical antifungals are preferred over oral antifungals in pregnant/lactating women.
- As with topical antibacterial drugs, avoid occlusive dressings as this may increase absorption.

The Three-Step Approach

Nursing management for patients receiving topical antibacterial or antifungal therapy includes these three steps. Be certain to pay particular attention to the type of drug being given, and personalize care accordingly.

Preadministration

(Recognize and analyze cues)

- Establish baseline assessment of the affected site before therapy begins and watch for significant changes. It is helpful to measure and record the size of the affected area so that accurate comparison can later be made.

 PHARM FACT ALERT

In neonates, avoid administering any antifungal drug containing benzyl alcohol, as it can cause a potentially fatal toxicity.

(Prioritize hypothesis)
- Skin integrity impairment
- Discomfort due to compromise of skin integrity

(Generate solutions)
- Infection will be eradicated.
- Discomfort will be eradicated or minimized to an acceptable level based on the patient's perception.

Medication administration

(Take action)
- Wear gloves when applying to prevent inadvertent exposure and absorption of drug.
- Promote measures to relieve itching (for example, cool compresses) and discomfort (for example, acetaminophen as prescribed).

Postadministration

(Evaluate outcomes)
- Conduct a follow-up assessment to determine if specific symptoms including infection and discomfort are alleviated.
- Provide teaching as included in *Teaching about use of topical drugs*, page 46. Additionally, teach patients who have been prescribed an antifungal drug for a vaginal infection to avoid vaginal intercourse, tampons, douches, spermicides, and other product use in or around the vagina during course of treatment.
- It is helpful to let patients know to monitor themselves closely, as fungal infections of the foot and groin often reoccur (Goldstein & Goldstein, 2021c; Lexicomp database, 2021).

Antivirals

Antiviral drugs are used to treat viral infections. For dermatological conditions, antiviral drugs are usually administered orally or topically; in certain cases, some are given intravenously (for example, acyclovir, Merck Manual Professional Version, 2021). Select examples of antiviral drugs include:

Antiviral drugs	Routes	Indications
Acyclovir (Zovirax)	Topical, oral, ophthalmic, buccal, intravenous	Herpesvirus infections
Valacyclovir (Valtrex)	Oral	Herpesvirus infections
Penciclovir (Denavir)	Topical	Herpes labialis
Docosanol (Abreva)—available over-the-counter	Topical	Herpes labialis

Pharmacokinetics

Similar to topical antibacterials and antifungals, when *topical* antivirals are applied to an affected area, most of the drug remains localized to that area. In contrast, *oral* acyclovir has poor bioavailability (10% to 20% in normal renal function), whereas *oral* valacyclovir has approximately 55% bioavailability once it has been converted to acyclovir by the intestinal and liver metabolism (Zachary, 2020). As antiviral drugs are not highly protein bound, they are able to penetrate tissue and fluid throughout the body. In patients with normal renal function, the peak time of acyclovir is 1.5 to 2 hours with oral formulation versus 1 hour with intravenous. As valacyclovir is a prodrug, its half-life is 30 minutes. Once valacyclovir is converted into acyclovir, then its half-life is the same as acyclovir (2.5 to 3.3 hours). Excretion of antivirals is mostly achieved renally. Renal failure may extend half-life to 20 hours.

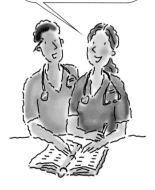

Remember that antivirals *do not cure* herpes viruses, but they can prevent or shorten outbreaks.

Pharmacodynamics

Antiviral drugs inhibit one of the stages of a virus' replication cycle.

Pharmacotherapeutics

Antiviral drugs are used to treat or prevent viral infections and reduce duration of infection. In dermatology, acyclovir and valacyclovir are commonly used to treat herpesvirus infections (for example, herpes simplex, varicella-zoster, cytomegalovirus). In addition to herpes labialis (orolabial herpes, known as cold sores), genital herpes, chickenpox, and shingles, antivirals are used to treat herpes simplex virus encephalitis or meningitis, prophylaxis after exposure to varicella, and suppressive therapy for herpes simplex. Systemic acyclovir has also been used off-label for prevention of herpes simplex virus and varicella zoster virus in immunocompromised patients and for treatment of herpes zoster ophthalmicus, acute retinal necrosis from varicella zoster virus, new onset Bell's palsy as an adjunctive or alternative therapy, cytomegalovirus prevention, herpes simplex esophagitis, or varicella zoster encephalitis.

PHARM FACT ALERT

Antiviral therapy can treat, prevent, or reduce duration of viral infection. However, the patient can still transmit the viral infection to others at certain times within the window of contagion. Make sure patients know how to protect themselves and others!

In contrast to broad uses of drugs like acyclovir and valacyclovir, penciclovir and docosanol are used for herpes labialis in people 12 years of age and older.

Drug interactions

There are multiple drug interactions between antivirals and other medications. Often, antivirals interact with other antivirals. Check the package insert or an agency's drug database for specific interactions based on the antiviral drug that has been prescribed. As an example, select antiviral drugs may interact with:

- cladribine, clozapine, foscarnet, mycophenolate, talimogene laherparepvec, tenofovir, theophylline, tizanidine, varicella virus vaccine, zidovudine, and zoster vaccine.

Adverse reactions

Adverse reactions associated with antiviral drugs by route of administration include:

Topical

- Common: local skin burning, itching, stinging, redness, or dryness, dry/cracked lips, headache.
- Specific: Buccal tablets have been associated with erythema, lethargy, aphthous stomatitis, gingival pain.
- Rare: contact dermatitis, angioedema, anaphylaxis.

Systemic

- Common: headache, fever, nasopharyngitis, abdominal pain, nausea, vomiting, diarrhea, leukopenia, increase in serum bilirubin, increase in blood urea nitrogen, menstrual pain, joint pain, depression, fatigue.
- Specific: With IV acyclovir, there is a risk for kidney and neurological toxicities. In patients infected with HIV-1 taking IV acyclovir, there have been reports of skin rash, neutropenia, thrombocytopenia, fatigue, and an increase in serum transaminases.
- Rare: anemia, leukocytosis, neutropenia, thrombocytopenia, increase in serum creatinine, severe allergic reaction, thrombotic microangiopathy, hemolytic-uremic syndrome, agitation/aggressive behavior, hallucinations, seizures, encephalopathy, tremor, dysarthria.

> Monitor renal function for patients taking acyclovir or valacyclovir.

Cautions

- Recognize that acyclovir is preferred over valacyclovir when treating a patient who is pregnant.
- Due to risk for acute kidney injury, caution is advised in older adults and those with renal impairment or receiving nephrotoxic agents.
- As with other topical applications, avoid occlusive dressings as these may increase drug absorption.

Lifespan Lightbulb

Older adults may be more likely to experience neurological adverse effects when taking an antiviral drug. Monitor for any change in neurologic status.

The Three-Step Approach

Nursing management for patients receiving topical antiviral therapy is similar to management of patients receiving topical antibacterial or antifungal therapy. Depending on the duration of therapy, the health care provider may request baseline laboratory data including a complete blood count, serum creatinine, blood urea nitrogen, urinalysis, and liver enzymes. If ordered, assure that these have been done, and continue to monitor these values throughout the duration of therapy.

Remind patients using topical therapy to avoid touching the site of infection and then touching their eyes or mucous membranes. Convey that they can still pass chickenpox or herpes to another person while taking this medication, and remind them to not allow infected areas to come in contact with others.

If IV administration is prescribed, monitor for dehydration and infuse over at least 1 hour to prevent nephrotoxicity. Monitor the peripheral intravenous site closely. If extravasation occurs, stop the infusion immediately, do not flush yet gently aspirate the extravasated solution from the catheter, and then remove catheter. The affected extremity should be elevated, and warm dry compresses should be applied. The prescribing provider should be notified for further orders; they may consider intradermal hyaluronidase to resolve the extravasation.

As with any drug administration, be certain to pay particular attention to the type of drug being given, teach about therapy (see *Teaching about use of topical drugs*, page 46) and personalize care accordingly.

Anti-inflammatories

There are several anti-inflammatory medications used to reduce dermatologic inflammation (for example, redness, swelling, heat, and pain). These include corticosteroids, nonsteroidal anti-inflammatory drugs (NSAIDs), topical calcineurin inhibitors, phosphodiesterase-4 (PDE4) inhibitors, and biologics.

Corticosteroids

Corticosteroids, also known as steroids or cortisones, are immunosuppressive and anti-inflammatory agents commonly used when treating dermatologic conditions. The routes of topical administration are ointment, cream, lotion, gel, spray, or foam. They may also be given orally, intramuscularly, or by intralesional injection right into a skin lesion (Mathes & Alguire, 2019). Select examples of the multitudes of products on the market (some of which are available over-the-counter) include:

- Alclometasone (no trade name at time of publication)
- Betamethasone dipropionate (Diprolene, Sernivo)
- Dexamethosone (Hemady)
- Hydrocortisone (Cortaid Maximum Strength, Cortef)
- Methylprednisolone (Medrol, DEPO-Medrol, SOLU-medrol)
- Prednisolone (Millipred, Pediapred)
- Prednisone (Rayos)

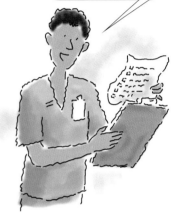

Be sure to clarify the names of medications! For example, prednisolone may be confused with prednisone, or hydrocortisone may be confused with hydrocodone.

Pharmacokinetics

Nearly every cell has receptors for cortisol, allowing for cortisol to have a myriad of different influences on the body: anti-inflammatory response, regulating metabolism, mediating stress response, glucose and blood pressure control, and more. Secretion of cortisol is controlled by the hypothalamus, pituitary gland, and the adrenal gland (also known as the HPA axis).

Corticosteroids are synthetic cortisol-like compounds. Corticosteroids administered systemically are rapidly absorbed, with peak time of onset of 1 to 2 hours (longer if taken with food), metabolized via the liver, and excreted via the kidneys with half-life of 2 to 4 hours.

Topical corticosteroids have varying potencies that are divided into seven groups according to the United States Classification System based on their level of potency (Jacob & Steele, 2006, in Gabros et al., 2021). Therapies should be potency appropriate and use the smallest amount for the shortest time period to avoid HPA axis suppression. Topical corticosteroids are localized to the site of application, but some of the medication can be absorbed via the skin depending on the integrity of the skin, medication formulation, age of the patient, frequency and duration of treatment, the amount of skin surface being treated, and location of treatment area. Use of an occlusive dressing can also influence absorption. Unlike systemic steroids, topical steroids have a half-life of 18 to 36 hours and are excreted via kidneys and intestines.

Pharmacodynamics

Corticosteroids suppress inflammation by binding to intracellular corticosteroid receptors, initiating a cascade of anti-inflammatory mediators. They also cause vasoconstriction in inflamed tissue and prevent macrophages and leukocytes from moving into the area.

Pharmacotherapeutics

Corticosteroids are used to relieve redness, swelling, warmth, pain, and itching in steroid-responsive disorders. Steroids are commonly used in treatment of the skin. Examples of conditions include eczema, psoriasis, contact dermatitis, seborrheic dermatitis, atopic dermatitis, urticaria, bullous dermatitis herpetiformis, bullous pemphigoid, erythema multiforme, Stevens-Johnson syndrome, severe psoriasis, mycosis fungoides, exfoliative erythroderma, exfoliative dermatitis, and more.

Drug interactions

- Corticosteroids (topical and systemic) may reduce the antineoplastic effect of aldesleukin.
- Systemic corticosteroids have *numerous* potential drug interactions. Be certain to reference a current drug database before administration to understand whether other medications your patient is taking may interact with the specific prescribed systemic corticosteroid.

Adverse reactions

While topical corticosteroids are safer than systemic corticosteroids, they are not without side effects. Assess for:
- Skin changes—localized redness, burning, itching, or irritation, thinning of skin, telangiectasia (spider veins), striae (stretch marks), dermatitis, purpura, changes in pigmentation, abnormal hair growth, folliculitis, maceration of the skin, secondary skin infection, xeroderma, and impaired wound healing.
- Kaposi sarcoma, which may occur with prolonged treatment.
- Immunosuppression, which also may occur with prolonged use. The risk for secondary infection, a masked acute infection, prolonged or worsened viral infections, or reduced efficacy to vaccines can happen.
- Withdrawal syndrome, also which occurs with prolonged use. (Days to weeks after stopping steroid therapy, erythema, a burning or stinging sensation, itching, pain, or facial hot flashes may occur.)
- Eye changes—Increased intraocular pressure, glaucoma, cataracts which can occur with prolonged use.
- Common occurrences with systemic therapy include headache, behavioral differences, sodium retention, weight gain (with prolonged therapy), and GI upset.

Cautions

- Use with careful caution in neonates, as some formulations may contain propylene glycol which, in large amounts, can lead to fatal toxicity.
- Do not use high potency topical corticosteroids on the face, as these can induce erythema, burning, itching, acneiform lesions, and telangiectasias (Sharma et al., 2017).
- There are limited data regarding the safety of corticosteroids in pregnant or lactating individuals. Systemic steroids are not the preferred first line of therapy for dermatologic disorders in this population, and they are generally not administered in the first trimester. If systemic steroids are required, prednisone or hydrocortisone is preferred. The lowest dose should be used for the shortest time possible.
- Systemic steroids may affect how the body absorbs and distributes some nutrients. Therefore, some may need to increase their dietary intact of pyridoxine, vitamin C, vitamin D, folate, calcium, phosphorus and decrease dietary intake of sodium and potassium.
- As with other topical applications, avoid occlusive dressings as they can increase the absorption and potency of topical corticosteroids up to 100-fold.

The Three-Step Approach

Nursing management for patients receiving topical antiviral therapy is similar to management of patients receiving other topical drug therapy. Monitor skin integrity throughout the duration of time of treatment. If systemic therapy is used over a duration, teach the patient to weigh themselves weekly and report any pattern of increasing weight to the health care provider.

Topical calcineurin inhibitors

Calcineurin inhibitors are a class of drugs used to suppress the immune system. Two topical calcineurin inhibitors used in treatment of dermatologic disorders include:

- Pimecrolimus (Elidel)
- Tacrolimus (Protopic)

Pharmacokinetics

Topical calcineurin inhibitors are poorly absorbed. Peak onset is 2 to 6 hours. Patients usually experience significant improvement of atopic dermatitis within 8 days of initiation of treatment.

Pharmacodynamics

Topical calcineurin inhibitors are immune modulators; they alter the immune system by stopping the enzyme calcineurin from activating

T cells and releasing inflammatory chemicals. Consequently, they reduce inflammation.

Pharmacotherapeutics

Topical calcineurin inhibitors are usually second-line therapy for atopic dermatitis (eczema) in nonimmunocompromised patients aged two and older.

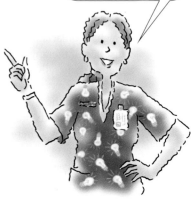

Topical calcineurin inhibitors increase the risk for infection, especially skin infections.

Drug interactions

- CYP3A4 inhibitors may decrease the metabolism of pimecrolimus.
- Topical calcineurin inhibitors may increase the adverse/toxic effect of immunosuppressants.
- Alcohol consumption while taking tacrolimus may cause skin flushing or burning sensation.

Adverse reactions

Most common adverse effects of topical calcineurin inhibitors are local irritation, flushing, burning, itching, pain, or redness. This usually occurs during the first few days of treatment and reduces as atopic dermatitis resolves. Use of alcohol can increase these integumentary effects. Rarely, severe allergic reaction, lymphadenopathy, malignant neoplasm, and skin discoloration have been reported.

Cautions

Caution is exercised if a topical calcineurin inhibitor is used in patients who are immunocompromised, since these drugs are immune modulators. These drugs are usually not used for neonates, as they may contain benzyl alcohol, which can be toxic.

The Three-Step Approach

Nursing management for patients receiving topical calcineurin inhibitor therapy is similar to management of patients receiving other topical drug therapy. Monitor skin integrity throughout the duration

Black Box Warning

Primecrolimus and Tacrolimus

Pimecrolimus topical (Elidel) and tacrolimus topical (Protopic) both have a Black Box Warning regarding the risk for malignancies and lymphoma, although evidence has not established a firm relationship between those drugs and conditions. Neither drug should be given to patients under the age of 2. Tacrolimus topical (Protopic) should be given only in the 0.03% strength for patients between 2 and 15 years of age.

of treatment, and recognize that these drugs are not used for long-term therapy. Additionally, teach the patient to limit sun exposure and use sun protection during treatment.

PDE4 inhibitors

PDE4 inhibitors are a type of anti-inflammatory drug class used to treat inflammatory skin and lung disease. Two PDE4 inhibitors used in treatment of dermatologic disorders include:
- Apremilast (Otezla)
- Crisaborole (Eucrisa)

Pharmacokinetics

Crisaborole is topical and is, therefore, poorly absorbed. Apremilast, on the other hand, is administered via oral route; it has a high bioavailability, is metabolized in the liver, and has a peak onset in 2.5 hours. It is excreted in urine and feces.

Pharmacodynamics

PDE4 inhibitors block the enzyme phosphodiesterase 4, resulting in the interruption of the inflammatory response, thereby reducing inflammation.

Pharmacotherapeutics

PDE4 inhibitors have multiple uses depending on the specific drug. Topical crisaborole is used to treat atopic dermatitis. Apremilast is used to treat psoriasis (including psoriatic arthritis) and oral ulcers caused by Behçet's disease.

Drug interactions

- CYP3A4 inducers (for example, dabrafenib, etc.) may decrease serum concentration of apremilast.
- PDE4 inhibitors may increase blood pressure, which can reduce the effect of riociguat.

Adverse reactions

Crisaborole
- Common adverse effects: local application site pain, swelling, or irritation
- Rare adverse effects: urticaria and allergic contact dermatitis

Apremilast
- Common adverse effects: weight loss, diarrhea, headache, and development of an upper respiratory infection
- Rare adverse effects: suicidal ideation, or exacerbation of psoriasis after discontinuing medication

Cautions

Apremilast is used with caution in those with renal impairments, on nephrotoxic agents, or with a history of depression or suicidal ideation. It is usually not used in pregnant women; studies on humans are limited, but animal studies indicate that use of this drug can increase the risk for pregnancy loss (Amgen, 2021).

The Three-Step Approach

Nursing management for patients undergoing treatment with a *topical* PDE4 inhibitor drug is similar to management of patients receiving other topical drug therapy. For patients who are prescribed apremilast, which is taken *orally*, follow all medication rights when administering this drug, and provide teaching about reporting any signs of suicidal ideation immediately to the health care provider. If the patient develops active suicidal ideation, 9-1-1 should be called and the patient should be taken to the nearest emergency department.

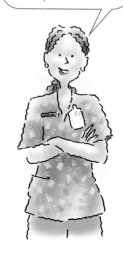

Carefully monitor renal function in patients taking apremilast.

Biologic agents and biosimilars

Biologic agents are often used for treatment of moderate to severe psoriasis, and moderate to severe atopic dermatitis. These types of drugs include tumor necrosis factor-alpha (TNF-alpha) inhibitors, interleukin 12 and 23 (IL-12, IL-23) inhibitors, interleukin 17 (IL-17) inhibitors, T-cell inhibitors, and interleukin 23 (IL-23) inhibitors. Depending on the specific drug, they may be administered by injection or intravenously. Biologic drugs include:

Tumor necrosis factor-alpha (TNF-alpha) inhibitors
- adalimumab (Humira)
- certolizumab pegol (Cimzia)
- etanercept (Enbrel)
- golimumab (Simponi or Simponi Aria)
- infliximab (Remicade)

Interleukin 12 and 23 (IL-12, IL-23) inhibitors
- ustekinumab (Stelara)

Interleukin 17 (IL-17) inhibitors
- brodalumab (Siliq)
- ixekizumab (Siliq)
- secukinumab (Cosentyx)

T-cell inhibitors
- abatacept (Orencia)

Interleukin 23 (IL-23) inhibitors
- guselkumab (Tremfya)
- risankizumab-rzaa (Skyrizi)
- tildrakizumab (Ilumya)

Biosimilar drugs are a type of biologic drug in the sense that they were modeled after an existing biologic (National Psoriasis Foundation, 2021). Also administered via injection or IV infusion, these drugs are indicated for individuals with more advanced disease processes. Although a number of biosimilar drugs have been approved, they are not all available on the market at time of publication. Reference a current electronic drug database the most immediate availability. Drugs that have been approved by the FDA include:

- Biosimilar drugs similar to adalimumab (Humira)
  - adalimumab-atto (Amjevita)
  - adalimumab-afzb (Abrilada)
  - adalimumab-adbm (Cyltezo)
  - adalimumab-bwwd (Hadlima)
  - adalimumab-fkjp (Hulio)
  - adalimumab-adaz (Hyrimoz)
- Biosimilar drugs similar to etanercept (Enbrel)
  - etanercept-szzs (Erelzi)
  - etanercept-ykro (Eticovo)
- Biosimilar drugs to infliximab (Remicade)
  - infliximab-axxq (Avsola)
  - infliximab-dyyb (Inflectra)
  - infliximab-qbtx (Ixifi)
  - infliximab-abda (Renflexis)

All the Pharmaco—info!

Because certain biosimilar products are not yet available, only biologics are discussed in this section. Each drug has its own unique pharmacokinetics; reference a current electronic drug database prior to administration for more information. Pharmacodynamics and pharmacotherapeutics include:

Biologics	TNF-alpha inhibitors	IL-12 and IL-23 inhibitors	IL-17 inhibitors	T-cell inhibitors	IL-23 inhibitors
Pharmacodynamics (how drugs act)	Blocks the TNF-alpha cytokine, which stops the inflammatory cycle	Targets cytokines IL-12 and IL-23 (which are associated with psoriatic inflammation)	Targets cytokine IL-17 (which is associated with psoriatic inflammation)	Targets T cells, inhibiting them from becoming activated, which reduces inflammation	Targets cytokine IL-23 (which are associated with psoriasis and psoriatic arthritis). This slows disease progression
Pharmacotherapeutics (how drugs are used)	These drugs are used for treatment of moderate to severe plaque psoriasis; some may be used for psoriatic arthritis or other types of psoriasis				

Drug interactions

There are multiple potential drug interactions when biologics (and, upon availability, biosimilars) are given with other drugs. Again, consult a current electronic drug database for very specific information. An important concept to recall when administering biologics is that when given with other immonusuppressive therapies, a synergistic effect can occur (Armanious & Vender, 2020). Although this is not a true drug interaction, it is important to recognize that this phenomenon can occur. It does not occur in every case of administration of multiple immunosuppressives as their mechanisms may have different pathways of action; however, it is a risk that should be evaluated so that the nurse can provide appropriate teaching about risks and protective actions (Armanious & Vender, 2020).

Adverse reactions

Most common adverse effect of biologics and biosimilars is a suppressed immune system.

Cautions

Caution is exercised when patients are prescribed more than one immunosuppressive drug.

The Three–Step Approach

Nursing management for patients undergoing treatment with a biologic (or eventually, a biosimilar) drug include these three steps.

Preadministration

(Recognize and analyze cues)
- Establish baseline assessment of the affected sites before therapy begins and watch for significant changes.
- Conditions like psoriasis often involve the patient's perception of degree of difficulty that the disorder inflicts on their life. Similar to conducting a pain assessment on a scale of 0 to 10, conduct

Black Box Warning

Biologic drugs

The majority of biologic drugs available have Black Box Warnings. Examples of conditions that can occur when taking certain biologics are serious infections (for example, tuberculosis, histoplasmosis, bacterial sepsis), or malignancy (for example, lymphoma), which are included on the Black Box Warning for Humira® (adalimumab) (AbbVie Inc, 2021). Check each drug carefully for specific Black Box Warning information.

a baseline evaluation, asking the patient to rate the level of impact that they feel the disorder creates.

- Assess for any underlying conditions or other medications the patient is taking that increases the risk for infection. If concerns are noted, collaborate with the health care provider.

(Prioritize hypothesis)
- Skin integrity impairment
- Alteration in self-perception

(Generate solutions)
- Skin condition will be improved.
- Impact on the patient's life will be eradicated or minimized to an acceptable level based on the patient's perception.
- Infection and malignancy will not develop.

Medication administration

(Take action)
- Carefully follow the rights of medication administration, giving the specific medication exactly as indicated. Remember that some of these drugs are given by injection and others are given by IV infusion.

Postadministration

(Evaluate outcomes)
- Conduct a follow-up assessment to determine if initial physical symptoms are alleviated.
- Conduct a follow-up assessment regarding the degree of impact the patient feels the disorder has on their life; compare this against the baseline determination and assess for improvement.
- Provide teaching about specific Black Box Warning information, which often includes the risk for infection or malignancy. Patients must be informed about signs and symptoms that they should immediately report to their health care provider.

Hair growth stimulant

The only FDA-approved topical hair growth stimulants for men and women pattern baldness are finasteride and minoxidil. Finasteride and minoxidil are available for oral administration; minoxidil is also available as a topical foam application.
- Finasteride (Propecia)
- Minoxidil (various Rogaine products, Theroxidil)

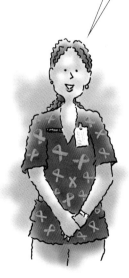

Many products claim to promote hair growth, but minoxidil and finasteride are the only drugs approved by the FDA for this purpose.

Pharmacokinetics

Systemic finasteride and minoxidil, taken orally, are readily absorbed. Topical minoxidil is poorly absorbed through skin.

Pharmacodynamics

Although the exact mechanism of action is unknown, it is thought that these drugs stimulate hair growth by causing vasodilation, which increases blood flow to the skin.

Pharmacotherapeutics

Finasteride and minoxidil are used to treat alopecia (baldness) of the scalp.

Drug interactions

Systemic cyclosporine may enhance the effect of topical minoxidil, resulting in hypertrichosis, excessive hair growth. Hypertrichosis can occur anywhere on the body. Cyclosporine and finasteride, when given together, do not have any known interactions.

Adverse reactions

Select adverse effects include:
- hair color and/or texture changes
- localized irritation, redness, burning, itching, dryness, or stinging
- unwanted facial/body hair growth
- worsening hair loss
- contact dermatitis, acne at the site of application, or increased hair loss (rare).

Caution

Caution should be exercised when these drugs are administered to patients with heart disease. Even the topical form of minoxidil may be systemically absorbed, leading to potential adverse effects. These include fluid retention, electrolyte changes, chest pain, flushing, elevated heart rate, rapid weight gain, headache, vision changes, and dizziness.

The Three-Step Approach

Nursing management for patients undergoing treatment with a *topical* hair growth stimulant drug is similar to management of patients receiving other topical drug therapy. For patients who are prescribed finasteride or minoxidil *orally*, follow all medication rights. See also information contained in *Teaching about use of topical drugs* (page 46) and *Teaching about topical minoxidil* (page 63). Finally, provide teaching about possible cardiac side effects to patients with heart disease.

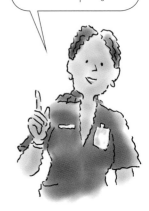

Apply minoxidil to the scalp only.

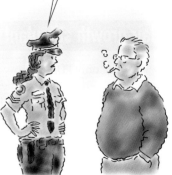

Topical minoxidil is flammable—Avoid fire/flame, smoking, or electric/heat sources while medication is drying.

Teaching about topical minoxidil

If a topical hair growth stimulant is prescribed, teach these points:
• Ensure hair and scalp are completely dry before application. Gently massage onto affected areas on scalp.
• Do not shampoo your hair for at least 4 hours after applying.
• Minoxidil can stain if the hair/scalp are not fully dry.
• Topical hair growth stimulants are flammable. Do not smoke and do not use a hairdryer or any other electric/heat sources while medication is drying (2 to 4 hours).
• Hair growth should be evident within 4 months of initiation of treatment. However, once initiated, the drug needs to be continued indefinitely, as hair loss will begin again within a few months after stopping treatment.

Antiacne drugs

Acne is a common skin condition that is treated with topical and/ or oral antiacne drugs. Often, both types of drugs are used in combination to treat acne depending on the patient's age, type of acne, and degree of severity. Two types of topical antiacne drugs that are covered in this chapter include keratolytics and retinoids. Oral antiacne drugs include antibiotics like benzoyl peroxide (see Chapter 16), combined oral contraceptives (Chapter 11), spironolactone (see Chapter 11), and isotretinoin, covered in this chapter. There are many different trade names of antiacne drugs that are available on the market. A very limited sample of these drugs used for acne treatment include:

Keratolytics
• Salicylic acid

Retinoids (vitamin A derivatives):
• Adapalene (Differin)
• Isotretinoin (Absorica, Claravis)
• Tazarotene (Tazorac)
• Tretinoin (Retin-A, Retin-A Micro)

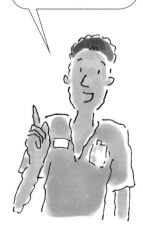

Avoid occlusive dressings with topical antiacne drugs as this may increase absorption of the drug.

Pharmacokinetics

Topical keratolytics are poorly absorbed. Onset of action depends on the condition being treated. In general, it takes approximately 2 to 8 weeks or more for treatment of acne, up to 6 months for treatment of wrinkles, 1 week for treatment of psoriasis, and 1 to 2 weeks for treatment of warts. Oral formulations are highly protein bound.

Pharmacodynamics

Keritolytics soften and loosen the outer layer of the skin, facilitating exfoliation. Retinoids interfere with the cohesion of hyperproliferative keratinocytes (Osteopathic College of Dermatology, 2021).

Pharmacotherapeutics

Topical keratolytics are commonly used to treat acne in those aged 8 years and older. Salicylic acid is used to treat calluses, corns, dandruff, seborrheic dermatitis, warts, and hyperkeratotic skin disorders. Retinoids are also used to fine wrinkles and other skin conditions, in addition to being used to treat acne.

Drug interactions

- Avoid using these drugs with other drying topical agent(s); combined use can cause severe drying or irritation of the skin.
- Avoid using these drugs with other medications that cause photosensitivity (for example, tetracyclines, fluoroquinolones, thiazides, phenothiazines, sulfonamides); sensitivity to the sun may increase.

Adverse reactions

- The most common adverse reactions include local burning, stinging, itching, redness, dryness, scaling, blistering, peeling, decreased skin pigmentation, and an increased sensitivity to sun or cold/wind.
- There is an increased risk for superinfection with prolonged use.
- Uncommonly, retinoids can cause acne flare, urticaria, angioedema, local dermatitis, hyperpigmentation, skin discoloration, and face swelling.
- Very rarely, salicylic acid use may lead to salicylic toxicity (nausea, vomiting, tinnitus, headache, confusion, febrile, tachypnea, metabolic acidosis, multiple organ failure).

Cautions

- Avoid use in neonates; do not use for children and adolescents with varicella or influenza, as salicylic acid may be associated with Reye syndrome.

 PHARM FACT ALERT

Tretinoin may be confused with isotretinoin, tenormin, triamcinolone, or trientine. As always, read labels extremely carefully.

- May cause severe irritation in those using a concomitant drying topical agent(s) or with those with eczema.
- Avoid excessive intake of vitamin A when taking a retinoid.
- Retinoids are avoided when treating people who are pregnant, plan to get pregnant, or are at high risk behaviors for pregnancy.
- Avoid prolonged use over large areas, in children, or in those with liver or kidney impairment, and when using other salicylates to prevent salicylic toxicity.

The Three-Step Approach

Nursing management for patients undergoing treatment with a topical antiacne drug is similar to management of patients receiving other topical therapy for a dermatologic concern.

Remind patients to avoid use of these products on moles, birthmarks, warts with hair growing from them, and genital/anal warts. Also provide teaching about the potential for increased photosensitivity. As with any drug administration, be certain to pay particular attention to the type of drug being given and personalize care and teaching.

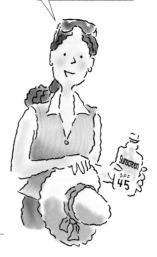

Remember to avoid direct exposure to the sun when using topical antiacne drugs.

Isotretinoin

Isotretinoin is a systemic retinoid utilized primarily for refractory severe cystic (nodular) acne. This treatment is usually only used when a patient has not had success with other therapies. Select examples of brand names include Absorica and Zenatane.

Pharmacokinetics

Systemic isotretinoin is administered orally. As isotretinoin is lipophilic, this medication should be taken with food or milk to increase its bioavailability. This drug is 99% to 100% bound to plasma proteins and is hepatically metabolized and excreted via urine and feces. Time to peak is approximately 3 hours if fasting and 5 to 6 hours if taken with a meal.

Pharmacodynamics

Isotretinoin reduces inflammation at a cellular level and decreases the size of sebaceous gland and the amount of facial oil produced, thereby decreasing follicular hyperkeratinization and suppressing the bacteria *Propionibacterium acnes*. Consequently, this reduces inflammation.

Pharmacotherapeutics

Isotretinoin is primarily used for the dermatologic condition of refractory severe acne in those 12 years of age and older.

Drug interactions

Several drug interactions can occur in patients taking isotretinoin:

- Alcohol consumption may increase the risk for elevated triglycerides.
- Photosensitizing agents may increase sensitivity to sun.
- Avoid excessive concurrent intake of vitamin A as this may increase the toxic effects of retinoic acid derivatives.
- Tetracyclines may increase adverse/toxic effects of isotretinoin (for example, development of pseudotumor cerebri).

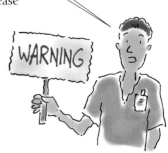

Isotretinoin has numerous and potentially severe adverse effects.

Adverse reactions

Isotretinoin is almost exclusively used as a last resort to treat acne due to the number of potential serious adverse effects. There are numerous potential adverse effects that impact every organ system. Refer to an electronic database for a complete listing. Common adverse effects include:

- increased triglycerides, cholesterol, creatinine phosphokinase, liver enzymes, and erythrocyte sedimentation rate
- decreased high-density lipoproteins, bone mineral density
- development of anemia, headaches, muscle or bone pain, facial redness, sun sensitivity, and dryness of skin and mucous membranes.

The Three-Step Approach

Nursing management for patients undergoing treatment with isotretinoin is similar to management of patients receiving other oral therapy for a dermatologic concern. Be certain to obtain baseline laboratory values as prescribed (for example, complete blood count with differential, sedimentation rate, glucose, creatine phosphokinase, lipid panel, liver function test). Special attention must be given to these three points:

- All patients regardless of gender must be registered in the iPLEDGE risk management program (Pile & Sadiq, 2021).

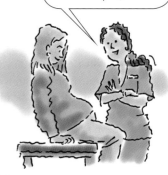

Isotretinoin must never be given to a patient who is pregnant or may become pregnant.

Black Box Warning

Isotretinoin

Isotretinoin is contraindicated during pregnancy or for use in people who may become pregnant due to the risk of development of severe, life-threatening birth defects. This drug can only be prescribed by certain prescribers and be dispensed by pharmacies who are registered with the iPLEDGE program, a restricted distribution program by the FDA (Pile & Sadiq, 2021).

- Two negative pregnancy tests taken 1 month apart are also recommended before starting therapy.
- Teach patients who may become pregnant to use two simultaneous forms of contraception for 1 month prior to therapy and throughout the duration of treatment. Progestin oral contraceptives should not be used, as isotretinoin reduces their efficacy.

   During therapy, ongoing pregnancy tests and ongoing laboratory monitoring may be required.

   As with any drug administration, be certain to pay particular attention to the type of drug being given and personalize care and teaching.

Other antiacne treatments

Anti-infectives

Topical clindamycin, erythromycin, dapsone, and azelaic acid are often used to treat acne. However, topical antibiotics are not recommended to be used alone. For moderate to severe acne, a tetracycline or a macrolide is used in combination with another treatment, such as benzoyl peroxide. Refer to Chapter 16.

Oral contraceptives

Oral contraceptives are often used to decrease acne breakouts. Refer to information about oral contraceptives in Chapter 11.

Spironolactone

This drug may be used to treat acne. Refer to Chapter 8.

Antiparasitics: scabicides, pediculicides, anthelmintics

Parasite infections, including scabies (infection caused by the mite *Sarcoptes scabiei*), pediculosis (skin infection caused by lice), and

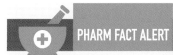

PHARM FACT ALERT

Historically, isotretinoin use has been associated with a higher risk for suicide risk. Current research including a study of 443,814 patients indicated that there was no evidence of a triggering effect of isotretinoin culminating in suicide attempt (Droitcourt et al., 2019). Until further research is conducted, risk management plans should still be initiated for patients prescribed isotretinoin.

helminths (parasitic worms), are common worldwide problems affecting people of all socioeconomic backgrounds. Select examples of commonly used antiparasitic medications include:

Topical antiparasitics	Indications
Benzyl alcohol (over-the-counter)	Head lice
Crotamiton (Eurax)	Scabies
Ivermectin lotion (Sklice—over-the-counter)	Head lice, rosacea
Malathion	Head lice and pubic lice (off-label)
Pyrethroids: Permethrin • Nix Combing Gel and Crème Rinse—over-the-counter • Nix Lice and Bedbug Killing Spray for Home	 Lice Lice and bedbugs
Spinosad (Natroba)	Head lice
Oral antiparasitic	**Indications**
Ivermectin	Parasitic worm infections

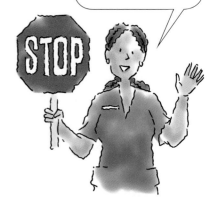

Read labels carefully! Benzyl alcohol may be confused with benzoyl peroxide.

Pharmacokinetics

Topical antiparasitics are minimally absorbed. Oral ivermectin is absorbed quickly on an empty stomach; bioavailability increases if taken after a fatty meal. Oral ivermectin is metabolized in the liver and excreted primarily in feces.

Pharmacodynamics

Most antiparasitics kill parasites by their neurotoxic effects to the pest. In contrast, benzyl alcohol kills lice by suffocation and crotamiton kills scabies via an unknown mechanism of action.

PHARM FACT ALERT

Lindane is topical scabicide not listed in the table above. It is available in the United States only by prescription and *very* rarely used due to the risk for neurotoxicity. It may be considered as a last line of treatment for patients who cannot tolerate other scabicides or who have not achieved eradication of scabies from other methods of treatment. It is restricted or banned in many countries. If it is prescribed for your patient, teach them to use nitrile, sheer vinyl, or latex gloves with neoprene (unless they have a latex allergy), as these are less permeable to lindane (U.S. Food and Drugs Administration, n.d.).

Pharmacotherapeutics

When selecting a medication to treat a parasite infection, the decision is based on the patient's age, location and type of parasite infestation, resistance patterns, treatment cost, and the drug's adverse effects profile. Pyrethroids are usually the preferred first-line therapy for lice (head, body, pubic) and scabies given that they are inexpensive, safe, and effective, with oral ivermectin being used to treat parasitic worms.

Drug interactions

Topical antiparasitics
- None known; consult an electronic database for evolving information

Oral ivermectin
- May decrease the therapeutic effect of vaccines
- May increase anticoagulant effect of vitamin k antagonists (for example, warfarin)

Adverse reactions

Topical antiparasitics
- Common adverse effects include redness, itching, pain, transient numbness/tingling, dryness, or swelling at application site.
- Rare adverse effects include dermatitis, rash, thermal injury, peeling skin, and hair thinning.
- Pyrethroids my cause breathing difficulties in patients with a ragweed allergy.
- Malathion has been associated with respiration depression (if accidentally ingested) in addition to chemical burns.

Oral ivermectin
- Common adverse effects include itching, swelling, hives, fever, joint pain/inflammation, and lymphadenitis.
- Other selected potential adverse effects include tachycardia, extremity or facial swelling, dizziness, orthostatic hypotension, nausea, diarrhea, elevated liver enzymes, elevated eosinophil count, decreased white blood cell count, and increased hemoglobin.

Cautions
- Avoid benzyl alcohol in neonates as it has been associated with potentially fatal toxicities.
- Avoid use in neonates and infants given the increased risk of systemic absorption.
- As pyrethroids are made from a natural chrysanthemum extract, those who are allergic to chrysanthemums should avoid this medication.
- Oral ivermectin should be avoided, if possible, in people who are pregnant or lactating, and in children weighing less than 15 kg.

The Three-Step Approach

Nursing management for patients being treated with topical antiparasitics is similar to management of patients receiving other topical drug therapy. Teach patients that household members should be evaluated and treatment as needed. Also teach to wash or dry clean all recently used clothes, hats, bedding, towels, combs/brushes, and hair accessorizes in hot water; items that cannot be washed should be sealed in a plastic bag for at least 2 weeks. Bed linens should be changed the day after application. As with any drug administration, be certain to pay particular attention to the type of drug being given, teach about therapy. Other specific information to teach includes (Lexicomp database, 2021; Goldstein & Goldstein, 2021a; Goldstein & Goldstein, 2021b):

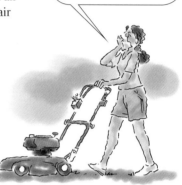

Pyrethroids may cause breathing difficulties in patients with a ragweed allergy.

- *For lice treatment*: Hair should be dry. Do not use hair conditioner prior to application as this may decrease the efficacy. Avoid fire/flame, smoking, or electric heat sources while medication drying. Rinse topical pediculicides over a sink to limit skin exposure. Avoid hot water to limit vasodilation and systemic absorption.
- *For scabies treatment*: Take a bath or shower and trim nails prior to application. Apply medication from the neck down to the toes, including under nails. After 8 to 14 hours of application, take a bath or shower to cleanse the body. (Of note, with crotamiton, a bath or shower is to be taken 48 hours after application.)

For patients receiving oral ivermectin, provide this teaching:

- Take as directed; guidelines state this drug is most effective when taken as a single dose with 8 oz of water before breakfast, although other experts state that taking it with a meal increases bioavailability (Centers for Disease Control and Prevention, 2019).
- Treatment may last up to 12 months.

Quick quiz

1. Which administration method will the nurse use when providing for treatment for scabies?
   A. Apply topical medication from neck down to toes, including under nails.
   B. Apply topical medication to hair and then rinse off over a sink.
   C. Gently massage topical medication onto affected areas on body.
   D. Administer an intradermal injection once weekly.

Answer: A. Scabies requires topical treatment from the neck down (including nails). Also, teach patients to refrain from bathing for 48 hours after application. Other methods of administration listed are incorrect.

2. Which laboratory data will the nurse assess as the **priority** before administering isotretinoin to a patient?
  A. Complete blood count
  B. Lipid panel
  C. C-reactive protein
  D. Latest pregnancy test

Answer: D. The nurse will assess the pregnancy test, as this medication is highly teratogenic. The other laboratory findings can be assessed but are not the priority.

3. What's the most common adverse reaction experienced with topical drugs used to address dermatologic problems?
  A. Nausea
  B. Headache
  C. Site reaction
  D. Hair loss

Answer: C. Local application site reaction is the most common adverse reaction to topical drugs, as these are placed directly on the skin. There are other side effects that are associated with these medications at a lesser frequent rate than site reactions.

Scoring

☆☆☆ If you answered all three questions correctly, magnificent! You've got it!

☆☆ If you answered two questions correctly, way to go! You're in the know about drugs that are used for dermatologic conditions!

☆ If you answered fewer than two questions correctly, stay calm. Another look at this chapter will be helpful.

Suggested References

AbbVie Inc. (2021). *Humira*. Retrieved from https://www.rxabbvie.com/pdf/humira.pdf

Amgen. (2021). *Otezla* (apremilast). Retrieved from www.otezla.com

Armanious, M., & Vender, R. (2020). A review of drug-drug interactions for biologic drugs used in the treatment of psoriasis. *Journal of Cutaneous Medicine and Surgery, 25*(1), 38–44.

Centers for Disease Control and Prevention. (2019). *Parasites – Scabies: Medications*. Retrieved from https://www.cdc.gov/parasites/scabies/health_professionals/meds.html

Droitcourt, C., et al. (2019). Risk of suicide attempt associated with isotretinoin: A nationwide cohort and nested case-time-control study. *International Journal of Epidemiology, 48*(5), 1623–1635.

Elidel (tacrolimus topical). (2021). *Epocrates database*. Retrieved from https://online.epocrates.com/drugs/268011/Elidel/Black-Box-Warnings

Gabros, S., Nessel, T. A., & Zito, P. M. (2021). Topical Corticosteroids. [Updated 2021 July 13]. In *StatPearls [Internet]*. Treasure Island, FL: StatPearls Publishing. Retrieved from https://www.ncbi.nlm.nih.gov/books/NBK532940/

Goldstein, A. O., & Goldstein, B. G. (2021a). Pediculosis pubis and pediculosis ciliaris. In R. Dellavalle, M. Levy, & T. Rosen (Eds.), *UpToDate*. Waltham, MA: UpToDate.

Goldstein, A. O., & Goldstein, B. G. (2021b). Scabies: Management. In R. Dellavalle, M. Levy, & T. Rosen (Eds.), *UpToDate*. Waltham, MA: UpToDate.

Goldstein, A. O., & Goldstein, B. G. (2021c). Dermatopyte (tinea) infections. In R. Dellavalle, M. Levy, & T. Rosen (Eds.), *UpToDate*. Waltham, MA: UpToDate.

Graber, E. (2021). Acne vulgaris: Overview of management. In R. Dellavalle, M. Levy, & C. Owen (Eds.), *UpToDate*. Waltham, MA: UpToDate.

Lexicomp database. (2021). Used to reference all drugs in this chapter.

Mathes, B., & Alguire, P. (2019). Intralesional corticosteroid injection. In Deliavalle, R. (Ed.), *UpToDate*. Waltham, MA.

Merck Manual Professional Version. (2021). *Drugs used to treat herpesvirus infections*. Retrieved from https://www.merckmanuals.com/professional/multimedia/table/v1019328

National Psoriasis Foundation. (2021). Biologics. Retrieved from https://www.psoriasis.org/biologics/

Osteopathic College of Dermatology. (2021). *Retinoids, topical*. Retrieved from https://www.aocd.org/page/Retinoidstopical

Pile, H., & Sadiq, N. (2021). Isotretinoin. In *StatPearls [Internet]*. Treasure Island, FL: StatPearls Publishing. Retrieved from https://www.ncbi.nlm.nih.gov/books/NBK525949/

Protopic (tacrolimus topical). (2021). *Epocrates database*. Retrieved from https://online.epocrates.com/drugs/234911/Protopic/Black-Box-Warnings

Ray P., Singh, S., & Gupta, S. (2019). Topical antimicrobial therapy: Current status and challenges. *Indian Journal of Medical Microbiology, 37*(3), 299–308.

Sharma, R., Abrol, S., & Wani, M. (2017). Misuse of topical corticosteroids on facial skin. A study of 200 patients. *Journal of dermatological case reports, 11*(1), 5–8. https://doi.org/10.3315/jdcr.2017.1240

U.S. Food and Drugs Administration. (n.d.). *Lindane lotion USP 1%*. Retrieved from https://www.accessdata.fda.gov/drugsatfda_docs/label/2003/006309lotionlbl.pdf

Williams, D. M. (2018). Clinical pharmacology of corticosteroids. *Respiratory Care, 63*(6), 655–670. doi: 10.4187/respcare.06314.

Zachary, K. C. (2020). Acyclovir: An overview. In M. Hirsch (Ed.), *UpToDate*. Waltham, MA: UpToDate.

Chapter 5

Pain medications

Just the facts

In this chapter, you'll learn:

◆ classes of drugs used to control pain

◆ uses and actions of these drugs

◆ absorption, distribution, metabolization, and excretion of these drugs

◆ drug interactions and adverse reactions to these drugs.

Drugs and pain control

Drugs used to control pain range from mild, over-the-counter (OTC) preparations, such as acetaminophen, to potent general anesthetics. Drug classes in this category include:

- nonopioid analgesics, antipyretics, and nonsteroidal anti-inflammatory drugs (NSAIDs)
- opioid agonist and antagonist drugs
- anesthetic drugs.

Nonopioid analgesics, antipyretics, and NSAIDs

Nonopioid analgesics, antipyretics, and NSAIDs are a broad group of pain medications. In addition to pain control, they produce antipyretic (fever control) and anti-inflammatory effects. They can be used alone or as adjuvant medications. These drugs have a ceiling effect, and no physical dependence is associated with them.

The drug classes included in this group are:

- salicylates (especially aspirin)
- acetaminophen, a para-aminophenol derivative
- NSAIDs (nonselective and selective)
- phenazopyridine hydrochloride, a urinary tract analgesic.

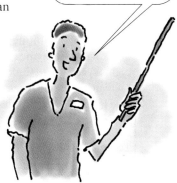

A ceiling effect is when the medication dose has reached its maximum effectiveness.

Salicylates

Salicylates are among the most commonly used pain medications. They're used to control pain and reduce fever and inflammation.

Cheap, easy, and reliable

Salicylates usually cost less than other analgesics and are readily available without a prescription. Aspirin is the most commonly used salicylate for anti-inflammatory drug therapy (Karch, 2020).

Other salicylates include:
- choline magnesium trisalicylate
- diflunisal
- olsalazine.

Pharmacokinetics

Taken orally, salicylates are primarily absorbed in the upper part of the small intestine and partially absorbed in the stomach. The pure and buffered forms of aspirin reabsorb readily, but sustained-release and enteric-coated salicylate preparations, food, or antacids in the stomach delay absorption. Enteric-coated products are slowly absorbed and are not suitable for acute effects. They cause less GI bleeding and may be better suited for long-term therapy, such as for rheumatoid or osteoarthritis (Karch, 2020). Absorption after rectal administration is slow and variable, depending on how long the suppository is retained.

Dynamite distribution, marvelous metabolism

Salicylates are distributed widely throughout body tissues and fluids, including breast milk. In addition, they easily cross the placenta. The liver metabolizes salicylates extensively into several metabolites. The kidneys excrete the metabolites along with some unchanged drug.

I'm great at metabolizing salicylates into metabolites!

Pharmacodynamics

The different effects of salicylates stem from their separate mechanisms of action. They relieve pain and inflammation primarily by inhibiting the synthesis of prostaglandin by blocking two enzymes known as cyclooxygenase-1 (COX-1) and cyclooxygenase-2 (COX-2). (Recall that prostaglandin is a chemical mediator that sensitizes nerve cells to pain.)

Half-life is 15 minutes to 12 hours depending on the salicylate (Karch, 2020).

Temperature goes down

Salicylates lower body temperature by inhibiting cyclooxygenase (COX-1 and COX-2), which blocks prostaglandin production and reduces fever (Abramson, 2021).

Bonus effects

One salicylate, aspirin, inhibits platelet aggregation (the clumping of platelets to form a clot) by interfering with the production of thromboxane A_2, a substance necessary for platelet aggregation. Unlike aspirin, NSAIDs' effects on platelet aggregation are temporary. As a result, aspirin can be used to enhance blood flow during myocardial infarction (MI) and to prevent an event such as recurrent MI or acute ischemic strokes (Abramson, 2021). In addition, recent trials have indicated that aspirin may help to prevent colorectal cancer (Spencer et al., 2021).

Pharmacotherapeutics

Salicylates are primarily used to relieve pain and reduce fever; however, they don't effectively relieve visceral pain (pain from the organs and smooth muscle) or severe pain from trauma. They can also be used to reduce an elevated body temperature in conjunction with relieving headache and muscle ache. When used to reduce inflammation in rheumatic fever, rheumatoid arthritis, or osteoarthritis, salicylates can provide considerable relief within 24 hours.

How low can you go?

No matter what the clinical indication, the main guideline of salicylate therapy is to use the lowest dose that provides relief. This reduces the likelihood of adverse reactions. (See *Preparing for practice: Topical anesthetics: Salicylate warning.*)

Drug interactions

Because salicylates are highly protein-bound, they can interact with many other protein-bound drugs by displacing those drugs from sites to which they normally bind. This increases the serum concentration of the unbound active drug, causing increased pharmacologic effects (the unbound drug is said to be *potentiated*). Here are some drug interactions that may occur:

- Oral anticoagulants (such as warfarin), heparin, methotrexate, oral antidiabetic agents, and insulin are among the drugs that have increased effects or risk of toxicity when taken with salicylates.
- Probenecid, sulfinpyrazone, and spironolactone may have decreased effects when taken with salicylates.
- Corticosteroids may decrease plasma salicylate levels and increase the risk of ulcers.
- Alkalizing drugs and antacids may reduce salicylate levels.
- The antihypertensive effects of angiotensin-converting enzyme (ACE) inhibitors and beta-adrenergic blockers (commonly called *beta-blockers*) may be reduced when these drugs are taken concomitantly with salicylates.
- NSAIDs may have reduced therapeutic effects and an increased risk of GI effects when taken with salicylates.

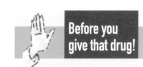

Before you give that drug!

Preparing for practice: Salicylate warning

Before administering salicylates to a patient, be aware of its risks to special populations:

- *Children and teenagers*: Avoid the use of aspirin and salicylates to treat chickenpox or flulike symptoms because Reye's syndrome may develop.
- *Surgical patients*: If possible, discontinue aspirin 1 week before surgery because of the risk of intraoperative and postoperative bleeding.
- *Asthmatics*: Be aware that these patients are more likely to develop bronchospasm, urticaria, angioedema, or shock when salicylates are administered.

Side effects/adverse reactions

The most common side effects/adverse reactions to salicylates include gastric distress, nausea, vomiting, and bleeding tendencies. (Choline magnesium is a salicylate that doesn't increase bleeding time.) Other adverse reactions include:

- hearing loss (when taken for prolonged periods)
- diarrhea
- increased thirst
- tinnitus
- confusion (especially in older adults)
- dizziness
- drowsiness (especially in children)
- impaired vision
- hyperventilation (rapid breathing)
- Reye's syndrome (when given to children with chickenpox or flulike symptoms)
- acute renal injury (Abramson, 2021).

Children with chickenpox or flulike symptoms shouldn't take salicylates because of the risk of Reye's syndrome.

The Three-Step Approach

Nursing management for the patient being treated with salicylates includes these three steps.

Preadministration

(Recognize and analyze cues)
- Assess the patient's vital signs and inspect for signs of inflammation before therapy begins.
- Ask the patient to rate the level of pain on a scale of 0 to 10 or use behavioral pain scales for children under 6. (Beltramini, Milojevic, & Pateron, 2017).
- Monitor the patient's ophthalmic and auditory function before beginning drug therapy and periodically thereafter to detect toxicity.
- Periodically monitor complete blood count (CBC), platelet count, prothrombin time (PT), and hepatic and renal function to detect abnormalities.

(Prioritize hypothesis—priority patient problems)
- Acute pain
- Chronic pain
- Injury risk
- Knowledge deficiency

(Generate solutions)
- The patient will acknowledge a reduction in pain or fever.
- The patient remains free from signs and symptoms of toxicity or other adverse reactions.
- The patient and family members will demonstrate an understanding of drug therapy.

Medication administration

(Take action)

- Give aspirin with food, milk, antacids, or a large glass of water to reduce GI symptoms.
- Withhold the dose and notify the prescriber if bleeding, salicylism (salicylate poisoning, characterized by tinnitus or hearing loss), or adverse GI reactions occur.
- Stop aspirin 5 to 7 days before elective surgery, as ordered.
- Monitor the patient for signs and symptoms of bleeding. Assess bleeding time if the patient is scheduled to undergo surgery.
- During long-term therapy, monitor serum salicylate levels. A therapeutic level in a patient with arthritis is 10 to 30 mg/mL.

A hard pill to swallow

- If the patient has trouble swallowing the drug, crush tablets or mix them with food or fluid. Do not crush enteric-coated aspirin.

Education edge

Teaching about salicylates

See Education edge: Teaching template in Chapter 3, page 38 for general teaching for all medications. Specific points to review with patients and family for salicylates:

- If receiving high-dose prolonged treatment, maintain adequate fluid intake and watch for petechiae, bleeding gums, and signs of GI bleeding. Use a soft toothbrush.
- Be aware that various OTC preparations contain aspirin. Because numerous drug interactions are possible when taking aspirin, check with the prescriber or pharmacist before taking herbal preparations or OTC medications containing aspirin.
- Avoid alcohol consumption during drug therapy.
- Restrict caffeine intake during drug therapy.

- Take the drug as directed to achieve the desired effect. Know that the benefits of drug therapy may not be noticeable for 2 to 4 weeks.
- Take the drug with food or milk to prevent GI upset.
- Notify the prescriber about severe or persistent adverse reactions.
- Be sure to safely store medications in the home. Aspirin ingestion is a leading cause of poisoning in children. Keep aspirin and other drugs out of children's reach. Use child-resistant containers in households with children.
- If salicylate therapy will be long term, be sure to follow the prescriber's orders for monitoring laboratory values, especially blood urea nitrogen and creatinine levels, liver function, and CBC.

Postadministration

(Evaluate outcomes)

- Evaluate drug effectiveness after administration.
- Observe and monitor for adverse reactions and drug interactions. Watch for bronchospasm in the patient with aspirin hypersensitivity, rhinitis or nasal polyps, or asthma.
- The patient remains free from adverse effects throughout drug therapy.
- The patient and family members state an understanding of drug therapy. (See *Teaching about salicylates*, page 77.)

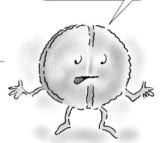

Be sure not to crush me before giving me to your patient because enteric-coated aspirins are made to protect the lining of the stomach.

Acetaminophen

Although the class of para-aminophenol derivatives includes two drugs—phenacetin and acetaminophen—only acetaminophen is available in the United States. Acetaminophen is an OTC drug that produces analgesic and antipyretic effects. Acetaminophen is also combined with several other medications, both prescription and OTC products, for treatment of pain and symptoms associated with colds and influenza. Acetaminophen comes in a variety of delivery modes: tablets, chewable tablets, capsules, liquid, rectal suppositories, injection, and IV.

Pharmacokinetics

Acetaminophen is absorbed rapidly and completely from the GI tract. It is irregularly absorbed from the mucous membranes of the rectum (Lexicomp, Inc., 2021). It's widely distributed in body fluids and readily crosses the placenta. After the liver metabolizes acetaminophen, it's excreted by the kidneys and, in small amounts, in breast milk.

Pharmacodynamics

Acetaminophen is classified as an analgesic and antipyretic, but unlike salicylates, it doesn't affect the inflammatory response or platelet function. It may potentiate the effects of warfarin and increase international normalized ratio (INR) values.

Pain and fever

The pain-control effects of acetaminophen works by inhibiting prostaglandin synthesis and reduces fever by acting directly on the heat-regulating center in the hypothalamus.

Acetaminophen and blood pressure?

Recent studies have shown that acetaminophen and NSAIDs can increase blood pressure (Townsend, 2021).

Pharmacotherapeutics

Acetaminophen is used to reduce fever and relieve headache, muscle ache, and general pain.

Child's play

Acetaminophen is the drug of choice to treat fever and flulike symptoms in children. The use of acetaminophen following some vaccinations is not recommended (Lexicomp, Inc., 2021).

Drug interactions

Acetaminophen can produce these drug interactions:
- It may slightly increase the effects of oral anticoagulants, such as warfarin, and thrombolytic drugs.
- The risk of liver toxicity is increased when phenytoin, barbiturates, carbamazepine, rifampin, and isoniazid are combined with acetaminophen. This risk is also increased with chronic alcohol use.
- The effects of loop diuretics and zidovudine may be reduced when taken with acetaminophen.

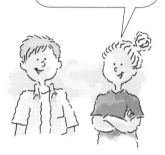

"Acetaminophen is commonly used to treat fever and flulike symptoms in children."

Side effects/adverse reactions

Most patients tolerate acetaminophen well. Unlike the salicylates, acetaminophen rarely causes gastric irritation or bleeding tendencies; however, it may cause liver toxicity, and the total daily dose should be monitored.

Other side effects/adverse reactions include:
- skin rash or other serious skin reactions
- nausea, vomiting, abdominal pain
- constipation
- hypoglycemia (with overdose)
- hematologic reaction: neutropenia, hemolytic anemia (with long-term use)
- injection site pain.

The Three-Step Approach

Nursing management for patients undergoing treatment with acetaminophen includes these three steps.

Preparing for practice: Acetaminophen

Hepatotoxicity
Factors influencing toxicity include current liver damage; concomitant use of alcohol, substance use, or other drugs; nutritional status; aging; some herbal products; and genetics (Burns et al., 2021).

Preadministration

(Recognize and analyze cues)
- Assess the patient's level of pain and inflammation before therapy begins.
- Analyze the patient's medication history. Many OTC products and combination prescription pain products contain acetaminophen and must be considered when calculating the total daily dosage.

(Prioritize hypothesis—priority patient problems)
- Acute pain
- Injury risk
- Knowledge deficiency

(Generate solutions)
- The patient will acknowledge a reduction in pain.
- No serious complications will occur while the patient is on drug therapy.
- The patient and family members will verbalize understanding of the purpose and intended effect of drug therapy.

Medication administration

(Take action)
- Administer the liquid form of the drug to children and other patients who have difficulty swallowing.
- Monitor the patient for adverse reactions and drug interactions, including hepatotoxicity, hypoglycemia, or Stevens-Johnson syndrome (a severe hypersensitivity reaction evidenced by reddened skin, rash, blisters, detachment of the epidermis, and even death).

Calculating the dosage

- When giving oral preparations, calculate the dosage based on the concentration of the drug because drops and elixir have different concentrations (for example, 80 versus 120 mg/mL).
- Use the rectal route in young children and other patients for whom oral administration isn't feasible.

Postadministration

(Evaluate outcomes)
- Evaluate drug effectiveness after administration.
- The patient remains free from adverse effects throughout drug therapy.
- The patient and family members state an understanding of drug therapy. (See *Teaching about acetaminophen*, page 81.)

> Check your patient's medication history for combination pain products that contain acetaminophen; you'll need to consider that when calculating the total daily acetaminophen dosage.

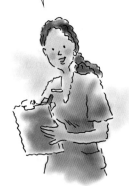

Teaching about acetaminophen

See Education edge: Teaching template in Chapter 3, page 38 for general teaching for all medications. Specific points to review with patients and family for acetaminophen medication:

• Consult a prescriber before giving the drug to children younger than age 2.

• Be aware that the drug is for short-term use only. A prescriber should be consulted if the drug is to be administered to children for more than 5 days or to adults for more than 10 days.

• Don't use the drug for marked fever (over 103.1°F [39.5°C]), fever persisting longer than 3 days, or recurrent fever, unless directed by a prescriber.

• Be aware that high doses or unsupervised long-term use can cause liver damage. Excessive ingestion of alcoholic beverages may increase the risk of hepatotoxicity.

• Keep track of daily acetaminophen intake, including OTC and prescription medications. Don't exceed the total recommended dose of acetaminophen per day because of the risk of hepatotoxicity.

• Stop use of the drug if a skin rash or reaction occurs and seek medical attention immediately.

• If pregnant, carefully consider taking any medications for pain and discuss use of medications with the health care provider **prior** to taking medications. Be aware that the drug is found in breast milk in low levels (less than 1% of the dose). The drug is safe for short-term therapy in breast-feeding women as long as the recommended dose isn't exceeded.

Nonselective NSAIDs

As their name suggests, NSAIDs are typically used to combat inflammation. Their anti-inflammatory action equals that of aspirin. They also have analgesic and antipyretic effects.

Nonselective NSAIDs inhibit prostaglandin synthesis by blocking COX-1 and COX-2. These drugs (called *COX-1* and *COX-2 inhibitors*) include indomethacin, ibuprofen, diclofenac, etodolac, fenoprofen, flurbiprofen, ketoprofen, ketorolac, mefenamic acid, meloxicam, nabumetone, naproxen, oxaprozin, and sulindac.

Selective NSAIDs selectively block COX-2 enzymes, thereby inhibiting prostaglandin synthesis. This selective inhibition of COX-2 produces the analgesic and anti-inflammatory effects without causing the adverse GI effects associated with COX-1 inhibition by nonselective NSAIDs. (See *NSAIDs: Ibuprofen*, page 82.)

Prototype pro

NSAIDs: Ibuprofen

Actions
- Interferes with the prostaglandins involved in pain; appears to sensitize pain receptors to mechanical stimulation or to other chemical mediators (such as bradykinin and histamine)
- Inhibits synthesis of prostaglandins peripherally and possibly centrally
- Inhibits prostaglandin synthesis and release during inflammation
- Suppresses prostaglandin synthesis in the CNS, causing an antipyretic effect

Indications
- Rheumatoid arthritis
- Dysmenorrhea
- Osteoarthritis
- Juvenile arthritis
- Mild to moderate pain
- Fever

Nursing considerations
- Monitor the patient for adverse effects, such as bronchospasm, Stevens-Johnson syndrome, hematologic disorders, and aseptic meningitis.
- Keep in mind that it may take 1 to 2 weeks to achieve full anti-inflammatory effects.
- Be aware that the drug may mask the signs and symptoms of infection.

Before you give that drug!

Nonselective NSAIDs warning

Before administering an NSAID to a patient, be aware of its risks to special populations:
- *Children:* Some NSAIDs aren't recommended for use in children.
- *Older adults:* The risk of ulcers increases with age.
- *Pregnant and lactating woman:* NSAIDs are contraindicated, and they have potential adverse effects on the neonate, and many NSAIDs are excreted in breast milk.
- *Patients undergoing coronary artery bypass graft surgery or have had recent heart attack or stroke.* The use of NSAIDs in these patients may increase their risk of heart attack or stroke.

Pharmacokinetics

All NSAIDs (nonselective and selective) are absorbed in the GI tract. They're mostly metabolized in the liver and excreted primarily by the kidneys.

Pharmacodynamics

Inflammatory disorders produce and release prostaglandins from cell membranes, resulting in pain. Nonselective NSAIDs produce their effects by inhibiting prostaglandin synthesis and cyclooxygenase activity. NSAIDs inhibit both isoenzymes of cyclooxygenase, COX-1 and COX-2, which convert arachidonic acid into prostaglandins. COX-1 produces prostaglandins that maintain the stomach lining, whereas COX-2 produces prostaglandins that mediate an inflammatory response; therefore, COX-1 inhibition is associated with NSAID-induced GI toxicity, whereas COX-2 inhibition alleviates pain and inflammation (Karch, 2020).

Pharmacotherapeutics

NSAIDs are primarily used to decrease inflammation. They're also used to relieve pain but are seldom prescribed to reduce fever. (See *Nonselective NSAIDs warning.*)

All in favor?

The following conditions respond favorably to treatment with NSAIDs:

- ankylosing spondylitis (an inflammatory joint disease that first affects the spine)
- moderate to severe rheumatoid arthritis (an inflammatory disease of peripheral joints)
- osteoarthritis (a degenerative joint disease) in the hip, shoulder, or other large joints
- osteoarthritis accompanied by inflammation
- acute gouty arthritis (urate deposits in the joints)
- dysmenorrhea (painful menstruation)
- migraines
- bursitis
- tendinitis
- mild to moderate pain.

Drug interactions

Many drugs can interact with NSAIDs, especially with indomethacin and sulindac. Because they're highly protein-bound, NSAIDs are likely to interact with other protein-bound drugs. Such drugs include fluconazole, phenobarbital, rifampin, ritonavir, and salicylates. NSAIDs affect oral anticoagulants, aminoglycosides, ACE inhibitors, beta-adrenergic blockers, digoxin, phenytoin, methotrexate, glucocorticoids, and others. Lithium toxicity can result when lithium is taken with ibuprofen.

Side effects/adverse reactions

All NSAIDs produce similar side effects or adverse reactions, which include:
- abdominal pain and bleeding
- anorexia
- diarrhea
- nausea
- ulcers
- liver toxicity
- drowsiness
- headache
- dizziness
- confusion
- tinnitus
- vertigo
- depression
- bladder infection
- blood in urine
- kidney necrosis
- hypertension
- heart failure
- pedal edema.

In addition, the use of NSAIDs can increase the risk for heart attack or stroke.

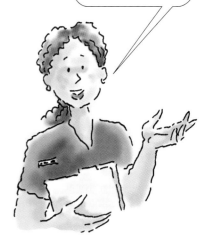

"NSAID toxicity symptoms include GI bleeding, hypertension, hepatotoxicity, and renal damage" (Ghlichloo & Gerriets, 2020).

The Three-Step Approach

Nursing management for the patient being treated with NSAIDs includes these three steps.

Preadministration

(Recognize and analyze cues)

- Obtain an assessment of the patient's underlying condition before starting drug therapy.
- Assess the patient's level of pain and inflammation before therapy begins.
- Assess bleeding time if the patient is expected to undergo surgery. Avoid use if the patient is undergoing cardiac surgery.
- Analyze the patient's medication history. Many OTC products and combination prescription pain products contain NSAIDs and must be considered when calculating the total daily dosage.
- Monitor the patient's ophthalmic and auditory function before and periodically during therapy to detect toxicity.
- Monitor CBC, platelet count, PT, and hepatic and renal function periodically to detect abnormalities.

(Prioritize hypothesis—priority patient problems)

- Acute pain
- Chronic pain
- Injury risk
- Knowledge deficiency

(Generate solutions)

- The patient will acknowledge a reduction in pain.
- No serious complications will occur while the patient is on drug therapy.
- The patient and family members will verbalize an understanding of the purpose and intended effect of drug therapy.

Medication administration

(Take action)

- Administer oral NSAIDs with 8 oz (240 mL) of water to ensure adequate passage into the stomach. Have the patient sit up for 15 to 30 minutes after taking the drug to prevent it from lodging in the esophagus.
- As needed, crush tablets or mix with food or fluid to aid swallowing.
- Evaluate drug effectiveness after administration.
- Monitor the patient for signs and symptoms of bleeding.
- Be alert for adverse reactions and drug interactions. Report GI bleeding and symptoms of anaphylactoid or anaphylactic reactions.

Stomach soothers

- Give the drug with meals or milk or administer it with antacids to reduce adverse GI reactions.
- Notify the prescriber if the drug is ineffective.
- Stop the drug and notify the prescriber if renal or hepatic abnormalities occur.

Postadministration

(Evaluate outcomes)

- The patient states that pain is relieved.
- Evaluate drug effectiveness after administration.
- The patient remains free from adverse effects throughout drug therapy.
- The patient and family members state an understanding of drug therapy. (See *Teaching about nonselective NSAIDs.*)

Education edge

Teaching about nonselective NSAIDs

See Education edge: Teaching template in Chapter 3, page 38 for general teaching for all medications. Specific points to review with patients and family for nonselective NSAIDs:

- Take the drug as directed to achieve the desired effect. Be aware that the benefits of some types of therapy may not be achieved for 2 to 4 weeks.
- Take the drug with meals or milk to reduce adverse GI effects.
- Don't exceed the recommended daily dosage, don't give the drug to children younger than age 12, and don't take the drug for extended periods without consulting a prescriber.
- Be aware that using the drug with aspirin, alcohol, or corticosteroids may increase the risk of adverse GI effects.

- Recognize and report signs and symptoms of GI bleeding, such as dark-colored stools, blood in urine, or unusual bleeding (for example, in the gums).
- Use sunblock, wear protective clothing, and avoid prolonged exposure to sunlight during therapy.
- If taking the medication as long-term therapy, check with the prescriber about the need for monitoring of laboratory values, especially blood urea nitrogen and creatinine levels, liver function, and CBC.
- Notify the prescriber about severe or persistent adverse reactions.
- Don't take other medications, OTC products, or herbal products without first consulting with the prescriber.

Selective NSAIDs

Prostaglandins produced by COX-2 are associated with pain and inflammation. The selective NSAIDs (also called *COX-2 inhibitors*) are NSAIDs that selectively block COX-2, relieving pain and inflammation. They produce fewer adverse effects, such as stomach damage, than do nonselective NSAIDs (Karch, 2020). The only currently available selective NSAID is celecoxib.

Pharmacokinetics

Celecoxib is highly protein-bound, primarily to albumin, and is extensively distributed into the tissues. Peak levels occur within 3 hours, and steady plasma states can be expected in 5 days, if given in multiple doses. Celecoxib is metabolized in the liver, with less than 3% unchanged, and excreted in urine and feces.

Pharmacodynamics

Celecoxib produces its effect by selectively blocking the COX-2 enzyme, thereby inhibiting prostaglandin synthesis.

Less than the rest

This selective inhibition of COX-2 produces analgesic and anti-inflammatory effects without the adverse GI effects associated with COX-1 inhibition by nonselective NSAIDs; however, some degree of COX-1 inhibition still occurs.

Pharmacotherapeutics

Celecoxib is primarily used to provide analgesia and to decrease inflammation. It's particularly useful in the treatment of osteoarthritis, rheumatoid arthritis, acute pain, primary dysmenorrhea, and familial adenomatous polyposis.

Drug interactions

Because celecoxib is metabolized by the liver, drug interactions have been identified. For example:
- Celecoxib decreases the clearance of lithium, which can result in lithium toxicity.
- It reduces the antihypertensive effects of ACE inhibitors and diuretics.
- When celecoxib is taken with warfarin, increased PT levels and bleeding complications can occur.
- Celecoxib interacts with herbal preparations that increase the risk of bleeding, such as dong quai, feverfew, garlic, ginger, ginkgo, horse chestnut, and red clover.

Side effects/adverse reactions

These side effects/adverse reactions may occur with celecoxib:
- dyspepsia

- abdominal pain
- nausea and vomiting
- GI ulcers (to a lesser degree than with nonselective NSAIDs)
- hypertension
- fluid retention
- peripheral edema
- dizziness
- headache
- rash.

The Three-Step Approach

Nursing management for the patient being treated with celecoxib (selective NSAIDs) includes these three steps.

Preadministration

(Recognize and analyze cues)
- Obtain an assessment of the patient's underlying condition before starting drug therapy.
- Avoid use if the patient has hypertension, edema, heart failure, or kidney disease because celecoxib can impair renal function.
- Obtain an accurate list of the patient's allergies. If allergic to or has anaphylactic reactions to sulfonamides, aspirin, or other NSAIDs, the patient may also be allergic to selective NSAIDs.
- Assess the patient's level of pain and inflammation before therapy begins.
- Monitor the patient's ophthalmic and auditory function before therapy and periodically thereafter to detect toxicity.

(Prioritize hypothesis—priority patient problems)
- Acute pain
- Chronic pain
- Injury risk
- Knowledge deficiency

(Generate solutions)
- The patient will acknowledge a reduction in pain.
- No serious complications will occur while the patient is on drug therapy.
- The patient and family members will verbalize an understanding of the purpose and intended effect of drug therapy.

Medication administration

- Although the drug can be given without regard to meals, food may decrease GI upset.
- Before starting treatment, be sure that the patient is well hydrated.
- Although the drug may be used with low aspirin dosages, monitor for increased risk of GI bleeding.
- NSAIDs such as celecoxib can cause fluid retention; closely monitor the patient who has hypertension, edema, or heart failure.

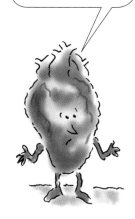

Woe is me! Celecoxib has been linked to a relatively high risk of heart attack.

- Notify the prescriber if the drug is ineffective.
- Monitor the patient for signs and symptoms of bleeding. Assess bleeding time if the patient requires surgery.
- Periodically monitor CBC, platelet count, PT, and hepatic and renal function to detect abnormalities.
- Closely monitor the patient on celecoxib for signs or symptoms of MI or other cardiovascular events. This drug has been linked to a relatively high risk of heart attacks and may increase the risk for stroke and other cardiovascular events. Celecoxib should be avoided in patients with known cardiac disease, recent heart surgery, hypertension, diabetes, and dyslipidemia.
- Evaluate the patient's and family's knowledge of drug therapy.

Postadministration

(Evaluate outcomes)
- The patient states pain is relieved.
- The patient remains free from adverse effects throughout drug therapy.
- The patient and family members state an understanding of drug therapy. (See *Teaching about selective NSAIDs.*)

Education edge

Teaching about selective NSAIDs

See Education edge: Teaching template in Chapter 3, page 38 for general teaching for all medications. Specific points to review with patients and family for selective NSAIDs or COX-2 drugs:

- Report a history of allergic reactions to sulfonamides, aspirin, or other NSAIDs before starting therapy.
- Immediately report to the prescriber signs of GI bleeding (such as bloody vomitus, blood in urine or stool, and black, tarry stools), chest pain, strokelike symptoms, rash, or unexplained weight gain or edema.
- Notify the prescriber if you become pregnant or are planning to become pregnant while taking this drug.
- Take the drug with food if stomach upset occurs.

- Be aware that all NSAIDs, including COX-2 inhibitors, may adversely affect the liver. Signs and symptoms of liver toxicity include nausea, fatigue, lethargy, itching, jaundice, right upper quadrant tenderness, and flulike symptoms. Stop therapy and seek immediate medical advice if any of these signs and symptoms develops.
- Be aware that it may take several days to feel consistent pain relief.
- Don't take other medications, OTC products, or herbal remedies unless first approved by the prescriber.
- Inform all health care providers that you're taking this medication.
- Avoid or minimize the use of alcoholic beverages because alcohol increases gastric irritation and the risk of bleeding.

Opioid agonists, agonists-antagonists, and antagonists

The word *opioid* refers to any derivative of the opium plant or any synthetic drug that imitates natural narcotics. Opioid agonists (also called *narcotic agonists*) include opium derivatives and synthetic drugs with similar properties. They're used to relieve or decrease pain without causing the person to lose consciousness. Some opioid agonists also have antitussive and antidiarrheal effects. (See *Opioid agonists: Morphine*, page 90.)

Opioid opponent

Opioid antagonists aren't pain medications. They block the effects of opioid agonists and are used to reverse adverse drug reactions, such as respiratory and CNS depression, produced by those drugs. Unfortunately, by reversing the analgesic effect, they also cause the patient's pain to recur. Opioid antagonists include naloxone and naltrexone (Karch, 2020).

Having it both ways

Some opioid analgesics, called *mixed opioid agonist-antagonists*, have agonist and antagonist properties. The agonist component relieves pain, and the antagonist component decreases the risk of toxicity and drug dependence. These mixed opioid agonist-antagonists reduce the risk of respiratory depression and drug abuse.

Opioid agonists

Opioid agonists include:
- codeine
- fentanyl citrate
- hydrocodone
- hydromorphone hydrochloride
- levorphanol tartrate
- meperidine hydrochloride
- methadone hydrochloride
- morphine sulfate
- oxycodone
- remifentanil
- tramadol.

Opioid agonists: Morphine

Actions
- Acts on opiate receptors in the CNS

Indications
- Moderate to severe pain

Nursing considerations
- Monitor the patient for adverse effects, such as sedation, euphoria, seizures, dizziness, nightmares, bradycardia, shock, cardiac arrest, nausea, constipation, vomiting, thrombocytopenia, and respiratory depression.
- Keep an opioid antagonist (naloxone) and resuscitation equipment available.

Pharmacokinetics

Opioid agonists can be administered by different routes, although inhalation administration is uncommon. Oral doses are absorbed readily from the GI tract. Transmucosal and intrathecal opiates are fast acting. Opioid agonists administered IV provide the most rapid (almost immediate) and reliable pain relief. The subcutaneous and IM routes may result in delayed absorption, especially in patients with poor circulation.

Opioid agonists are distributed widely throughout body tissues. They have a relatively low plasma protein-binding capacity (30% to 35%).

Liver lovers

These drugs are metabolized extensively in the liver. For example, meperidine is metabolized to normeperidine, a toxic metabolite with a longer half-life than meperidine. This metabolite accumulates in renal failure and may lead to CNS excitation (Yasaei et al., 2021).

Metabolites are excreted by the kidneys. A small amount is excreted in feces through the biliary tract.

Pharmacodynamics

Opioid agonists reduce pain by binding to opiate receptor sites (mu receptors or kappa receptors) in the peripheral and central nervous system. When these drugs stimulate the opiate mu receptors, analgesia, respiratory depression, euphoria, sedation, and physical dependence occurs, whereas stimulation of the kappa receptors

Pharm function

How opioid agonists control pain

Opioid agonists inhibit pain transmission by mimicking the body's natural pain control mechanisms.

Where neurons meet
Peripheral pain neurons meet CNS neurons in the dorsal horn of the spinal cord. At the synapse, the pain neuron releases substance P (a pain neurotransmitter). This agent helps transfer pain impulses to the CNS neurons that carry the impulses to the brain.

Taking up space
In theory, the spinal interneurons respond to stimulation from the descending neurons of the CNS by releasing endogenous opiates. These opiates bind to the peripheral pain neuron to inhibit release of substance P and to retard the transmission of pain impulses.

Stopping substance P
Synthetic opiates supplement this pain-blocking effect by binding with free opiate receptors to inhibit the release of substance P. Opiates also alter consciousness of pain, but how this mechanism works remains unknown.

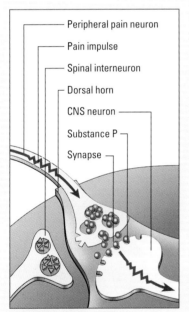

Peripheral pain neuron
Pain impulse
Spinal interneuron
Dorsal horn
CNS neuron
Substance P
Synapse

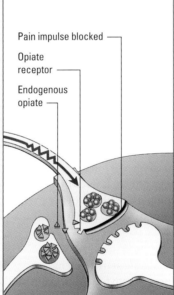

Pain impulse blocked
Opiate receptor
Endogenous opiate

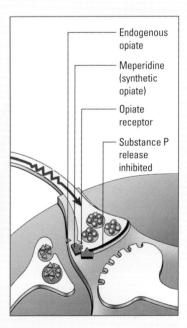

Endogenous opiate
Meperidine (synthetic opiate)
Opiate receptor
Substance P release inhibited

produces analgesia, sedation, dysphoria, and decreased GI motility. Receptor site binding is what produces the therapeutic effects of analgesia and cough suppression as well as adverse reactions, such as respiratory depression and constipation. (See *How opioid agonists control pain.*)

Smooth operator

Besides reducing pain, opioid agonists, especially morphine, affect the smooth muscle of the GI and genitourinary tracts (the organs of the reproductive and urinary systems). This causes contraction of the bladder and ureters and slows intestinal peristalsis (rhythmic contractions that move food along the digestive tract), resulting in constipation, a common adverse reaction to opiates (Yasaei et al., 2021).

A fine line

These drugs also cause blood vessels to dilate, especially in the face, head, and neck. In addition, they suppress the cough center in the brain, producing antitussive effects and causing constriction of the bronchial muscles. Any of these effects can become adverse reactions if produced in excess. For example, if the blood vessels dilate too much, hypotension can occur.

Pharmacotherapeutics

Opioid agonists are prescribed to relieve severe pain in acute, chronic, and terminal illnesses. They're sometimes prescribed to control diarrhea and suppress coughing. Methadone is used for temporary maintenance of opioid addiction. Opioids such as fentanyl and remifentanil are used for the induction and maintenance of general anesthesia. Fentanyl may be prescribed for breakthrough pain in patients with cancer and can be delivered via buccal table, nasal spray, sublingual, or transdermal patch routes (Karch, 2020).

Cardio-assistance

Morphine reduces myocardial oxygen demand by decreasing heart rate, blood pressure, and venous return. It does this by dilating peripheral blood vessels, keeping more blood in the periphery, and decreasing cardiac preload (Murphy et al., 2020).

Drug interactions

Drugs that can affect opioid analgesic activity include amitriptyline, protease inhibitors, phenytoin, diazepam, and rifampin. Taking tricyclic antidepressants, phenothiazines, or anticholinergics with opioid agonists may cause severe constipation and urine retention. Drugs that may be affected by opioid analgesics include carbamazepine, warfarin, beta-adrenergic blockers, and calcium channel blockers. Meperidine can interact with MAO inhibitors to cause seizures, coma, and death.

The use of opioid agonists with other substances that decrease respiration, such as alcohol, sedatives, hypnotics, and anesthetics, increases the patient's risk of severe respiratory depression.

(See *Opioid agonists warning*, page 93.)

"Meperidine should be avoided in older adults and those who have taken in the past 14 days or currently taking a monoamine oxidase inhibitor (MAOI)."

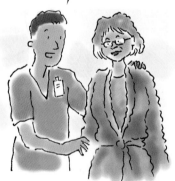

Side effects/adverse reactions

One of the most common side effects/adverse reactions to opioid agonists is decreased rate and depth of breathing that worsens as the dose of narcotic is increased. This may cause periodic irregular breathing or trigger asthmatic attacks in a susceptible patient.

Other adverse reactions include:
- flushing
- orthostatic hypotension
- pupil constriction
- central nervous system depression
- nausea and vomiting.

With meperidine administration, these side effects/adverse reactions can occur:
- tremors
- palpitations
- tachycardia
- delirium
- serotonin syndrome
- seizures
- life-threatening respiratory failure with first dose.

The Three–Step Approach

Nursing management for the patient being treated with opioid agonist medications includes these three steps.

Preadministration

(Recognize and analyze cues)
- Obtain a baseline assessment of the patient's pain and reassess frequently to determine drug effectiveness.

When breathing easy is hard work

- Evaluate the patient's respiratory status before each dose; watch for a respiratory rate below the patient's baseline level and for restlessness, which may be compensatory signs of hypoxia. Respiratory depression may last longer than the analgesic effect.

(Prioritize hypothesis—priority patient problems)
- Acute pain
- Altered breathing pattern risk
- Knowledge deficiency

(Generate solutions)
- The patient will acknowledge a reduction in pain.

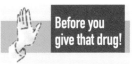

Opioid agonists warning

Before administering medications, be aware that morphine sulfate (MSO$_4$) can be confused with magnesium sulfate (MgSO$_4$). Verify abbreviations or, better yet, spell out the medication to avoid confusion.

Most opioid agonists appear in breast milk; most doctors recommend waiting 4 to 6 hours after ingestion to breast-feed.

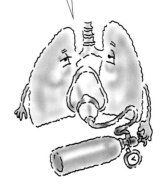

Watch for a respiratory rate below the patient's baseline and for restlessness, possible signs of hypoxia. A little more oxygen, please.

- Throughout therapy, the patient will maintain adequate breathing function.
- The patient and family members will verbalize an understanding of the purpose and intended effect of drug therapy.

Medication administration
(Take action)
- Keep resuscitative equipment and a narcotic antagonist (naloxone) available.
- Give the IV form of the drug by slow injection, preferably in diluted solution. Rapid IV injection increases the risk of adverse effects.
- Give IM or subcutaneous injections cautiously to a patient with a decreased platelet count and to a patient who's chilled, hypovolemic, or in shock; decreased perfusion may lead to drug accumulation and toxicity. Rotate injection sites to avoid induration.
- Carefully note the strength of the solution when measuring a dose. Oral solutions of varying concentrations are available.
- For maximum effectiveness, give the drug on a regular dosage schedule rather than as needed.
- Institute safety precautions.
- Encourage a postoperative patient to turn, cough, and breathe deeply every 2 hours to avoid atelectasis.
- If GI irritation occurs, give oral forms of the drug with food.
- Monitor the patient for other adverse reactions.
- Monitor the patient for tolerance and dependence. The first sign of tolerance to opioids is usually a shortened duration of effect.
- Be aware that withdrawal symptoms, including tremors, agitation, nausea, and vomiting, may occur if the drug is stopped abruptly. Monitor the patient with these signs and symptoms carefully and provide supportive therapy.

Postadministration
(Evaluate outcomes)
- The patient states that pain is relieved.
- Evaluate drug effectiveness after administration.
- The patient maintains adequate ventilation, such as normal respiratory rate and rhythm and pink skin color.
- The patient and family state an understanding of drug therapy. (See *Teaching about opioid agonists*, page 95)

Teaching about opioid agonists

See Education edge: Teaching template in Chapter 3, page 38 for general teaching for all medications. Specific points to review with patients and family for opioid agonist medications:

• Take the drug exactly as prescribed. Call the prescriber if you don't experience the desired effect or if you experience significant adverse reactions.

• Be careful when getting out of bed and walking. Avoid hazardous activities until the drug's effects are known.

• Avoid alcohol while taking opioid agonists because it causes additive CNS depression.

• To prevent constipation, increase fiber in the diet and use a stool softener.

• Breathe deeply, cough, and change position every 2 hours to avoid respiratory complications.

• Report continued pain.

Mixed opioid agonist-antagonists

Mixed opioid agonist-antagonists are given to relieve pain while reducing toxic effects and dependency. Examples include:

• buprenorphine hydrochloride
• butorphanol tartrate
• nalbuphine hydrochloride
• pentazocine hydrochloride combined with naloxone hydrochloride and/or acetaminophen.

A mixed bag

Originally, mixed opioid agonist-antagonists appeared to have less misuse potential than the pure opioid agonists; however, butorphanol and pentazocine have reportedly caused dependence. This class of drugs isn't recommended for use in patients with chronic pain who are taking other opioid agonists.

Pharmacokinetics

Absorption of mixed opioid agonist-antagonists occurs rapidly from parenteral sites. These drugs are distributed to most body tissues and cross the placenta. They're metabolized in the liver and excreted primarily by the kidneys, although more than 10% of a butorphanol dose and a small amount of a pentazocine dose are excreted in stool.

Pharmacodynamics

The exact mechanism of action of mixed opioid agonist-antagonists isn't known; however, researchers believe that these drugs weakly antagonize the effects of morphine, meperidine, and other opiates at one of the opioid receptors. They also exert agonistic effects at other opioid receptors.

In no rush

Buprenorphine binds with receptors in the CNS, altering the perception of and the emotional response to pain through an unknown mechanism. It seems to release slowly from binding sites, producing a longer duration of action than the other drugs in this class.

Don't get emotional

The site of action of butorphanol may be opiate receptors in the limbic system (part of the brain involved in emotion). Like pentazocine, butorphanol also acts on pulmonary circulation, increasing pulmonary vascular resistance (resistance in the blood vessels of the lungs that the right ventricle must pump against). Both drugs also increase blood pressure and the workload of the heart and, therefore, should be used with caution or avoided in patients with a history of MI.

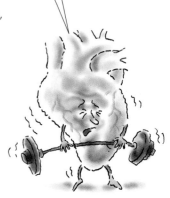

Ack! Pentazocine and butorphanol increase my workload. I'm already doing enough heavy lifting!

Pharmacotherapeutics

Mixed opioid agonist-antagonists are used as analgesia during childbirth as well as postoperatively; however, nalbuphine has been shown to cause serious side effects in the fetus and neonate, so it's use should be avoided during labor and delivery.

Independence day

Mixed opioid agonist-antagonists are sometimes prescribed in place of opioid agonists because they have a lower risk of drug dependence. Mixed opioid agonist-antagonists also are less likely to cause respiratory depression and constipation, although they can produce some adverse reactions.

Drug interactions

Increased CNS depression and an additive decrease in respiratory rate and depth may result if mixed opioid agonist-antagonists are administered to a patient taking other CNS depressants, such as barbiturates and alcohol.

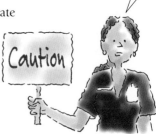

A patient with a history of opioid misuse shouldn't receive opioid agonist-antagonists. Withdrawal symptoms may result.

Clean and sober?

The patient with a history of opioid misuse shouldn't receive the mixed opioid agonist-antagonists pentazocine, nalbuphine, and butorphanol because they can cause withdrawal symptoms; however, sublingual preps of buprenorphine have been approved for to prevent withdrawal symptoms and manage opioid dependence.

Side effects/adverse reactions

The most common adverse reactions to opioid agonist-antagonists include nausea, vomiting, light-headedness, sedation, and euphoria.

The Three-Step Approach

Nursing management for patients undergoing treatment with mixed opioid agonist-antagonist medications includes these three steps.

Preadministration
(Recognize and analyze cues)
- Obtain a baseline assessment of the patient's pain and reassess frequently to determine the drug's effectiveness.
- Evaluate the patient's respiratory status before each dose; watch for a respiratory rate below the baseline level and watch for restlessness, which may be a compensatory sign of hypoxemia. Respiratory depression may last longer than the analgesic effect.

(Priority hypothesis—priority patient problems)
- Acute pain
- Altered breathing pattern risk
- Knowledge deficiency

(Generate solutions)
- The patient will acknowledge a reduction in pain.
- Throughout therapy, the patient will maintain an adequate breathing pattern.
- The patient and family will state an understanding of the purpose and intended effect of drug therapy.

Medication administration
(Take action)
- Keep resuscitative equipment and an opioid antagonist (naloxone) available. Naloxone won't completely reverse respiratory depression caused by buprenorphine overdose; mechanical ventilation may be necessary. Doxapram and larger-than-usual doses of naloxone may also be ordered.
- Monitor the patient for other adverse reactions.
- Monitor the patient for tolerance and dependence. The first sign of tolerance to opioids is usually a shortened duration of effect.

Take it slow
- Give the IV form of the drug by slow injection, preferably in diluted solution. Rapid IV injection increases the risk of adverse effects (Karch, 2020).
- Institute safety precautions.
- Encourage a postoperative patient to turn, cough, and breathe deeply every 2 hours to avoid atelectasis.

Withdrawal warning

- Be aware that the drug may precipitate withdrawal syndrome in an opioid-dependent patient. Withdrawal symptoms—including tremors, agitation, nausea, and vomiting—may occur if the drug is stopped abruptly. If dependence occurs, withdrawal symptoms may appear up to 14 days after the drug is stopped. Monitor a patient with these symptoms carefully and provide supportive therapy.

Postadministration

(Evaluate outcomes)
- The patient states that pain is relieved.
- The patient maintains adequate ventilation, such as normal respiratory rate and rhythm and pink skin color.
- The patient and family state an understanding of drug therapy.

Opioid antagonists

Opioid antagonists attach to opiate receptors, but don't stimulate them, and have a greater attraction for opiate receptors than opioids do. As a result, they prevent opioid drugs, enkephalins, and endorphins from producing their effects.

Opioid antagonists include:
- naloxone hydrochloride
- naltrexone hydrochloride
- methylnaltrexone.

Pharmacokinetics

Naloxone is administered IM, subcutaneous, or IV. Naltrexone is administered orally. Both drugs are metabolized by the liver and excreted by the kidneys.

Pharmacodynamics

In a process known as *competitive inhibition*, opioid antagonists block the effects of opioids by occupying the opiate receptor sites, displacing opioids attached to opiate receptors and blocking further opioid binding at these sites.

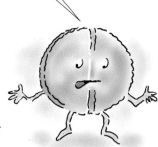

It's tough out there for us opioids. The competitive inhibition of opioid antagonists can keep me from doing my job.

Pharmacotherapeutics

Naloxone is the drug of choice for managing an opioid overdose. It reverses respiratory depression and sedation and helps stabilize the patient's vital signs within seconds after administration.

Because naloxone also reverses the analgesic effects of opioid drugs, a patient who was given an opioid drug for pain relief may experience pain or even experience withdrawal symptoms.

Methylnaltrexone is used to treat opioid-induced constipation not responsive to laxatives in patients who are taking opioids continuously for pain.

Kicking the habit

Naltrexone is used along with psychotherapy or counseling to treat drug misuse. It's given only, however, to a patient who has gone through a detoxification program to remove all opioids from the body. A patient who still has opioids in the body may experience acute withdrawal symptoms if given naltrexone.

Drug interactions

Naloxone produces no significant drug interactions. Naltrexone will cause withdrawal symptoms if given to a patient who is receiving an opioid agonist or who is misusing opioids.

Side effects/adverse reactions

Naltrexone can cause several side effects/adverse reactions, including:
- edema
- hypertension
- palpitations
- phlebitis
- shortness of breath
- anxiety
- depression
- disorientation
- dizziness
- headache
- nervousness
- anorexia
- diarrhea or constipation
- nausea and vomiting
- thirst
- urinary frequency
- liver toxicity.

Methylnaltrexone can cause several side effects/adverse reactions, including:
- abdominal pain
- flatulence
- nausea
- dizziness
- diarrhea.

Watch the wake-up

Naloxone may cause nausea, vomiting, and, occasionally, hypertension and tachycardia. An unconscious patient returned

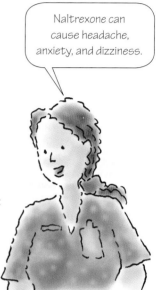

Naltrexone can cause headache, anxiety, and dizziness.

to consciousness abruptly after naloxone administration may hyperventilate and experience tremors.

The Three-Step Approach

Nursing management for the patient receiving treatment with opioid antagonist medications includes these three steps.

Preadministration

(Recognize and analyze cues)
- Assess the patient's opioid use before therapy.
- Assess the drug's effectiveness regularly throughout therapy.

(Priority hypothesis—priority patient problems)
- Risky health behavior
- Dehydration risk
- Knowledge deficiency

(Generate solutions)
- The patient will demonstrate improved health as evidenced by maintenance of vital signs within normal parameters.
- The patient will maintain adequate hydration as evidenced by adequate urine output.
- The patient and family will verbalize an understanding of the purpose and intended effect of drug therapy.

Medication administration

(Take action)
- Provide oxygen, ventilation, and other resuscitation measures when the drug is used in the management of acute opiate overdose and when the patient has severe respiratory depression.
- Keep in mind that these drugs are effective in reversing respiratory depression only when it's caused by opioids. When they're used for this purpose, monitor the patient for tachypnea.
- Be prepared to give continuous IV naloxone infusion to control adverse effects of epidural morphine.
  Monitor the patient's respiratory depth and rate. The duration of the opioid may exceed that of naloxone, causing relapse into respiratory depression.
- Monitor the patient's hydration status if adverse GI reactions occur.
- Evaluate the patient's and family's knowledge of drug therapy.

Postadministration

(Evaluate outcomes)
- The patient responds well to drug therapy.
- The patient maintains adequate hydration.
- The patient and family state an understanding of drug therapy.

Anesthetic drugs

Anesthetic drugs can be divided into three groups—general anesthetics, local anesthetics, and topical anesthetics.

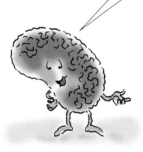

My high blood flow means that anesthetics can make their way to me more quickly.

Inhale or inject?

General anesthetic drugs are further subdivided into two main types, those given by inhalation and those given IV.

Inhalation anesthetics

The most commonly used general anesthetics given by inhalation include:
- desflurane
- sevoflurane
- halothane
- isoflurane
- nitrous oxide (Miller et al., 2021).

Pharmacokinetics

The absorption and elimination rates of anesthetics are governed by their solubility in blood. Inhalation anesthetics enter the blood from the lungs and are distributed to other tissues. Distribution is most rapid to organs with high blood flow, such as the brain, liver, kidneys, and heart.

Leaving? Try the lungs

Inhalation anesthetics are eliminated primarily by the lung.

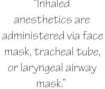

"Inhaled anesthetics are administered via face mask, tracheal tube, or laryngeal airway mask."

Pharmacodynamics

Inhalation anesthetics work primarily in the CNS, producing loss of consciousness, loss of responsiveness to sensory stimulation (including pain), and muscle relaxation. They can also affect other organ systems such as the cardiovascular system.

Pharmacotherapeutics

Inhalation anesthetics are most commonly used for surgery because they offer more precise and rapid control of depth of anesthesia than injection anesthetics. These anesthetics, which are liquids at room temperature, require a vaporizer and special delivery system for safe use.

Stop signs
Inhalation anesthetics are contraindicated in a patient with known hypersensitivity to the drug, a liver disorder, or malignant hyperthermia (a potentially fatal complication of anesthesia characterized by skeletal muscle rigidity and high fever). They require cautious use in a pregnant or breast-feeding patient.

Drug interactions
The most important drug interactions involving inhalation anesthetics are with other CNS, cardiac, or respiratory-depressant drugs. These drug combinations can cause CNS depression, cardiac arrhythmias, or respiratory depression, resulting in compromised patient status.

Side effects/adverse reactions
The most common adverse reaction to inhalation anesthetics is an exaggerated patient response to a normal dose. Malignant hyperthermia, characterized by a sudden and usually lethal increase in body temperature, is a serious and unexpected reaction to inhalation anesthetics. It occurs in the genetically susceptible patient only and may result from a failure in calcium uptake by muscle cells. The skeletal muscle relaxant dantrolene is used to treat this condition.

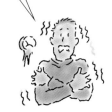

After surgery, a patient may experience reactions similar to those seen with other CNS depressants, including confusion, sedation, and—brrr!— hypothermia.

Waking up woes
After surgery, a patient may experience reactions similar to those seen with other CNS depressants, including depression of breathing and circulation, confusion, sedation, nausea, vomiting, ataxia, and hypothermia.

The Three-Step Approach
Nursing management for patients undergoing treatment with inhaled anesthetic medications includes these three steps.

Preadministration
(Recognize and analyze cues)
- Assess the patient's use of prescription, nonprescription, and herbal remedies, especially those taken within the past 3 days.
- Assess drug allergies and risk factors for complications of anesthesia and surgery (cigarette smoking; obesity; limited exercise or activity; and chronic cardiovascular, respiratory, renal, or other disease processes).
- Assess the patient's vital signs, laboratory data, and physical condition to establish baseline measurements for monitoring changes.
- Assess medical and family history for evidence of malignant hyperthermia.

(Prioritize hypothesis—priority patient problems)
- Injury risk
- Altered breathing pattern risk
- Knowledge deficiency

(Generate solutions)
- The risk of injury to the patient will be minimized.
- While under anesthesia, the patient will maintain adequate ventilation and breathing patterns.
- The patient and family will verbalize an understanding of the purpose and intended effect of drug therapy.

Medication administration
(Take action)
- Explain the preoperative and expected postoperative phases of the recovery period.
- Review postoperative recovery requirements, such as deep breathing exercises, coughing, leg exercises, early ambulation, maintaining fluid balance, and urine output.
- Monitor the patient's vital signs, level of consciousness (LOC), respiratory and cardiovascular status, and laboratory results, as indicated.
- Monitor the patient's response to the medication.

Postadministration
(Evaluate outcomes)
- The patient remains free from complications.
- The patient maintains adequate ventilation.
- The patient and family state an understanding of anesthetic drug therapy.

IV anesthetics

IV anesthetics are usually used as general anesthesia when anesthesia is needed for only a short period, such as with outpatient surgery. They're also used to promote rapid induction of anesthesia or to supplement inhalation anesthetics.

A "knockout" bunch

The drugs most commonly used as IV anesthetics are:
- barbiturates (methohexital)
- benzodiazepines (midazolam, diazepam, lorazepam)
- dissociatives (ketamine)
- hypnotics (etomidate, propofol)
- opiates (fentanyl, sufentanil, alfentanil, remifentanil) (Smith et al., 2020).

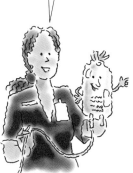

IV administration promotes rapid induction of anesthesia.

Pharmacokinetics

IV anesthetic agents are lipid-soluble and are well distributed throughout the body, crossing the placenta and entering breast milk. These drugs are metabolized in the liver and excreted in urine.

Pharmacodynamics

Opiates work by occupying sites on specialized receptors scattered throughout the CNS and modifying the release of neurotransmitters from sensory nerves entering the CNS. Ketamine appears to induce a profound sense of dissociation from the environment by acting directly on the cortex and limbic system of the brain.

You're getting sleepy

Barbiturates, benzodiazepines, and etomidate appear to enhance responses to the CNS neurotransmitter gamma-aminobutyric acid (GABA). This inhibits the brain's response to stimulation of the reticular activating system, the area of the brainstem that controls alertness. Barbiturates also depress the excitability of CNS neurons.

Pharmacotherapeutics

Because of the short duration of action of IV anesthetics, they're used in shorter surgical procedures, including outpatient surgery. Barbiturates are used alone in surgery that isn't expected to be painful and as adjuncts to other drugs in more extensive procedures.

Benzodiazepines produce sedation and amnesia but not pain relief. Etomidate is used to induce anesthesia and to supplement low-potency inhalation anesthetics such as nitrous oxide. The opiates provide pain relief and supplement other anesthetic drugs.

Drug interactions

IV anesthetics, particularly ketamine, can produce many drug interactions:
- Verapamil enhances the anesthetic effects of etomidate, producing respiratory depression and apnea.
- Giving ketamine and nondepolarizing drugs together increases neuromuscular effects, resulting in prolonged respiratory depression.

A longer road to recovery

- Using barbiturates or opioids with ketamine may prolong recovery time after anesthesia.
- Ketamine plus theophylline may promote seizures.
- Ketamine and thyroid hormones may cause hypertension and tachycardia (rapid heart rate).

Side effects/adverse reactions

- Adverse reactions to injection anesthetics vary by drug.

Ketamine

Ketamine that induces anesthesia and provides intense analgesia can produce these side effects/adverse reactions:

- prolonged recovery
- irrational behavior
- excitement
- distortion of sight/sound perceptions including hallucinations and disorientation
- feelings of detachment from self
- increased heart rate
- hypertension
- excess salivation
- tearing
- shivering
- seizures.

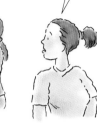

"How sad. Ketamine can cause excessive tearing and salivation and feelings of detachment."

Propofol

Propofol has a rapid-onset, short-duration, and minimal residual sedation effect but can cause these side effects/adverse reactions:

- respiratory depression
- bradycardia
- hiccups
- coughing
- muscle twitching
- hypotension
- pain at the injection site
- propofol infusion syndrome: severe metabolic acidosis, rhabdomyolysis, hyperkalemia, kidney injury, cardiovascular collapse.

Etomidate

Etomidate, used for induction of anesthesia only, can cause these side effects/adverse reactions:

- hiccups
- coughing
- muscle twitching
- apnea
- nausea and vomiting
- pain and phlebitis at the injection site.

Fentanyl

Fentanyl, used as an IV anesthetic, can cause these side effects/adverse reactions:

- CNS and respiratory depression
- hypoventilation
- arrhythmias.

Midazolam

Midazolam, used commonly as a preoperative sedative, promotes anxiolysis, sedation, and amnesia but can cause these side effects/adverse reactions:

- CNS and respiratory depression
- hypotension
- dizziness
- cardiac arrest.

The Three-Step Approach

Nursing management for the patient being treated with IV anesthetic medications includes these three steps.

Preadministration

(Recognize and analyze cues)

- Assess the use of prescription, nonprescription, and herbal remedies, especially those taken within the past 3 days.
- Assess the patient's drug allergies and risk factors for complications of anesthesia and surgery (cigarette smoking; obesity; limited exercise or activity; and chronic cardiovascular, respiratory, renal, or other disease processes).
- Assess the patient's vital signs, laboratory data, and physical condition to establish baseline measurements for monitoring changes.

(Prioritize hypothesis—priority patient problems)

- Injury risk
- Altered breathing pattern
- Knowledge deficiency

(Generate solutions)

- The risk of injury to the patient will be minimized.
- While under anesthesia, the patient will maintain adequate ventilation and breathing patterns.
- The patient and family will verbalize an understanding of the purpose and intended effect of drug therapy.

Medication administration

(Take action)

- Explain expectations for the preoperative and postoperative phases of the recovery period.
- Review postoperative recovery requirements, such as deep breathing exercises, coughing, leg exercises, early ambulation, maintaining fluid balance, and urine output.
- Monitor the patient's vital signs, LOC, respiratory and cardiovascular status, and laboratory results, as indicated.
- Monitor the patient's response to pain medication.

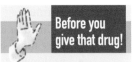

Opiates warning

Fentanyl is 100 times more potent than morphine sulfate.

Sufentanil is 1,000 times more potent than morphine sulfate.

Postadministration

(Evaluate outcomes)
- The patient remains free from major complications.
- The patient maintains adequate ventilation.
- The patient and family members state an understanding of drug therapy.

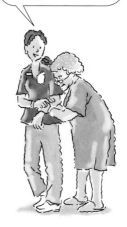

Local anesthetics are typically a safer choice than general anesthesia for elderly patients.

Local anesthetics

Local anesthetics are administered to prevent or relieve pain in a specific area of the body. In addition, these drugs are commonly used as an alternative to general anesthesia for older adults or patients who are debilitated.

Molecular chains?

Local anesthetics may be classified as:
- amide drugs (with nitrogen in the molecular chain, such as bupivacaine, ropivacaine, lidocaine, levobupivacaine, mepivacaine, dibucaine, and prilocaine)
- ester drugs (with oxygen in the molecular chain, such as procaine, chloroprocaine, and tetracaine).
  (See *Amide and ester examples*.)

Amide and ester examples

Amide anesthetics are local anesthetics that have nitrogen as part of their molecular makeup. They include:
- bupivacaine hydrochloride
- levobupivacaine
- lidocaine hydrochloride
- mepivacaine hydrochloride
- ropivacaine hydrochloride.

Give them oxygen

Ester anesthetics have oxygen, not nitrogen, as part of their molecular makeup. They include:
- chloroprocaine hydrochloride
- procaine hydrochloride
- tetracaine hydrochloride.

Pharmacokinetics

Absorption of local anesthetics varies widely, but distribution occurs throughout the body. Esters and amides undergo different types of metabolism, but both yield metabolites that are excreted in urine.

Pharmacodynamics

Local anesthetics block nerve impulses at the point of contact in all kinds of nerves. For example, they can accumulate and cause the nerve cell membrane to expand. As the membrane expands, the cell loses its ability to depolarize, which is necessary for impulse transmission.

Pharmacotherapeutics

Local anesthetics are used to prevent and relieve pain caused by medical procedures, diseases, or injuries. They're used for severe pain that topical anesthetics or analgesics can't relieve.

When a general won't do

Local anesthetics are usually preferred to general anesthetics for surgery in older adults or in patients with disorders that affect respiratory function, such as chronic obstructive pulmonary disease and myasthenia gravis.

Combining and coordinating

For some procedures, a local anesthetic is combined with a drug, such as epinephrine, that constricts blood vessels. Vasoconstriction helps control local bleeding and reduces absorption of the anesthetic. Reduced absorption prolongs the anesthetic's action at the site and limits its distribution and CNS effects (Garmon & Huecker, 2020).

Drug interactions

Local anesthetics produce few significant interactions with other drugs but can produce side effects/adverse reactions.

Side effects/adverse reactions

Dose-related CNS reactions include metallic taste, restlessness, confusion, dizziness, blurred vision, tremors, twitching, shivering, and seizures. Dose-related cardiovascular reactions may include myocardial depression, bradycardia, arrhythmias, hypotension, cardiovascular collapse, and cardiac arrest.

An array of effects

Local anesthetic solutions that contain vasoconstrictors, such as epinephrine, can also produce CNS and cardiovascular reactions, including anxiety, dizziness, headache, restlessness, tremors, palpitations, tachycardia, angina, and/or hypertension.

The Three-Step Approach

Nursing management for the patient being treated with local anesthetic medications includes these three steps.

Preadministration

(Recognize and analyze cues)

- Assess the patient's drug allergies and risk factors for complications of anesthesia and surgery (cigarette smoking; obesity; limited exercise or activity; and chronic cardiovascular, respiratory, renal, or other disease processes).
- Assess the patient's vital signs, laboratory data, and physical condition to establish baseline measurements for monitoring changes.

(Prioritize hypothesis—priority patient problems)

- Injury risk
- Acute pain
- Knowledge deficiency

(Generate solutions)

- The risk of injury to the patient will be minimized.
- The patient will acknowledge a reduction in pain.
- The patient and family will verbalize an understanding of the purpose and intended effect of drug therapy.

Medication administration

(Take action)

- Explain the purpose of therapy and its intended effect.
- Monitor the patient's vital signs, level of pain, respiratory and cardiovascular status, and laboratory results, as indicated.
- Monitor the patient's response to medication.

Postadministration

(Evaluate outcomes)

- The patient remains free from complications.
- The patient has reduced pain.
- The patient and family state an understanding of drug therapy.

Topical anesthetics

Topical anesthetics are applied directly to intact skin or mucous membranes. All topical anesthetics are used to prevent or relieve minor pain.

All together now

Some injectable local anesthetics, such as lidocaine and tetracaine, also are effective topically. In addition, some topical anesthetics, such as lidocaine, are combined in products.

Other topical anesthetics include:
- benzocaine *(See Preparing for practice: Topical anesthetics)*
- procaine
- dyclonine

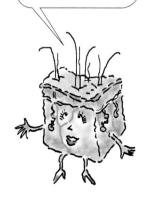

Topical anesthetics are meant to be applied directly to intact skin or dye mucous membranes.

- ethyl chloride
- menthol (methyl salicylate)
- benzyl alcohol.

Pharmacokinetics

Topical anesthetics produce little systemic absorption, except for the application of procaine to mucous membranes; however, systemic absorption may occur if the patient receives frequent or high-dose applications to the eye or large areas of burned or injured skin.

Tetracaine and other esters are metabolized extensively in the blood and to a lesser extent in the liver. Lidocaine and other amides are metabolized primarily in the liver. Both types of topical anesthetics are excreted in urine.

Pharmacodynamics

Benzocaine, procaine, and dyclonine produce topical anesthesia by blocking nerve impulse transmission. They accumulate in the nerve cell membrane, causing it to expand and lose its ability to depolarize, thus blocking impulse transmission. Lidocaine and tetracaine may block impulse transmission across nerve cell membranes.

Drowning out input

The aromatic compounds, such as benzyl alcohol and clove oil, appear to stimulate nerve endings. This stimulation causes counterirritation that interferes with pain perception.

Putting on the deep freeze

Ethyl chloride spray superficially freezes the tissue, stimulating the cold sensation receptors and blocking the nerve endings in the frozen area. Menthol selectively stimulates the sensory nerve endings for cold, causing a cool sensation and some local pain relief.

Pharmacotherapeutics

Topical anesthetics are used to:
- relieve or prevent pain, especially minor burn pain
- relieve itching and irritation
- anesthetize an area before an injection is given
- numb mucosal surfaces before a tube, such as a urinary catheter, is inserted
- alleviate sore throat or mouth pain when used in a spray or solution.

Tetracaine also is used as a topical anesthetic for the eye.

Drug interactions

Few interactions with other drugs occur with topical anesthetics because they aren't absorbed well into the systemic circulation.

Before you give that drug!

Local anesthetics warning

Local anesthetics should be used with caution. The FDA is requiring all prescribed local anesthetic products to warn users about methemoglobinemia. Over-the-counter oral products containing benzocaine should not be used especially on infants and children under 2 years of age.

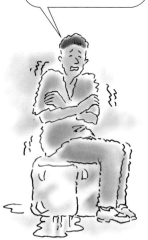

Some topical anesthetics stimulate a c-c-cooling sensation to initiate local pain relief.

Adverse reactions

Topical anesthetics can cause several adverse reactions, depending on the specific drug:

- Any topical anesthetic can cause a hypersensitivity reaction, including a rash, itching, hives, swelling of the mouth and throat, and breathing difficulty.
- Benzyl alcohol can cause topical reactions such as skin irritation.
- Refrigerants, such as ethyl chloride, may produce frostbite at the application site.

The Three-Step Approach

Nursing management for the patient being treated with topical anesthetic medications includes these three steps.

Preadministration

(Recognize and analyze cues)

- Assess the patient's underlying condition and need for drug therapy.
- Assess the patient's vital signs, laboratory data, level of pain, and physical condition to establish baseline measurements for monitoring changes.

(Prioritize hypothesis—priority patient problems)

- Injury risk
- Acute pain
- Knowledge deficiency

(Generate solutions)

- The risk of injury to the patient will be minimized.
- The patient will acknowledge a reduction in pain.
- The patient and family will verbalize an understanding of the purpose and intended effect of drug therapy.

Medication administration

(Take action)

- Explain the purpose of therapy and its intended effect.
- Monitor the patient's vital signs, level of pain, respiratory and cardiovascular status, and laboratory results, as indicated.
- Monitor the patient's response to pain medication.
- Apply topical anesthetic as directed. (See *Teaching about topical anesthetics*, page 112).

Postadministration

(Evaluate outcomes)

- The patient remains free from major complications.
- The patient states pain is lessened with drug therapy.
- The patient and family state an understanding of drug therapy.

Education edge

Teaching about topical anesthetics

See Education edge: Teaching template in Chapter 3, page 38 for general teaching for all medications. Specific points to review with the patient and family for topical anesthetic medications:

• Use the preparation only on the part of the body for which it was prescribed and the condition for which it was prescribed.

• Apply the topical anesthetic to clean areas.

• Apply the medication only as often as directed to avoid local irritation, rash, or hives.

• If a spray is being used, don't inhale the vapors, spray near food, or store near a heat source.

• Notify the prescriber if the medication isn't effective.

• Inform health care providers of any allergies to medications or local anesthetic drugs.

Quick quiz

1.   A nurse is given a report on a patient for a patient experiencing side effects of general anesthesia. Which finding would the nurse anticipate? Select all that apply.

    A.   Seizures
    B.   Cyanosis
    C.   Tachypnea
    D.   Increased heart rate
    E.   Nausea and vomiting

Answer: E. After surgery involving general anesthesia, a patient is most likely to experience side effects/adverse reactions similar to those produced by other CNS-depressant drugs, including nausea and vomiting.

2.   A nurse administered buprenorphine hydrochloride as prescribed to a patient who had denied opioid misuse. After administration of the medication, which finding would indicate that the patient is misusing opioids?

    A.   Constipation
    B.   Urinary incontinence
    C.   Withdrawal symptoms
    D.   Hypersensitivity reaction

Answer: C. Because they can counteract the effects of opioid agonists, mixed opioid agonist-antagonists can cause withdrawal symptoms in the patient who's dependent on opioid agonists.

3. A nurse is caring for a patient with an opioid overdose. Which medication would the nurse prepare to administer?
   A.   Naloxone
   B.   Nalbuphine
   C.   Pentazocine
   D.   Butorphanol

Answer: A. Naloxone is the drug of choice for managing an opioid overdose.

4. A nurse is teaching a family about medication safety in the use of aspirin. Which common side effect/adverse reaction would the nurse include in the teaching?
   A.   Bladder infection
   B.   Dizziness and vision changes
   C.   Nausea, vomiting, and GI distress
   D.   Increased rate and depth of respirations

Answer: C. Aspirin most commonly produces adverse GI reactions, such as nausea, vomiting, and GI distress.

5. A patient asks the nurse, "Why are you applying this topical anesthetic?" Which response would the nurse make?
   A.   "Topical anesthetics are used to prevent or relieve muscle pain."
   B.   "We are using this to numb a mucosal surface before tube insertion."
   C.   "This is used as an alternative to general anesthesia for older adults."
   D.   "The medication is used when anesthesia is needed for only a short time."

Answer: A. Topical anesthetics are used to numb mucosal surfaces as well as relieve or prevent pain, relieve itching and irritation, anesthetize an area for an injection, and alleviate sore throat or mouth pain.

Scoring

⭐⭐⭐   If you answered all five questions correctly, bravo! You're a pain medication powerhouse.

⭐⭐   If you answered four questions correctly, fabulous! For you, this chapter was painless.

⭐   If you answered fewer than four questions correctly, hey, don't give up! Remember you can review!

Suggested References

Abramson, S. (2021). Aspirin: Mechanism of action, major toxicities, and use in rheumatic diseases. In D. Furst & P. Romain. (Eds.), *UpToDate Waltham, MA: UpToDate.*

Beltramini, A., Milojevic, K., & Pateron, D. (2017). Pain assessment in newborns, infants, and children. *Pediatric Annuals, 46*(10), e387–e395. doi: 10.3928/19382359-20170921-03.

Burns, M., Friedman, S., & Larson, A. (2021). Acetaminophen (paracetamol) poisoning in adults: Pathophysiology, presentation, and evaluation. In S. Truab & J. Grayzel. (Eds.), *UpToDate*. Waltham, MA: UpToDate.

Garmon, E., & Huecker, M. (2020). Topical, local, and regional anesthesia and anesthetics. In *StatPearls*. Treasure Island, FL: StatPearls Publishing. Retrieved from https://www.ncbi.nlm.nih.gov/books/NBK430894/

Ghlichloo, I., & Gerriets, V. (2020). Nonsteroidal antiinflammatory drugs (NSAIDs). In *StatPearls*. Treasure Island, FL: StatPearls Publishing. Retrieved from https://www.ncbi.nlm.nih.gov/books/NBK547742/

Karch, A. (2020). *Focus on nursing pharmacology* (8th ed.). Philadelphia, PA: Wolters Kluwer.

Lexicomp, Inc. (2021). Acetaminophen (paracetamol): Drug information. In S. Truab & J. Grayzel (Eds), *UpToDate*. Waltham, MA: UpToDate.

Miller, A., Theodore, D., & Widrich, J. (2021). Inhaled anesthetics. In *StatPearls*. Treasure Island, FL: StatPearls Publishing. Retrieved from https://www.ncbi.nlm.nih.gov/books/NBK554540/

Murphy, P., Bechmann, S., & Barrett, M. (2020). Morphine. In *StatPearls*. Treasure Island, FL: StatPearls Publishing. Retrieved from https://www.ncbi.nlm.nih.gov/books/NBK526115/

Smith, G., D'Cruz, J., Rondeau, B., & Goldman, J. (2020). General anesthesia. In *StatPearls*. Treasure Island, FL: StatPearls Publishing. Retrieved from https://www.ncbi.nlm.nih.gov/books/NBK493199/

Spencer, F., Guyatt, G., Tampi, M., & Golemiec, B. (2021). Aspirin in the primary prevention of cardiovascular disease and cancer. In J. Elmore & P. Cannon (Eds.), *UpToDate*. Waltham, MA:UpToDate.

Townsend, R. (2021). NSAIDs and acetaminophen: Effects on blood pressure and hypertension. In R. Sterns & G. Bakris (Eds.), *UpToDate*. Waltham, MA: UpToDate.

U. S. Food and Drug Administration. (2019). *Medication guide for NSAIDs*. Retrieved from https://www.accessdata.fda.gov/drugsatfda_docs/label/2019/020998s054lbl.pdf#page=21

Yasaei, R., Rosani, A., & Saadabadi, A. (2021). Meperidine. In *StatPearls*. Treasure Island, FL: StatPearls Publishing. Retrieved from https://www.ncbi.nlm.nih.gov/books/NBK470362/

Chapter 6

Autonomic nervous system drugs

Just the facts

In this chapter, you'll learn:

◆ classes of drugs that affect the autonomic nervous system

◆ uses and actions of these drugs

◆ absorption, distribution, metabolization, and excretion of these drugs

◆ drug interactions, side effects, and adverse reactions to these drugs.

Drugs and the autonomic nervous system

The peripheral nervous system is divided into two smaller systems: somatic and autonomic. The somatic nervous system innervates the voluntary movement, while the autonomic nervous system regulates the body's involuntary functions. The focus of this chapter is on the autonomic nervous system, which regulates homeostasis including heart rate, respiratory rate, and digestion. The autonomic nervous system works by balancing its two main components, the sympathetic and parasympathetic nervous systems.

The sympathetic nervous system is the "flight or fight" response to stress. The parasympathetic nervous system restores the body to normal homeostasis. The types of drugs used to treat disorders of the autonomic nervous system include:

• cholinergic drugs
• anticholinergic drugs
• adrenergic drugs
• adrenergic blocking drugs.

Pharm function

How cholinergic drugs work

Cholinergic drugs fall into one of two major classes: cholinergic agonists and anticholinesterase drugs. Here is how these drugs achieve their effects.

Cholinergic agonists (direct-acting drugs)

When a neuron in the parasympathetic nervous system is stimulated, the neurotransmitter acetylcholine is released. Acetylcholine crosses the synapse and interacts with receptors in an adjacent neuron. Cholinergic agonist drugs work by stimulating cholinergic receptors, mimicking the action of acetylcholine.

Anticholinesterase drugs (indirect-acting drugs)

After acetylcholine stimulates the cholinergic receptor, acetylcholine is destroyed by the enzyme acetylcholinesterase. Anticholinesterase drugs produce their effects by inhibiting acetylcholinesterase. As a result, acetylcholine isn't broken down and begins to accumulate; therefore, the effects of acetylcholine are prolonged.

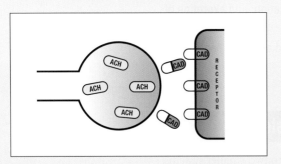
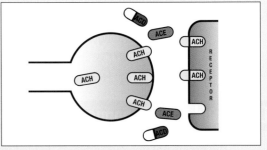

Key:

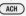 Acetylcholine   Cholinergic agonist drug   Acetylcholinesterase   Anticholinesterase drug

Cholinergic drugs

Cholinergic stimulant drugs promote the action of the neurotransmitter acetylcholine. These drugs are also called *parasympathomimetic drugs* because they produce effects that imitate parasympathetic nerve stimulation.

Mimic or inhibit

There are two major classes of cholinergic drugs:
- *Cholinergic agonists* mimic the action of the neurotransmitter acetylcholine.
- *Anticholinesterase drugs* work by inhibiting the destruction of acetylcholine at cholinergic receptor sites. (See *How cholinergic drugs work.*)

> Simon says, "Act like an acetylcholine neurotransmitter!"

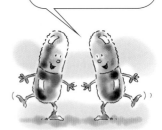

Cholinergic agonists

By directly stimulating cholinergic receptors, cholinergic agonists mimic the action of the neurotransmitter acetylcholine. They include such drugs as:

- acetylcholine chloride (not to be confused with the neurotransmitter)
- bethanechol
- carbachol
- cevimeline
- pilocarpine.

Pharmacokinetics

The action and metabolism of cholinergic agonists vary widely and depend on the affinity of the individual drug to their muscarinic or nicotinic receptors. For example, the drug acetylcholine chloride poorly penetrates the central nervous system (CNS), and its effects are primarily peripheral, with a widespread parasympathetic action. The drug is rapidly destroyed in the body. Bethanechol, on the other hand, binds to muscarinic receptors and stimulates smooth muscles in the urinary tract, bronchi, and biliary and intestinal tracts.

The "eyes" (and the mouth, and the skin) have it!

Cholinergic agonists are usually administered:

- topically, such as eye drops
- orally
- by subcutaneous injection.

Subcutaneous injections begin to work more rapidly than oral doses.

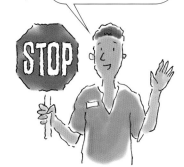

Giving cholinergic agonists IM or IV can cause cholinergic crisis.

N-O to IM or IV

The cholinergic agonists rarely are administered by IM or IV injection because they're almost immediately broken down by acetylcholinesterase in the interstitial spaces between tissues and inside the blood vessels. They work rapidly and can cause a *cholinergic crisis* (a drug overdose resulting in extreme muscle weakness and possible paralysis of the muscles used in respiration).

Fast operators

Cholinergic agonists are absorbed rapidly and reach peak levels within 2 hours. Food decreases their absorption. Less than 20% of a cholinergic agonist is protein bound.

All cholinergic agonists are metabolized by cholinesterase:

- at the muscarinic and nicotinic receptor sites
- in the plasma (the liquid portion of the blood)
- in the liver.

These drugs are excreted by the kidneys.

Pharmacodynamics

Cholinergic agonists work by mimicking the action of acetylcholine on the neurons in certain organs of the body, called *target organs*. When they combine with receptors on the cell membranes of target organs, they stimulate the muscle and produce:

- salivation
- bradycardia (a slow heart rate)
- dilation of blood vessels
- constriction of the pulmonary bronchioles
- increased activity of the GI tract (secretions and motility)
- increased tone and contraction of the muscles of the bladder
- constriction of the pupils (Karch, 2020).

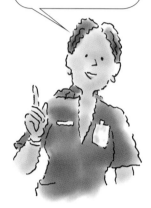

Cholinergic agonists stimulate the muscles of target organs, causing such effects as pupil constriction.

Pharmacotherapeutics

Cholinergic agonists are used to:

- treat atonic (weak) bladder conditions and postoperative and postpartum urinary retention
- treat GI disorders, such as postoperative abdominal distention and GI atony
- reduce eye pressure in patients with glaucoma and during eye surgery
- treat salivary gland hypofunction caused by radiation therapy and Sjögren's syndrome.

Drug interactions

Cholinergic agonists have specific interactions with other drugs. Here are some examples:

- Other cholinergic drugs, particularly anticholinesterase drugs, such as pyridostigmine, boost the effects of cholinergic agonists and increase the risk of toxicity.
- Anticholinergic drugs (such as atropine, homatropine, methscopolamine, and scopolamine) reduce the effects of cholinergic drugs.
- Quinidine reduces the effectiveness of cholinergic agonists.

Side effects and adverse reactions of cholinergic agonists include nausea and vomiting, cramps and diarrhea, and blurred vision.

Side effects/adverse reactions

Because they bind with receptors in the parasympathetic nervous system, cholinergic agonists can produce side effects and adverse reactions in any organ innervated by the parasympathetic nerves.

I'm not feeling well…

Side effects and adverse reactions of cholinergic agonists can include:

- nausea and vomiting
- abdominal cramps and diarrhea
- blurred vision
- decreased heart rate and low blood pressure
- shortness of breath

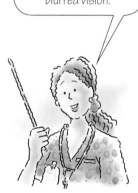

- urinary frequency
- increased salivation and sweating.

The Three-Step Approach

Nursing management for patients undergoing treatment with cholinergic agonists includes these three steps.

Preadministration

(Recognize and analyze cues)
- Assess for disorders in which cholinergic agonists are used, such as glaucoma or neurogenic atony of the bladder.
- Assess for urinary retention and bladder distention; determine the patient's fluid intake and time and amount of last urination.
- Assess mucous membranes for moisture and changes in vision or eye pain.
- Monitor blood pressure and cardiac output during treatment.
- Monitor for side effects, adverse reactions, and drug interactions during treatment.
- Assess the patient and family or caregiver's knowledge of drug therapy.

(Prioritize hypothesis—priority patient problems)
- Impaired gas exchange risk
- Urinary retention risk
- Hypotension risk
- Injury risk
- Knowledge deficiency

(Generate solutions)
- The patient will maintain effective oxygenation of tissues.
- The patient will regain usual patterns of urinary and bowel elimination.
- The patient will be free from injury and free from side effects and adverse reactions associated with cholinergic drugs.
- The patient and family member or caregiver will demonstrate correct drug administration.

Medication administration

(Take action)
- Administer cholinergic drugs on an empty stomach to prevent nausea and vomiting.
- Teach patient how to administer ophthalmic drops as prescribed.
- Perform measures to promote adequate gas exchange, such as deep breathing and coughing, suctioning, and proper positioning of the patient.
- Prevent injury associated with side effects and adverse reactions associated with the cholinergic drug.

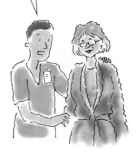

Before giving cholinergic agonists, check for disorders such as Alzheimer's disease that may be aggravated by these drugs.

Teaching about cholinergic drugs

See Education Edge: Teaching template in Chapter 3, page 38 for general teaching for all medications. Specific points to review with patients and family for cholinergic treatment:

• Take oral cholinergic drugs on an empty stomach to increase the drug's absorption.

• If diarrhea or vomiting occurs, ensure adequate fluid intake.

• Cholinergic drugs for urinary retention act within 60 minutes of taking them. Make sure bathroom facilities are available.

• If taking a cholinergic drug long term, such as for bladder problems, wear or carry medical alert identification.

• Report abdominal cramping, diarrhea, or excessive salivation to the health care provider.

• If dizziness or syncope occurs, lie down and rest, then get up gradually. Ambulation should be supervised.

• Do not take over-the-counter drugs or herbal preparations without first consulting with the health care provider because interactions may occur.

- Monitor urinary output.
- Provide patient teaching. (See *Teaching about cholinergic drugs*.)

Postadministration

(Evaluate outcomes)
- Patient maintains normal gas exchange.
- Patient is free from urinary retention, injury, side effects, and adverse reactions during drug treatment.
- Patient and family or caregiver demonstrates understanding of drug therapy and administration.

Anticholinesterase drugs

Anticholinesterase drugs block the action of the enzyme acetylcholinesterase at cholinergic receptor sites (muscarinic and nicotinic), preventing the breakdown of the neurotransmitter acetylcholine. As acetylcholine builds up, it continues to stimulate the cholinergic receptors.

Anticholinesterase drugs are divided into two categories— reversible and irreversible.

The short...

Reversible anticholinesterase drugs have a short duration of action and include:
- donepezil
- galantamine
- neostigmine
- pyridostigmine
- rivastigmine.

... and the long of it

Irreversible anticholinesterase drugs have long-lasting effects and are used primarily as toxic insecticides and pesticides or as nerve gas agents in chemical warfare. The antidote for irreversible anticholinesterase drugs is pralidoxime (Karch, 2020).

Pharmacokinetics

Here's a brief rundown of how anticholinesterase drugs move through the body.

Ready to be readily absorbed

Many of the anticholinesterase drugs are readily absorbed from the GI tract, subcutaneous tissue, and mucous membranes.

Poorly absorbed but packs some action

Because neostigmine is poorly absorbed from the GI tract, the patient needs a higher dose when taking this drug orally. The duration of action for an oral dose is longer, however, so the patient doesn't need to take it as frequently.

Need it now?

When a rapid effect is needed, such as reversing nondepolarizing neuromuscular blocking agents, the anticholinesterase drug should be given by the IM or IV route (Lexicomp, 2021b).

Diverse delivery

The distribution of anticholinesterase drugs varies. Donepezil is highly bound to plasma proteins, whereas rivastigmine is 40% bound, and galantamine is 18% bound.

Most anticholinesterase drugs are metabolized in the body by enzymes in the plasma and excreted in the urine. Donepezil, galantamine, and rivastigmine, however, are metabolized in the liver but are still excreted in urine.

Pharmacodynamics

Anticholinesterase drugs, like cholinergic agonists, promote the action of acetylcholine at receptor sites. Depending on the site and the drug's dose and duration of action, they can produce a stimulant or depressant effect on cholinergic receptors.

How long do the effects go on?

Reversible anticholinesterase drugs block the breakdown of acetylcholine for minutes to hours. The blocking effect of irreversible anticholinesterase drugs can last for days or weeks.

Now, I want you anticholinesterase drugs to go out there and block the acetylcholinesterase enzymes from breaking down the neurotransmitter acetylcholine. Got it?

Pharmacotherapeutics

Anticholinesterase drugs have various therapeutic uses. They're used to treat patient with:

- dementia associated with Alzheimer's (donepezil, galantamine, and rivastigmine)
- myasthenia gravis (pyridostigmine and neostigmine) (See *Use of anticholinesterase drugs in patients with myasthenia gravis,* page 124)
- postoperative urinary retention
- neuromuscular blockade (pyridostigmine and neostigmine).

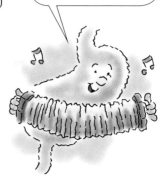

Anticholinesterase drugs improve tone and peristalsis through the GI tract. I'd say my tone is improving already!

Drug interactions

These interactions can occur with anticholinesterase drugs:

- Other cholinergic drugs, particularly cholinergic agonists (such as bethanechol, carbachol, and pilocarpine), increase the risk of toxic effects when taken with anticholinesterase drugs.
- Carbamazepine, dexamethasone, rifampin, phenytoin, and pentobarbital may increase the elimination rate of donepezil.
- Beta-blockers and other drugs resulting in bradycardia or arrhythmias should be used with caution.
- Corticosteroids increase the effects of anticholinesterase drugs contributing the potential for cholinergic crisis.

Covering up a cholinergic crisis

- Aminoglycoside antibiotics, anesthetics, anticholinergic drugs (such as atropine, propantheline, and scopolamine), magnesium, and antiarrhythmic drugs (such as procainamide and quinidine) can reduce the effects of anticholinesterase drugs and can mask early signs of a cholinergic crisis.
- Other drugs with cholinergic blocking properties, such as tricyclic antidepressants, bladder relaxants, and antipsychotics, can counteract the effects of anticholinesterase drugs. Rivastigmine may increase the neurotoxic effect of antipsychotics.
- The effects of donepezil and galantamine may be increased when combined with known inhibitors of cytochrome P-450 (CYP450), such as cimetidine and erythromycin.

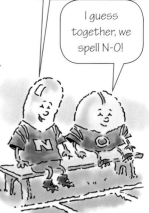

Giving cholinergic agonists with anticholinesterase drugs increases the risk of toxic effects.

I guess together, we spell N-O!

Side effects/adverse reactions

Most of the side effects and adverse reactions to anticholinesterase drugs result from increased action of acetylcholine at receptor sites. Side effects and adverse reactions associated with anticholinesterase drugs include:

- cardiac arrhythmias including prolonged QT (donepezil) and bradycardia
- nausea, vomiting, abdominal pain, diarrhea
- weight loss (galantamine and donepezil)

Preparing for Practice: Cholinergic Crisis

Excessive acetylcholine is an adverse reaction to cholinergic drugs. It is most often seen when treating myasthenia gravis and includes symptoms best remembered using the acronym SLUDGE: **s**alivation, **l**acrimation, **u**rinary incontinence, **d**iarrhea, **G**I cramps, and **e**mesis (Lilley et al., 2020, p. 317). Recognizing early signs of cholinergic toxicity is an important role of the nurse, with the goal of avoiding severe consequences of overdose, including circulatory collapse, shock, and cardiac arrest. Use of a cholinergic antagonist, such as atropine, can reverse the adverse symptoms. Epinephrine (an adrenergic agonist) may be indicated for treatment of cardiovascular or pulmonary complications.

- tremors and extrapyramidal effects (rivastigmine) or twitching (pyridostigmine)
- syncope
- CNS depression (rivastigmine)
- skin reactions (especially rivastigmine)
- urinary frequency and nocturia
- uterine irritability and induction of preterm labor (when given IV to pregnant women near term)
- shortness of breath, wheezing, or tightness in the chest
- cholinergic crisis. (See *Preparing for Practice—Cholinergic crisis.*)

The Three-Step Approach

Nursing management for patients undergoing treatment with anticholinesterase drugs includes these three steps.

Preadministration

(Recognize and analyze cues)

- Assess for disorders in which anticholinesterase drugs are used, such as myasthenia gravis, Alzheimer's disease, and urinary retention.
- Evaluate the patient's medical history for contraindications of the prescribed anticholinesterase drugs including peptic ulcer disease, chronic obstructive pulmonary disease, asthma, seizures, urinary obstruction, glaucoma, and seizure disorders.
- Perform a complete physical assessment to determine baseline, effectiveness of treatment, or occurrence of side effects and adverse reactions.

Use of anticholinesterase drugs in patients with myasthenia gravis

A diagnosis of myasthenia gravis is confirmed by testing serum levels of AChR antibody and/or by EMG-electromyography (Rubin, 2020). According to Bird (2020), the initial treatment of patients with mild to moderate myasthenia gravis typically begins with using the anticholinesterase drug pyridostigmine. The goal of therapy is to reduce symptoms with minimal to no medication side effects. To evaluate the efficacy of pyridostigmine, a thorough evaluation of neurological function and deficits should be completed prior to initiation of therapy. From this baseline, therapeutic responses can be monitored as medications and dosages are adjusted. Dosing levels for patients with myasthenia gravis vary and must be individualized according to the specific symptom relief needed and the limitation of cholinergic side effects. Considerations include the patient's:

• symptom severity, including time of day that symptoms are more severe
• individual response to pyridostigmine
• tolerance to side effects.

- Determine patient and family member or caregiver's understanding of drug therapy and administration.
- Assess for urinary retention and bladder distention, determine the patient's fluid intake, and find out the time and amount of the patient's last urination.
- Assess for possible paralytic ileus by checking for bowel sounds and abdominal distention and determining the patient's elimination patterns.

(Prioritize hypothesis—priority patient problems)
- Impaired gas exchange
- Altered tissue integrity risk
- Injury
- Knowledge deficiency

(Generate solutions)
- The patient will maintain effective oxygenation of tissues.
- The patient will maintain skin integrity during treatment.
- The patient will be free from injury, side effects, and adverse reaction associated with the underlying condition and drug therapy.
- The patient and family or caregiver will demonstrate understanding of drug therapy and correct drug administration.

Medication administration

(Take action)
- Administer drugs before or at meals unless otherwise directed.
- Monitor for side effects and adverse reactions including cholinergic crisis and myasthenia crisis.
- Assess for signs of respiratory adequacy and perform measures to promote adequate gas exchange, such as deep breathing and coughing, suctioning, and proper positioning of the patient.
- Monitor EKG for changes in rhythm.

Education edge

Teaching about anticholinesterase drugs

See Education Edge: Teaching template in Chapter 3, page 38 for general teaching for all medications. Specific points to review with patients and family for anticholinesterase therapy:

• The drug doesn't alter underlying degenerative disease but can alleviate symptoms.
• Memory improvement may be subtle. A more likely result of therapy is a slower decline in memory loss.
• When used for myasthenia gravis, these drugs relieve ptosis, double vision, difficulty chewing and swallowing, and trunk and limb weakness.
• The drug may have to be taken for life.
• If you have myasthenia gravis, wear or carry medical alert identification. If taking an anticholinesterase drug long term, such as for myasthenia gravis, bladder problems, or Alzheimer's disease, wear or carry medical alert identification.
• Immediately report significant adverse effects or changes in overall health status.
• Report the use of anticholinesterase drugs to the health care team before receiving anesthesia.
• Report episodes of nausea, vomiting, or diarrhea. If indicated, record symptoms of myasthenia gravis and the effects of the drug in a journal, especially if the dosage is adjusted.

• If taking anticholinesterase drugs for myasthenia gravis, plan rest periods between activities and space activities throughout the day. The goal of therapy is to obtain optimal benefit from the drug using the lowest possible dose with fewest adverse effects. If activity increases, the dosage may need to be increased. Report increased muscle weakness, difficulty breathing, recurrence of myasthenia gravis symptoms, and other adverse reactions to the prescriber.
• Do not take over-the-counter drugs or herbal preparations without first consulting with the health care provider because interactions may occur. For example, remedies such as St. John's wort alter the blood levels of donepezil.
• Take rivastigmine with meals.
• Avoid activities that require mental alertness until the effect of the drug is known due to CNS depression (rivastigmine).
• Avoid abrupt withdrawal of donepezil to prevent withdrawal symptoms: agitation, insomnia, hallucinations, and rapid mood changes.

• Assess for orthostatic hypotension and take actions to prevent syncope.
• Ensure atropine is available when administering IV pyridostigmine or neostigmine to maintain heart rate.
• Provide patient teaching. (See *Teaching about anticholinesterase drugs.*)

Postadministration

(Evaluate outcomes)
• The patient maintains adequate gas exchange.
• The patient maintains skin integrity.
• The patient remains free from injury, side effects, and adverse reactions associated with the underlying condition and drug therapy.
• The patient and family or caregiver demonstrates understanding of drug therapy and correct administration of drug.

Assess for signs of respiratory adequacy and perform measures to promote adequate gas exchange.

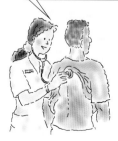

Anticholinergic drugs

Anticholinergic drugs (also called *cholinergic blockers*) interrupt parasympathetic nerve impulses in the CNS and autonomic nervous system. They also prevent acetylcholine from stimulating cholinergic receptors.

For muscarinic sites only

Anticholinergic (or *parasympatholytic*) drugs don't block all cholinergic receptors, just the muscarinic receptor sites. They do not block the nicotinic receptors (Karch, 2020). The major anticholinergic drug is atropine, a belladonna alkaloid.

Anticholinergic drugs are prescribed for many different conditions. They are listed below with their labeled use/s within the various body systems.

Respiratory agents (See *Respiratory chapter for more details,* page 314)
- Aclidinium—chronic obstructive pulmonary disease (COPD) with chronic bronchospasms
- Atropine (See *Anticholinergic drugs: Atropine,* page 127.)
- Glycopyrrolate—COPD, neuromuscular blockade, and to decrease secretions for surgery
- Ipratropium—COPD and rhinitis (nasal spray)
- Tiotropium and umeclidinium—COPD

Gastrointestinal agents (See *Gastrointestinal chapter for more details,* page 344)
- Dicyclomine—irritable bowel
- Meclizine—nausea and vomiting and prevention of motion sickness
- Methscopolamine—adjunctive treatment for peptic ulcer disease
- Scopolamine—prevention of motion sickness, decrease secretions, dilate pupils for testing

Genitourinary agents (See *Genitourinary chapter for more details,* page 401)
- Darifenacin, fesoterodine, oxybutynin, solifenacin, tolterodine, and trospium—overactive bladder
- Flavoxate—conditions associated with dysuria and incontinence

Neurological agents (See *Neuromuscular chapter for more details,* page 159)
- Benztropine and trihexyphenidyl—extrapyramidal effects caused by drugs or Parkinsonism

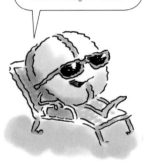

I prefer muscarinic receptor sites to other receptor sites. I'm really quite selective, you know.

Prototype pro

Anticholinergic drugs: Atropine

Actions
• Competitively antagonizes the actions of acetylcholine and other cholinergic agonists at the muscarinic receptors

Indications
• Symptomatic bradycardia
• Preoperative reduction of secretions
• Antidote for cholinergic drugs, muscarine containing mushroom poisoning, and anticholinesterase poisoning (Lexicomp, 2021a)

Nursing considerations
• Monitor for side effects and adverse reactions, such as headache, tachycardia, restlessness, dizziness, blurred vision, dry mouth, urinary hesitancy, and constipation.
• Monitor vital signs, cardiac rhythm, urine output, and vision for signs of impending toxicity.
• Provide stool softeners or bulk laxatives as ordered for constipation.

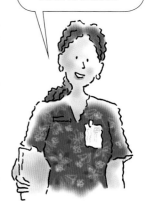

Each type of drug has its own benefits. For example, the belladonna alkaloids are absorbed more readily through the GI tract and distributed widely, but tertiary amines have fewer adverse effects.

Effects of anticholinergic drugs
The effects of anticholinergic drugs are opposite of the cholinergic drugs and include:
• pupil dilation (mydriasis) and cycloplegia (decrease ability of lens to accommodate)
• decrease secretions—tears, saliva, and GI secretions
• decrease GI motility
• increase heart rate, conduction, and contractility
• increase bladder sphincter constriction.

Pharmacokinetics
The belladonna alkaloids are absorbed from the eyes, GI tract, mucous membranes, and skin. Others are absorbed primarily through the GI tract, although not as readily as the belladonna alkaloids.

Instant gratification
When administered IV, anticholinergic drugs such as atropine begin to work immediately. The belladonna alkaloids are distributed more widely throughout the body than other anticholinergic drugs. The alkaloids readily cross the blood-brain barrier; the other drugs in this class don't.

Ready and able

The belladonna alkaloids have low to moderate binding with serum proteins and are only slightly to moderately protein bound. This means that a moderate to high amount of the drug is active and available to produce a therapeutic response. They're metabolized in the liver and excreted by the kidneys as unchanged drug and metabolites.

Pharmacodynamics

Anticholinergic drugs can have paradoxical effects on the body, depending on the dosage, the condition being treated, and the target organ. For example, anticholinergic drugs can produce a stimulating or depressing effect. In the brain, they do both—low drug levels stimulate and high drug levels depress.

Disorder-related dynamics

A patient's disorder can also impact the effects of a drug. Parkinsonism, for example, is characterized by low dopamine levels that intensify the stimulating effects of acetylcholine. Cholinergic blockers, however, depress this effect. In other disorders, these same drugs stimulate the CNS.

Pharmacotherapeutics

Here's how anticholinergic drugs are used in various GI situations:
- All anticholinergic drugs are used to treat spastic or hyperactive conditions of the GI and urinary tracts because they relax muscles and decrease GI secretions. However, for bladder relaxation and urinary incontinence, oxybutynin, fesoterodine, and tolterodine are preferred.
- The belladonna alkaloids are used with morphine to treat biliary colic (pain caused by stones in the bile duct).
- Anticholinergic drugs are given by injection before some diagnostic procedures, such as endoscopy or sigmoidoscopy, to relax the GI smooth muscle.

Preop purposes

Anticholinergic drugs such as atropine are given before surgery to:
- reduce oral, gastric, and respiratory secretions
- prevent a drop in heart rate caused by vagal nerve stimulation during anesthesia.

Brain games

The belladonna alkaloids can affect the brain. For example, when given with the pain medication morphine or meperidine, scopolamine causes drowsiness and amnesia. It's also used to treat motion sickness.

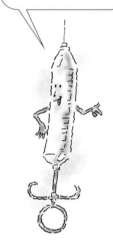

Giving anticholinergics by injection before diagnostic procedures relaxes GI smooth muscle.

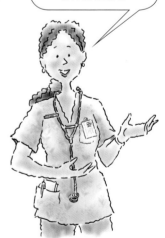

Belladonna alkaloids have therapeutic effects on the heart.

Heart matters

The belladonna alkaloids also have therapeutic effects on the heart. Atropine is the drug of choice to treat:

- symptomatic sinus bradycardia—when the heart beats too slowly, causing low blood pressure or dizziness (See *How atropine speeds heart rate*.)
- arrhythmias resulting from anesthetics, choline esters, or succinylcholine.

In your eyes

Anticholinergic drugs are also used as cycloplegics, which means they paralyze the ciliary muscles of the eye (used for fine focusing) and alter the shape of the lens of the eye. Furthermore, anticholinergic

Pharm function

How atropine speeds heart rate

To understand how atropine affects the heart, first consider how the heart's electrical conduction system functions.

Without the drug
When the neurotransmitter acetylcholine is released, the vagus nerve stimulates the sinoatrial (SA) node (the heart's pacemaker) and atrioventricular (AV) node, which controls conduction between the atria and ventricles of the heart. This inhibits electrical conduction and causes the heart rate to slow down.

With the drug
When a patient receives atropine, a cholinergic blocking drug, it competes with acetylcholine for binding with the cholinergic receptors on the SA and AV nodes. By blocking acetylcholine, atropine speeds up the heart rate.

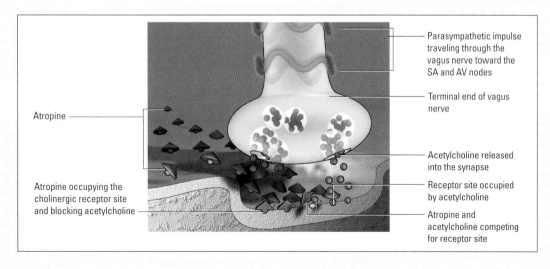

drugs act as mydriatics to dilate the pupils of the eye, making it easier to measure refractive errors during an eye examination or to perform surgery on the eye.

Antidote-i-ful

The belladonna alkaloids, particularly atropine, are effective antidotes to cholinergic and anticholinesterase drugs. Atropine is the drug of choice to treat poisoning from organophosphate pesticides. Atropine also counteracts the effects of the neuromuscular blocking drugs by competing for the same receptor sites.

Drug interactions

Because anticholinergic drugs slow the passage of food and drugs through the stomach, drugs remain in prolonged contact with the mucous membranes of the GI tract. This increases the amount of the drug that's absorbed and, therefore, increases the risk of side effects and adverse effects.

Effect boosters

Drugs that increase the effects of anticholinergic drugs include:
- antidyskinetics (such as amantadine)
- antiemetics and antivertigo drugs (such as diphenhydramine)
- antipsychotics (such as haloperidol, phenothiazines, and thioxanthenes)
- cyclobenzaprine
- disopyramide
- orphenadrine
- tricyclic and tetracyclic antidepressants.

Effect busters

Drugs that decrease the effects of anticholinergic drugs include:
- anticholinesterase drugs (such as neostigmine)
- cholinergic agonists (such as bethanechol).

And there's more

Here are other drug interactions that can occur:
- The risk of digoxin toxicity increases when digoxin is taken with an anticholinergic drug.
- Opiate-like analgesics further enhance the slow movement of food and drugs through the GI tract when taken with cholinergic blockers.
- The absorption of nitroglycerin tablets placed under the tongue is reduced when taken with a cholinergic blocker.

Side effects/adverse reactions

Side effects and adverse reactions of anticholinergic drugs are closely related to drug dose. The difference between a therapeutic and a toxic dosage is small with these drugs.

Side effects and adverse reactions may include:

- dry mouth
- reduced bronchial secretions
- increased heart rate
- blurred vision
- decreased sweating
- confusion
- delirium
- cognitive decline (See *Preparing for Practice—Anticholinergics*).

The Three–Step Approach

Nursing management for patients undergoing treatment with anticholinergic drugs include these three steps.

Preadministration

(Recognize and analyze cues)

- Assess for conditions in which anticholinergic drugs would be used, such as bradycardia, heart block (a delay or interruption in the conduction of electrical impulses between the atria and ventricles), diarrhea, and peptic ulcer disease.
- Assess for conditions in which anticholinergic drugs would be contraindicated, such as glaucoma, myasthenia gravis, prostatic hyperplasia, reflux esophagitis, or GI obstructive disease.

(Prioritize hypothesis—priority patient problems)

- Urinary retention
- Constipation
- Injury risk
- Knowledge deficiency

(Generate solutions)

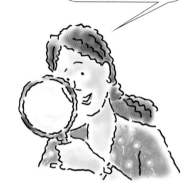

You can clearly see you'll need to monitor vital signs, cardiac rhythm, urine output, and vision for potential drug toxicity.

Preparing for Practice: Anticholinergics

Adverse effects of confusion, cognitive decline, and even delirium have been a potential concern for elderly patients taking anticholinergic drugs. However, the effects of anticholinergics are not associated with cognitive decline in children. It is hypothesized that the adverse effects of anticholinergics on older adults may be related to long years of exposure to anticholinergics, polypharmacy, or possibly that early (undiagnosed) dementia is responsible for the association of anticholinergic use and cognitive decline in older adults (Ghezzi et al., 2021).

- The patient will experience normal urinary and bowel patterns.
- The patient will remain free from injury from the underlying condition, side effects, and adverse reactions.
- The patient and family or caregiver will demonstrate understanding of drug therapy and administration.

Medication administration

(Take action)

- Administer drugs with meals as directed.
- Monitor vital signs, cardiac rhythm, urine output, and vision for potential drug toxicity.
- Monitor for side effects and adverse reactions, such as dry mouth, increased heart rate, and blurred vision.
- Have emergency equipment available to treat new cardiac arrhythmias.
- Help alleviate symptoms if side effects or adverse reactions occur. For example, provide lozenges and frequent mouth care for patients experiencing dry mouth.
- Provide patient teaching. (See *Teaching about anticholinergic drugs.*)

Postadministration

(Evaluate outcomes)

- The patient maintains normal bladder and bowel patterns.

Education edge

Teaching about anticholinergic drugs

See Education Edge: Teaching template in Chapter 3, page 38 for general teaching for all medications. Specific points to review with patients and family for anticholinergic therapy:

- Avoiding taking any other drugs with the anticholinergic unless prescribed.
- Avoid hazardous tasks if dizziness, drowsiness, or blurred vision occurs.
- The drug may increase sensitivity to high temperatures, resulting in dizziness.
- Avoid alcohol because it may have additive CNS effects.
- Drink plenty of fluids and eat a high-fiber diet to prevent constipation.
- Obtain regular dental care to help manage periodontal (gum) disease and dental caries that may occur from dry mouth side effects from anticholinergic drugs.
- Notify the prescriber promptly if confusion, rapid or pounding heartbeat, dry mouth, blurred vision, rash, eye pain, a significant change in urine volume, pain on urination, or difficulty urinating occur.
- Women should report planned or known pregnancy.

- The patient remains free from injury from the underlying condition, side effects, and adverse reactions.
- The patient and family or caregiver demonstrates understanding of drug therapy and administration.

Adrenergic drugs

Adrenergic drugs are also called *sympathomimetic drugs* because they produce effects similar to those produced by the sympathetic nervous system neurotransmitters norepinephrine, epinephrine, and dopamine.

Sort by chemical…

Adrenergic drugs are classified into two groups based on their chemical structure: catecholamines (naturally occurring as well as synthetic) and noncatecholamines.

… or by action

Adrenergic drugs are also divided by how they act. They can be:
- *direct-acting*, in which the drug acts directly on the organ or tissue innervated (supplied with nerves or nerve impulses) by the sympathetic nervous system
- *indirect-acting*, in which the drug triggers the release of a neurotransmitter, usually norepinephrine
- *dual-acting*, in which the drug has direct and indirect actions. (See *How adrenergics work*, page 134.)

Catecholamines

Because of their common basic chemical structure, catecholamines share certain properties—they stimulate the nervous system, constrict peripheral blood vessels, increase heart rate, and dilate the bronchi. They can be manufactured in the body or in a laboratory. Common catecholamines include:
- dobutamine
- dopamine
- epinephrine, epinephrine bitartrate, and epinephrine hydrochloride
- norepinephrine
- isoproterenol hydrochloride.

Pharmacokinetics

Here's an overview of how catecholamines move through the body.

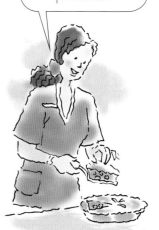

Catecholamines can't be taken orally because they're destroyed by digestive enzymes. I'll let those digestive enzymes work on this pie instead!

Pharm function

How adrenergics work

Adrenergic drugs are distinguished by how they achieve their effect. The illustrations below show the action of direct-, indirect-, and dual-acting adrenergics.

Direct-acting adrenergic action
Direct-acting adrenergic drugs directly stimulate adrenergic receptors.

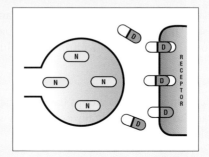

Indirect-acting adrenergic action
Indirect-acting adrenergic drugs stimulate the release of norepinephrine from nerve endings into the synapse.

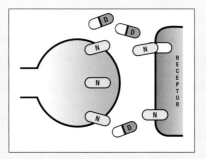

Dual-acting adrenergic action
Dual-acting adrenergic drugs stimulate both adrenergic receptor sites and the release of norepinephrine from nerve endings.

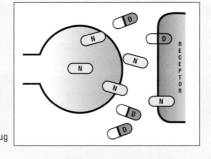

Key:
(N) Norepinephrine (D) Adrenergic drug

No P.O.

Catecholamines can't be taken orally because they're destroyed by digestive enzymes. In contrast, when these drugs are given sublingually or inhalation, they are rapidly absorbed through the mucous membranes. Any sublingual drug not completely absorbed is rapidly metabolized by swallowed saliva.

Subcutaneous versus IM

Absorption by the subcutaneous route is slowed because catecholamines cause the blood vessels around the injection site to constrict. IM absorption is more rapid because less constriction of local blood vessels occurs.

Catecholamines are widely distributed in the body. They're metabolized and inactivated predominantly in the liver but can also be metabolized in the GI tract, lungs, kidneys, plasma, and tissues.

On the way out

Catecholamines are excreted primarily in urine.

Pharmacodynamics

Catecholamines are primarily direct-acting. When catecholamines combine with alpha-adrenergic receptors or beta-adrenergic receptors, they cause either an excitatory or inhibitory effect. Typically, activation of alpha-adrenergic receptors generates an excitatory response except for intestinal relaxation. Activation of the beta-adrenergic receptors mostly produces an inhibitory response, except in the cells of the heart, where norepinephrine produces excitatory effects.

Workin' the heart

The clinical effects of catecholamines depend on the dosage and the route of administration. Catecholamines are potent inotropes—they make the heart contract more forcefully. As a result, the ventricles of the heart empty more completely with each heartbeat, increasing the workload of the heart and the amount of oxygen it needs to do this harder work.

Kickin' up the beat

Catecholamines also produce a positive chronotropic effect, which means they cause the heart to beat faster. That's because pacemaker cells in the SA node of the heart depolarize at a faster rate. As catecholamines cause blood vessels to constrict and blood pressure to rise, heart rate can fall as the body tries to compensate and prevent an excessive rise in blood pressure.

All fired up

Catecholamines can cause the Purkinje fibers (an intricate web of fibers that carry electrical impulses into the ventricles of the heart) to fire spontaneously, possibly producing abnormal heart rhythms, such as premature ventricular contractions and fibrillation. Epinephrine is more likely than norepinephrine to produce this spontaneous firing.

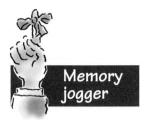

Memory jogger

To help you remember the effects of catecholamines on alpha and beta receptors, remember that **A** stands for **a**lpha (and **a**ctivation, suggesting an excitatory response) and **B** stands for **b**eta (or **b**anished, which suggests an inhibitory effect).

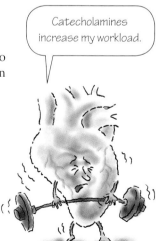

Catecholamines increase my workload.

Pharmacotherapeutics

How adrenergic drugs are used depends on which receptors they stimulate and to what degree. Adrenergic drugs can affect:
- alpha-adrenergic receptors
- beta-adrenergic receptors
- dopamine receptors. (See *Pharm function: Alpha, Beta, and Dopamine.*)

Most adrenergics produce their effects by stimulating alpha- and beta-adrenergic receptors. These drugs mimic the action of norepinephrine and epinephrine.

Of the catecholamines:
- norepinephrine has the most nearly pure alpha activity
- dobutamine and isoproterenol have only beta-related therapeutic uses
- epinephrine stimulates alpha- and beta-adrenergic receptors and is used to treat bronchospasms, croup, anaphylaxis, shock, and cardiac arrest

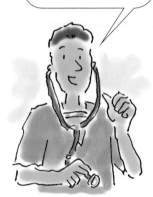

Catecholamines that stimulate alpha-adrenergic receptors are used to treat hypotension.

Pharm function

Alpha, beta, and dopamine

	Alpha	Beta	Dopamine
Function	Stimulates effector cells	Relaxes effector cells	Stimulates dopamine receptors
Location	Vascular smooth muscle and effector tissues	Bronchial, heart, and uterine muscles	Brain, pituitary, kidney, and retina
Types	Alpha 1—vasoconstriction, decreased bronchial secretions Alpha 2—vasoconstriction	Beta 1—positive chronotropic response and positive inotropic response Beta 2—vasodilator, inhibits mast cell release, decreasing histamine release	Dopamine 1—vasodilation in cerebral, coronary, and renal vessels Dopamine 2—inhibits norepinephrine release and in high doses stimulates Alpha 1 and 2
Drug examples and uses	Norepinephrine (Alpha$_1$ and Alpha$_2$)—used to treat hypotension	Isoproterenol—(Beta$_1$ and Beta$_2$)—used to treat bronchospasms, hypotension, shock, and cardiac arrest. Dobutamine (Beta$_1$ and Beta$_2$)—used to treat low cardiac output and decompensated heart failure	Dopamine (D$_1$ and D$_2$)– used to treat hypotension and low cardiac output due to major systems' illnesses and failure

- dopamine primarily exhibits dopaminergic activity (it acts on sympathetic nervous system receptors that are stimulated by dopamine).

Helping hypotension

Catecholamines that stimulate alpha-adrenergic receptors are used to treat low blood pressure (hypotension). As a rule, catecholamines work best when used to treat hypotension caused by:
- relaxation of the blood vessels (also called a *loss of vasomotor tone*)
- blood loss (such as from hemorrhage).

Rhythm makers

Catecholamines that stimulate beta$_1$-adrenergic receptors are used to treat:
- bradycardia
- heart block
- low cardiac output.

Increasing response

Because they're believed to make the heart more responsive to defibrillation (using an electrical current to terminate a deadly arrhythmia), beta$_1$-adrenergic drugs are used to treat:
- ventricular fibrillation (quivering of the ventricles resulting in no pulse)
- asystole (no electrical activity in the heart)
- cardiac arrest.

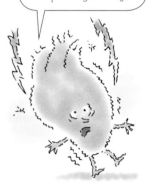

Beta$_1$-adrenergic drugs make the heart more responsive to defibrillation. Yikes! I'm responding already!

Breathing better with beta$_2$ activity

Catecholamines that exert beta$_2$-adrenergic activity are used to treat:
- acute and chronic bronchial asthma
- emphysema
- bronchitis
- acute hypersensitivity (allergic) reactions to drugs.

More blood for the kidneys

Dopamine, which stimulates dopaminergic receptors, is used in low doses to improve blood flow to the kidneys because it dilates the renal blood vessels.

Drug interactions

Drug interactions involving catecholamines can be serious:
- Alpha-adrenergic blockers, such as phentolamine, used with catecholamines can produce hypotension.
- Because the catecholamine epinephrine may cause hyperglycemia, diabetic patients receiving epinephrine may require an increased dose of insulin or drugs.

- Beta-adrenergic blockers, such as propranolol, used with catecholamines can lead to bronchial constriction, especially in patients with asthma.

Adding it all up
- Other adrenergic drugs can produce additive effects, such as hypertension and arrhythmias, and enhance adverse effects.
- Tricyclic antidepressants used with catecholamines can lead to hypertension.

Side effects/adverse reactions

Side effects and adverse reactions to catecholamines include:
- restlessness
- anxiety
- dizziness
- headache
- palpitations
- cardiac arrhythmias
- hypotension
- hypertension and hypertensive crisis
- stroke
- angina
- increased glucose levels.

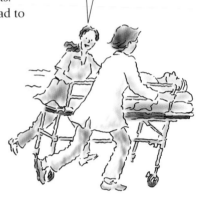

Catecholamines can cause a number of adverse reactions, including hypertensive crisis and stroke.

The Three–Step Approach

Nursing management for patients undergoing treatment with catecholamines includes these three steps.

Preadministration
(Recognize and analyze cues)

Preparing for Practice: Catecholamines

• Dopamine and epinephrine have a Black Box Warning for extravasation (if a catecholamine administered by IV leaks into the surrounding tissue). If tissue necrosis and sloughing, stop the infusion. Phentolamine diluted in normal saline can be infiltrated into the affected area (Skidmore-Roth, 2021).
• Epinephrine concentrations must be carefully checked for accuracy because death has occurred from concentration errors.

- Assess the patient's condition before and during therapy and regularly thereafter.
- Analyze the patient's medical history and physical assessment data for changes in condition.
- Continuously monitor electrocardiogram (ECG), blood pressure, pulmonary artery wedge pressure, cardiac condition, and urine output.
- Monitor electrolyte levels.
- Throughout therapy, assess for side effects, adverse reactions, drug interactions, and acidosis, which decrease effectiveness of dopamine.
- After dopamine is stopped, watch closely for a sudden drop in blood pressure.
- Assess the patient and family or caregivers' knowledge of drug therapy.

(Prioritize hypothesis—priority patient problems)
- Altered cardiac output
- Altered tissue perfusion
- Hypovolemia
- Injury risk
- Knowledge deficiency related to drug therapy

(Generate solutions)
- The patient will maintain effective cardiac output.
- The patient will maintain an adequate blood pressure and maintain tissue perfusion.
- The risk for injury will be minimized.
- The patient and family or caregiver will demonstrate an understanding of the purpose and intended effect of therapy.

Medication administration
(Take action)
- Before starting catecholamines, correct hypovolemia with plasma volume expanders.
- Give cardiac glycosides before catecholamines; cardiac glycosides increase AV node conduction, and patients with atrial fibrillation may develop rapid ventricular rate.
- Administer drug using a central venous catheter or large peripheral vein. Adjust the infusion according to the prescriber's order and the patient's condition. Use an infusion pump.
- Dilute the concentrate for injection before administration, according to pharmacy guidelines.
- Watch for irritation and infiltration; extravasation can cause an inflammatory response.
- Don't give catecholamines in the same IV line as other drugs; be aware of incompatibilities. For example, dobutamine is

incompatible with heparin, hydrocortisone sodium succinate, penicillin, and ethacrynate sodium.
- Don't mix dobutamine or dopamine with sodium bicarbonate injection or phenytoin because the drug is incompatible with alkaline solutions.
- Change IV sites regularly to avoid phlebitis.
- Provide patient teaching.

Postadministration
(Evaluate outcomes)
- Patient maintains adequate cardiac output.
- Patient maintains adequate cerebral, cardiopulmonary, and renal tissue perfusion.
- Patient maintains adequate blood pressure.
- Patient remains free from injury.
- Patient and family or caregiver demonstrates understanding of drug therapy.

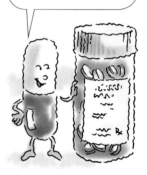

Sometimes, the order of drug administration matters. For example, cardiac glycosides should be given before catecholamines.

Noncatecholamines

Noncatecholamines are adrenergic drugs that do not contain catechol. Unlike catecholamines which are direct-acting adrenergic drugs, noncatecholamines can be direct-acting, indirect-acting, or dual-acting. Noncatecholamines also differ from catecholamines in that they can be used orally and have a longer half-life. Noncatecholamines have many therapeutic uses because of the various effects these drugs can have on the body, including:
- local or systemic constriction of blood vessels (phenylephrine)
- nasal and eye decongestion and dilation of the bronchioles (albuterol, ephedrine, formoterol, isoproterenol, metaproterenol, salmeterol, and terbutaline)
- smooth muscle relaxation (terbutaline).
  Dilation of the bronchioles is the most common use of this type of drug.

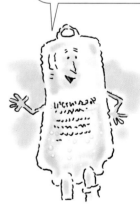

Don't mix me up! Catecholamines shouldn't be administered in the same IV line as other drugs.

Pharmacokinetics

Absorption of noncatecholamines depends on the route of administration:

Breathe deep...
- Inhaled drugs, such as albuterol, are gradually absorbed from the bronchi of the lungs and result in lower drug levels in the body.

Open wide...

- Oral drugs are absorbed well from the GI tract and are distributed widely in the body fluids and tissues.
- Some noncatecholamine drugs (such as ephedrine) cross the blood-brain barrier and can be found in high concentrations in the brain and cerebrospinal fluid.

Metabolism and inactivation of noncatecholamines occur primarily in the liver but can also occur in the lungs, GI tract, and other tissues.

Exit time varies

These drugs and their metabolites are excreted primarily in urine. Some, such as inhaled albuterol, are excreted within 24 hours; others, such as oral albuterol, are excreted within 3 days. Acidic urine increases excretion of many noncatecholamines; alkaline urine slows excretion.

Pharmacodynamics

Noncatecholamines can be direct-, indirect-, or dual-acting.

- Direct-acting noncatecholamines that stimulate alpha-adrenergic receptors include phenylephrine. Those that selectively stimulate beta$_2$-adrenergic receptors include albuterol, metaproterenol, and terbutaline.
- Indirect-acting noncatecholamines exert their effect by indirect action on adrenergic receptors.
- Dual-acting noncatecholamines include ephedrine.

Pharmacotherapeutics

Noncatecholamines stimulate the sympathetic nervous system and produce various effects on the body. It's important to become familiar with each individual drug, including its indication, route, dose, and administration technique. Monitor the patient closely for therapeutic effect and tolerance.

Drug interactions

Here are a few examples of how other drugs may interact with noncatecholamines:

- General anesthetics can cause arrhythmias when used with noncatecholamines.
- Hypotension can occur when noncatecholamines have predominantly beta$_2$ activity, such as terbutaline.

A deadly combo: noncatecholamines and....

- Monoamine oxidase inhibitors can cause severe hypertension and death.

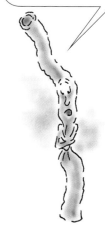

Noncatecholamines have several therapeutic effects, including local or systemic constriction of blood vessels. I must say, this doesn't feel terribly therapeutic!

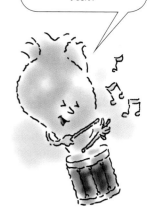

Keep in mind that using noncatecholamines with tricyclic antidepressants can cause arrhythmias. Gotta make sure I maintain my steady beat!

- Tricyclic antidepressants can cause severe hypertension and arrhythmias.
- Oxytocic drugs that stimulate uterine contraction can be inhibited with terbutaline. When taken with other noncatecholamines, hypertensive crisis or a stroke can occur.
- Urine alkalizers slow excretion of noncatecholamines, prolonging their action. Read labels for sodium bicarbonate.

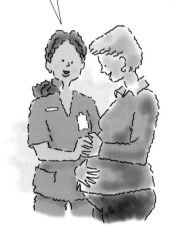

Keep in mind that noncatecholamines can change heart rate and blood pressure in a pregnant woman and her fetus.

Side effects/adverse reactions

Side effects and adverse reactions to noncatecholamines may include:
- headache
- restlessness
- anxiety or euphoria
- irritability
- trembling
- drowsiness or insomnia
- light-headedness
- incoherence
- seizures
- hypertension or hypotension
- palpitations
- bradycardia or tachycardia
- irregular heart rhythm
- cardiac arrest
- cerebral hemorrhage
- tingling or coldness in the arms or legs
- pallor or flushing
- angina
- changes in heart rate and blood pressure in a pregnant woman and her fetus. (See *Preparing for Practice—Noncatecholamines*, page 143.)

The Three-Step Approach

Nursing management for patients undergoing treatment with noncatecholamines includes these three steps.

Preadministration

(Recognize and analyze cues)
- Obtain a baseline assessment of the patient's respiratory status and assess it frequently throughout therapy.
- Analyze the patient's medical history and physical assessment for contraindications or special needs associated with noncatecholamine therapy.
- Assess for side effects, adverse reactions, and drug interactions.
- Assess the patient's and/or caregivers' knowledge of drug therapy.

(Prioritize hypothesis—priority patient problems)
- Ineffective airway clearance

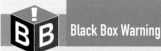

Preparing for Practice: Noncatecholamines

Paradoxical bronchospasm has been known to occur with albuterol. If it occurs, instruct patient to discontinue the drug and contact prescriber.

Black Box Warnings

• Formoterol and salmeterol for asthma-related death or severe asthma exacerbations. Immediate medical attention should be obtained if an acute asthma attack is not relieved when using the drug (Skidmore-Roth, 2021, pp. 581 and 1129.)

• Salmeterol for asthma-related deaths in children less than 4 years of age. Additionally, use of a single-ingredient long-acting beta agonist for treatment of asthma is not recommended (Skidmore-Roth, 2021, pp. 1128–1129).

• Terbutaline for use during maternal labor, as it can inhibit uterine contractions. It should also be avoided in breastfeeding mothers (Skidmore-Roth, 2021, p. 1206).

- Injury risk related
- Knowledge deficiency

(Generate solutions)
- The patient will maintain effective airway clearance.
- The risk of injury will be minimized.
- The patient and family or caregiver will demonstrate understanding of the purpose and intended effect of drug therapy.

Medication administration

(Take action)
- If using the inhalation route, wait at least 2 minutes between doses if more than one dose is ordered. If a corticosteroid inhaler also is used, first have the patient use the bronchodilator, wait for 5 minutes, and then have the patient use the corticosteroid inhaler. This permits the bronchodilator to open air passages for maximum corticosteroid effectiveness.
- Give the injectable form (terbutaline) in the lateral deltoid area. Protect the injection from light. Don't use the drug if it's discolored.
- Notify the prescriber immediately if bronchospasms develop during therapy.
- Instruct the patient to use the aerosol form 15 minutes before exercise to prevent exercise-induced bronchospasm as indicated.
- Provide patient teaching. (See *Teaching about noncatecholamines,* page 144.)

Postadministration

(Evaluate outcomes)
- The patient has effective airway clearance.

Teaching about noncatecholamines

See Education Edge: Teaching template in Chapter 3, page 38 for general teaching for all medications. Specific points to review with patients and family for noncatecholamine therapy:

- Stop the drug immediately if paradoxical bronchospasm occurs.
- Follow these instructions for using a metered-dose inhaler:
  - Clear the nasal passages and throat.
  - Breathe out, expelling as much air from the lungs as possible.
  - Place the mouthpiece well into the mouth and inhale deeply as the dose is released.
  - Hold your breath for several seconds, remove the mouthpiece, and exhale slowly.
  - Wait at least 2 minutes before repeating the procedure if more than one inhalation is ordered.
- Avoid accidentally spraying the inhalant form into the eyes; doing so may temporarily blur vision.
- Reduce intake of foods and herbs containing caffeine, such as coffee, cola, and chocolate, when using a bronchodilator.
- Check pulse rate before and after using the bronchodilator. Call the prescriber if pulse rate increases more than 20 to 30 beats/minute.

- The patient is free from injury.
- The patient and family or caregiver demonstrates understanding of drug therapy.

Adrenergic blocking drugs

Adrenergic blocking drugs, also called *sympatholytic drugs,* are used to disrupt sympathetic nervous system function. These drugs work by blocking impulse transmission (and thus sympathetic nervous system stimulation) at adrenergic neurons or adrenergic receptor sites. Their action at these sites can be exerted by:
- interrupting the action of adrenergic drugs
- reducing available norepinephrine
- preventing the action of cholinergic drugs.

We're adrenergic blocking drugs. We block impulse transmissions from adrenergic neurons and receptor sites. It's quite a job, but we're up to it!

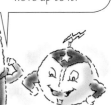

Classified information

Adrenergic blocking drugs are classified according to their site of action as:
- alpha-adrenergic blockers (also called *alpha blockers*)
- beta-adrenergic blockers (also called *beta blockers*).

Alpha-adrenergic blockers

Alpha-adrenergic blockers work by interrupting the actions of the catecholamines epinephrine and norepinephrine at alpha receptors. This results in:
- relaxation of the smooth muscle in the blood vessels
- increased dilation of blood vessels
- reduced peripheral vascular resistance, resulting in decreased blood pressure.

Drugs in this class include:
- ergoloid mesylates
- ergotamine
- phenoxybenzamine
- phentolamine
- terazosin
- doxazosin
- prazosin (See *Alpha-adrenergic blockers: Prazosin.*)
- tamsulosin.

Two actions in one

Ergotamine is a mixed alpha agonist and antagonist; at high doses, it acts as an alpha-adrenergic blocker.

Pharmacokinetics

Most alpha-adrenergic blockers are absorbed erratically when given orally and more rapidly and completely when given sublingually. Alpha-adrenergic blockers vary considerably in their onset of action, peak concentration levels, and duration of action.

Pharmacodynamics

Alpha-adrenergic blockers work in one of two ways:

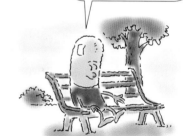

My job is to block alpha-receptor sites so that catecholamines can't occupy them. Sorry, catecholamine, this seat is taken.

Prototype pro

Alpha-adrenergic blockers: Prazosin

- Monitor for side effects and adverse reactions, such as dizziness, first-dose syncope, palpitations, or nausea.
- Monitor pulse rate and blood pressure frequently.
- Advise the patient to rise slowly and to avoid abrupt position changes.
- Use cautiously with older adults due to risk of orthostatic hypotension (Lilley et al., 2020).

- They interfere with or block the synthesis, storage, release, and reuptake of norepinephrine by neurons.
- They antagonize epinephrine, norepinephrine, or adrenergic drugs at alpha-receptor sites.

Alpha-adrenergic blockers include drugs that block stimulation of alpha₁ receptors and drugs that may block alpha₂ stimulation.

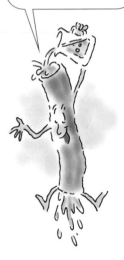

Thanks, alpha-adrenergic blockers, for helping me dilate!

More flow, less pressure

Alpha-adrenergic blockers occupy alpha-receptor sites on the smooth muscle of blood vessels. (See *How alpha-adrenergic blockers affect peripheral blood vessels.*) This prevents catecholamines from occupying and stimulating the receptor sites. As a result, blood vessels dilate, increasing local blood flow to the skin and other organs. The decreased peripheral vascular resistance helps to decrease blood pressure.

Watch your patient's tone

The therapeutic effect of an alpha-adrenergic blocker depends on the sympathetic tone (the state of partial constriction of blood vessels) in the body before the drug is administered. For instance, when the drug is given with the patient lying down, only a small change in blood

---

Pharm function

How alpha-adrenergic blockers affect peripheral blood vessels

By occupying alpha-receptor sites, alpha-adrenergic blocking drugs cause blood vessel walls to relax. This leads to dilation of blood vessels and reduced peripheral vascular resistance (the pressure that blood must overcome as it flows in a vessel).

One result: orthostatic hypotension

These effects can cause orthostatic hypotension, a drop in blood pressure that occurs when changing position from lying down to standing. Redistribution of blood to the dilated blood vessels of the legs causes hypotension.

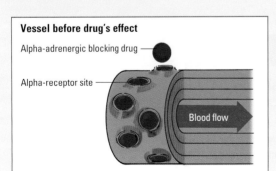

Vessel before drug's effect

Alpha-adrenergic blocking drug

Alpha-receptor site

Blood flow

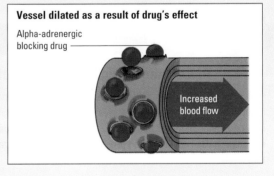

Vessel dilated as a result of drug's effect

Alpha-adrenergic blocking drug

Increased blood flow

pressure occurs. In this position, the sympathetic nerves release very little norepinephrine.

On the other hand, when a patient stands up, norepinephrine is released to constrict the veins and shoot blood back up to the heart. If the patient receives an alpha-adrenergic blocker, however, the veins can't constrict and blood pools in the legs. Because blood return to the heart is reduced, blood pressure drops. This drop in blood pressure that occurs when a person stands up is called *orthostatic hypotension*.

Pharmacotherapeutics

Because alpha-adrenergic blockers cause smooth muscles to relax and blood vessels to dilate, they increase local blood flow to the skin and other organs and reduce blood pressure. As a result, they are used to treat:

- hypertension
- peripheral vascular disorders (disease of the blood vessels of the extremities), especially those in which spasm of the blood vessels causes poor local blood flow, such as Raynaud's disease (characterized by intermittent pallor, cyanosis, or redness of the fingers), acrocyanosis (characterized by symmetrical mottled cyanosis [bluish color] of the hands and feet), and frostbite
- pheochromocytoma (a catecholamine-secreting tumor causing severe hypertension)
- vascular headaches (treated with ergoloid mesylates, ergotamine)
- benign prostatic hypertrophy (treated with tamsulosin, terazosin, prazosin).

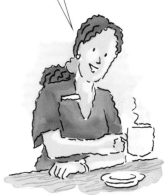

Taking caffeine with ergotamine can increase ergotamine's effects. I'll stick with decaf!

Treatment of PTSD

Patients who experience post-traumatic stress disorder (PTSD) frequently report recurring and persistent nightmares, which negatively impact sleep quality and increase anxiety. Use of the alpha-adrenergic blocker called prazosin has been associated with improving nightmare symptoms (Zhang et al., 2020).

Drug interactions

Many drugs interact with alpha-adrenergic blockers, producing a synergistic or exaggerated effect that may lead to such conditions as severe hypotension or vascular collapse.

Here are some examples of interactions that can occur:

- Prazosin taken with diuretics, propranolol, or other beta-adrenergic blockers results in increased frequency of syncope with loss of consciousness.
- Doxazosin or terazosin taken with clonidine results in decreased clonidine effects.

- Terazosin taken with antihypertensives may cause excessive hypotension.

  These effects are specific to ergoloid mesylates and ergotamine:
- Caffeine and macrolide antibiotics can increase the effects of ergotamine.
- Dopamine increases the pressor (rise in blood pressure) effect.
- Nitroglycerin can produce hypotension due to excessive dilation of blood vessels.
- Adrenergic drugs, including many over-the-counter drugs, can increase the stimulating effects on the heart. Hypotension with rebound hypertension can occur.

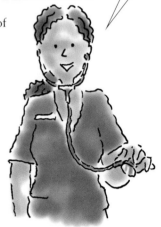

The patient's blood pressure indicates whether fluid volume is adequate.

Side effects/adverse reactions

Most side effects and adverse reactions associated with alpha-adrenergic blockers are caused primarily by dilation of the blood vessels. They include:
- orthostatic hypotension or severe hypertension
- bradycardia or tachycardia
- edema
- difficulty breathing
- light-headedness
- flushing
- arrhythmias
- angina or heart attack
- spasm of the blood vessels in the brain
- a shock-like state.

The Three-Step Approach

Nursing management for patients undergoing treatment with alpha-adrenergic blockers includes these three steps.

Preadministration

(Recognize and analyze cues)
- Assess vital signs, especially blood pressure before, during, and after therapy.
- Analyze the patient's medical history and physical assessment data to determine contraindications or special needs in relation to taking alpha-adrenergic blockers.
- Assess the patient for side effects, adverse reactions, and drug interactions.
- Assess the patient and family or caregiver's knowledge of drug therapy.

(Prioritize hypothesis—priority patient problems)
- Hypotension
- Hypertension

- Altered peripheral tissue perfusion
- Acute pain (vascular headache)
- Knowledge deficiency

(Generate solutions)
- The patient will maintain normal blood pressure.
- The patient will have adequate tissue perfusion as evidenced by adequate circulatory checks and pulses.
- The patient will state that pain is decreased.
- The patient, family, or caregiver will demonstrate understanding of drug therapy and correct drug administration.

Medication administration
(Take action)
- Give drugs at bedtime to minimize dizziness or light-headedness.
- Begin therapy with a small dose to avoid syncope with the first dose.
- Give ergotamine during the prodromal stage of a headache or as soon as possible after onset.
- Avoid giving sublingual tablets with food or drink.
- Provide patient teaching.

Postadministration
(Evaluate outcomes)
- The patient maintains normal blood pressure.
- The patient has adequate tissue perfusion throughout therapy.
- The patient has headache relief.
- The patient and family or caregiver demonstrate understanding of drug therapy and performs correct drug administration. (See *Teaching about alpha-adrenergic blocker*, page 150.)

Beta-adrenergic blockers

Beta-adrenergic blockers, the most widely used adrenergic blockers, prevent stimulation of the sympathetic nervous system by inhibiting the action of catecholamines at beta-adrenergic receptors.

Some are picky, others aren't
Beta-adrenergic blockers are either selective or nonselective. Nonselective beta-adrenergic blockers affect:
- $beta_1$-receptor sites (located mainly in the heart)
- $beta_2$-receptor sites (located in the bronchi, blood vessels, and uterus).

Nonselective beta-adrenergic blocking drugs include carvedilol (has $alpha_1$ blocking activity too), labetalol (has $alpha_1$ blocking activity too), nadolol, pindolol, propranolol, and sotalol.

Teaching about alpha-adrenergic blockers

See Education Edge: Teaching template in Chapter 3, page 38 for general teaching for all medications. Specific points to review with patients and family for alpha-adrenergic blocker therapy:

- Rise slowly when moving from a lying or sitting position.
- Avoid hazardous tasks that require mental alertness until the full effects of the drug are known.
- Keep in mind that alcohol, excessive exercise, prolonged standing, and heat exposure intensify side effects and adverse reactions.

- Report dizziness or irregular heartbeat.
- Avoid eating, drinking, or smoking while the sublingual tablet is dissolving.
- Avoid increasing the drug dosage without first consulting the prescriber.
- Avoid prolonged exposure to cold weather whenever possible. Cold may increase adverse reactions to ergotamine.
- If receiving long-term ergotamine therapy, check for and report coldness in the limbs or tingling in the fingers or toes. Severe vasoconstriction may result in tissue damage.

Selective beta-adrenergic blockers primarily affect just the beta$_1$-adrenergic sites. They include acebutolol, atenolol, betaxolol, bisoprolol, esmolol, and metoprolol tartrate and metoprolol succinate.

Part blocker, part stimulator

Some beta-adrenergic blockers, such as pindolol and acebutolol, also have intrinsic sympathetic activity. This means that instead of attaching to beta receptors and blocking them, these beta-adrenergic blockers attach to beta receptors and stimulate them. These drugs are sometimes classified as *partial agonists*.

Pharmacokinetics

Beta-adrenergic blockers are usually absorbed rapidly from the GI tract. They are protein bound to some extent. Some beta-adrenergic blockers are absorbed more completely than others.

Reach the peak faster: Go IV

The onset of action of beta-adrenergic blockers is primarily dose- and drug-dependent. The time it takes to reach peak concentration levels depends on the route of administration. Beta-adrenergic blockers given IV reach peak levels much more rapidly than when given by mouth.

Beta-adrenergic blockers are distributed widely in body tissues, with the highest concentrations found in the heart, liver, lungs, and saliva.

The liver delivers

Except for nadolol and atenolol, beta-adrenergic blockers are metabolized in the liver. They are excreted primarily in urine, as metabolites or in unchanged form, but can also be excreted in feces and bile, with some secretion in breast milk.

Pharmacodynamics

Beta-adrenergic blockers have widespread effects in the body because they produce their blocking action not only at adrenergic nerve endings but also in the adrenal medulla.

Happenings in the heart

Effects on the heart include increased peripheral vascular resistance, decreased blood pressure, decreased force of heart contractions, decreased oxygen consumption by the heart, slowed conduction of

Pharm function

How beta-adrenergic blockers work

By occupying beta-receptor sites, beta-adrenergic blockers prevent catecholamines (norepinephrine and epinephrine) from occupying these sites and exerting their stimulating effects. This illustration shows the effects of beta-adrenergic blockers on the heart, lungs, and blood vessels.

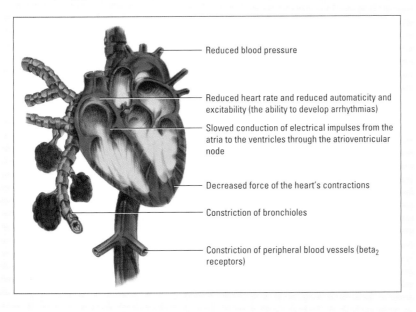

Reduced blood pressure

Reduced heart rate and reduced automaticity and excitability (the ability to develop arrhythmias)

Slowed conduction of electrical impulses from the atria to the ventricles through the atrioventricular node

Decreased force of the heart's contractions

Constriction of bronchioles

Constriction of peripheral blood vessels (beta$_2$ receptors)

impulses between the atria and ventricles of the heart, and decreased cardiac output. (See *How beta-adrenergic blockers work*, page 151.)

Choosy blockers choose beta$_1$ receptors...

Some of the effects of beta-adrenergic blocking drugs depend on whether the drug is classified as selective or nonselective. Selective beta-adrenergic blockers, which preferentially block beta$_1$-receptor sites, reduce stimulation of the heart. They are commonly referred to as *cardioselective beta-adrenergic blockers*.

Nonselective beta-adrenergic blockers, which block both beta$_1$- and beta$_2$-receptor sites, not only reduce stimulation of the heart but also cause the bronchioles of the lungs to constrict. Therefore, nonselective beta-adrenergic blockers can cause bronchospasm in patients with chronic obstructive lung disorders. This adverse effect isn't seen when nonselective beta-adrenergic blockers are given at lower doses.

The most selective beta-adrenergic blockers have the good taste to choose me over you!

Pharmacotherapeutics

Beta-adrenergic blockers are used to treat many conditions and are under investigation for use in many more. As mentioned earlier, their clinical usefulness is based largely (but not exclusively) on how they affect the heart.

Taken to heart

Beta-adrenergic blockers have been found to lower the risk of a heart attack when administered in the acute phase after a heart attack (Safi et al., 2019, December 17). It is also used to treat:
- angina (chest pain)
- hypertension
- hypertrophic cardiomyopathy (a disease of the heart muscle)
- supraventricular arrhythmias (irregular heartbeats that originate in the atria, SA node, or AV node).

Very versatile

Beta-adrenergic blockers are also used to treat:
- anxiety
- cardiovascular symptoms associated with thyrotoxicosis (overproduction of thyroid hormones)
- essential tremor
- migraine headaches
- open-angle glaucoma
- pheochromocytoma.

Drug interactions

Many drugs can interact with beta-adrenergic blockers to cause potentially dangerous effects. Some of the most serious effects include cardiac depression, arrhythmias, respiratory depression, severe bronchospasm, and severe hypotension that can lead to vascular collapse. Here are some others:

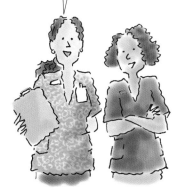

Beta-adrenergic blockers may affect how much antidiabetic drug you need.

- Increased effects or toxicity can occur when digoxin, calcium channel blockers (primarily verapamil), and cimetidine are taken with beta-adrenergic blockers.
- Decreased effects can occur when antacids, calcium salts, barbiturates, anti-inflammatories (such as indomethacin and salicylates), and rifampin are taken with beta-adrenergic blockers.
- The requirements for insulin and oral antidiabetic drugs can be altered when taken with beta-adrenergic blockers.
- Potential lidocaine toxicity can occur when taken with beta-adrenergic blockers.
- The ability of theophylline to produce bronchodilation is impaired by nonselective beta-adrenergic blockers.
- Clonidine taken with a nonselective beta-adrenergic blocker can result in life-threatening hypertension during clonidine withdrawal.
- Sympathomimetics and nonselective beta-adrenergic blockers can cause hypertension and reflex bradycardia.

Side effects/adverse reactions

Beta-adrenergic blockers generally cause few side effects or adverse reactions; however, when they occur, it is dose- and drug-dependent. The side effects and adverse reactions can include:

- hypotension
- bradycardia
- peripheral vascular insufficiency
- AV block
- heart failure
- bronchospasm
- diarrhea or constipation
- nausea
- vomiting
- abdominal discomfort
- anorexia
- flatulence
- rash
- fever with sore throat
- spasm of the larynx
- respiratory distress (allergic response). (See *Preparing for Practice— Beta-adrenergic blockers*, page 154.)

Black Box Warning

Preparing for Practice: Beta-adrenergic Blockers

• Labetalol, nadolol, propranolol, and sotalol have Black Box Warnings against abrupt discontinuation. The drug needs to be discontinued over 2 weeks to avoid life-threatening cardiac symptoms (Skidmore-Roth, 2021, p. 725, 890, 1055, 1163).
• Sotalol has additional Black Box Warnings for congenital or acquired long QT syndromed, increased QT prolongation with several drug interactions, use of specialized care setting so that patient can be closely monitored, and against use in cardiogenic shock and acute pulmonary edema (Skidmore-Roth, 2021, pp. 1162–1163).

The Three-Step Approach

Nursing management for patients undergoing treatment with beta-adrenergic blockers includes these three steps.

Preadministration

(Recognize and analyze cues)
- Assess the patient's condition before therapy and regularly thereafter.
- Assess respiratory status, especially in a patient with chronic obstructive pulmonary disease or asthma, because of the potential risk of bronchospasm.
- Check apical pulse rate daily; alert the prescriber about extremes, such as a pulse rate below 60 beats/minute.
- Monitor blood pressure, ECG, and heart rate and rhythm frequently; be alert for progression of AV block or bradycardia.
- If the patient has heart failure, weigh the patient regularly and watch for weight gain of more than 5 lb (2.3 kg) per week.
- Observe the diabetic patient for sweating, fatigue, and hunger. Signs of hypoglycemia such as tachycardiac and tremors may be masked.
- Be alert for side effects, adverse reactions, and drug interactions.
- Assess the patient's and/or caregiver's knowledge of drug therapy.

(Prioritize hypothesis—priority patient problems)
- Injury risk
- Fluid overload risk
- Altered cardiac output
- Knowledge deficiency

(Generate solutions)
- The patient's chances for injury will be diminished.

- The patient will experience normal fluid volume as shown by adequate urine output and blood pressure.
- The patient will maintain an adequate cardiac output.
- The patient and family or caregiver will demonstrate understanding of drug therapy and correct drug administration.

Medication administration

(Take action)
- Before any surgical procedure, notify the anesthesiologist that the patient is taking a beta-adrenergic blocker.
- Keep glucagon nearby in case it's prescribed to reverse beta-adrenergic blocker overdose.
- Check the apical pulse before giving the drug; if it's slower than 60 beats/minute, withhold the drug and call the provider.
- Give the drug with meals because food may increase absorption.
- For IV use, give the drug undiluted and by direct injection, unless recommended otherwise by a pharmacy.

Postadministration

(Evaluate outcomes)
- The patient remains free from injury.
- The patient maintains normal fluid volume.
- The patient maintains an adequate cardiac output.
- The patient and family or caregiver demonstrates understanding of drug therapy and correct drug administration. (See *Teaching about beta-adrenergic blockers*.)

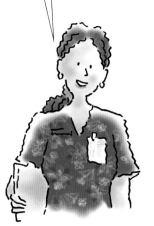

If your patient is undergoing surgery, make sure you tell the anesthesiologist that the patient is taking a beta-adrenergic blocker.

Education edge

Teaching about beta-adrenergic blockers

See Education Edge: Teaching template in Chapter 3, page 38 for general teaching for all medications. Specific points to review with patients and family for beta-adrenergic blocking drug therapy:
- Take the drug exactly as prescribed, even if signs or symptoms are relieved.
- Don't stop the drug suddenly. This can worsen angina or precipitate myocardial infarction and cause tachycardia.
- Take the oral form of the drug with meals to enhance absorption.
- Don't take over-the-counter drugs or herbal remedies without medical consent.
- Avoid performing hazardous activities until CNS effects of the drug are known.

Quick quiz

1. The nurse is caring for a patient taking an anticholinesterase drug for myasthenia gravis. Which finding would the nurse anticipate if the drug is effective?

    A. Reduce peristalsis
    B. Reduced bladder tone
    C. Increased eye pressure
    D. Increased muscle contraction ability

Answer: D. Effects of anticholinesterase drugs include reduction in eye pressure, increased bladder tone, improved peristalsis, and promotion of muscle contraction in patients with myasthenia gravis.

2. A patient is undergoing a surgery that will require general anesthesia. Which drug would the nurse expect to administer to the patient to reduce preoperative secretions?

    A. Atropine
    B. Terazosin
    C. Dopamine
    D. Propranolol

Answer: A. Atropine is commonly prescribed for preoperative reduction of secretions. Dopamine, an adrenergic agonist is used for hypotension while terazosin and propranolol are used for hypertension.

3. A patient is being treated for shock with the adrenergic drug dobutamine. Which assessment finding by the nurse indicates an adverse reaction is occurring?

    A. Diarrhea
    B. Tachycardia
    C. Hallucinations
    D. Decreased glucose levels

Answer: B. Adverse reactions to catecholamines include palpitations, restlessness, anxiety, dizziness, headache, cardiac arrhythmias, hypotension, hypertension and hypertensive crisis, stroke, angina, and increased glucose levels. Hallucinations and diarrhea are not documented side effects or adverse reactions for dobutamine.

4. A patient who is in therapy for PTSD tells the nurse about having recurrent nightmares. Which drug would the nurse anticipate being prescribed as treatment?

    A. Prazosin
    B. Albuterol
    C. Clonidine
    D. Labetalol

Answer: A. Prazosin is commonly prescribed for the treatment of nightmares associated with PTSD. Albuterol (beta$_2$ blocker) treats bronchospasms, clonidine (alpha adrenergic agonist) treats hypertension, and labetalol (alpha$_1$ and beta$_{1\&2}$ blockers) treats hypertension.

5. The nurse is caring for a patient being treated for cardiac dysrhythmia with the beta-blocker, carvedilol (Coreg). What priority action would the nurse take before administering this medication?
   A. Assess blood glucose.
   B. Monitor patient's weight.
   C. Count apical heart rate for 60 seconds.
   D. Teach patient to avoid abruptly discontinuing the drug.

Answer: C. The nurse would assess the apical heart rate. Beta-blockers should not be given if heart rate is less than 60 beats/minute. Teaching the patient to avoid abruptly stopping the medication is important; however, it is not the priority action to take before administering the drug. Monitoring the patient's weight and blood glucose are not priority actions.

Scoring

☆☆☆ If you answered all five questions correctly, super!

☆☆ If you answered four questions correctly, good work! You have no reason to be nervous about working with autonomic nervous system drugs.

☆ If you answered three or fewer questions correctly, assess your trouble spots and plan some time for review.

Suggested References

Bird, S. J. (2020, April 3). Overview of the treatment of myasthenia gravis. In *UpToDate*. Retrieved from https://www.uptodate.com/contents/overview-of-the-treatment-of-myasthenia-gravis?search=drug%20toxicity%20with%20myasthenia%20gravis&source=search_result&selectedTitle=1~150&usage_type=default&display_rank=1

Ghezzi, E., Chan, M., Kalish Elleet, L. M., Ross, T. J., Richardson, K., Ni Ho, J., …Keage, H. A. D. (2021, January 8). The effects of anticholinergic medications on cognition in children: A systematic review and meta-analysis. *Scientific Reports, 11*(1), 1–15. doi: 10.1038/s41598-020-80211-6.

Karch, A. (2020). *Focus on nursing pharmacology* (8th ed.). Philadelphia, PA: Wolters Kluwer.

Lexicomp. (2021a). Atropine (systemic) and pralidoxime: Drug information. In *UpToDate*.

Lexicomp. (2021b). Pyridostigmine: Drug information. In *UpToDate*.

Lilley, L. L., Rainforth Collins, S., & Snyder, J. S. (2020). *Pharmacology and the nursing process* (9th ed.). St. Louis, MO: Elsevier, Inc.

Rubin, M. (2020, December). Myasthenia gravis. In *Merck Manual Professional Version*. Retrieved from https://www.merckmanuals.com/professional/neurologic-disorders/peripheral-nervous-system-and-motor-unit-disorders/myasthenia-gravis?query=anticholinesterase drugs

Safi, S., Sethi, N. J., Nielsen, E., Feinberg, J., Gluud, C., & Jakobsen, J. C. (2019, December 17). Beta-blockers versus placebo or no intervention for patients with suspected or diagnosed myocardial infarction (review). *Cochrane Database of Systematic Reviews*, (12), 1–3. doi: 10.1002/14651858.CD012484. pub2.

Skidmore-Roth, L. (2021). *Mosby's 2021 nursing drug reference*. St. Louis, MO: Elsevier Inc.

Zhang, Y., Ren, R., Sanford, L. D., Yang, L., Ni, Y., Zhou, J., …Tang, X. (2020, March). The effects of prazosin on sleep disturbances in post-traumatic sleep disorder: A systematic review and meta-analysis. *Sleep Medicine, 67*, 225–231. http://dx.doi.org.me.opal-libraries.org/10.1016/j.sleep.2019.06.010

Chapter 7

Neurologic and neuromuscular drugs

Just the facts

In this chapter, you will learn:

♦ classes of drugs used to treat neurologic and neuromuscular disorders

♦ uses and actions of these drugs

♦ absorption, distribution, metabolization, and excretion of these drugs

♦ drug interactions, side effects, and adverse reactions to these drugs.

Drugs and the neurologic and neuromuscular systems

The neurologic, or nervous, system includes the central nervous system (CNS) (brain and spinal cord) and the peripheral nervous system (somatic and autonomic nervous systems). The neuromuscular system consists of the muscles of the body and the nerves that supply them. Several types of drugs are used to treat disorders of these two major systems, including:

• skeletal muscle relaxants
• neuromuscular blocking drugs
• antiparkinsonian drugs
• anticonvulsant drugs
• antimigraine drugs.

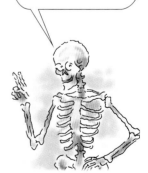

This chapter reviews drugs that are used to treat two major body systems—the neurologic and the neuromuscular.

Skeletal muscle relaxants

Skeletal muscle relaxants relieve musculoskeletal pain or spasms and severe musculoskeletal spasticity (stiff, awkward movements). They're used to treat acute, painful musculoskeletal conditions and muscle spasticity associated with multiple sclerosis (MS), a progressive demyelination of the white matter of the brain and spinal cord that causes widespread neurologic dysfunction; cerebral palsy, a motor function disorder caused by neurologic damage; stroke, the death of brain cells caused by a reduced supply of oxygen to the brain, which can result in neurologic deficits; and spinal cord injuries, which can result in paralysis or death. This section discusses centrally acting, direct-acting, and other skeletal muscle relaxants.

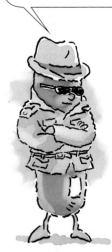

Skeletal muscle relaxants like me can help control your spasticity.

Centrally acting agents

Centrally acting skeletal muscle relaxants are used to treat acute muscle spasms caused by such conditions as anxiety, inflammation, pain, and trauma. They also treat spasticity from such conditions as MS and cerebral palsy.

Examples of these drugs include:
- carisoprodol (Soma)
- chlorzoxazone
- cyclobenzaprine (Amrix)
- metaxalone (Skelaxin)
- methocarbamol (Robaxin)
- orphenadrine (Orphenadrine Citrate, Orphengesic Forte)
- tizanidine hydrochloride (Zanaflex).

Pharmacokinetics

Much is still unknown about how centrally acting skeletal muscle relaxants circulate within the body. In general, these drugs are absorbed from the GI tract, widely distributed in the body, metabolized in the liver, and excreted by the kidneys.

Cyclobenzaprine sticks around

When administered orally, these drugs can take from 30 minutes to 1 hour to be effective. Although the duration of action of most of these drugs varies from 4 to 6 hours, cyclobenzaprine has the longest duration of action at 12 to 25 hours.

I'm an agent of the CAA: Centrally Acting Agency.

Pharmacodynamics

Although their precise mechanism of action is unknown, the centrally acting drugs do not relax skeletal muscles directly or depress neuronal conduction, neuromuscular transmission, or muscle excitability. Rather, centrally acting drugs are known to be CNS depressants. The skeletal muscle relaxant effects that they cause are likely related to their sedative effects.

Pharmacotherapeutics

Patients receive centrally acting skeletal muscle relaxants to treat acute, painful musculoskeletal conditions. They're usually prescribed along with rest, physical therapy or modalities such as chiropractic care, and often intermittent ice or heat application.

Drug interactions

Centrally acting skeletal muscle relaxants interact with other CNS depressants (including alcohol, opioids, barbiturates, anticonvulsants, tricyclic antidepressants, and antianxiety drugs), causing increased sedation, impaired motor function, and respiratory depression. In addition, some of these drugs have other interactions, such as those listed here:

- Cyclobenzaprine interacts with monoamine oxidase (MAO) inhibitors (for example, isocarboxazid, phenelzine, selegiline, and tranylcypromine) and can result in a high body temperature, excitation, and seizures.
- Cyclobenzaprine can decrease the antihypertensive effects of the blood pressure–lowering drug clonidine.
- Orphenadrine and cyclobenzaprine sometimes enhance the effects of cholinergic blocking drugs.
- Orphenadrine can reduce the antipsychotic effects of phenothiazines.

Add it up!

- Methocarbamol can antagonize the cholinergic effects of the anticholinesterase drugs used to treat myasthenia gravis.
- Tizanidine combined with diuretics, central alpha-adrenergic agonists, or antihypertensives may increase hypotensive drug effects.
- Concurrent use of tizanidine with other CNS depressants may cause additive CNS depression.
- Hormonal contraceptive agents may reduce the clearance of tizanidine, necessitating a dose reduction.

Side effects/Adverse reactions

Long-term use of centrally acting muscle relaxants can result in physical and psychological dependence. Abrupt cessation of these drugs can cause severe withdrawal symptoms.

Adverse reactions can also occur when a patient is taking these drugs. Common reactions include dizziness and drowsiness. Severe reactions include allergic reactions, arrhythmias, and bradycardia. Less common reactions include abdominal distress, ataxia, constipation, diarrhea, heartburn, nausea, and vomiting. Extreme caution needs to be used when considering use of centrally acting muscle relaxants in geriatric patients. When compared to patients who did not take these medications, the risk of emergency department visits following a fall or fracture has been shown to increase by 2.25 times in geriatric patients, with subsequent increased likeliness of hospitalization (Trueman et al., 2020).

The Three-Step Approach

Nursing management for patients needing centrally acting skeletal muscle relaxants includes these three steps:

Preadministration

(Recognize and analyze cues)

- Obtain an initial history of the patient's pain and/or muscle spasms and reassess regularly thereafter.
- Evaluate the patient's and family's understanding of the intended purpose of this drug therapy and their expectations of results.

(Prioritize hypothesis—priority patient problems)

- Safety
- Fall risk
- Impaired comfort
- Knowledge deficiency

(Generate solutions)

- The patient's safety will be maintained.
    - The patient's risk for falls will be minimized.
    - The patient will acknowledge and exhibit decreased discomfort after administration of medication.
    - The patient and family will verbalize an understanding of the medication's purpose and intended effect.

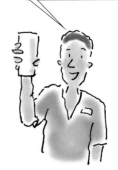

Give oral forms of centrally acting agents with meals or milk to prevent GI distress. Bottoms up!

Medication administration

(Take action)

- Institute safety precautions as needed.
- Give oral forms of these drugs with meals or milk to prevent GI distress.
- Obtain an order for mild analgesics to relieve drug-induced headache.
- Avoid abrupt discontinuation to reduce risk of experiencing withdrawal symptoms, such as returning or worsening spasticity, hypotension, paresthesia, and muscle rigidity.
- After long-term therapy (unless the patient has severe adverse reactions), avoid stopping carisoprodol abruptly to prevent withdrawal symptoms, such as insomnia, headache, nausea, and abdominal pain.

Postadministration

(Evaluate outcomes)

- Observe for injury, including falls, because of drug-induced drowsiness.
- Evaluate pain and muscle spasms following administration of medication.

- Monitor ongoing adherence to therapy regimen.
- Evaluate the patient's and family's understanding of drug therapy. (See *Teaching about skeletal muscle relaxants*.)
- Monitor for hypersensitivity reactions.
- Assess the degree of relief obtained to help the prescriber determine when the dosage can be reduced.
- Closely monitor complete blood count (CBC) results.
- In a patient receiving cyclobenzaprine, monitor platelet counts (thrombocytopenia can occur).

That fainting feeling

- Monitor vital signs, especially for orthostatic hypotension in a patient receiving methocarbamol.
- In a patient receiving long-term chlorzoxazone therapy, monitor hepatic function and urinalysis results.
- Assess compliance of a patient receiving long-term therapy with any of these agents.
- Promote measures to relieve discomfort.

Education edge

Teaching about skeletal muscle relaxants

If skeletal muscle relaxants are prescribed, review these points with the patient and caregivers:

- Take the drug exactly as prescribed. Don't stop baclofen or carisoprodol suddenly after long-term therapy to avoid withdrawal symptoms.
- Avoid hazardous activities that require mental alertness until the CNS effects of the drug are known. Drowsiness is usually transient.
- Avoid alcohol or other depressants during therapy.
- Follow the prescriber's advice regarding rest and physical therapy.
- Try to spread out activities throughout the day and allow rest periods to avoid fatigue, weakness, and drowsiness. If adverse effects become too severe, consult with the prescriber.
- Change positions slowly to help avoid dizzy spells. If dizziness occurs, avoid driving, operating dangerous machinery, or performing delicate tasks.
- Take the drug with food or milk to prevent GI distress.
- Report urinary hesitancy with cyclobenzaprine or baclofen therapy.
- Be aware that urine may be discolored when taking methocarbamol or chlorzoxazone.
- Make sure you keep regular medical follow-up appointments to evaluate the effects of this drug.

Direct-acting agents

Dantrolene sodium (Dantrium, Revonto, Ryanodex) is the only direct-acting skeletal muscle relaxant. Although dantrolene has therapeutic effects similar to those of the centrally acting drugs, it works through a different mechanism of action.

Head case

Dantrolene is most effective for spasticity of cerebral origin. Because the drug produces muscle weakness, the benefits of dantrolene administration in a patient with borderline strength are questionable.

Pharmacokinetics

Although the peak drug concentration of dantrolene occurs within about 5 hours of ingestion, the patient may not notice any therapeutic benefit for a week or more (given regular use). Dantrolene is absorbed slowly and incompletely (but consistently) from the GI tract and is highly plasma protein bound. This means that only a small portion of the drug is available to produce a therapeutic effect.

Hiking up the half-life

Dantrolene is metabolized by the liver and excreted in urine. Its elimination half-life in a healthy adult is about 9 hours. Because dantrolene is metabolized in the liver, its half-life can be prolonged in a patient with impaired liver function.

Pharmacodynamics

Dantrolene is chemically and pharmacologically unrelated to other skeletal muscle relaxants. It acts directly on muscle to interfere with calcium ion release from the sarcoplasmic reticulum and weaken the force of contractions. At therapeutic concentrations, dantrolene has little effect on cardiac or intestinal smooth muscle.

Pharmacotherapeutics

Dantrolene can be used to help manage several types of spasticity but is most effective in patients with:
- cerebral palsy
- multiple sclerosis (MS)
- spinal cord injury
- stroke.

Anesthesia antidote

Dantrolene is also used to treat and prevent malignant hyperthermia. This rare but potentially fatal complication of anesthesia is characterized by skeletal muscle rigidity and high fever. (See *How dantrolene reduces muscle rigidity*, page 165.)

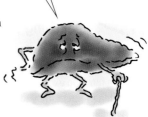

Dantrolene has a half-life of about 9 hours in a healthy adult, but impaired liver function can prolong that half-life. I think I'll need a little extra time to metabolize…

Pharm function

How dantrolene reduces muscle rigidity

Dantrolene appears to decrease the number of calcium ions released from the sarcoplasmic reticulum (a structure in muscle cells that controls muscle contraction and relaxation by releasing and storing calcium). The lower the calcium level in the muscle plasma or myoplasm, the less energy produced when calcium prompts interaction of the muscle's actin and myosin filaments (responsible for muscle contraction). Less energy means a weaker muscle contraction.

Reducing rigidity, halting hyperthermia
By promoting muscle relaxation, dantrolene prevents or reduces the rigidity that contributes to the life-threatening body temperatures of malignant hyperthermia.

Drug interactions

CNS depressants can increase the depressive effects of dantrolene and result in sedation, lack of coordination, and respiratory depression. In addition, dantrolene may have other drug interactions:

- Estrogens, when given with dantrolene, can increase the risk of liver toxicity.
- IV verapamil shouldn't be administered if giving dantrolene because it may result in arrhythmias and cardiovascular collapse.
- Alcohol may increase CNS depression when used with dantrolene.

Side effects/Adverse reactions

Because its major effect is on the muscles, dantrolene has a lower incidence of adverse CNS reactions than other skeletal muscle relaxants. However, high therapeutic doses are toxic to the liver. Common adverse effects of dantrolene include drowsiness, dizziness, malaise, and muscle weakness. More serious adverse effects include bleeding, seizures, and hepatitis.

The Three-Step Approach

Nursing management for patients needing dantrolene includes these three steps:

Preadministration

(Recognize and analyze cues)
- Obtain a history of the patient's pain and muscle spasms before therapy.

(Prioritize hypothesis—priority patient problems)
- Injury risk

- Impaired comfort
- Knowledge deficiency

(Generate solutions)
- The patient's injury risk will be minimized.
- The patient will acknowledge and demonstrate increased comfort after administration of medication.
- The patient and family will verbalize an understanding of the medication's purpose and intended effect. (See *Teaching about skeletal muscle relaxants*, page 163.)
- The patient will adhere to pharmacological therapy regimen.

Medication administration
(Take action)
- Institute safety precautions as needed.
- If hepatitis, severe diarrhea, severe weakness, or sensitivity reactions occur, withhold the dose and notify the prescriber.
- Give the oral form of the drug with meals or milk to prevent GI distress.
- Obtain an order for a mild analgesic to relieve drug-induced headache.
- Avoid abrupt discontinuation to prevent the return of symptoms, such as spasticity, paresthesia, and muscle rigidity.
- Assess for immediate adverse reactions and drug interactions.

Postadministration
(Evaluate outcomes)
- Monitor the patient for hypersensitivity reactions.
- Assess the degree of relief obtained to help the prescriber determine when the dosage can be reduced.
- Monitor lab results, including CBC and liver function tests.
- Assess adherence to treatment regimen, especially in patients receiving long-term therapy.
- Evaluate the patient's and family's understanding of drug therapy.

Other skeletal muscle relaxants

Two additional drugs used as skeletal muscle relaxants are diazepam (Diastat, Valium) and baclofen (Lioresal). Because diazepam is primarily used as an antianxiety drug, this section discusses only baclofen. (See *Diazepam as a skeletal muscle relaxant*, page 167.)

Diazepam as a skeletal muscle relaxant

Diazepam is a benzodiazepine drug that is used to treat acute muscle spasms as well as spasticity caused by chronic disorders. It seems to work by promoting the inhibitory effect of the neurotransmitter gamma-aminobutyric acid (GABA) on muscle contraction. Other uses of diazepam include treating anxiety, alcohol withdrawal, and seizures.

The negatives: Sedation and tolerance

Diazepam can be used alone or in conjunction with other drugs to treat spasticity, especially in patients with spinal cord lesions and, occasionally, in patients with cerebral palsy. It's also helpful in patients with painful, continuous muscle spasms who aren't too susceptible to the drug's sedative effects. Unfortunately, the use of diazepam is limited by the CNS effects and the tolerance that develops with prolonged use.

Pharmacokinetics

Baclofen is absorbed rapidly from the GI tract. It's distributed widely (with only small amounts crossing the blood-brain barrier), undergoes minimal liver metabolism, and is excreted primarily unchanged in urine.

A long wait

It can take hours to weeks before the patient notices the beneficial effects of baclofen. The elimination half-life of baclofen is $2\frac{1}{2}$ to 4 hours.

Pharmacodynamics

It isn't known exactly how baclofen works. Chemically similar to the neurotransmitter GABA, baclofen probably acts in the spinal cord. It reduces nerve impulses from the spinal cord to skeletal muscle, decreasing the number and severity of muscle spasms and the associated pain.

A choice drug

Because baclofen produces less sedation than diazepam and less peripheral muscle weakness than dantrolene, it's the drug of choice to treat spasticity.

Pharmacotherapeutics

Baclofen's major clinical use is for paraplegic or quadriplegic patients with spinal cord lesions, most commonly caused by MS or trauma. For these patients, baclofen significantly reduces the number and severity of painful flexor spasms. Unfortunately, however, baclofen doesn't improve stiff gait, manual dexterity, or residual muscle function.

Baclofen can be administered intrathecally for patients who are unresponsive to oral baclofen or who experience intolerable adverse effects. After a positive response to a bolus dose, an implantable port for chronic therapy can be placed. Extreme caution should be taken to avoid abrupt discontinuation of intrathecal baclofen.

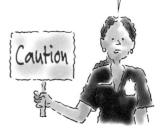

Avoid abrupt discontinuation of intrathecal baclofen treatment.

No abrupt endings

Abrupt withdrawal of intrathecal baclofen has resulted in high fever, altered mental status, exaggerated rebound spasticity, and muscle rigidity that, in rare cases, has progressed to rhabdomyolysis, multiple organ system failure, and death. (See *Skeletal muscle relaxants: Baclofen.*)

Prototype pro

Skeletal muscle relaxants: Baclofen

Actions
- Unknown
- Appears to reduce the transmission of impulses from the spinal cord to skeletal muscle
- Relieves muscle spasms

Indications
- Spasticity in MS and spinal cord injury
- Management of severe spasticity in the patient who doesn't respond to or can't tolerate oral baclofen therapy (intrathecal baclofen)

Nursing considerations
- Give oral baclofen with meals or milk to prevent GI distress.
- Avoid abrupt discontinuation of intrathecal baclofen because this can result in high fever, altered mental status, exaggerated rebound spasticity, and muscle rigidity that, in rare cases, may progress to rhabdomyolysis, multiple organ system failure, and death.
- If intrathecal baclofen is delayed, treatment with a GABA agonist or IV benzodiazepines may prevent potentially fatal sequelae.

Drug interactions

Baclofen has few drug interactions:

- The most significant drug interaction is an increase in CNS depression when baclofen is administered with other CNS depressants, including alcohol.
- Analgesia can be prolonged when fentanyl and baclofen are administered together.
- Lithium carbonate (Lithobid) and baclofen taken together can aggravate hyperkinesia (an abnormal increase in motor function or activity).
- Tricyclic antidepressants and baclofen taken together can increase muscle relaxation.

Side effects/Adverse reactions

The most common adverse reaction to baclofen is transient drowsiness. Some less common effects include nausea, fatigue, vertigo, hypotonia, muscle weakness, depression, and headache.

The Three-Step Approach

The nursing management for patients who are prescribed the skeletal muscle relaxant baclofen includes these three steps:

Preadministration

(Recognize and analyze cues)

- Obtain a history of the patient's pain and muscle spasms before administration of therapy.

(Prioritize hypothesis—priority patient problems)

- Injury risk
- Acute pain
- Knowledge deficiency

(Generate solutions)

- The patient's injury risk will be minimized.
- The patient will acknowledge and demonstrate decreased pain after administration of the medication
- The patient and family will verbalize an understanding of the medication's purpose and intended effect.

Medication administration

(Take action)

- Institute safety precautions as needed.
- Watch for an increased risk of seizures in the patient with a seizure disorder. Seizures have been reported during overdose and withdrawal of intrathecal baclofen as well as in patients maintained on therapeutic doses. Monitor the patient carefully and institute seizure precautions.
- Give the oral forms of the drug with meals or milk to prevent GI distress.

Warning! Wrong way

- Don't administer an intrathecal injection by the IV, IM, subcutaneous, or epidural route.
- Avoid an abrupt discontinuation of intrathecal baclofen. Early symptoms of baclofen withdrawal include return of baseline spasticity, pruritus, hypotension, and paresthesia. Symptoms that have occurred include high fever, altered mental status, exaggerated rebound spasticity, and muscle rigidity that—in rare cases—has advanced to rhabdomyolysis, multiple organ system failure, and death.
- Assess for immediate adverse reactions to drug administration.

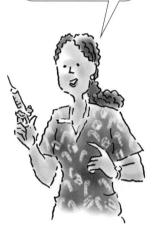

Make sure you don't administer intrathecal baclofen by the IV, IM, subcutaneous, or epidural route.

Postadministration

(Evaluate outcomes)

- Monitor for injury, including falls, following drug administration (primarily related to drug-induced drowsiness).
- Evaluate status of muscle spasms.
- Monitor the patient for hypersensitivity reactions.
- Assess the degree of pain relief obtained; communicate with the prescriber in order to properly adjust dosage.
- Monitor pertinent labs, including CBC.
- Assess adherence to treatment regimen, especially in patients receiving long-term therapy.
- Evaluate the patient's and family's ongoing understanding of the goals and benefits of drug therapy. (See *Teaching about skeletal muscle relaxants*, page 163.)

Neuromuscular blocking drugs

Neuromuscular blocking drugs relax skeletal muscles by disrupting the transmission of nerve impulses at the motor end plate (the branching terminals of a motor nerve axon). (See *How neuromuscular blocking drugs work*, page 171.)

Relax, reduce, and manage

Neuromuscular blockers have three major clinical indications:

- to relax skeletal muscles during surgery
- to reduce the intensity of muscle spasms in drug-induced or electrically induced seizures
- to manage patients who are fighting the use of a ventilator to help with breathing.

Pharm function

How neuromuscular blocking drugs work

The motor nerve axon divides to form branching terminals called *motor end plates*. These are enfolded in muscle fibers but separated from the fibers by the synaptic cleft.

Competing with contraction

A stimulus to the nerve causes the release of acetylcholine into the synaptic cleft. There, acetylcholine occupies receptor sites on the muscle cell membrane, depolarizing the membrane and causing muscle contraction. Neuromuscular blocking agents act at the motor end plate by competing with acetylcholine for the receptor sites or by blocking depolarization.

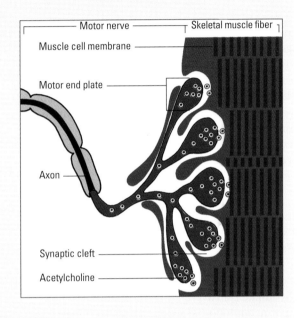

Polar opposites

There are two main classes of natural and synthetic drugs used as neuromuscular blockers—nondepolarizing and depolarizing.

Nondepolarizing blocking drugs

Nondepolarizing blocking drugs, also called *competitive* or *stabilizing* drugs, are derived from curare alkaloids and synthetically similar compounds. They include:

- atracurium besylate
- cisatracurium besylate
- pancuronium bromide
- rocuronium bromide
- vecuronium bromide.

Pharmacokinetics

Because nondepolarizing blockers are poorly absorbed from the GI tract, they're administered parenterally. The IV route is preferred because the action is more predictable.

Fast movers

Nondepolarizing blockers are distributed rapidly throughout the body. Some drugs, such as pancuronium, rocuronium, and vecuronium, are partially metabolized in the liver. After IV administration, atracurium undergoes rapid metabolism by a physiologic process known as *Hofmann elimination* and by enzymatic hydrolysis; it's also partially metabolized in the liver. Mivacurium is hydrolyzed by plasma pseudocholinesterase.

These drugs are excreted primarily in urine, and some, such as cisatracurium and vecuronium, are also excreted in feces.

Pharmacodynamics

Nondepolarizing blockers compete with acetylcholine at the cholinergic receptor sites of the skeletal muscle membrane. This blocks acetylcholine's neurotransmitter action, preventing the muscle from contracting.

The effect can be counteracted by anticholinesterase drugs, such as neostigmine methylsulfate (Bloxiverz) or pyridostigmine bromide (Mestinon, Regonol), which inhibit the action of acetylcholinesterase, the enzyme that destroys acetylcholine.

Paralysis pattern

The initial muscle weakness produced by these drugs quickly changes to a flaccid (loss of muscle tone) paralysis that affects the muscles in a specific sequence. The first muscles to exhibit flaccid paralysis are those of the eyes, face, and neck. Next, the limb, abdomen, and trunk muscles become flaccid. Finally, the intercostal muscles (between the ribs) and diaphragm (the breathing muscle) are paralyzed. Recovery from the paralysis usually occurs in the reverse order.

Conscious—and anxious

Because these drugs don't cross the blood-brain barrier, the patient remains conscious and able to feel pain. Although the patient is paralyzed, they are aware of what is happening and can experience extreme anxiety. However, they can't communicate their feelings. For this reason, an analgesic or antianxiety drug should be administered along with a neuromuscular blocker.

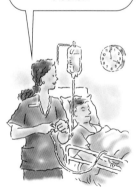

Remember, an anti-anxiety medication should be administered with a neuromuscular blocker.

Pharmacotherapeutics

Nondepolarizing blockers are used for intermediate or prolonged muscle relaxation to:

- ease the passage of an endotracheal (ET) tube (a tube placed in the trachea)
- decrease the amount of anesthetic required during surgery
- facilitate realigning broken bones and dislocated joints
- paralyze the patient who needs ventilatory support but who resists the ET tube and mechanical ventilation due to agitation and restlessness
- prevent muscle injury during electroconvulsive therapy (ECT) (passage of an electric current through the brain to treat depression) by reducing the intensity of muscle spasms.

Drug interactions

Several drugs alter the effects of nondepolarizing neuromuscular blockers:

- Aminoglycoside antibiotics and anesthetics potentiate or exaggerate the neuromuscular blockade.

That's so intense…

- Drugs that alter serum levels of the electrolytes calcium, magnesium, and potassium also alter the effects of nondepolarizing blockers.
- Anticholinesterases (neostigmine methylsulfate, pyridostigmine bromide) antagonize nondepolarizing blockers are used as antidotes.
- Drugs that can increase the intensity and duration of paralysis when taken with a nondepolarizing blocking drug include inhalation anesthetics, aminoglycosides, clindamycin, polymyxin, verapamil, quinine derivatives, ketamine, lithium, nitrates, thiazide diuretics, tetracyclines, and magnesium salts.
- Drugs that can cause decreased neuromuscular blockade when taken with a nondepolarizing blocking drug include carbamazepine (Tegretol), hydantoin anticonvulsant (for example, phenytoin sodium or Dilantin, Fosphenytoin sodium or Cerebyx), ranitidine (Zantac), and theophylline. Concurrent corticosteroid use may result in prolonged muscle weakness.

Side effects/Adverse reactions

A patient taking nondepolarizing drugs may experience these adverse reactions:

- apnea
- hypotension
- skin reactions
- bronchospasm
- excessive bronchial and salivary secretions.

A patient taking pancuronium may also experience tachycardia, cardiac arrhythmias, and hypertension.

Additional short-term or long-term complications of using neuromuscular blocking agents in the inpatient setting include extended ICU stay, need for prolonged mechanical ventilatory support, increased risk of venous thromboembolism, integumentary changes (skin tears and ulcerations), infection, decreased mobility leading to muscle weakness, and resultant increased recovery time (Gustafson & Brown, 2017).

The Three-Step Approach

Nursing management of patients requiring treatment with nondepolarizing muscle relaxants includes these three steps:

Preadministration

(Recognize and analyze cues)
- Assess the patient's neuromuscular condition before administration of therapy.

(Prioritize hypothesis—priority patient problems)
- Altered health maintenance
- Altered breathing pattern
- Knowledge deficiency

(Generate solutions)
- The patient's vital signs will remain within normal parameters while on drug therapy.
- The patient will maintain respiratory function as evidenced by adequate arterial blood gas (ABG) values and ventilatory parameters.
- The patient and family will verbalize an understanding of the medication's purpose and intended effect.

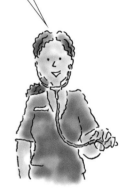

The patient's vital signs should remain normal while on drug therapy.

Medication administration

(Take action)
- Administer sedatives or general anesthetics before neuromuscular blockers. Neuromuscular blockers don't reduce consciousness or alter the pain threshold. Give analgesics for pain. Note that general anesthetics should be administered only by qualified personnel, such as nurse-anesthetists or anesthesiologists.
- Keep in mind that neuromuscular blockers should be used only by personnel skilled in airway management.
- Mix the drug only with fresh solutions; precipitates form if alkaline solutions, such as barbiturate solutions, are used. Vecuronium may be given by rapid IV injection or diluted to be titrated in a drip form. Store reconstituted solutions in the refrigerator.

- Allow succinylcholine (depolarizing blocking) effects to subside before giving pancuronium.
- Store the drug in a refrigerator. Don't store the drug in plastic containers or syringes, although plastic syringes may be used for administration.
- Have emergency respiratory support equipment (ET equipment, ventilator, oxygen, atropine, edrophonium, epinephrine, and neostigmine) immediately available.
- Provide skin care and turning to prevent skin breakdown.
- Provide eye care, such as administering lubricating eyedrops and patching and taping eyelids, during neuromuscular blockade.
- When spontaneous recovery starts, drug-induced neuromuscular blockade may be reversed with an anticholinesterase (such as neostigmine or edrophonium), usually given with an anticholinergic such as atropine.
- Monitor the patient's baseline electrolyte levels (electrolyte imbalance can increase neuromuscular effects) and vital signs.
- Measure the patient's fluid intake and output; renal dysfunction may prolong the duration of action because 25% of the drug is unchanged before excretion.
- As ordered, provide nerve stimulator and train-of-four monitoring (a procedure in which electrodes are applied to the skin and electrical stimulation is delivered to measure the degree of neuromuscular blockade) to confirm the antagonism of neuromuscular blockade and recovery of muscle strength. Before attempting pharmacologic reversal with neostigmine, you should see some evidence of spontaneous recovery.

Postadministration

(Evaluate outcomes)
- Observe the patient for improvement in condition.
- Monitor the patient's respirations closely until there is full recovery from the neuromuscular blockade, and maintain mechanical ventilation assistance.
- Assess the patient's skin per facility protocol for pressure areas and breakdown.
- Assess for incomplete closure of the eyelids (neuromuscular blockade results in loss of corneal reflex and blocks the action of eye muscles).
- Assess for immediate adverse reactions and drug interactions.
- Evaluate the patient's and family's understanding of drug therapy. (See *Teaching about neuromuscular blocking drugs*, page 176.)

Teaching about neuromuscular blocking drugs

If neuromuscular blocking drugs are prescribed, make sure to tell the patient what you're going to do before administering care. Review these points with the patient and caregivers:

• The drug causes complete paralysis; therefore, expect to be unable to move or speak while receiving the drug. This experience can be very frightening.

• Expect to be unable to breathe (assistance will be provided).

• Expect to be aware of what's going on. The drug doesn't affect level of consciousness.

A reassuring word

The patient will be able to see, hear, and feel and will be aware of their surroundings. Make sure to explain all events and reassure the patient and family.

• Tell the patient that someone will be with them at all times to try to anticipate their needs and explain what's going on.

• Assure the patient that they will be monitored at all times.

• Tell the patient that pain and antianxiety medication will be provided, if appropriate.

• Tell the patient that eyedrops will be administered or their eyes may be covered to prevent drying of the corneas.

Depolarizing blocking drugs

Succinylcholine chloride (Anectine) is the only therapeutic depolarizing blocking drug. Although it's like the nondepolarizing blockers in its therapeutic effect, its mechanism of action differs. Succinylcholine acts like acetylcholine, but it isn't inactivated by cholinesterase. It's the drug of choice when short-term muscle relaxation is needed.

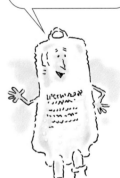

Because succinylcholine is absorbed poorly from the GI tract, the IV route is used most often.

Pharmacokinetics

Because succinylcholine is absorbed poorly from the GI tract, the IV route is the preferred administration method; the IM route can also be used if necessary.

Succinylcholine is hydrolyzed in the liver and plasma by the enzyme pseudocholinesterase, producing a metabolite with a nondepolarizing blocking action. It's excreted by the kidneys; a small amount is excreted unchanged.

Pharmacodynamics

After administration, succinylcholine is rapidly metabolized, although at a slower rate than acetylcholine. As a result, succinylcholine remains attached to receptor sites on the skeletal muscle membrane for a longer period. This prevents repolarization of the motor end plate and results in muscle paralysis.

Pharmacotherapeutics

Succinylcholine is the drug of choice for short-term muscle relaxation such as that needed during intubation and ECT.

Drug interactions

The action of succinylcholine is potentiated by several anesthetics and antibiotics. In contrast to their interaction with nondepolarizing blockers, anticholinesterases increase succinylcholine blockade.

Side effects/Adverse reactions

The primary adverse reactions to succinylcholine are hypotension and prolonged apnea.

Genetics: Raising the risk

The risk associated with succinylcholine is increased with certain genetic predispositions, such as a low pseudocholinesterase level and the tendency to develop malignant hyperthermia.

The Three-Step Approach

Nursing management for patients receiving treatment with succinylcholine includes the following three steps:

Preadministration

(Recognize and analyze cues)
- Assess the patient's baseline condition before initiating therapy.

(Prioritize hypothesis—priority patient problems)
- Altered health maintenance
- Altered breathing pattern
- Knowledge deficiency

(Generate solutions)
- The patient's vital signs will remain within normal parameters while they are on drug therapy.
- The patient will maintain respiratory function as evidenced by adequate ABG values and ventilatory parameters.
- The patient and family will verbalize an understanding of the medication's purpose and intended effect.

Medication administration

(Take action)
- Succinylcholine is the drug of choice for short procedures (less than 3 minutes) and for orthopedic manipulations; use caution in the treatment of fractures or dislocations.
- Administer sedatives or general anesthetics before neuromuscular blockers. Neuromuscular blockers don't reduce consciousness or alter pain threshold. Give analgesics for pain. Note that

general anesthesia and succinylcholine should be administered only by personnel skilled in airway management, such as nurse-anesthetists and anesthesiologists.

- Allow succinylcholine effects to subside before giving pancuronium.
- Have emergency respiratory support equipment (ET equipment, ventilator, oxygen, atropine, epinephrine) available for immediate use.
- For IV use, to evaluate the patient's ability to metabolize succinylcholine, give a test dose after they have been anesthetized. A normal response (no respiratory depression or transient depression for up to 5 minutes) indicates that the drug may be given. Don't give subsequent doses if the patient develops respiratory paralysis sufficient to permit ET intubation.
- For IM use, give deep IM, preferably high into the deltoid.

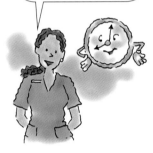

Succinylcholine is the drug of choice for short procedures— less than 3 minutes.

The storage situation

- Store the injectable form in a refrigerator. Store the powder form at room temperature in a tightly closed container and use it immediately after reconstitution. Don't mix with alkaline solutions (thiopental sodium, sodium bicarbonate, or barbiturates).
- Reversing drugs shouldn't be used. Unlike what happens with nondepolarizing drugs, giving neostigmine or edrophonium with succinylcholine may worsen neuromuscular blockade.
- Continuous infusions of succinylcholine are not advised; this may reduce response or prolong muscle relaxation and apnea.

Postadministration

(Evaluate outcomes)

- Assess for improvement in patient's condition.
- Monitor the patient's ventilatory status, while maintaining mechanical assistance as needed.
- Monitor the patient's baseline electrolyte determinations (electrolyte imbalance can increase neuromuscular effects) and vital signs.
- Measure the patient's fluid intake and output; renal dysfunction may prolong the duration of action because 10% of the drug is unchanged before excretion.
- As ordered, provide nerve stimulator and train-of-four monitoring to confirm the antagonism of the neuromuscular blockade and recovery of muscle strength.

Testing, testing...

- Monitor the patient's respirations closely until the patient fully recovers from the neuromuscular blockade, as evidenced by tests of muscle strength (handgrip, head lift, and ability to cough).
- Be alert for adverse reactions and drug interactions.
- Evaluate the patient's and family's knowledge of drug therapy. (See *Teaching about neuromuscular blocking drugs*, page 176.)

Antiparkinsonian drugs

Drug therapy is an important part of the treatment of Parkinson's disease, a progressive neurologic disorder characterized by four cardinal features:
- muscle rigidity (inflexibility)
- akinesia (loss of voluntary muscle movement)
- tremors at rest
- disturbances of posture and balance.

Upsetting the balance

Reduction of dopamine in the corpus striatum disturbs the normal balance between two neurotransmitters, acetylcholine and dopamine. When nerve cells in the brain become impaired, they can no longer produce dopamine. This results in a relative excess of acetylcholine. The excessive excitation caused by cholinergic activity creates the movement disorders of Parkinson's disease.

Defect in the dopamine pathway

Parkinson's disease affects the extrapyramidal system, which influences movement. The extrapyramidal system includes the corpus striatum, globus pallidus, and substantia nigra of the brain. In Parkinson's disease, dopamine deficiency occurs in the basal ganglia, the dopamine-releasing pathway that connects the substantia nigra to the corpus striatum.

Other culprits

Parkinsonism can also result from drugs, encephalitis, neurotoxins, trauma, arteriosclerosis, or other neurologic disorders and environmental factors.

Bringing back balance

The goal of drug therapy is to provide symptom relief and maintain the patient's independence and mobility. This can be achieved by correcting the imbalance of neurotransmitters in one of several ways, including:
- inhibiting cholinergic effects (with anticholinergic drugs)
- enhancing the effects of dopamine (with dopaminergic drugs)
- inhibiting catechol-O-methyltransferase (COMT) with COMT-inhibiting drugs.

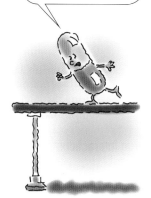

Drug therapy to correct the imbalance of neurotransmitters in patients with Parkinson's disease can help maintain mobility.

Anticholinergic drugs

Anticholinergic drugs are sometimes called *parasympatholytic drugs* because they inhibit the action of acetylcholine at special receptors in the parasympathetic nervous system. Anticholinergics used to treat Parkinson's disease include synthetic tertiary amines, such as benztropine mesylate (Cogentin) and trihexyphenidyl hydrochloride.

Pharmacokinetics

Typically, anticholinergic drugs are well absorbed from the GI tract and cross the blood-brain barrier to their action site in the brain. Most are metabolized in the liver, at least partially, and are excreted by the kidneys as metabolites or unchanged drug. The exact distribution of these drugs is unknown.

Benztropine is a long-acting drug with a duration of action of up to 24 hours in some patients. For most anticholinergics, half-life is undetermined.

Pharmacodynamics

High acetylcholine levels produce an excitatory effect on the CNS, which can cause parkinsonian tremors. Patients with Parkinson's disease take anticholinergic drugs to inhibit the action of acetylcholine at receptor sites in the central and autonomic nervous systems, thus reducing tremors.

Pharmacotherapeutics

Anticholinergics are used to treat all forms of parkinsonism. They're most commonly used in the early stages of Parkinson's disease, when symptoms are mild and don't have a major impact on the patient's lifestyle.

Playing the percentages

These drugs effectively control sialorrhea (excessive flow of saliva) and are about 20% effective in reducing the incidence and severity of akinesia and rigidity.

Anticholinergics can be used alone or with amantadine hydrochloride (Gocovri, Osmolex ER) in the early stages of Parkinson's disease. Anticholinergics can be given with levodopa during the later stages of Parkinson's disease to further relieve symptoms.

Drug interactions

Interactions can occur when certain medications are taken with anticholinergics:

- Amantadine can cause increased anticholinergic adverse effects.

- The absorption of levodopa can be decreased, which can lead to worsening of parkinsonian signs and symptoms.
- Antipsychotics (such as phenothiazines, thiothixene, haloperidol [Haloperidol Decanoate, Haldol], and loxapine [Loxapine Succinate, Adasuve]) and anticholinergics taken together decrease the effectiveness of both drugs. The incidence of anticholinergic adverse effects can also increase.
- Over-the-counter cough and cold preparations, diet aids, and analeptics (drugs used to stay awake) increase anticholinergic effects.
- Alcohol increases CNS depression.

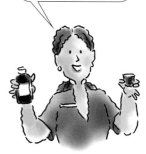

Over-the-counter cough and cold preparations, diet aids, and analeptics—which, unfortunately, include caffeine—increase anticholinergic effects.

Side effects/Adverse reactions

Mild, dose-related adverse reactions to anticholinergics are seen in 30% to 50% of patients. Dry mouth may be a dose-related reaction to trihexyphenidyl. While older adults tend to experience significant cognitive and other adverse events associated with anticholinergic drugs, a higher anticholinergic burden is associated with cognitive impairment and freezing of gait (FOG) even in younger patients with PD (Rajan et al., 2020).

Cataloging common concerns

Some common adverse reactions to anticholinergic drugs include:
- confusion
- restlessness
- agitation and excitement
- drowsiness or insomnia
- tachycardia
- palpitations
- constipation
- nausea and vomiting
- urine retention
- increased intraocular pressure (IOP), blurred vision, pupil dilation, and photophobia.
  Sensitivity-related reactions to anticholinergics can include hives and allergic rashes.

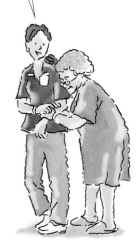

Older adult patients may have an increased sensitivity to anticholinergic drugs.

Senior sensitivity

Among elderly patients, increased sensitivity to anticholinergic drugs may occur. Signs and symptoms include mental confusion, agitation, freezing of gait and, possibly, psychotic symptoms such as hallucinations (Rajan et al., 2020).

The Three-Step Approach

Nursing management for patients undergoing treatment with anticholinergic drugs includes these three steps:

Preadministration

(Recognize and analyze cues)
- Obtain a baseline assessment of the patient's impairment.

(Prioritize hypothesis—priority patient problems)
- Altered mobility
- Injury risk
- Urinary retention
- Knowledge deficiency

(Generate solutions)
- The patient will exhibit improved mobility with a reduction in muscle rigidity, akinesia, and tremors.
- The patient's injury risk will be reduced.
- The patient's voiding pattern will be maintained.
- The patient and family will state an understanding of drug therapy.

Medication administration

(Take action)
- Administer the drug with food to prevent GI irritation.
- Adjust the dosage according to the patient's response and tolerance.
- Assess for immediate adverse reactions and drug interactions.
- Never withdraw the drug abruptly; reduce the dosage gradually.
- Institute safety precautions.

Care for a drink? Candy? Gum?

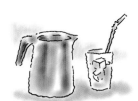

- Provide ice chips, drinks, or sugarless hard candy or gum to relieve dry mouth. Increase fluid and fiber intake to prevent constipation as appropriate.
- Notify the prescriber about urine retention and be prepared to catheterize the patient if necessary.
- Administer the drug at bedtime if the patient receives a single daily dose.

Postadministration

(Evaluate outcomes)
- Monitor drug effectiveness by regularly checking body movements for signs of improvement; keep in mind that the full effect of the drug may take several days.
  - ○ Promote measures to encourage mobility and maintain proper techniques.
  - ○ Monitor voiding patterns and notify the prescriber of any adverse changes.
  - ○ Evaluate the patient and family's ongoing understanding of drug therapy. (See *Teaching about antiparkinsonian drugs*, page 183.)
  - ○ Monitor the patient for adverse reactions and be alert for drug interactions. Some adverse reactions may result from atropinelike toxicity and are dose related.
  - ○ Monitor the patient's vital signs, especially during dosage adjustments.

Teaching about antiparkinsonian drugs

If antiparkinsonian drugs are prescribed, review these points with the patient and caregivers:

• Take the drug exactly as prescribed and don't stop the drug suddenly.

• Take the drug with food to prevent GI upset. Don't crush or break tablets, especially COMT inhibitors, and take them at the same time as carbidopa-levodopa.

• To relieve dry mouth, suck on ice chips, take sips of water, suck on sugarless candy, or chew sugarless gum.

• Avoid hazardous tasks if adverse CNS effects occur. Also avoid alcohol use during therapy.

• Use caution when standing after a prolonged period of sitting or lying down because dizziness may occur, especially early in therapy.

• Report severe or persistent adverse reactions. Also report any uncontrolled movements of the body, chest pain, palpitations, depression or mood changes, difficulty voiding, or severe or persistent nausea or vomiting. With COMT inhibitors, hallucinations, increased dyskinesia, nausea, and diarrhea may occur.

• Don't take vitamins, herbal products, or over-the-counter preparations without consulting a health care provider.

• Be aware that COMT inhibitors may cause urine to turn brownish orange.

• Tell all health care providers about the drug therapy.

• Schedule frequent rest periods to prevent overexertion and fatigue.

• Obtain regular medical follow-up, which is necessary to evaluate the effects of this drug.

Dopaminergic drugs

Dopaminergics include drugs that are chemically unrelated. These drugs increase the effects of dopamine at receptor sites and are useful in treating symptoms of Parkinson's disease. Examples include:

• levodopa (Sinemet), the metabolic precursor to dopamine

• carbidopa-levodopa, a combination drug composed of carbidopa and levodopa

• amantadine, an antiviral drug with dopamine activity

• bromocriptine (Cycloset, Parlodel), an ergot-type dopamine agonist

• ropinirole (Requip) and pramipexole dihydrochloride (Mirapex), two non–ergot-type dopamine agonists

• selegiline hydrochloride (Emsam, Zelapar), a type B MAO inhibitor.

Pharmacokinetics

Like anticholinergic drugs, dopaminergic drugs are absorbed from the GI tract into the bloodstream and delivered to their action site in the brain. The body absorbs most levodopa, carbidopa-levodopa, pramipexole, and amantadine from the GI tract after oral administration, but only about 28% of bromocriptine is absorbed.

Absorption of levodopa is slowed and reduced when it's ingested with food. In some patients, levodopa can significantly interact with foods. Dietary amino acids can decrease levodopa's effectiveness by competing with it for absorption from the intestine and slowing its transport to the brain. About 73% of an oral dose of selegiline is absorbed.

Levodopa is widely distributed in body tissues, including those in the GI tract, liver, pancreas, kidneys, salivary glands, and skin. Carbidopa-levodopa and pramipexole (Mirapex) are also widely distributed. Amantadine is distributed in saliva, nasal secretions, and breast milk. Bromocriptine is highly protein bound. The distribution of selegiline is unknown.

Would you prefer the liver or the kidneys?

Dopaminergic drugs are metabolized extensively in various areas of the body and are eliminated by the liver, the kidneys, or both. Here are more specifics about the metabolism and excretion of dopaminergic drugs:

- Large amounts of levodopa are metabolized in the stomach and during the first pass through the liver. It's metabolized extensively and excreted by the kidneys.
- Carbidopa isn't metabolized extensively. The kidneys excrete approximately one third of it unchanged within 24 hours. (See *Antiparkinsonian drugs: carbidopa and levodopa*, page 185.)
- Amantadine, ropinirole, and pramipexole are excreted by the kidneys largely unchanged.
- Almost all of a bromocriptine dose is metabolized by the liver to pharmacologically inactive compounds and primarily eliminated in feces; only a small amount is excreted in urine.
- Selegiline is metabolized to amphetamine, methamphetamine, and *N*-desmethylselegiline (the major metabolite), which are eliminated in urine.

Pharmacodynamics

Dopaminergic drugs act in the brain to improve motor function in one of two ways: by increasing the dopamine concentration or by enhancing the neurotransmission of dopamine.

Two is better than one

Levodopa is inactive until it crosses the blood-brain barrier and is converted to dopamine by enzymes in the brain, increasing dopamine concentrations in the basal ganglia. Carbidopa enhances levodopa's effectiveness by blocking the peripheral conversion of L-dopa, thus permitting more levodopa to be transported to the brain.

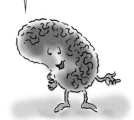

Dopaminergic drugs act in the brain to improve motor function by increasing dopamine concentration or enhancing the neurotransmission of dopamine. I'm feeling better already!

Antiparkinsonian drugs: Carbidopa and levodopa

Actions
• Improves voluntary movement

Levodopa
• Chemical effect of levodopa unknown; thought to be carboxylated to dopamine, countering depletion of striatal dopamine in extrapyramidal centers

Carbidopa
• Inhibits peripheral decarboxylation of levodopa without affecting levodopa's metabolism within the CNS, making more levodopa available to be decarboxylated to dopamine in the brain

Indications
• Idiopathic Parkinson's disease
• Postencephalitic parkinsonism
• Symptomatic parkinsonism resulting from carbon monoxide or manganese intoxication

Nursing considerations
• If the patient is being treated with levodopa, discontinue the drug at least 8 hours before starting carbidopa-levodopa.
• The dosage should be adjusted according to the patient's response and tolerance.
• Withhold the dose and notify the prescriber if the patient's vital signs or mental status changes significantly. A reduced dosage or discontinuation may be necessary.
• Monitor the patient for adverse effects, such as choreiform, dystonic, or dyskinetic movements; involuntary grimacing; head movements; myoclonic jerks; ataxia; suicidal tendencies; hypotension; dry mouth; nausea and vomiting; signs and symptoms of hematologic disorders; and hepatotoxicity.
• A patient on long-term therapy should be tested for acromegaly and diabetes.

The other dopaminergic drugs have various mechanisms of action:
• Amantadine's mechanism of action isn't clear. It's thought to release dopamine from intact neurons, but it may also have nondopaminergic mechanisms.
• Bromocriptine, ropinirole, and pramipexole stimulate dopamine receptors in the brain, producing effects similar to those of dopamine.
• Selegiline can increase dopaminergic activity by inhibiting type B MAO activity or by other mechanisms.

Pharmacotherapeutics
The choice of therapy is highly individualized and is determined by the patient's symptoms and level of disability. A patient with mild Parkinson's disease with predominantly symptoms of tremor is commonly given anticholinergics or amantadine. Selegiline is

indicated for extending the duration of levodopa by blocking its breakdown; it has also been used in early Parkinson's disorder because of its neuroprotective properties and potential to slow the progression of parkinsonism. Usually, dopaminergic drugs are used to treat the patient with severe Parkinson's disease or the patient who doesn't respond to anticholinergics alone.

Levodopa is the most effective drug used to treat Parkinson's disease. When fluctuations in response to levodopa occur, dosage adjustments and increased frequency of administration may be tried. Variables such as the patient's genetic sex may have an effect on dosage response. There have been studies that have demonstrated a need for higher levodopa equivalent daily dose (LEdD) in men than in women (Meoni et al., 2020). Alternatively, adjunctive therapy, such as dopamine agonists, selegiline, amantadine, or a COMT inhibitor, may be added. Controlled-release formulations of carbidopa-levodopa may be helpful in managing the wearing-off effect or delayed-onset motor fluctuations.

Add carbidopa, reduce levodopa

When carbidopa is given with levodopa, the dosage of levodopa can be reduced, decreasing the risk of GI and cardiovascular adverse effects. Levodopa is almost exclusively combined with carbidopa as the standard therapy for Parkinson's disease.

Tapered treatment

Some dopaminergic drugs, such as amantadine, levodopa, pramipexole, and bromocriptine, must be gradually tapered to avoid precipitating parkinsonian crisis (sudden marked clinical deterioration) and possible life-threatening complications (including a syndrome with muscle rigidity, elevated body temperature, tachycardia, mental changes, and increased serum creatine kinase [CK], resembling neuroleptic malignant syndrome).

Drug interactions

Dopaminergic drugs can interfere with many other drugs, causing potentially fatal reactions. Here are some examples:
- The effectiveness of levodopa can be reduced when taking pyridoxine (vitamin B_6), phenytoin, benzodiazepines, reserpine, and papaverine.
- Concomitant use with a type A MAO inhibitor, such as tranylcypromine, increases the risk of hypertensive crisis.
- Antipsychotics, such as phenothiazines, thiothixene, haloperidol, and loxapine, can reduce the effectiveness of levodopa.
- Amantadine may potentiate anticholinergic adverse effects of anticholinergic drugs, such as confusion and hallucinations, and can reduce the absorption of levodopa.
- Meperidine taken with selegiline at higher-than-recommended doses can cause a fatal reaction.

Side effects/Adverse reactions

Side effects/adverse reactions to dopaminergic drugs vary with the drug prescribed.

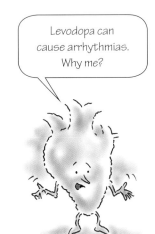

Levodopa can cause arrhythmias. Why me?

Levodopa

Side effects/adverse effects of levodopa include:
- nausea and vomiting
- orthostatic hypotension
- anorexia
- neuroleptic malignant syndrome
- arrhythmias
- irritability
- confusion.

Amantadine

Side effects/adverse effects of amantadine include orthostatic hypotension and constipation.

Bromocriptine

Side effects/adverse effects of bromocriptine include:
- persistent orthostatic hypotension
- ventricular tachycardia
- bradycardia
- worsening angina.

Selegiline

Side effects/adverse effects of selegiline include:
- headache
- insomnia
- dizziness
- nausea
- arrhythmias.

Ropinirole and pramipexole

Side effects/adverse effects of ropinirole and pramipexole include:
- orthostatic hypotension
- dizziness
- confusion
- insomnia.

The Three-Step Approach

Nursing management for patients needing dopaminergic drugs includes these three steps:

Preadministration

(Recognize and analyze cues)
- Assess the patient's baseline status before starting therapy.

(Prioritize hypothesis—priority patient problems)
- Altered mobility
- Injury risk
- Knowledge deficiency

(Generate solutions)
- The patient will exhibit improved mobility with reduction in muscle rigidity, akinesia, and tremors.
- The patient will not experience injury.
- The patient and family will demonstrate an understanding of drug therapy. (See *Teaching about antiparkinsonian drugs*, page 183.)

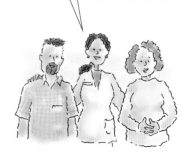

Patient and family understanding is important with any type of drug therapy.

Medication administration

(Take action)
- Administer the drug (except levodopa) with food to prevent GI irritation.
- The dosage should be adjusted by the prescriber according to the patient's response and tolerance.
- Never withdraw the drug abruptly; reduce the dosage gradually.
- Withhold the dose and notify the prescriber if the patient's vital signs or mental status change significantly. A reduced dosage or discontinuation may be necessary.
- Institute safety precautions.
- Provide ice chips, drinks, or sugarless hard candy or gum to relieve dry mouth. Increase fluid and fiber intake to prevent constipation as appropriate.

Better at bedtime
- Give the drug at bedtime if the patient receives a single daily dose.
- If the patient is being treated with levodopa, discontinue the drug at least 8 hours before starting carbidopa-levodopa.
- Treat a patient with open-angle glaucoma with caution. Monitor closely and watch for a change in IOP and arrange for periodic eye examinations.
- A patient receiving long-term therapy should be tested regularly for diabetes and acromegaly and should have periodic tests of liver, renal, and hematopoietic function.
- Assess for immediate adverse reactions and drug interactions.

Postadministration

(Evaluate outcomes)
- Assess the patient's underlying condition before therapy and regularly thereafter; therapeutic response usually follows each dose and disappears within 5 hours but may vary considerably.

- Monitor drug effectiveness by regularly checking body movements for signs of improvement; the full effect of the drug may take several days.

The tell-tale twitch

- Monitor the patient for adverse reactions and be alert for drug interactions. Some adverse reactions may result from atropinelike toxicity and are dose related. Immediately report muscle twitching and blepharospasm (twitching of the eyelids), which may be early signs of drug overdose.
- Monitor the patient's vital signs, especially during dosage adjustments.
- Evaluate the patient's and family's understanding of drug therapy.

COMT inhibitors

COMT inhibitors are used as adjunctive treatments to carbidopa-levodopa in the management of a patient with Parkinson's disease who experiences "wearing off" at the end of the dosing interval.

Choice of two

Two COMT inhibitors are currently available:
- tolcapone (Tasmar)
- entacapone (carbidopa, levodopa, and entacapone; Comtan, Stalevo).

Pharmacokinetics

Tolcapone and entacapone are rapidly absorbed by the GI tract, and absolute bioavailability of each agent is 65% and 35%, respectively. Food decreases bioavailability 10% to 20%. Both drugs are highly bound to albumin and, therefore, have limited distribution to the tissues. They're almost completely metabolized in the liver to inactive metabolites and are excreted in urine.

Pharmacodynamics

Tolcapone and entacapone are selective and reversible inhibitors of COMT, the major metabolizing enzyme for levodopa in the presence of a decarboxylase inhibitor such as carbidopa. Inhibition of COMT alters the pharmacokinetics for levodopa, leading to sustained plasma levels of levodopa. This results in more sustained dopaminergic stimulation in the brain and improvement in the signs and symptoms of Parkinson's disease.

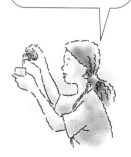

Combining COMT inhibitors with carbidopa-levodopa may reduce wearing-off effects at the end of a dosing interval.

Pharmacotherapeutics

Tolcapone or entacapone may be added to carbidopa-levodopa in a patient who experiences a wearing-off effect at the end of a dosing interval or random on-off fluctuations in response to carbidopa-levodopa. COMT inhibitors have no antiparkinsonian effect when used alone and should always be combined with carbidopa-levodopa. Addition of a COMT inhibitor commonly necessitates a decrease in the dose of carbidopa-levodopa, particularly in the patient receiving a levodopa dose of more than 800 mg.

Not so fast!

Rapid withdrawal of COMT inhibitors may lead to parkinsonian crisis and may cause a syndrome of muscle rigidity, high fever, tachycardia, confusion, and elevated serum CK similar to neuroleptic malignant syndrome. A slow tapering of the dosage is suggested to avoid rapid withdrawal.

Drug interactions

COMT inhibitors can interfere with many drugs. Here are some examples:
- COMT inhibitors shouldn't be used concurrently with type A MAO inhibitors but may be used with selegiline.
- Significant arrhythmias may result when COMT inhibitors are combined with catecholamine drugs (such as dopamine, dobutamine, epinephrine, methyldopa, and norepinephrine).
- The use of COMT inhibitors with CNS depressants (benzodiazepines, tricyclic antidepressants, antipsychotics, ethanol, opioid analgesics, and other sedative-hypnotics) may cause additive CNS effects.
- Entacapone chelates iron and, therefore, iron absorption may be decreased.
- Because of MAO inhibition, COMT inhibitors shouldn't be taken concomitantly with linezolid.
- Fibrotic complications have been associated with the use of entacapone and bromocriptine.
- Drugs that interfere with glucuronidation (erythromycin, rifampin, cholestyramine, and probenecid) may decrease entacapone elimination.
- When using COMT inhibitors for a patient on dopaminergic therapy, the potential for orthostatic hypotension may be increased.

Side effects/Adverse reactions

Common adverse reactions to COMT inhibitors include:
- nausea
- dyskinesia

- diarrhea
- brown-orange urine discoloration (entacapone)
- hyperkinesia or hypokinesia.
  Less common adverse reactions include:
- orthostatic hypotension
- syncope
- dizziness
- fatigue
- abdominal pain
- constipation
- vomiting
- dry mouth
- back pain
- diaphoresis.

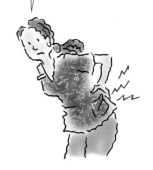

Thank goodness back pain is one of the less common adverse reactions to COMT inhibitors!

You bet your life!

Life-threatening reactions to COMT inhibitors include acute liver failure. Because of this risk, tolcapone should be used only in a patient with Parkinson's disease who experiences fluctuations in levodopa response and doesn't respond to or isn't an appropriate candidate for other adjunctive therapies. The patient should be advised of the risks of liver injury, and written informed consent should be obtained before drug administration. Liver function tests should be obtained at baseline and every 2 weeks for the first year, every 4 weeks for the next 3 months, and every 8 weeks thereafter.

The Three-Step Process

Nursing management for patients needing treatment with COMT inhibitors includes these three steps:

Preadministration

(Recognize and analyze cues)
- Assess the patient's baseline functioning before starting therapy.

(Prioritize hypothesis—priority patient problems)
- Altered mobility
- Visual impairment
- Knowledge deficiency

(Generate solutions)
- The patient's physical mobility will improve.
- The patient will be alert and able to verbalize orientation adequately.
- The patient and family will verbalize an understanding of drug therapy. (See *Teaching about antiparkinsonian drugs*, page 183.)

Medication administration

(Take action)

- Give the drug with immediate or sustained-release carbidopa-levodopa as ordered, with or without food.
- Assess the patient's hepatic and biliary function before starting therapy.
- Check to see that the drug is used only with carbidopa-levodopa; no antiparkinsonian effects will occur when the drug is given as monotherapy.
- Keep in mind that carbidopa-levodopa dosage requirements are usually lower when given with entacapone; the carbidopa-levodopa dosage should be lowered, or the dosing interval should be increased to avoid adverse effects.
- Keep in mind that the drug may cause or worsen dyskinesia despite a reduced levodopa dosage.
- Watch the patient for onset of diarrhea, which usually begins 4 to 12 weeks after therapy starts but may begin as early as the first week or as late as many months.
- Keep in mind that rapid withdrawal or abrupt reduction in the dosage could lead to signs and symptoms of Parkinson's disease; it may also lead to hyperpyrexia and confusion, a symptom complex resembling neuroleptic malignant syndrome. Discontinue the drug slowly and monitor the patient closely. Adjust other dopaminergic treatments.
- Observe for urine discoloration.
- Watch for signs of rhabdomyolysis, which can rarely occur with drug use.
- Assess for immediate adverse reactions and drug interactions

Postadministration

(Evaluate outcomes)

- Monitor the patient's blood pressure closely. Watch for orthostatic hypotension.
- Monitor the patient for hallucinations.
- Evaluate the patient's and family's knowledge of drug therapy.
- Monitor for improved physical mobility.
  - Assess the patient's thought processes frequently; notify the prescriber of any acute changes.
  - The patient and family state an understanding of drug therapy.

Anticonvulsant drugs

Anticonvulsant drugs inhibit neuromuscular transmission. They can be prescribed for:
- long-term management of chronic epilepsy (recurrent seizures)
- short-term management of acute isolated seizures not caused by epilepsy, such as seizures after trauma or brain surgery.

In addition, some anticonvulsants are used in the emergency treatment of status epilepticus (a continuous seizure state).

Try one, then another, before together

Treatment of epilepsy should begin with a single drug, increasing the dosage until seizures are controlled or adverse effects become problematic. Generally, a second alternative should be tried as monotherapy before considering combination therapy. Choice of drug treatment depends on the seizure type, the drug's characteristics, and the patient's preferences.

Class discussion

Anticonvulsants can be categorized into several major classes:
- hydantoins
- barbiturates
- iminostilbenes
- benzodiazepines
- carboxylic acid derivatives
- 1-(aminomethyl) cyclohexaneacetic acid
- phenyltriazine
- carboxamide
- sulfamate-substituted monosaccharides
- succinimides
- sulfonamides.

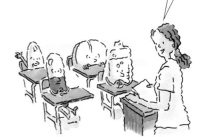

Anticonvulsants can be categorized into several major classes.

Hydantoins

The two most prescribed anticonvulsant drugs—phenytoin (Dilantin) and phenytoin sodium (Cerebyx, Phenytek)—belong to the hydantoin class. Another hydantoin is fosphenytoin (Sesquient).

Pharmacokinetics

The pharmacokinetics of hydantoins varies from drug to drug.

Phenytoin: Slow start, fast finish

Phenytoin is absorbed slowly after oral and IM administration. It's distributed rapidly to all tissues and is highly (90%) protein bound. Phenytoin is metabolized in the liver. Inactive metabolites are excreted in bile and then reabsorbed from the GI tract. Eventually, however, they're excreted in urine.

Fosphenytoin: A short-term solution

Fosphenytoin is indicated for short-term IM or IV administration. It's widely distributed throughout the body, is highly (90%) protein bound, and is metabolized by the liver and excreted in urine.

Pharmacodynamics

In most cases, the hydantoin anticonvulsants stabilize nerve cells to keep them from getting overexcited. Phenytoin appears to work in the motor cortex of the brain, where it stops the spread of seizure activity. The pharmacodynamics of fosphenytoin is thought to mimic those of phenytoin.

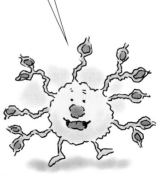

Hydantoins stabilize nerve cells to keep us from getting overexcited!!! Okay, calming down, now...

Pharmacotherapeutics

Because of its effectiveness and relatively low toxicity, phenytoin is the most prescribed anticonvulsant and one of the drugs of choice to treat:
- complex partial seizures (also called *psychomotor* or *temporal lobe seizures*)
- tonic-clonic seizures.

The enzyme system responsible for the metabolism of phenytoin is saturable. A change in dose can result in disproportional changes in serum concentration. (See *Anticonvulsants: Phenytoin*, page 195.)

Resistance is futile

Phenytoin and fosphenytoin are the long-acting anticonvulsants of choice to treat status epilepticus after initial IV benzodiazepines.

Drug interactions

Hydantoins interact with several drugs. Here are some drug interactions of major to moderate clinical significance:
- The effect of phenytoin is reduced when taken with phenobarbital, diazoxide, theophylline, carbamazepine, rifampin, antacids, and sucralfate.

Prototype pro

Anticonvulsants: Phenytoin

Actions
• Stabilizes neuronal membranes and limits seizure activity by either increasing efflux or decreasing influx of sodium ions across cell membranes in the motor cortex during generation of nerve impulses

Indications
• Control of tonic-clonic and complex partial seizures
• Status epilepticus
• Prevention of and treatment for seizures during neurosurgery

Nursing considerations
• Monitor the patient for adverse effects, such as ataxia, slurred speech, mental confusion, nystagmus, blurred vision, gingival hyperplasia, nausea, vomiting, hematologic disorders, hepatitis, Stevens-Johnson syndrome, and hirsutism.
• Don't withdraw the drug suddenly; seizures may occur.
• Monitor drug levels as ordered; therapeutic levels range from 10 to 20 mcg/mL.

Oral interference

- Enteral tube feedings may interfere with the absorption of oral phenytoin. Stop feedings for 2 hours before and after phenytoin administration.
- The effect of phenytoin is increased, and the risk of toxicity increases when phenytoin is taken with allopurinol, cimetidine, disulfiram, fluconazole, isoniazid, omeprazole, sulfonamides, oral anticoagulants, chloramphenicol, valproic acid, or amiodarone.
- The effect of the following drugs is reduced when taken with a hydantoin anticonvulsant: oral anticoagulants, levodopa, amiodarone, corticosteroids, doxycycline, methadone, metyrapone, quinidine, theophylline, thyroid hormone, hormonal contraceptives, valproic acid, cyclosporine, and carbamazepine.

Side effects/Adverse reactions

Side effects/adverse reactions to hydantoins include:
- drowsiness
- ataxia
- irritability and restlessness
- headache
- nystagmus
- dizziness and vertigo
- dysarthria

- nausea and vomiting
- abdominal pain
- anorexia
- depressed atrial and ventricular conduction
- ventricular fibrillation (in toxic states)
- bradycardia, hypotension, and cardiac arrest (with IV administration)
- hypersensitivity reactions.

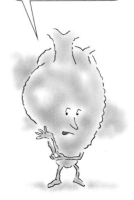

Bradycardia, hypotension, and cardiac arrest can occur with IV administration of hydantoins.

The Three-Step Approach

Nursing management for patients needing treatment with hydantoin anticonvulsant drugs includes these three steps.

Preadministration

(Recognize and analyze cues)
- Assess the patient's baseline status prior to starting therapy.

(Prioritize hypothesis—priority patient problems)
- Injury risk
- Mobility impairment
- Knowledge deficiency
- Nonadherence

(Generate solutions)
- The patient will not sustain injury related to seizure activity.
- The patient will be able to perform activities of daily living (ADLs).
- The patient and family will verbalize an understanding of drug therapy. (See *Teaching about anticonvulsants*, page 197.)
- The patient will use support systems to help modify nonadherent behavior.

Medication administration

(Take action)
- Administer oral forms with food to reduce GI irritation.
- Phenytoin binds with tube feedings, thus decreasing the absorption of the drug. Turn off tube feedings for 2 hours before and after giving phenytoin, according to your facility's policy.

Forecast: Chance of precipitation

- If using as an infusion, don't mix the drug with dextrose 5% in water (D₅W) because phenytoin will precipitate. Clear IV tubing first with normal saline solution. Mix with normal saline solution if necessary and infuse over 30 to 60 minutes with an in-line filter.
- Avoid giving phenytoin by IV push into veins on the back of the hand to avoid discoloration known as *purple glove syndrome*. Inject into larger veins or a central venous catheter, if available.

- Discard any unused drug 4 hours after preparation for IV administration.
- Don't give phenytoin IM unless dosage adjustments are made. The drug may precipitate at the site, cause pain, and be erratically absorbed.
- Expect to adjust the dosage according to the patient's response.
- Assess for immediate adverse reactions and drug interactions.
- Administer safety precautions if the patient has an adverse CNS reaction.

Postadministration
(Evaluate outcomes)
- Monitor for the anticipated response to the prescribed drug.
- Assess the patient's condition before therapy and regularly thereafter.
- Monitor the patient's blood levels; the therapeutic level for phenytoin is 10 to 20 mcg/mL.
- Monitor additional labs including CBC and calcium level every 6 months; monitor hepatic function periodically as well.

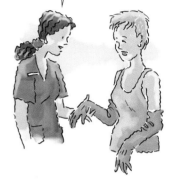

No, I don't think this is what is meant by a case of purple glove syndrome...

Education edge

Teaching about anticonvulsants

If anticonvulsants are prescribed, review these points with the patient and caregivers:
- Take the drug exactly as prescribed and don't stop the drug without medical supervision. The drug must be taken regularly to be effective.
- Take the drug with food to reduce GI upset and loss of appetite. Eating small, frequent meals can help.
- Don't change brands or dosage forms.
- Avoid hazardous activities that require mental alertness if adverse CNS reactions occur.
- Wear or carry medical identification at all times.
- Record and report any seizure activity while taking the drug.
- Don't stop the drug abruptly. If for some reason you can't continue taking the drug, notify the health care provider at once; the drug must be slowly withdrawn when it's discontinued.

- Try to space activities throughout the day and allow rest periods to avoid fatigue, weakness, and drowsiness. Take safety precautions and avoid driving or operating dangerous machinery if these conditions occur.
- Report persistent or bothersome adverse effects to the health care provider.
- Perform oral hygiene and see a dentist for regular examinations, especially if taking phenytoin or its derivatives.
- Be aware that phenytoin may discolor urine pink, red, or red brown.
- Don't take over-the-counter medications or herbal preparations without first consulting your health care provider.
- Be aware that heavy alcohol use may diminish the drug's benefit.
- Make sure you have regular medical follow-up, possibly including blood tests, to help evaluate the effects of the drug.

- Assess the patient's vital signs, including blood pressure, and electrocardiography (ECG) during IV administration.
- Monitor the patient for adverse reactions.
- Assess the patient's compliance with therapy at each follow-up visit.
- Monitor the patient for increased seizure activity; certain viral illnesses (including mononucleosis) may cause a decrease in the phenytoin level.

Barbiturates

Formerly one of the most widely used anticonvulsants, the long-acting barbiturate phenobarbital is now used less frequently because of its sedative effects. Phenobarbital is sometimes used for long-term treatment of epilepsy and is prescribed selectively for treatment of status epilepticus if hydantoins aren't effective.

Other options

Primidone (Mysoline), a structural analog of phenobarbital that's closely related chemically to the barbiturate-derivative anticonvulsants, is also used in the chronic treatment of epilepsy.

Pharmacokinetics

Each barbiturate has a slightly different set of pharmacokinetic properties.

Phenobarbital for the long haul

Although absorbed slowly, phenobarbital is well absorbed from the GI tract. Peak plasma concentration levels occur 8 to 12 hours after a single dose. The drug is 20% to 45% bound to serum proteins and to a similar extent to other tissues, including the brain. The liver metabolizes about 75% of a phenobarbital dose, and 25% is excreted unchanged in urine.

Primidone evens out

Approximately 60% to 80% of a primidone dose is absorbed from the GI tract, and it's distributed evenly among body tissues. The drug is protein bound to a small extent in the plasma. Primidone is metabolized by the liver to two active metabolites, phenobarbital and phenylethylmalonamide (PEMA). From 15% to 25% of primidone is excreted unchanged in urine, 15% to 25% is metabolized to phenobarbital, and 50% to 70% is excreted in urine as PEMA.

Pharmacodynamics

Barbiturates exhibit anticonvulsant action at doses below those that produce hypnotic effects. For this reason, the barbiturates usually don't produce addiction when used to treat epilepsy. Barbiturates elevate the seizure threshold by decreasing postsynaptic excitation.

Pharmacotherapeutics

The barbiturate anticonvulsants are effective alternative therapy for:
- partial seizures
- tonic-clonic seizures
- febrile seizures.

Barbiturates can be used alone or with other anticonvulsants. IV phenobarbital is also used to treat status epilepticus. The major disadvantage of using phenobarbital for status epilepticus is a delayed onset of action when an immediate response is needed. Barbiturate anticonvulsants are ineffective in treating absence seizures.

"Ph" before "pr"

Primidone has no advantage over phenobarbital and is used when the patient can't tolerate phenobarbital's adverse effects. In general, because of monitoring, costs, and dosing frequency, phenobarbital is tried before primidone. Primidone may be effective in a patient who doesn't respond to phenobarbital.

Drug interactions

Here are some drug interactions of barbiturates:
- The effects of barbiturates can be reduced when taken with rifampin.
- The risk of toxicity increases when phenobarbital is taken with CNS depressants, valproic acid, chloramphenicol, felbamate, cimetidine, or phenytoin.
- The metabolism of corticosteroids, cimetidine, or phenytoin can be enhanced with phenobarbital therapy, leading to decreased effects. Evening primrose oil may increase anticonvulsant dosage requirements.

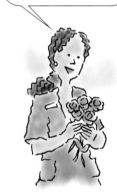

Evening primrose oil may increase anticonvulsant dosage requirements.

Reduced rates

In addition, the effects of many drugs can be reduced when taken with a barbiturate, including such drugs as beta-adrenergic blockers, corticosteroids, digoxin, estrogens, doxycycline, oral anticoagulants, hormonal contraceptives, quinidine, phenothiazine, metronidazole, tricyclic antidepressants, theophylline, cyclosporine, carbamazepine, felodipine, and verapamil.

Side effects/Adverse reactions

Side effects/adverse reactions to phenobarbital include:
- drowsiness
- lethargy
- dizziness
- nystagmus, confusion, and ataxia (with large doses)
- laryngospasm, respiratory depression, and hypotension (when administered IV).

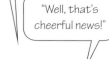

"When given IV, phenobarbital can sometimes cause respiratory depression."

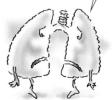

"Well, that's cheerful news!"

And then some

Primidone can cause the same CNS and GI adverse reactions as phenobarbital. It can also cause acute psychoses, hair loss, impotence, and osteomalacia.

As a group

All three barbiturate anticonvulsants can produce hypersensitivity rashes and other rashes, lupuslike syndrome (an inflammatory disorder), and enlarged lymph nodes.

The Three-Step Approach

Nursing management for patients requiring treatment with barbiturate anticonvulsant drugs includes these three steps:

Preadministration

(Recognize and analyze cues)
- Assess the patient's condition, establishing a baseline, before initiating therapy.

(Prioritize hypothesis—priority patient problems)
- Injury risk
- Mobility impairment
- Nonadherence

(Generate solutions)
- Risk of injury to the patient will be minimized.
- The patient will be able to perform ADLs.
- The patient will verbalize factors that contribute to noncompliance.
- The patient and family will demonstrate an understanding of drug therapy.

Medication administration

(Take action)
- Administer oral forms of the drug with food to reduce GI irritation.
- IV phenobarbital is reserved for emergency treatment; monitor the patient's respirations closely and don't give more than 60 mg/minute. Have resuscitation equipment available.
- Don't stop the drug abruptly because seizures may worsen. Call the prescriber immediately if adverse reactions occur.

Nothing superficial about it

- Give the IM injection deeply. Superficial injection may cause pain, sterile abscess, and tissue sloughing.
- Assess for immediate adverse reactions and drug interactions.
- Expect to adjust the dosage according to the patient's response.
- Administer safety precautions if the patient has adverse CNS reactions.

Postadministration
(Evaluate outcomes)

- Monitor the patient's response to the prescribed drug and serum levels, as indicated.
- Assess the patient's condition regularly after initiating therapy.
- Monitor the patient for adverse reactions.
- Assess the patient's compliance with therapy at each follow-up visit.
- Promote measures that help increase safe mobility.

Iminostilbenes

Carbamazepine (Carbatrol, Tegretol) is the most commonly used iminostilbene anticonvulsant. It effectively treats:

- partial and generalized tonic-clonic seizures
- mixed seizure types
- complex partial seizures (first choice of treatment).

Pharmacokinetics

Carbamazepine is absorbed slowly from the GI tract, is metabolized in the liver by the cytochrome P-450 isoform 3A4 (CYP3A4), and is excreted in urine. Carbamazepine is distributed rapidly to all tissues; 75% to 90% is bound to plasma proteins. The half-life varies greatly.

Pharmacodynamics

Carbamazepine's anticonvulsant effect is similar to that of phenytoin. The anticonvulsant action of the drug can occur because of its ability to inhibit the spread of seizure activity or neuromuscular transmission in general.

Pharmacotherapeutics

Carbamazepine is the drug of choice, in adults and children, for treating:

- generalized tonic-clonic seizures
- simple and complex partial seizures.

Neutralizes neuralgia, benefits bipolar

Carbamazepine also relieves pain when used to treat trigeminal neuralgia (tic douloureux, characterized by excruciating facial pain along the trigeminal nerve) and may be useful in some psychiatric disorders, such as bipolar affective disorder and intermittent explosive disorder. Carbamazepine may increase absence or myoclonic seizures and isn't recommended for treatment for these types of seizures.

Drug interactions

Carbamazepine can reduce the effects of several drugs, including oral anticoagulants, haloperidol, bupropion, lamotrigine, tricyclic antidepressants, hormonal contraceptives, doxycycline, felbamate, theophylline, and valproic acid.

Other drug interactions can also occur:

- Increased carbamazepine levels and toxicity can occur with cimetidine, danazol, diltiazem, erythromycin, isoniazid, selective serotonin reuptake inhibitors (SSRIs), propoxyphene, troleandomycin, ketoconazole, valproic acid, and verapamil.
- Lithium and carbamazepine taken together increase the risk of toxic neurologic effects.
- Carbamazepine levels can decrease when taken with barbiturates, felbamate, or phenytoin.
- Plantain may inhibit GI absorption of carbamazepine.

Side effects/Adverse reactions

Occasionally, serious hematologic toxicity occurs. Because carbamazepine is related structurally to the tricyclic antidepressants, it can cause similar toxicities and affect behaviors and emotions. Hives and Stevens-Johnson syndrome (a potentially fatal inflammatory disease) can occur. Rashes are the most common hypersensitivity response.

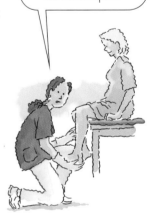

Rashes are the most common hypersensitivity response to carbamazepine.

The Three–Step Approach

Nursing management for patients requiring treatment with iminostilbene anticonvulsant drugs includes these three steps:

Preadministration

(Recognize and analyze cues)

- Assess the patient's seizure disorder or trigeminal neuralgia before therapy.

(Prioritize hypothesis—priority patient problems)

- Injury risk
- Mobility impairment
- Nonadherence

(Generate solutions)
- Risk of injury to the patient will be minimized.
- The patient will maintain physical mobility.
- The patient will be able to perform ADLs.
- The patient will exhibit behaviors that demonstrate willingness to comply with the health care regimen.
- The patient and family will demonstrate an understanding of drug therapy.

Medication administration

(Take action)
- Administer oral forms with food to reduce GI irritation. Give the drug in divided doses when possible to maintain a consistent blood level.

Shake it up!

- Shake an oral suspension well before measuring the dose.
- When giving the drug by nasogastric tube, mix the dose with an equal volume of water, normal saline solution, or D_5W. Flush the tube with 100 mL of diluent after administering the dose.
- Expect to adjust the dosage according to the patient's response.
- Administer safety precautions if the patient has adverse CNS reactions.
- Never suddenly discontinue the drug when treating seizures or status epilepticus.
- Assess for immediate adverse reactions and drug interactions.
- Notify the prescriber immediately if adverse reactions occur.

Postadministration

(Evaluate outcomes)
- Observe the patient for delayed reactions to the therapy.
- Monitor the patient's mobility and eliminate barriers to safe and efficient mobility. Monitor for seizure activity.
- Obtain baseline determinations of urinalysis, blood urea nitrogen level, liver function, CBC, platelet and reticulocyte counts, and iron level. Reassess regularly.
- Monitor drug level and drug effects closely; the therapeutic level ranges from 4 to 12 mcg/mL.
- Monitor the patient's response to the prescribed drug and serum levels, as indicated.
- Monitor the patient for adverse reactions.
- Assess the patient's adherence to therapy at each follow-up visit.

Benzodiazepines

The four benzodiazepine drugs that provide anticonvulsant effects are:
- diazepam (in the parenteral form) (Diastat, Valium)
- clonazepam (Klonopin)
- clorazepate (Tranxene)
- lorazepam (Ativan).

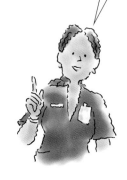

There's only one benzodiazepine recommended for the long-term treatment of epilepsy—clonazepam.

Only one for ongoing treatment

Only clonazepam is recommended for long-term treatment of epilepsy. Diazepam is restricted to acute treatment of status epilepticus and rectally for repetitive seizures. IV lorazepam is considered the drug of choice for acute management of status epilepticus. Clorazepate is prescribed as an adjunct in treating partial seizures.

Pharmacokinetics

The patient can receive benzodiazepines orally, parenterally, or, in special situations, rectally. These drugs are absorbed rapidly and almost completely from the GI tract but are distributed at different rates. Protein binding of benzodiazepines ranges from 85% to 90%.

Benzodiazepines are metabolized in the liver to multiple metabolites and are then excreted in urine. The benzodiazepines readily cross the placenta and are excreted in breast milk.

Pharmacodynamics

Benzodiazepines act as:
- anticonvulsants
- antianxiety agents
- sedative-hypnotics
- muscle relaxants.

Their mechanism of action is poorly understood.

Pharmacotherapeutics

Each of the benzodiazepines can be used in slightly different ways:
- Clonazepam is used to treat absence (petit mal), atypical absence (Lennox-Gastaut syndrome), atonic, and myoclonic seizures.
- IV lorazepam is currently considered the benzodiazepine of choice for status epilepticus.
- IV diazepam is used to control status epilepticus. Because diazepam provides only short-term effects of less than 1 hour, the patient must also be given a long-acting anticonvulsant, such as phenytoin or phenobarbital, during diazepam therapy.

Reining in repetitive seizures

- Diazepam rectal gel is approved for the treatment of repetitive seizures and has reduced the incidence of recurrent seizures in children.
- Diazepam isn't recommended for long-term treatment because of its potential for addiction and the high serum concentrations required to control seizures.
- Clorazepate is used with other drugs to treat partial seizures.

Drug interactions

When benzodiazepines are taken with CNS depressants, sedative and other depressant effects become enhanced. This can cause motor skill impairment, respiratory depression, and even death at high doses.

Cimetidine and hormonal contraceptives taken with a benzodiazepine drug can also cause excessive sedation and CNS depression.

Side effects/Adverse reactions

The most common adverse reactions to benzodiazepines include:

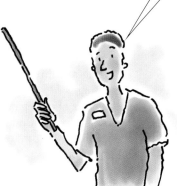

These are the most common adverse reactions to benzodiazepines.

- drowsiness
- confusion
- ataxia
- weakness
- dizziness
- nystagmus
- vertigo
- fainting
- dysarthria
- headache
- tremor
- glassy-eyed appearance.

Comin' round the less common bend

Less common adverse reactions include respiratory depression and decreased heart rate (with high doses and with IV diazepam) as well as rash and acute hypersensitivity reactions.

The Three-Step Approach

Nursing management for patients undergoing treatment with benzodiazepine anticonvulsant drugs includes these three steps:

Preadministration

(Recognize and analyze cues)
- Obtain a history of the patient's underlying condition before therapy.

(Prioritize hypothesis—priority patient problems)
- Injury risk
- Mobility impairment
- Nonadherence
- Knowledge deficiency

(Generate solutions)
- Risk of injury to the patient will be minimized.
- The patient will be able to perform ADLs.
- The patient will verbalize factors that contribute to noncompliance.
- The patient and family will verbalize an understanding of drug therapy.

Medication administration

(Take action)
- Administer oral forms of the drug with food to reduce GI irritation. If an oral concentrate solution is used, dilute the dose immediately before administering. Use water, juice, or carbonated beverages or mix with semisolid foods, such as applesauce or pudding.
- Avoid use of diazepam rectal gel for more than five episodes per month or one episode every 5 days.
- If giving the IV form of diazepam, administer no more than 5 mg/minute and inject directly into a vein.
- Have emergency resuscitation equipment and oxygen at the bedside when giving these drugs IV.
- Use IM forms only when the IV and oral routes aren't applicable; IM forms aren't recommended because absorption is variable, and injection is painful.
- Don't store parenteral diazepam solutions in plastic syringes.
- Assess for immediate adverse reactions and drug interactions.
- Expect to adjust the dosage according to the patient's response.
- Administer safety precautions if the patient has adverse CNS reactions.

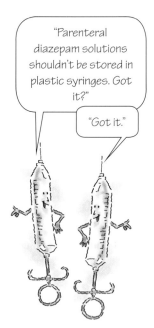

"Parenteral diazepam solutions shouldn't be stored in plastic syringes. Got it?"

"Got it."

Postadministration

(Evaluate outcomes)
- Observe the patient for adverse reactions after administration of medication.
- Assess physical mobility frequently.
- Assess the patient's adherence with therapy, including at each follow-up.
- Observe for, and ask about, seizure activity.
- Evaluate the patient's and family's ongoing understanding of drug therapy.
- Monitor the patient's respiratory rate every 5 to 15 minutes and before each repeated IV dose.
- Periodically monitor liver, kidney, and hematopoietic function studies in a patient receiving repeated or prolonged therapy.
- Monitor the patient's response to prescribed drug and serum levels as indicated.

Carboxylic acid derivatives

The drugs in this class are:
- valproate (Valproate Sodium)
- valproic acid
- divalproex (Depakote).

Pharmacokinetics

Valproate is converted rapidly to valproic acid in the stomach. Divalproex is a precursor of valproic acid that separates into valproic acid in the GI tract. Valproic acid is a hepatic enzyme inhibitor. It's absorbed well, strongly protein bound, and metabolized in the liver. Metabolites and unchanged drug are excreted in urine.

Valproic acid readily crosses the placental barrier and also appears in breast milk.

Pharmacodynamics

The mechanism of action for valproic acid remains unknown. It's thought to increase levels of GABA, an inhibitory neurotransmitter, as well as having a direct membrane-stabilizing effect. (See *Happy accident*, page 208.)

Pharmacotherapeutics

Valproic acid is prescribed for long-term treatment of:
- absence seizures
- myoclonic seizures
- tonic-clonic seizures
- partial seizures.

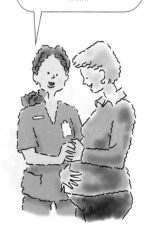

Keep in mind that valproic acid crosses the placental barrier and appears in breast milk.

Baby blues

Valproic acid may also be useful for neonatal seizures. However, it must be used cautiously in children younger than age 2, particularly those receiving multiple anticonvulsants, those with congenital metabolic disorders or hepatic disease, those with severe seizures and mental retardation, and those with organic brain disease. For these patients, the drug carries a risk of potentially fatal liver toxicity (usually within the first 6 months of treatment). This risk limits the use of valproic acid as a drug of choice for seizure disorders.

Drug interactions

Here are the most significant drug interactions associated with valproic acid:

- Cimetidine, aspirin, erythromycin, and felbamate may increase levels of valproic acid.
- Carbamazepine, lamotrigine, phenobarbital, primidone, phenytoin, and rifampin may decrease levels of valproic acid.
- Valproic acid may decrease the effects of lamotrigine, phenobarbital, primidone, benzodiazepines, CNS depressants, warfarin, and zidovudine.

Side effects/Adverse reactions

Rare, but deadly, liver toxicity has occurred with valproic acid use. The drug should be used with caution in the patient who has a history of liver disease. Pediatric patients younger than age 2 are at considerable risk for developing hepatotoxicity. Most other adverse reactions to valproic acid are tolerable and dose related. These include:

- nausea and vomiting
- diarrhea or constipation
- sedation
- dizziness
- ataxia
- headache
- muscle weakness
- increased blood ammonia level.

The Three-Step Approach

Nursing management for patients receiving treatment with carboxylic acid–derivative anticonvulsant drugs includes these three steps:

Preadministration

(Recognize and analyze cues)
- Assess the patient's condition before initiating therapy.

(Prioritize hypothesis—priority patient problems)
- Injury risk

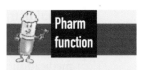

Pharm function

Happy accident

The anticonvulsant properties of valproic acid were discovered when it was being used as a vehicle for other compounds being tested for anticonvulsant properties. Structurally, valproic acid is unlike other anticonvulsants. Its mechanism of action isn't completely understood.

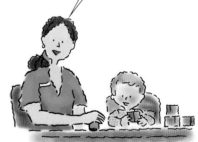

The use of valproic acid for seizures in children age 2 and younger should be limited due to the risk of potentially fatal liver toxicity.

- Mobility impairment
- Nonadherence

(Generate solutions)
- The injury risk to the patient will be minimized.
- The patient will be able to perform ADLs.
- The patient and family will demonstrate an understanding of drug therapy.
- The patient will verbalize factors that contribute to noncompliance.

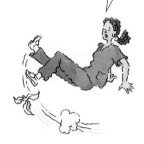

Reducing the patient's injury risk is an important planning goal. In fact, I think I'll make that one of my *own* planning goals! Yikes!

Mediation administration
(Take action)
- Administer oral forms of the drug with food to reduce GI irritation. Don't give the syrup form to a patient who needs sodium restriction. Check with the prescriber.
- Dilute the drug with at least 50 mL of a compatible diluent (D_5W, saline solution, lactated Ringer's solution) if injecting IV and give over 1 hour. Don't exceed 20 mg/minute.
- Avoid sudden withdrawal, which may worsen seizures.
- Expect to adjust the dosage according to the patient's response. In elderly patients, a reduced starting dose is suggested, with slower dosage increases.
- Administer safety precautions if the patient has adverse CNS reactions to the drug.
- Monitor closely for hepatotoxicity because it may follow nonspecific symptoms, such as malaise, fever, and lethargy.
- Assess for immediate adverse reactions and drug interactions.

Postadministration
(Evaluate outcomes)
- Monitor the level of the drug in the blood (therapeutic level is 50 to 100 mcg/mL).
- Monitor liver function studies, platelet counts, and prothrombin time before starting the drug and periodically thereafter.
- Monitor the patient's response to the drug, especially for adverse reactions.
- Be aware that the drug may produce false-positive test results for ketones in urine.
- Evaluate the patient's adherence to therapy at each follow-up visit.
- Promote measures that help the patient maintain physical mobility.

1-(Aminomethyl) cyclohexaneacetic acid

The 1-(aminomethyl) cyclohexaneacetic acid drug class includes the drug gabapentin (Neurontin). This drug was designed to be a GABA agonist, but its exact mechanism of action is unknown. It's approved as adjunctive therapy for partial seizures in adults with epilepsy and in children age 3 and older. Gabapentin has also been used for the treatment of pain from diabetic neuropathy and postherpetic neuralgia, tremors associated with MS, bipolar disorder, migraine prophylaxis, and Parkinson's disease.

Pharmacokinetics

Gabapentin is readily absorbed in the GI tract. Bioavailability isn't dose proportional, as the dose increases, the bioavailability decreases.

An exclusive deal

Gabapentin isn't metabolized and is excreted exclusively by the kidneys. The patient with renal impairment requires dosage reduction.

Pharmacodynamics

The exact mechanism of action of gabapentin isn't known.

Gabbing on about GABA

Originally designed as a GABA agonist, gabapentin doesn't appear to act at the GABA receptor, affect GABA uptake, or interfere with GABA transaminase. Rather, it appears to bind to a carrier protein and act at a unique receptor, resulting in elevated GABA in the brain.

Pharmacotherapeutics

Gabapentin is used as adjunctive therapy in adults and children age 3 and older with partial and secondary generalized seizures. Gabapentin also appears effective as monotherapy. Like carbamazepine, gabapentin may worsen myoclonic seizures.

Drug interactions

Antacids and cimetidine may affect gabapentin concentration.

Side effects/Adverse reactions

Side effects/adverse reactions to gabapentin commonly include:
- fatigue
- somnolence
- dizziness
- ataxia
- leukopenia.
  Some less common reactions include:
- edema
- weight gain
- hostility
- emotional lability
- nausea and vomiting
- bronchitis
- viral infection
- fever

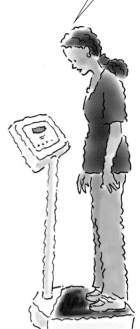

Weight gain is one of the less common adverse effects of gabapentin.

- nystagmus
- rhinitis
- diplopia
- tremor.

The Three-Step Approach

Nursing management for patients undergoing treatment with 1-(aminomethyl) cyclohexaneacetic acid anticonvulsant drugs includes these three steps:

Preadministration

(Recognize and analyze cues)
- Assess the patient's disorder before therapy.

(Prioritize hypothesis—priority patient problems)
- Injury risk
- Mobility impairment
- Nonadherence

(Generate solutions)
- The risk to the patient will be minimized.
- The patient will be able to perform ADLs.
- The patient will verbalize factors that contribute to noncompliance.
- The patient and family will demonstrate an understanding of drug therapy.

Medication administration

(Take action)
- Administer oral forms of the drug with food to reduce GI irritation.
- Expect to adjust the drug dosage according to the patient's response.
- Assess for immediate adverse reactions and drug interactions
- Administer safety precautions if the patient has adverse CNS reactions to the drug. Administer the first dose at bedtime to minimize the effect of drowsiness, dizziness, fatigue, and ataxia.
- Withdraw the drug gradually over 1 week to minimize seizure risk. Don't suddenly withdraw other anticonvulsants in the patient starting gabapentin therapy.

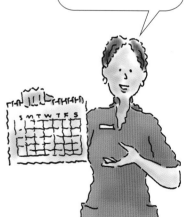

Withdraw gabapentin gradually over 1 week to minimize seizure risk.

Postadministration

(Evaluate outcomes)
- Assess for injury, including those related to adverse reactions.
- Assess physical mobility.
- Promote measures that encourage safe and effective mobility.

- Assess patient adherence with therapy, including at each follow-up visit.
- Monitor the patient's serum levels and response to the prescribed drug, as indicated.
- Monitor the patient for adverse reactions.

Phenyltriazine

Lamotrigine (Lamictal) belongs to the phenyltriazine drug class and is chemically unrelated to other anticonvulsants.

Stamp of approval

Lamotrigine is U.S. Food and Drug Administration (FDA) approved for adjunctive therapy in adults with partial seizures and in children older than age 2 with generalized seizures or Lennox-Gastaut syndrome.

Pharmacokinetics

Lamotrigine is well absorbed by the body at a rapid rate. It's metabolized by the liver and excreted by the kidneys. Clearance increases in the presence of other enzyme-inducing anticonvulsant drugs. The drug isn't significantly bound to plasma proteins.

Pharmacodynamics

The precise mechanism of action of lamotrigine is unknown, but it is thought to involve a use-dependent blocking effect on sodium channels, resulting in inhibition of the release of excitatory neurotransmitters, glutamate, and aspartate.

Pharmacotherapeutics

Lamotrigine is approved for adjunctive therapy in adults and children older than age 2 with generalized seizures or Lennox-Gastaut syndrome. It may also be used for conversion to monotherapy in adults. Lamotrigine appears effective for many types of generalized seizures but can worsen myoclonic seizures. Lamotrigine may also lead to improvement in the patient's mood.

Drug interactions

- Carbamazepine, phenytoin, phenobarbital, primidone, and acetaminophen may result in decreased lamotrigine effects.
- Valproic acid may decrease the clearance of lamotrigine and the steady-state level of lamotrigine.
- Lamotrigine may produce additive effects when combined with folate inhibitors.

Side effects/Adverse reactions

Side effects/adverse reactions to lamotrigine commonly include:
- dizziness

- ataxia
- somnolence
- headache
- diplopia
- nausea
- vomiting
- rash.

Don't be rash

Several types of rash may occur with lamotrigine use, including Stevens-Johnson syndrome. This generalized, erythematous, morbilliform rash usually appears in the first 3 to 4 weeks of therapy and is usually mild to moderate but may be severe. The drug now carries a "black box" warning regarding the rash, and the manufacturer recommends discontinuing the drug at the first sign of a rash. The risk of rash may be increased by starting at high doses, by rapidly increasing doses, or by using the drug with valproate.

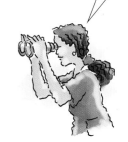

Discontinue lamotrigine at the first sight of a rash.

The Three-Step Approach

Nursing management for patients undergoing treatment with phenyltriazine anticonvulsant drugs includes these three steps:

Preadministration
(Recognize and analyze cues)
- Obtain a history of the patient's seizure disorder before therapy.

(Prioritize hypothesis—priority patient problems)
- Injury risk
- Mobility impairment
- Nonadherence

(Generate solutions)
- Risk to the patient will be minimized.
- The patient will be able to perform ADLs.
- The patient will exhibit behaviors that demonstrate willingness to comply with long-term therapy.
- The patient and family will demonstrate an understanding of drug therapy.

Medication administration
(Take action)
- Administer oral forms of the drug with food to reduce GI irritation.
- Expect the dosage to be lowered if the drug is added to a multidrug regimen that includes valproic acid.
- Expect that a lowered maintenance dosage will be used in a patient with severe renal impairment.

Come to a slow, steady stop

- Don't stop the drug abruptly. Abrupt withdrawal increases the risk of seizures. Instead, drug withdrawal should be tapered over at least 2 weeks.
- A rash may be life threatening. Notify the prescriber at the first sign of a rash.
- Administer safety precautions if the patient has adverse CNS reactions.
- Assess for immediate adverse reactions and drug interactions.

Postadministration

(Evaluate outcomes)
- Monitor the patient's physical mobility.
- Promote measures that encourage and maintain safe and efficient mobility.
- Evaluate the patient for reduction in seizure frequency and duration after therapy begins. Check the adjunct anticonvulsant's level periodically.
- Monitor the patient's serum levels and response to the prescribed drug as indicated.
- Monitor the patient for adverse reactions.
- Assess the patient's adherence with therapy at each follow-up visit.

Carboxamide

Oxcarbazepine, a carboxamide, is chemically similar to carbamazepine but causes less induction of liver enzymes. Oxcarbazepine is useful in adults as adjunctive therapy or monotherapy for partial seizures and in children as adjunctive therapy for partial seizures.

Pharmacokinetics

Oxcarbazepine (Oxtellar XR, Trileptal) is completely absorbed and extensively metabolized via liver enzymes to the 10-monohydroxy metabolite (MHD) that's responsible for its pharmacologic activity. It's excreted primarily by the kidneys. The half-life of MHD is about 9 hours. Unlike carbamazepine, oxcarbazepine doesn't induce its own metabolism.

Pharmacodynamics

The precise mechanism of oxcarbazepine and MHD is unknown, but antiseizure activity is thought to occur through blockade of sodium-sensitive channels, which prevents seizure spread in the brain.

Pharmacotherapeutics

Oxcarbazepine is FDA approved for adjunctive therapy of partial seizures in adults and children older than age 4 and for monotherapy in adults. As with carbamazepine, it's also effective for generalized seizures but may worsen myoclonic and absence seizures.

Drug interactions

Carbamazepine, phenytoin, phenobarbital, valproic acid, and verapamil may decrease the levels of active MHD. Oxcarbazepine may decrease the effectiveness of hormonal contraceptives and felodipine.

A dip in the dosage

Reduced dosages are necessary in the patient with renal impairment (clearance less than 30 mL/minute) and in the patient at risk for renal impairment (such as an older adult patient).

Side effects/Adverse reactions

Side effects/adverse reactions to oxcarbazepine commonly include:
- somnolence
- dizziness
- diplopia
- ataxia
- nausea
- vomiting
- abnormal gait
- tremor
- aggravated seizures
- abdominal pain.
  Some less common reactions include:
- agitation
- confusion
- hypotension
- hyponatremia
- rhinitis
- speech disorder
- back pain
- upper respiratory tract infection.
  About 20% to 30% of patients who have had an allergic reaction to carbamazepine will experience a hypersensitivity reaction to oxcarbazepine.

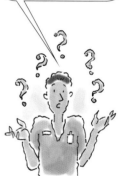

Quiz the patient about a history of hypersensitivity to carbamazepine.

The Three-Step Approach

Nursing management for patients undergoing treatment with carboxamide anticonvulsant drugs includes these three steps:

Preadministration

(Prioritize and analyze cues)
- Obtain a history of the patient's seizure disorder before therapy.

(Prioritize hypothesis—priority patient problems)
- Injury risk

- Mobility impairment
- Nonadherence

(Generate solutions)
- Risk to the patient will be minimized.
- The patient will be able to perform ADLs.
- The patient will exhibit behaviors that demonstrate willingness to comply with long-term therapy.
- The patient and family will demonstrate an understanding of drug therapy.

Medication administration
(Take action)
- Withdraw the drug gradually to minimize the risk of increased seizure frequency.
- Correct hyponatremia as needed.

A "shaky" situation
- For an oral suspension, shake well before administration. It can be mixed with water or may be swallowed directly from the syringe. It can be taken without regard to food. Oral suspensions and tablets may be interchanged at equal doses.
- Expect to adjust the dosage according to the patient's response.
- Assess for immediate adverse reactions and drug interactions.
- Administer safety precautions if the patient has adverse CNS reactions.

Postadministration
(Evaluate outcomes)
- Assess the patient's physical mobility.
- Promote measures that encourage safe and efficient mobility.
- Question the patient about a history of hypersensitivity reactions to carbamazepine.
- Obtain a history of the patient's underlying condition before therapy and reassess it regularly thereafter.
- Monitor the patient's serum levels and response to the prescribed drug as indicated.
- Monitor the patient for adverse reactions.
- Assess the patient's compliance with therapy at each follow-up visit.

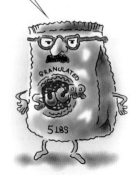

These sulfamate-substituted monosaccharides may be derived from the natural monosaccharide D-fructose, but I bet I taste sweeter.

Sulfamate-substituted monosaccharides

Sulfamate-substituted monosaccharides are structurally distinct from other anticonvulsant drug classes. The effect is to block the spread of seizures rather than to raise the threshold (like other anticonvulsant drugs). This class of drugs is derived from the natural monosaccharide D-fructose. Topiramate (Topamax) is an anticonvulsant drug in this class.

Pharmacokinetics

Topiramate is rapidly absorbed by the body. It's partially metabolized in the liver and excreted mostly unchanged in urine. For the patient with renal impairment (creatinine clearance less than 70 mL/minute), the dosage of topiramate is reduced.

Pharmacodynamics

Topiramate is believed to act by blocking voltage-dependent sodium channels, enhancing the activity of GABA receptors and antagonizing glutamate receptors.

Pharmacotherapeutics

Topiramate is approved as adjunctive therapy for partial and primary generalized tonic-clonic seizures in adults and children older than age 2 and for children with Lennox-Gastaut syndrome. The drug may also prove beneficial for other types of seizures and as monotherapy.

Drug interactions

Carbamazepine, phenytoin, and valproic acid may cause decreased topiramate levels. Topiramate may decrease the efficacy of hormonal contraceptives and may decrease valproic acid levels. CNS depressants may be potentiated when combined with topiramate.

Side effects/Adverse reactions

Psychomotor slowing, difficulty finding words, impaired concentration, and memory impairment are common and may require stopping the drug. Low starting doses and slow titration may minimize these effects.

Other common adverse reactions to topiramate include:

- drowsiness
- dizziness
- headache
- ataxia
- nervousness
- confusion
- paresthesia
- weight gain
- diplopia.

Serious but uncommon adverse reactions include:

- anemia
- liver failure
- hypohidrosis
- hyperthermia
- heatstroke
- renal calculi.

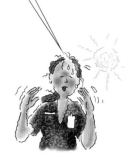

Serious but uncommon adverse reactions to topiramate include hyperthermia and heatstroke. Whew! Is it getting hotter, or is it just me?

The Three-Step Approach

Nursing management for patients undergoing treatment with sulfamate-substituted monosaccharide anticonvulsant drugs includes these three steps:

Preadministration

(Recognize and analyze cues)
- Assess the patient's seizure disorder before therapy.

(Prioritize hypothesis—priority patient problems)
- Injury risk
- Mobility impairment
- Nonadherence

(Generate solutions)
- Risk to the patient will be minimized.
- The patient will be able to perform ADLs.
- The patient will exhibit behaviors that demonstrate a willingness to comply with long-term drug therapy.
- The patient and family will demonstrate an understanding of drug therapy.

Medication administration

(Take action)
- Administer oral forms of the drug with food to reduce GI irritation.
- Expect to adjust the dosage according to the patient's response.
- Administer safety precautions if the patient has adverse CNS reactions.

Dial up the dose for hemodialysis

- The patient with renal insufficiency requires a reduced dosage. For the patient on hemodialysis, supplemental doses may be needed to avoid rapid drops in drug levels during prolonged treatment.
- Discontinue the drug if an ocular adverse event occurs, characterized by acute myopia and secondary angle-closure glaucoma.
- Assess for immediate adverse reactions and drug interactions.

Postadministration

(Evaluate outcomes)
- Monitor the patient for injury.
- Assess the patient's physical mobility.
- Promote measures that encourage safe and efficient mobility.
- Carefully monitor the patient taking topiramate in conjunction with other antiepileptic drugs; dosage adjustments may be needed to achieve an optimal response.
- Monitor the patient's serum levels and response to the prescribed drug as indicated.

- Monitor the patient for adverse reactions.
- Monitor the patient's body temperature, especially during the summer, because hyperthermia can occur resulting in heatstroke.
- Assess the patient's compliance with therapy, including at each follow-up visit.

Succinimides

The succinimide, ethosuximide (Zarontin), is used for the management of absence seizures. Ethosuximide is considered the drug of choice for this indication.

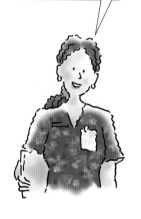

> Ethosuximide is considered the drug of choice for absence seizures.

Pharmacokinetics

The succinimides are readily absorbed from the GI tract, metabolized in the liver, and excreted in urine. Metabolites are believed to be inactive. The elimination half-life of ethosuximide is about 60 hours in adults and 30 hours in children.

Pharmacodynamics

Ethosuximide raises the seizure threshold; it suppresses the characteristic spike-and-wave pattern by depressing neuronal transmission in the motor cortex and basal ganglia. It's indicated for absence seizures.

Pharmacotherapeutics

The only indication for ethosuximide is the treatment of absence seizures. It's the treatment of choice for this type of seizure disorder but may be used in combination with valproic acid for difficult-to-control absence seizures.

Drug interactions

Ethosuximide may interact with concurrently administered anticonvulsant drugs. It can also elevate serum phenytoin levels. Carbamazepine may induce the metabolism of ethosuximide. Valproic acid may increase or decrease levels of ethosuximide.

Side effects/Adverse reactions

Ethosuximide is generally well tolerated and causes few adverse reactions. The most common effects include anorexia, nausea, and vomiting (in up to 40% of cases). Other common adverse effects include:
- drowsiness and fatigue
- lethargy
- dizziness
- hiccups
- headaches
- mood changes.

Rarely, blood dyscrasias, rashes (including Stevens-Johnson syndrome, erythema multiforme, and lupuslike syndrome), and psychotic behavior can occur.

The Three-Step Approach

Nursing management for patients undergoing treatment with succinimide anticonvulsant drugs includes these three steps:

Preadministration

(Recognize and analyze cues)
• Assess the patient's seizure disorder before therapy.

(Prioritize hypothesis—priority patient problems)
• Injury risk
• Mobility impairment
• Nonadherence

(Generate solutions)
• The risk to the patient will be minimized.
• The patient will be able to perform ADLs.
• The patient will exhibit behaviors that demonstrate a willingness to comply with long-term therapy.
• The patient and family will demonstrate an understanding of drug therapy.

Medication administration

(Take action)
• Administer oral forms of the drug with food to reduce GI irritation.
• Expect to adjust the dosage according to the patient's response.
• Administer safety precautions if the patient has adverse CNS reactions.
• Assess for immediate adverse reactions and drug interactions.

Postadministration

(Evaluate outcomes)
• Assess the patient for injury.
• Assess the patient's physical mobility.
• Promote measures that encourage safe and efficient mobility.
• Monitor the patient's serum levels and response to the prescribed drug as indicated.
• Monitor the patient for adverse reactions.
• Assess the patient's compliance with therapy at each follow-up visit.

Sulfonamides

Sulfonamides are a group of compounds consisting of amides of sulfanilic acid. They're known for their bacteriostatic effects; they interfere with the functioning of the enzyme necessary for bacteria metabolism, growth, and multiplication. Zonisamide (Zonegran), a sulfonamide, is approved for the adjunctive treatment of partial seizures in adults.

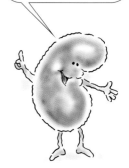

Start zonisamide at a low dose in older patients because of the possibility of renal impairment.

Pharmacokinetics

Peak concentrations of zonisamide occur within 2 to 6 hours of administration. The drug is widely distributed and is extensively bound to erythrocytes. Zonisamide is metabolized by the CYP3A4 enzyme in the liver and is excreted in urine, primarily as the parent drug and the glucuronide metabolite. Low doses should be initiated in elderly patients because of the possibility of renal impairment.

Pharmacodynamics

The precise mechanism of zonisamide is unknown, but it's believed to involve stabilization of neuronal membranes and suppression of neuronal hypersensitivity.

Pharmacotherapeutics

Zonisamide is approved only as adjunctive therapy for partial seizures in adults. Despite its limited indication, it has demonstrated usefulness in other types of seizure activity (infantile spasms and myoclonic, generalized, and atypical absence seizures).

Drug interactions

Drugs that induce liver enzymes (such as phenytoin, carbamazepine, or phenobarbital) increase the metabolism and decrease the half-life of zonisamide. Concurrent use of zonisamide with drugs that inhibit or induce CYP3A4 can be expected to increase or decrease the serum concentration of zonisamide. Zonisamide isn't an inducer of CYP3A4, so it's unlikely to affect other drugs metabolized by the CYP3A4 system.

Side effects/Adverse reactions

Common adverse reactions to zonisamide include:
- somnolence
- dizziness
- confusion
- anorexia
- nausea
- diarrhea
- weight loss
- rash.

Slow she goes

Slow titration of the dosage and administration with meals may decrease the incidence of adverse reactions.

Serious sides

More serious adverse reactions that have been associated with zonisamide include:

- Stevens-Johnson syndrome
- toxic epidermal necrolysis
- psychosis
- aplastic anemia
- agranulocytosis
- oligohidrosis, hyperthermia, and heatstroke (in children). Zonisamide is contraindicated in patients with allergies to sulfonamides. Zonisamide should be avoided in pregnancy and its disposition in breastmilk is unknown and its disposition in breast milk is unknown. The safety and effectiveness of the drug in children younger than age 16 hasn't been established. The use of zonisamide in patients with renal clearances of less than 50 mL/minute isn't recommended.

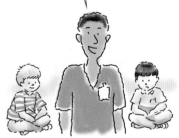

The safety and effectiveness of zonisamide in children younger than age 16 hasn't been established.

The Three-Step Approach

Nursing management for patients undergoing treatment with sulfonamide anticonvulsant drugs includes the following three steps:

Preadministration

(Recognize and analyze cues)
- Obtain a history of the patient's underlying condition before therapy.

(Priority hypothesis—priority patient problems)
- Injury risk
- Mobility impairment
- Nonadherence

(Generate solutions)
- Risk to the patient will be minimized.
- The patient will be able to perform ADLs.
- The patient will exhibit behavior that demonstrate a willingness to comply with drug therapy.
- The patient and family will demonstrate an understanding of drug therapy.

Medication administration

(Take action)
- The drug may be taken with or without food. Tell the patient not to bite or break the capsule.
- Use cautiously in the patient with hepatic or renal disease; the patient may need slower adjustments and more frequent

monitoring. If the patient's glomerular filtration rate is less than 50 mL/minute, don't use the drug.

- Reduce the dosage or discontinue the drug gradually; abrupt withdrawal of the drug may cause increased frequency of seizures or status epilepticus.
- Increase the patient's fluid intake to help increase urine output and help prevent renal calculi, especially if the patient has predisposing factors.
- Expect to adjust the drug dosage according to the patient's response.
- Assess for immediate adverse reactions and drug interactions.
- Administer safety precautions if the patient has adverse CNS reactions.

Postadministration

(Evaluate outcomes)

- Assess the patient for injury.
- Assess the patient's physical mobility.
- Promote measures that encourage safe and efficient mobility.
- Monitor the patient's body temperature, especially during the summer, because decreased sweating may occur (especially in children ages 17 and younger), resulting in heatstroke and dehydration.
- Monitor the patient's renal function periodically.
- Monitor the patient's serum levels and response to the prescribed drug as indicated.
- Monitor the patient for hypersensitivity or adverse reactions.
- Assess the patient's adherence with therapy, including at each follow-up visit.

Antimigraine drugs

A migraine, an episodic headache disorder, is one of the most common primary headache disorders, affecting an estimated 24 million people in the United States. A migraine is usually described as a unilateral headache pain that's pounding, pulsating, or throbbing. It may be preceded by an aura. Other symptoms typically associated with a migraine are sensitivity to light or sound, nausea, vomiting, and constipation or diarrhea.

Current theories suggest that the symptoms of migraines are due to vasodilation or to the release of vasoactive and proinflammatory substances from nerves in an activated trigeminal system.

So many choices

Treatment for acute migraines is targeted at altering an attack after it's under way (abortive and symptomatic treatment) or preventing the attack before it begins (such as in chronic migraines). The choice of therapy depends on the severity, duration, frequency, and degree of disability the headache creates as well as the patient's characteristics. Abortive treatments may include analgesics (aspirin and acetaminophen), nonsteroidal anti-inflammatory drugs (NSAIDs), ergotamine (Cafergot), 5-HT agonists, and other miscellaneous agents (such intranasal butorphanol, metoclopramide [Reglan], and corticosteroids). Prophylactic therapy includes beta-adrenergic blockers, tricyclic antidepressants, valproic acid, and NSAIDs, to name a few. Additionally, several pharmacological modalities are employed for the long-term treatment of chronic migraines. When determining which specific modality is used, factors such as efficacy and patient-specific risk factors help determine where to begin. Beta-blockers, antidepressants, and anticonvulsant medications are most cited as first-line agents in the treatment of chronic migraines. Among these classes, the specific medications commonly used for first-line treatment include propranolol, amitriptyline, topiramate, and valproic acid (Urits et al., 2020).

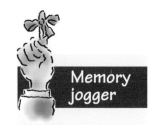

Memory jogger

How can you tell if it's a migraine or a headache? Look at the **PAIN** to see if the patient has these key symptoms:

Pain
Aura
Irritated by light
Nausea.

5-HT agonists

The 5-HT agonists, commonly known as the *triptans*, are the treatment of choice for moderate to severe migraine. Drugs in this class include:
- almotriptan (Almotriptan Malate)
- eletriptan (Relpax)
- frovatriptan (Frova)
- naratriptan (Amerge)
- rizatriptan (Maxalt)
- sumatriptan (Imitrex)
- zolmitriptan (Zomig).

Pharmacokinetics

When comparing the triptans, key pharmacokinetic features are onset of effect and duration of action. Most triptans have a half-life of approximately 2 hours; almotriptan and eletriptan have half-lives of 3 to 4 hours, naratriptan has a half-life of about 6 hours, and frovatriptan has the longest half-life (25 hours) and the most delayed onset of action.

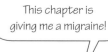

This chapter is giving me a migraine!

Freedom of choice

All of the triptans are available in an oral formulation. Rizatriptan is available in a rapid-dissolve tablet, and sumatriptan is also available in injectable and intranasal formulations. The injectable form of sumatriptan has the most rapid onset of action.

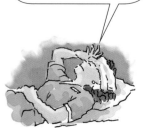

Pharmacodynamics

Triptans are specific serotonin 5-HT$_1$ receptor agonists that result in cranial vessel constriction as well as inhibition and reduction of the inflammatory process along the trigeminal nerve pathway. These actions may abort or provide symptomatic relief for a migraine. Triptans are effective in controlling the pain, nausea, and vomiting associated with migraines.

Pharmacotherapeutics

The choice of a triptan depends on patient preferences for dosage form (if nausea and vomiting are present), presence of recurrent migraine, and formulary restrictions. A patient experiencing nausea and vomiting may prefer injectable or intranasal sumatriptan. Recurrent migraines may respond better to triptans with longer half-lives, such as frovatriptan and naratriptan; however, these drugs have delayed onset of effects. Two newer triptans, almotriptan and eletriptan, have rapid onset and an intermediate half-life.

Triptans have many contraindications and should not be used in patients with certain conditions. (See *Contra-triptans.*)

Before you give that drug!

Contra-triptans

Before administering triptans to a patient, be aware of these contraindications:

A hearty no

Triptans are contraindicated in patients with ischemic heart disease (such as angina pectoris, history of myocardial infarction, or documented silent ischemia) and in patients who have symptoms or findings consistent with ischemic heart disease, coronary artery vasospasm (including Prinzmetal's variant angina), or other significant underlying cardiovascular conditions.

No strokes allowed

Triptans shouldn't be prescribed for patients with cerebrovascular syndromes (such as strokes of any type or transient ischemic attacks) or for patients with peripheral vascular disease, including, but not limited to, ischemic bowel disease. Triptans also shouldn't be given to patients with uncontrolled hypertension or to patients with hemiplegic or basilar migraines.

Not for the faint of heart

Triptans aren't recommended for use in the patient who has coronary artery disease (CAD) or risk factors for CAD (such as hypertension, hypercholesterolemia, smoking, obesity, diabetes, a strong family history of CAD, or age [risk increases in surgically or physiologically menopausal women and in men over age 40]) unless a cardiovascular evaluation provides satisfactory evidence that the patient is reasonably free from underlying cardiovascular disease. If a triptan is used for a patient who has any of these risk factors, it's strongly recommended that the first dose be administered in a doctor's office or other medically staffed and equipped facility.

It's further suggested that intermittent, long-term users of 5-HT agonists or those who have or acquire risk factors undergo periodic cardiac evaluation.

More than 3 in 30

The safety of treating an average of more than three migraine attacks in a 30-day period hasn't been established.

Drug interactions

These drug interactions are possible when taking triptans:
- The administration of a triptan within 24 hours of treatment with another 5-HT$_1$ agonist ergotamine-containing or ergot-type medication (such as dihydroergotamine) may cause prolonged vasospastic reactions. The use of ergot-containing medications and 5-HT agonists within 24 hours of each other should be avoided.

A timely warning

- Eletriptan shouldn't be used within at least 72 hours of treatment with the following potent CYP3A4 inhibitors: ketoconazole, itraconazole, nefazodone, clarithromycin, ritonavir, and nelfinavir, or other drugs that have demonstrated potent CYP3A4 inhibition.
- Almotriptan, rizatriptan, sumatriptan, and zolmitriptan shouldn't be used with or within 2 weeks of discontinuing an MAO inhibitor.
- Although rare, SSRIs, such as citalopram, fluoxetine, fluvoxamine, paroxetine, and sertraline, have been reported to cause weakness, hyperreflexia, and incoordination when coadministered with 5-HT$_1$ agonists. Monitor the patient closely if concomitant treatment with a triptan and an SSRI is clinically warranted. This reaction has also been reported with coadministration of a triptan and sibutramine.
- The bioavailability of frovatriptan is 30% higher in a patient taking oral forms of hormonal contraceptives.
- Propranolol increases the bioavailability of zolmitriptan, rizatriptan, frovatriptan, and eletriptan.

Side effects/Adverse reactions

Side effects/adverse reactions to triptans include:
- tingling
- warm or hot sensations or flushing
- nasal and throat discomfort
- visual disturbances
- paresthesia
- dizziness
- weakness and fatigue
- somnolence
- chest pain or pressure
- neck or throat pain
- jaw pain or pressure
- dry mouth
- dyspepsia
- nausea

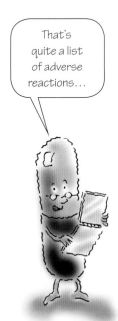

That's quite a list of adverse reactions...

- sweating
- injection site reaction (subcutaneous sumatriptan)
- taste disturbances (intranasal sumatriptan).

The heart takes part

Serious cardiac events, including acute myocardial infarction, arrhythmias, and death, have been reported within a few hours after taking triptans. However, the incidence of these events is considered extremely low.

The Three-Step Approach

Nursing management for patients undergoing treatment with triptans includes the following three steps:

Preadministration
(Recognize and analyze cues)
- Assess the patient's condition to establish a baseline before drug therapy.
- Obtain a list of the patient's medication intake within the previous 24 hours to prevent drug interactions.
- Use caution when giving the drug to a patient who is taking an MAO inhibitor or a CYP4503A4 or CYP4502D6 inhibitor.
- Don't give the drug with other serotonin agonist or ergotamine derivatives.

(Prioritize hypothesis—priority patient problems)
- Acute pain
- Injury risk
- Knowledge deficiency

(Generate solutions)
- The patient will state that pain is decreased.
- Risk of injury to the patient will be reduced.
- The patient and family will verbalize an understanding of drug therapy.

Medication administration
(Take action)
- Give the dose as soon as the patient complains of migraine symptoms.
- Reduce the dosage in a patient with poor renal or hepatic function.
- Repeat the dose as ordered and as needed, and monitor the patient for effect.
- Don't give more than two doses within 24 hours.
- Assess for immediate adverse reactions and drug interactions.
- These drugs aren't intended for the patient with ischemic heart disease or hemiplegic or basilar migraines.

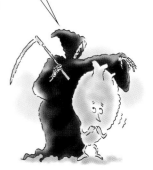

I don't like the sound of these "serious cardiac events" that triptans may trigger. Thank goodness they're rare!

Teaching about migraine drugs

If migraine drugs are prescribed, review these points with the patient and caregivers:

• Take the drug exactly as prescribed, such as only when you're having a migraine, and repeat the dosage as per the prescriber's orders. Don't exceed the prescribed dosage.

• Avoid possible migraine triggers, such as cheese, chocolate, citrus fruits, caffeine, and alcohol.

• Don't take other medicines, over-the-counter preparations, or herbal preparations without first consulting with your prescriber. Drug interactions can occur.

• Immediately report adverse reactions (chest, throat, jaw, or neck tightness; pain; or heaviness) to the prescriber and discontinue use of the drug until further notice.

• Use caution when driving or operating machinery while taking migraine drugs.

Postadministration

(Evaluate outcomes)

• Assess the patient's symptoms, including pain.
• Evaluate the patient's and family's knowledge of drug therapy. (See *Teaching about migraine drugs.*)
• Monitor closely for adverse reactions.
• Monitor the ECG in a patient with risk factors for CAD or with symptoms like those of CAD, such as chest or throat tightness, pain, and heaviness.

Ergotamine preparations

Ergotamine and its derivatives may be used as abortive or symptomatic therapy for migraines.

Common preparations used for migraines include:

• ergotamine—sublingual or oral tablet or suppository (combined with caffeine) (Cafergot, Migranal)
• dihydroergotamine—injectable or intranasal (Embolex).

Pharmacokinetics

Ergotamine is incompletely absorbed from the GI tract. The intranasal form of dihydroergotamine is rapidly absorbed. Peak plasma concentrations, following subcutaneous injection, occur within 45 minutes, and 90% of the dose is plasma protein bound. Ergotamine is metabolized in the liver, and 90% of the metabolites are excreted in bile; traces of unchanged drug are excreted in urine.

Pharmacodynamics

Ergotamine-derivative antimigraine effects are believed to be due to a blockade of neurogenic inflammation. These drugs also act as partial agonists or antagonists at serotonin, dopaminergic, and alpha-adrenergic receptors, depending on their site. Ergotamine preparations commonly need to be prescribed with antiemetic preparations when used for migraines.

Dihydroergotamine, a hydrogenated form of ergotamine, differs mainly in the degree of activity. It has less vasoconstrictive action than ergotamine and much less emetic potential.

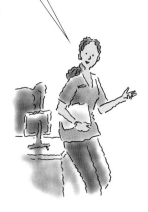

When prescribed for migraines, an ergotamine preparation is commonly accompanied by an antiemetic.

Pharmacotherapeutics

Ergotamine preparations are used to prevent or treat vascular headaches, such as migraines, migraine variants, and cluster headaches. Dihydroergotamine is used when rapid control of migraines is desired or when other routes are undesirable.

Drug interactions

These drug interactions can occur in a patient taking ergotamine preparations:

Getting cold feet

- Propranolol and other beta-adrenergic blockers close the natural pathway for vasodilation in the patient receiving ergotamine preparations, resulting in excessive vasoconstriction and cold extremities.
- The patient may be at increased risk for weakness, hyperflexion, and incoordination when ergotamine preparations are used with SSRIs.
- Sumatriptan may cause an additive effect when taken with ergotamine derivatives, increasing the risk of coronary vasospasm. An ergotamine preparation shouldn't be given within 24 hours of administration of a triptan.
- Drugs inhibiting CYP3A4 enzymes (such as erythromycin, clarithromycin, troleandomycin, ritonavir, nelfinavir, indinavir, and azole-derivative antifungal agents) may alter the metabolism of ergotamine, resulting in increased serum concentrations of ergotamine. This increases the risk of vasospasm and cerebral or peripheral ischemia. These drugs shouldn't be used together.
- Vasoconstrictors may cause an additive effect when given with ergotamine preparations, increasing the risk of high blood pressure.

Side effects/Adverse reactions

Side effects/adverse reactions to ergotamine derivatives include:
- nausea

- vomiting
- numbness
- tingling
- muscle pain
- leg weakness
- itching.

Prolonged administration of ergotamine derivatives may result in ergotism, gangrene, and rebound headaches.

The Three-Step Approach

Nursing management for patients undergoing treatment with ergotamine preparations includes the following three steps:

Preadministration

(Recognize and analyze cues)
- Assess the patient's baseline condition before initiating drug therapy.

(Prioritize hypothesis—priority patient problems)
- Acute pain
- Injury risk
- Knowledge deficiency

(Generate solutions)
- The patient will acknowledge a decrease in pain.
- Injury risk to the patient will be reduced.
- The patient and family will verbalize an understanding of drug therapy.

Medication administration

(Take action)
- Give the dose as soon as the patient reports migraine symptoms.
- Avoid prolonged administration and don't exceed the recommended dosage.
- Tell the patient to withhold food and drink while the sublingual tablets are dissolving. Sublingual tablets are preferred during the early stage of an attack because of their rapid absorption.
- Assess for immediate adverse reactions or drug interactions.
- Monitor the patient for signs of vasoconstriction and report them to the prescriber.
- Assess the patient for coronary, cerebral, or peripheral vascular disease; hypertension; and liver or kidney disease. These are contraindications to the use of ergotamine preparations.

Postadministration

(Evaluate outcomes)
- Assess the patient's symptoms frequently.

- Evaluate for the development of serious complications from drug interactions.
- Evaluate the patient's and family's understanding of drug therapy.
- Be alert for adverse reactions and drug interactions.

On the rebound

- Be alert for ergotamine rebound or an increase in the frequency and duration of headaches, which may occur if the drug is discontinued suddenly.
- Monitor the ECG in a patient with risk factors for CAD or with symptoms similar to those of CAD, such as chest or throat tightness, pain, and heaviness.

Quick quiz

1. Which assessment data are associated with abrupt discontinuation of intrathecal baclofen? **Select all that apply**.
   A. Altered mental status
   B. Lowered body temperature
   C. Muscle rigidity
   D. Exaggerated rebound spasticity
   E. Pupillary dilation

Answer: A, C, D. Abrupt cessation of intrathecal baclofen may result in altered mental status, high fever (not lowered body temperature), muscle rigidity, and exaggerated rebound spasticity. Pupil dilation is not affected by abrupt discontinuation of intrathecal baclofen.

2. An 83-year-old patient with partial seizures and a history of chronic kidney disease has been prescribed oxcarbazepine. Which information will the nurse consider prior to administration of this medication?
   A. Reduced doses are necessary in patients with actual or risk of impaired renal function.
   B. Increased safety measures should be put in place as this medication is known to cause insomnia in some patients.
   C. Serum levels are not required to be monitored with this medication.
   D. This medication does not require a slow taper to stop therapy; it can be stopped abruptly.

Answer: A. When administered to patients with altered kidney function or kidney disease (actual) or those at increased risk of altered kidney function or kidney disease (such as the elderly), reduced dosing is necessary.

3. A 48-year-old patient has been prescribed phenytoin to treat seizure disorder. When teaching about this medication, which patient statement requires further nursing intervention?

    A. "I will take this medication exactly as prescribed and won't stop without medical supervision."

    B. "It is ok to switch between the generic and brand names of this medication if the prescription changes."

    C. "I know that my urine may become discolored with this medication."

    D. "I need to have good oral hygiene while taking this medication."

Answer: B. The patient should NOT change brands or dosage forms of this medication. It is important to take the same brand to avert any unwanted adverse reactions or decreased efficacy of the medication.

4. Which medication can alter the effectiveness of nondepolarizing neuromuscular blockers?

    A. Aspirin

    B. Cephalosporin antibiotics

    C. Anesthetics

    D. Acetaminophen

Answer: C. The concomitant use of anesthetics may potentiate or exaggerate the neuromuscular blockade of this medication. Additionally, concomitant aminoglycoside antibiotic use may have the same effect.

Scoring

☆☆☆ If you answered all four questions correctly, marvelous! Your knowledge has a rapid onset and long duration.

☆☆ If you answered three questions correctly, congrats! You obviously answered these questions about neurologic drugs logically.

☆ If you answered two or less questions correctly, don't worry. Just give yourself another dose of this chapter and recheck the results.

Suggested References

Gustafson, K., & Brown, A. (2017). Neuromuscular blocking agents: Use and controversy in the hospital setting. *U.S. Pharmacist, 42*(1), HS16–HS20.

Meoni, S., Macerollo, A., & Moro, E. (2020). Sex differences in movement disorders. *Nature Reviews Neurology, 16*(2), 84–96. https://doi-org.echo.louisville.edu/10.1038/s41582-019-0294-x

Rajan, R., Saini, A., Verma, B., Choudhary, N., Gupta, A., & Vishnu, V., et al. (2020). Anticholinergics may carry significant cognitive and Gait burden in

Parkinson's Disease. *Movement Disorders Clinical Practice, 7*(7), 803–809. https://doi.org/10.1002/mdc3.13032

Trueman, C., Castillo, S., O'Brien, K., & Hoie, E. (2020). Inappropriate use of skeletal muscle relaxants in geriatric patients. *U.S. Pharmacist, 45*(1), 25–29.

Urits, I., Gress, K., Charipova, K., Zamarripa, A., Patel, P., & Lassiter, G., et al. (2020). Pharmacological options for the treatment of chronic migraine pain. *Best Practice & Research: Clinical Anaesthesiology, 34*(3), 383–407.

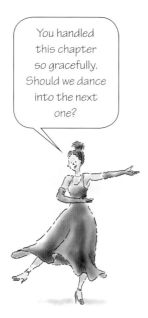

Chapter 8

Cardiovascular drugs

Just the facts

In this chapter, you'll learn:

◆ classes of drugs used to treat cardiovascular disorders

◆ uses and varying actions of these drugs

◆ absorption, distribution, metabolization, and excretion of these drugs

◆ drug interactions and adverse reactions to these drugs

Drugs and the cardiovascular system

Components of the cardiovascular system include the heart, arteries, capillaries, veins, and lymphatics. These structures transport life-supporting oxygen and nutrients to cells, remove metabolic waste products, and carry hormones from one part of the body to another. Because this system performs such vital functions, any problem with the heart or blood vessels can seriously affect a person's health.

Types of drugs used to improve cardiovascular function include:
- inotropic drugs
- antiarrhythmic drugs
- antianginal drugs
- antihypertensive drugs
- diuretics (See Chapter 11, Genitourinary drugs, for a full discussion.)
- antilipemic drugs.

Inotropic drugs

Inotropic drugs influence the strength or contractility of muscle tissue. As a result, they increase the force of the heart's contractions (this is known as a *positive inotropic effect*). Cardiac glycosides (digoxin), phosphodiesterase (PDE) inhibitors (milrinone), and beta adrenergic receptor agonists (dobutamine, epinephrine) are types of inotropic drugs. Digoxin is the only oral form of positive inotropic drug available.

In slow motion

Cardiac glycosides also slow the heart rate (a negative chronotropic effect) and slow electrical impulse conduction through the atrioventricular (AV) node (a negative dromotropic effect). This action is useful for patients who have atrial fibrillation; it can help to control their heart rate and to prevent the heart rate from becoming too fast.

Increased perfusion of the tissues improves function and helps decrease interstitial fluid buildup (edema).

Inotropic agents may also prevent remodeling of the left or right ventricle (called *cardiac* or *ventricular remodeling*) that occurs in heart failure.

> Digoxin gives me a real boost.

Cardiac glycosides

Cardiac glycosides are a group of drugs derived from digitalis, a substance that occurs naturally in foxglove plants. The most commonly used cardiac glycoside is digoxin. (See *Cardiac glycosides: Digoxin.*) Prior to evidence-based practice heart failure guidelines, digoxin was a mainstay in the treatment of heart failure. Over the years, studies have demonstrated that digoxin is effective at reducing morbidity and readmission rates for patients (Ponikowski et al., 2016). However, mortality has not decreased and in some cases, actually increased. Nevertheless, digoxin can be considered as a

Prototype pro

Cardiac glycosides: Digoxin (Lanoxin)

Actions
- Inhibits sodium-potassium–activated adenosine triphosphatase, an enzyme that regulates the amount of sodium and potassium inside the cell, resulting in increased intracellular levels of sodium and calcium
- Promotes movement of calcium from extracellular to intracellular cytoplasm and strengthens myocardial contraction
- Acts on the central nervous system (CNS) to enhance vagal tone, slowing contractions through the sinoatrial (SA) and AV nodes and providing an antiarrhythmic effect

Indications
- Heart failure
- Atrial fibrillation and flutter
- Supraventricular tachycardia

Nursing considerations
- Monitor the patient for adverse effects, such as fatigue, agitation, hallucinations, arrhythmias, anorexia, nausea, and diarrhea.
- Withhold the drug if the apical pulse is less than 60 beats/minute and notify the prescriber.
- Periodically monitor serum potassium and digoxin levels.
- Assess renal function because digoxin is excreted by the kidneys.

recommendation for heart failure treatment especially with those patients that have atrial fibrillation (Yancey et al., 2017).

Pharmacokinetics

The intestinal absorption of digoxin varies greatly. Capsules are absorbed most efficiently, followed by the elixir form, and then tablets. Digoxin is distributed widely throughout the body with highest concentrations in the heart muscle, liver, and kidneys. Digoxin is poorly bound to plasma proteins.

Going out the way it came in

In most patients, a small amount of digoxin is metabolized in the liver and gut by bacteria. This effect varies and may be substantial in some people. Most of the drug is excreted by the kidneys unchanged.

Pharmacodynamics

Digoxin is used to treat heart failure because it boosts intracellular calcium at the cell membrane, enabling stronger heart contractions. Digoxin may also enhance the movement of calcium into the myocardial cells and stimulate the release or block the reuptake of norepinephrine at the adrenergic nerve terminal.

What nerve!

Digoxin acts on the CNS to slow the heart rate, thus making it useful for treating supraventricular arrhythmias (an abnormal heart rhythm that originates above the bundle branches of the heart's conduction system), such as atrial fibrillation and atrial flutter. It also increases the refractory period (the period when the cells of the conduction system can't conduct an impulse).

Pharmacotherapeutics

In addition to treating heart failure and supraventricular arrhythmias, digoxin is used to treat paroxysmal atrial tachycardia (an arrhythmia marked by brief periods of tachycardia that alternate with brief periods of sinus rhythm) and atrial fibrillation. (See *Load that dose*.)

Drug interactions

Many drugs can interact with digoxin:
- Rifampin, barbiturates, cholestyramine, antacids, kaolin and pectin, sulfasalazine, neomycin, and metoclopramide reduce the therapeutic effects of digoxin.
- Calcium preparations, quinidine, verapamil, cyclosporine, tetracycline, nefazodone, clarithromycin, propafenone, amiodarone, spironolactone, hydroxychloroquine, erythromycin, itraconazole, and omeprazole increase the risk of digoxin toxicity.
- Amphotericin B, potassium-wasting diuretics, and steroids taken with digoxin may cause hypokalemia (low potassium levels) and increase the risk of digoxin toxicity.

Load that dose

Because digoxin (Lanoxin) has a long half-life, a loading dose must be given to a patient who requires immediate drug effects, as in supraventricular arrhythmia. By giving a larger initial dose, a minimum effective concentration of the drug in the blood may be reached faster. *Note:* Loading doses should be avoided in patients with heart failure to prevent toxicity.

- Beta-adrenergic blockers and calcium channel blockers taken with digoxin may cause an excessively slow heart rate and arrhythmias.
- Neuromuscular-blocking drugs, such as succinylcholine (Anectine), and thyroid preparations, such as levothyroxine (Synthroid), increase the risk of arrhythmias when taken with digoxin.

When herbs spice things up too much

- The herbal preparations St. John's wort and ginseng can increase levels of digoxin and increase the risk of toxicity. (See *Digoxin toxicity.*)

Side effects/Adverse reactions

Because cardiac glycosides have a narrow therapeutic index (margin of safety), they may produce digoxin toxicity. To prevent digoxin toxicity, the dosage should be individualized based on the patient's serum digoxin concentration.

Signs and symptoms of digoxin toxicity include:
- nausea and vomiting
- abdominal pain
- diarrhea
- headache
- irritability
- depression
- insomnia
- confusion
- vision changes (blurred or yellow vision)
- arrhythmias (bradycardia)
- complete heart block.

The Three-Step Approach

Preadministration
(Recognize and analyze cues)
- Obtain a history of the underlying condition before therapy.
- Monitor digoxin levels (therapeutic blood levels range from 0.5 to 2 ng/mL). Obtain blood for digoxin levels 8 hours after the last dose by mouth (PO).
- Closely monitor potassium levels.

Pay attention to the pulse

- Before giving the drug, take the patient's apical pulse for 1 full minute. Record and report to the prescriber significant changes (a sudden increase or decrease in pulse rate, pulse deficit, irregular beats, and regularization of a previously irregular rhythm). If these changes occur, check the patient's blood pressure and obtain a 12-lead ECG.

Digoxin toxicity

Digoxin (Lanoxin) has a narrow therapeutic index, so a dose adequate to produce therapeutic effects may produce signs of toxicity. Individuals with hypokalemia can develop digoxin toxicity even when their digoxin levels aren't elevated. Signs of digoxin toxicity include:
- slow to rapid ventricular rhythms
- nausea and vomiting
- blurred vision
- anorexia
- abdominal discomfort
- mental changes.

Antidote

Digoxin immune Fab is an antigen-binding fragment (Fab) derived from specific anti-digoxin antibodies. Dosage is determined by the serum digoxin level or the estimated amount of digoxin ingested.

- Withhold the drug and notify the prescriber if the pulse rate slows to 60 beats/minute or less.

(Prioritize hypothesis—priority patient problems)
- Altered tissue perfusion
- Electrolyte imbalance risk
- Knowledge deficiency

(Generate solutions)
- The patient will maintain tissue perfusion and electrolyte balance as demonstrated by vital signs, urine output, and level of consciousness.
- The patient will demonstrate correct drug administration and will verbalize correct symptoms of digoxin toxicity.

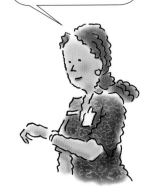

Before giving digoxin, take the patient's apical pulse for 1 full minute.

Medication administration

(Take action)
- Monitor drug effectiveness by taking the patient's apical pulse for 1 minute before each dose. Evaluate the electrocardiogram (ECG) when ordered and regularly assess the patient's cardiopulmonary status for signs of improvement.
- Be alert for adverse reactions and drug interactions.
- Patients with hypothyroidism are extremely sensitive to cardiac glycosides and may need lower doses. Reduce the dosage in patients with impaired renal function.
- Before giving a loading dose, obtain baseline data (heart rate and rhythm, blood pressure, and electrolyte levels) and question the patient about recent use of cardiac glycosides (within the previous 3 weeks). The loading dose is always divided over the first 24 hours unless the clinical situation indicates otherwise.
- Infuse the IV form of the drug slowly over at least 5 minutes.
- Withhold the drug for 1 to 2 days before elective cardioversion. Adjust the dose after cardioversion.
- Remember that colestipol and cholestyramine bind with the drug in the intestine.
- Treat arrhythmias with lidocaine IV and treat potentially life-threatening toxicity with specific antigen-binding fragments (such as digoxin immune Fab, Digibind).
- Teach the patient about digoxin, including signs and symptoms of digoxin toxicity.

Postadministration

(Evaluate outcomes)
- Evaluate for adequate tissue perfusion and fluid balance.
- Monitor closely for signs of digoxin toxicity.
- Evaluate patient's and family's understanding of drug therapy. (See *Teaching about digoxin*, page 239.)

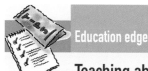

Teaching about digoxin (Lanoxin)

If digoxin is prescribed, review these points with the patient and caregivers:

• Digoxin helps strengthen the heartbeat and relieve ankle swelling, shortness of breath, and fatigue, which can accompany a heart problem.

• Take digoxin and other heart medications as prescribed, usually once daily, at the same time each day.

• Don't miss any doses of the medication.

• Don't take a double dose of the medication if a dose is missed.

• Don't take any over-the-counter (OTC) medications or herbal remedies without first consulting with your prescriber.

• You will need to have periodic physical examinations, ECGs, and blood tests (for digoxin as well as electrolyte levels) to see whether changes in dosages are needed.

• Report adverse effects, such as changes in heart rate or rhythm, nausea, vomiting, or vision problems, to your prescriber. These signs and symptoms may mean that your dosage needs to be changed.

• Limit salt intake and be sure to get enough potassium. Follow the diet set by your prescriber and don't take salt substitutes, such as potassium chloride, without first consulting with your prescriber.

• Use the same brand and type of digoxin all the time because forms and concentrations are different and aren't interchangeable.

• Take your pulse as instructed by your prescriber; count your pulse before each dose. If it's less than 60 beats/minute, call your prescriber.

• Don't crush digoxin capsules. Tablets may be crushed and can be taken with or after meals.

• If taking the liquid form of digoxin, measure accurately to prevent overdosage.

Antiarrhythmic drugs

Antiarrhythmic drugs are used to treat arrhythmias (disturbances in the normal heart rhythm).

For better or worse?

Unfortunately, many antiarrhythmic drugs can also worsen or cause the very arrhythmias they're supposed to treat. Therefore, the benefits of this therapy must always be weighed against its risks.

Antiarrhythmics are categorized into four classes:

• I (which includes classes IA, IB, and IC)
• II
• III
• IV.

Class I antiarrhythmics, the largest group of antiarrhythmic drugs, consist of sodium channel blockers. Class I agents are usually subdivided into classes IA, IB, and IC. One drug, adenosine (an AV

> Because many antiarrhythmic drugs can actually worsen the arrhythmias they're supposed to treat, the benefits must always be weighed against the risks.

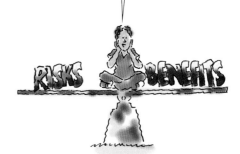

nodal-blocking agent used to treat paroxysmal supraventricular tachycardia [PSVT]), doesn't fall into any of these classes.

The mechanisms of action of antiarrhythmic drugs vary widely, and a few drugs exhibit properties common to more than one class.

Class IA antiarrhythmics

Class IA antiarrhythmics are used to treat a wide variety of atrial and ventricular arrhythmias. Class IA antiarrhythmics include:
- disopyramide phosphate (Norpace)
- procainamide hydrochloride
- quinidine (sulfate, gluconate)—not widely used.

Pharmacokinetics

When administered orally, class IA drugs are rapidly absorbed and metabolized. Because they work so quickly, sustained-release forms of these drugs are available to help maintain therapeutic levels.

The brainy one

These drugs are distributed through all body tissues. Quinidine, however, is the only one that crosses the blood-brain barrier.

All class IA antiarrhythmics are metabolized in the liver and are excreted unchanged by the kidneys. Acidic urine increases the excretion of quinidine.

Pharmacodynamics

Class IA antiarrhythmics control arrhythmias by altering the myocardial cell membrane and interfering with autonomic nervous system control of pacemaker cells. (See *How class I antiarrhythmics work*, page 241.)

No (para)sympathy

Class IA antiarrhythmics also block parasympathetic stimulation of the SA and AV nodes. Because stimulation of the parasympathetic nervous system causes the heart rate to slow down, drugs that block the parasympathetic nervous system increase the conduction rate of the AV node.

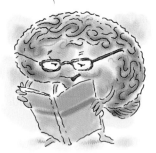

Quinidine is the only class IA antiarrhythmic that crosses the blood-brain barrier. Even I learn something new every day!

Pharm function

How class I antiarrhythmics work

All class I antiarrhythmics suppress arrhythmias by blocking the sodium channels in the cell membrane during an action potential, thereby interfering with the conduction of impulses along adjacent cardiac cells and producing a more membrane-stabilizing effect. The cardiac action potential, as illustrated below, occurs in five phases (0 through 4). Class I antiarrhythmics exert their effects during different phases of the action potential, binding quickly to sodium channels that are open or inactivated before repolarization occurs in the cell; they're most effective on tachycardia-type rhythms.

Phase 0: During this phase, sodium enters the cell and rapid depolarization takes place. Class IA and IB antiarrhythmics slow this phase of the action potential; class IC antiarrhythmics markedly slow the phase.

Phase 1: During this phase, sodium channels are inactivated.

Phase 2: During this plateau phase, sodium levels are equalized.

Phase 3: This marks when potassium leaves the cell and repolarization occurs. Class IA antiarrhythmics work during this phase to block sodium channels. Active transport via the sodium-potassium pump begins restoring potassium to the inside of the cell and sodium to the outside of the cell.

Phase 4: By this phase, potassium has left the cell, the cell membrane is impermeable to sodium, and the resting potential is restored. Then the cycle begins again.

Action potential curve: Pacemaker

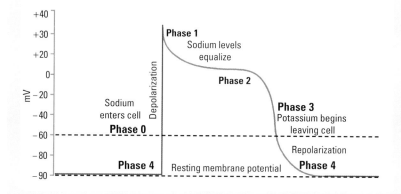

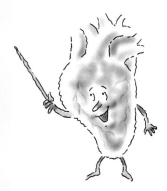

Prototype pro

Class IA antiarrhythmics

Black Box Warning: Increased mortality in treatment of non–life-threatening arrhythmia; increased risk if there is underlying structural heart disease ∎

Actions
- Causes direct and indirect effects on cardiac tissue
- Decreases automaticity, conduction velocity, and membrane responsiveness
- Prolongs effective refractory period

Indications (when other medications have failed)
- Atrial fibrillation, flutter, and tachycardia
- Premature atrial and ventricular contractions
- PSVT

Nursing considerations
- Monitor for adverse effects, such as vertigo, headache, arrhythmias, ECG changes (specifically, a widening QRS complex and prolonged QT interval), hypotension, heart failure, tinnitus, diarrhea, nausea, vomiting, hematologic disorders, hepatotoxicity, respiratory arrest, angioedema, fever, and temporary hearing loss.
- Frequently monitor pulse and blood pressure.
- Keep in mind that anticoagulation may be performed before treatment.

A chain reaction

This increase in conduction rate can produce dangerous increases in ventricular heart rate if rapid atrial activity is present, as in a patient with atrial fibrillation. In turn, the increased ventricular heart rate can offset the ability of the antiarrhythmics to convert atrial arrhythmias to a regular rhythm.

Pharmacotherapeutics

Class IA antiarrhythmics are used to treat certain arrhythmias, such as premature ventricular contractions, ventricular tachycardia, atrial fibrillation, atrial flutter, and paroxysmal atrial tachycardia. (See *Class IA antiarrhythmics.*)

Drug interactions

Class IA antiarrhythmics can interact with other drugs in various ways:
- Disopyramide (Norpace) taken with macrolide antibiotics, such as clarithromycin and erythromycin, increases the risk of QT interval prolongation, which may lead to an increased risk of arrhythmias, especially polymorphic ventricular tachycardia.
- Disopyramide (Norpace) plus verapamil may produce added myocardial depression and should be avoided in patients with heart failure.

- Class IA antiarrhythmics combined with other antiarrhythmics, such as beta-adrenergic blockers, increase the risk of arrhythmias, particularly bradycardia.
- Quinidine plus neuromuscular blockers cause increased skeletal muscle relaxation.
- Quinidine increases the risk of digoxin toxicity.
- Rifampin, phenytoin, and phenobarbital can reduce the effects of quinidine and disopyramide.
- Sodium bicarbonate and cimetidine may increase the level of quinidine, thiazide diuretics, and carbonic anhydrase inhibitors.
- Azole antifungals may increase the risk of cardiovascular events when used with quinidine; they shouldn't be used together.
- Grapefruit may delay the metabolism of quinidine.
- Verapamil significantly decreases hepatic clearance.

Side effects/Adverse reactions

Class IA antiarrhythmics, especially quinidine, commonly produce GI signs and symptoms, such as diarrhea, cramping, nausea, vomiting, anorexia, and bitter taste.

Good news, bad news

Ironically, not only do class IA antiarrhythmics treat arrhythmias, but they can also induce arrhythmias, especially conduction delays that may worsen existing heart blocks.

The Three-Step Approach

Nursing management for patients needing antiarrhythmic drugs includes these three steps.

Preadministration
(Recognize and analyze cues)

- Assess the patient's arrhythmia before therapy and regularly thereafter.
- Monitor the ECG continuously when therapy starts and when the dosage is adjusted. Specifically, monitor for ventricular arrhythmias and ECG changes (widening QRS complexes and a prolonged QT interval).
- Monitor the patient's vital signs frequently and assess for signs of toxicity.
- Measure apical pulse rate and blood pressure before giving the drug.
- Monitor serum drug levels as indicated.
- Monitor blood studies, such as liver function tests, as indicated.
- Be alert for adverse reactions and drug interactions.
- Evaluate the patient's and family's knowledge of drug therapy.

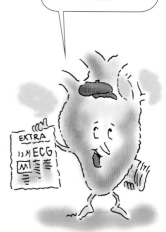

Have you heard the news? Class IA antiarrhythmics can induce arrhythmias as well as treat them.

- Monitor the patient's intake and output.
- Evaluate the patient's serum electrolyte levels.

(Prioritize hypothesis—priority patient problems)
- Altered tissue perfusion
- Hypotension risk
- Injury risk
- Knowledge deficiency

(Generate solutions)
- The patient will demonstrate sustained sinus rhythm without ectopy. Rhythm stability will contribute toward improved cardiac output and tissue perfusion as demonstrated by stable blood pressure, cardiac monitoring, and adequate urine output.
- The nurse will monitor closely for potential injury risks associated with complications from adverse reactions.
- The patient and family will demonstrate understanding of drug therapy.

Medication administration

(Take action)
- Don't crush sustained-release tablets.
- Notify the prescriber about adverse reactions.
- Use IV forms of these drugs to treat acute arrhythmias.

Postadministration

(Evaluate outcomes)
- Evaluate vital signs, mentation, urine output, skin color, and temperature to promptly recognize any alterations in tissue perfusion.
- The patient will not experience any serious adverse reactions.
- Evaluate patient's and family's understanding of drug therapy. (See *Teaching about antiarrhythmics*, page 245.)

Class IB antiarrhythmics

Class IB antiarrhythmics include mexiletine and lidocaine (Xylocaine); the latter is used to treat acute ventricular arrhythmias. Mexiletine is available as an oral medication, and lidocaine is available both as an intravenous (IV) form and oral form. Lidocaine can also be used as a topical, intrathecal, and intradermal anesthetic.

Pharmacokinetics

Mexiletine is absorbed well from the GI tract after oral administration.

Black Box Warning: Increased mortality: Restrict use to life-threatening ventricular arrhythmias. ∎

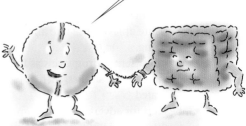

Don't worry! Plasma proteins like him can keep some antiarrhythmics occupied, but my "unbound" portion will still get the job done.

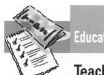

Teaching about antiarrhythmics

If antiarrhythmics are prescribed, review these points with the patient and caregivers:

• Antiarrhythmic drug therapy helps stop irregular beats in the heart and helps it to beat more effectively.

• It's important to take the drug exactly as prescribed. You may need to use an alarm clock or other reminders if the medication needs to be taken at odd hours around the clock.

• Take your pulse before each dose. Notify your prescriber if your pulse is irregular or less than 60 beats/minute.

• Avoid hazardous activities that require mental alertness if adverse CNS reactions occur.

• Limit fluid and salt intake if the prescribed drug causes fluid retention.

• Quinidine and disopyramide should be taken with food if GI upset occurs.

• Verapamil should be taken on an empty stomach or 1 to 2 hours after a meal.

• Some medications, such as quinidine, require you to limit intake of such foods as citrus juices, milk, and vegetables as well as avoid OTC drugs (such as antacids) that make urine alkaline.

• Report adverse effects, such as constipation or diarrhea, chest pain, difficulty breathing, ringing in the ears, swelling, unusually slow or fast pulse, sudden irregular pulse, or rash, to your prescriber.

• If tiredness occurs, space activities throughout the day and take periodic rest periods to help conserve energy.

• If nausea, vomiting, or loss of appetite occurs, eat small, frequent meals, or take the drug with meals, if appropriate.

• Some medications, such as disopyramide, may make you more sensitive to light, so avoid sunburn.

• Avoid OTC medications as well as herbal products unless approved by your prescriber. Many of these drugs and preparations can interfere with the action of antiarrhythmics.

• It's important to follow up with the prescriber to help evaluate heart rhythm and response to the drug.

• Don't stop taking the medication on your own; talk to your prescriber regarding any concerns.

It's (un)bound to happen

Lidocaine (Xylocaine) is distributed widely throughout the body, including the brain. Lidocaine and mexiletine are moderately bound to plasma proteins. (Remember, only the portion of a drug that's unbound can produce a response.)

Class IB antiarrhythmics are metabolized in the liver and excreted in the urine. Mexiletine also is excreted in breast milk.

Pharmacodynamics

Class IB drugs work by blocking the rapid influx of sodium ions during the depolarization phase of the heart's depolarization-repolarization cycle. This results in a decreased refractory period, which reduces the risk of arrhythmias.

Make an IB line for the ventricle

Because class IB antiarrhythmics affect the Purkinje fibers (fibers in the conduction system of the heart) and myocardial cells in the ventricles, they're only used to treat ventricular arrhythmias. (See *Class IB antiarrhythmics: Lidocaine,* page 246.)

Prototype pro

Class IB antiarrhythmics: Lidocaine

Actions
• Decreases depolarization, automaticity, and excitability in the ventricles during diastole by direct action on the tissues, especially the Purkinje network

Indications
• Life-threatening ventricular arrhythmias

Nursing considerations
• Monitor for adverse effects, such as confusion, tremor, restlessness, seizures, hypotension, new arrhythmias, cardiac arrest, tinnitus, blurred vision, respiratory depression, and anaphylaxis.
• Monitor serum lidocaine levels for toxicity.
• Monitor electrolyte, blood urea nitrogen (BUN), and creatinine levels.

Pharmacotherapeutics

Class IB antiarrhythmics are used to treat ventricular ectopic beats, ventricular tachycardia, and ventricular fibrillation.

Drug interactions

Class IB antiarrhythmics may exhibit additive or antagonistic effects when administered with other antiarrhythmics, such as phenytoin, propranolol, procainamide, and quinidine.
In addition:
• Rifampin may reduce the effects of mexiletine.
• Theophylline plasma levels are increased when theophylline is given with mexiletine.
• Use of a beta-adrenergic blocker or disopyramide with mexiletine may reduce the contractility of the heart.

> Stop! In the name of rhythm… Combining class IB antiarrhythmics with other antiarrhythmics can cause additive or antagonistic effects. And that would totally throw our rhythm off!

Side effects/Adverse reactions

Side effects/adverse reactions to class IB antiarrhythmics include:
• drowsiness
• light-headedness
• paresthesias
• sensory disturbances
• hypotension
• bradycardia.

Side effects/adverse reactions to mexiletine also include hypotension, AV block, bradycardia, confusion, ataxia, double vision, nausea, vomiting, tremors, and dizziness.

In addition, lidocaine toxicity can cause seizures and respiratory and cardiac arrest.

The Three-Step Approach

Nursing management for patients needing class IB antiarrhythmics includes these three steps.

Preadministration

(Recognize and analyze cues)
- Assess the patient's arrhythmia before therapy and regularly thereafter.
- Measure apical pulse rate and blood pressure before giving the drug.
- Monitor serum drug levels as indicated. Therapeutic levels for lidocaine are 2 to 5 mcg/mL.
- Monitor blood studies as indicated, such as liver function tests and BUN and creatinine levels.
- Assess the patient's and family's knowledge of drug therapy.

(Prioritize hypothesis—priority patient problems)
- Altered tissue perfusion
- Injury risk
- Knowledge deficiency

(Generate solutions)
- The patient's tissue perfusion will improve as demonstrated by stable blood pressure, cardiac monitoring, and adequate urine output.
- The patient will remain free of injury from adverse reactions.
- The patient will verbalize an understanding of drug therapy.

Medication administration

(Take action)
- Monitor the ECG continuously when therapy starts and when the dosage is adjusted. A patient receiving the drug via infusion must be on continuous cardiac monitoring with close observation.
- Monitor the patient's vital signs frequently, especially blood pressure.
- Assess for adverse reactions and signs of toxicity. As blood levels of lidocaine increase, nervousness, confusion, dizziness, tinnitus, somnolence, paresthesia, and circumoral numbness may occur. Acute toxicity may result in seizures, cardiovascular collapse, and respiratory arrest.

- Use an infusion control device to administer the infusion. Administer slowly as a faster rate greatly increases the risk of toxicity, especially over time. It can also precipitate ringing in the ears and cause a flushing response.
- If administering the drug via the IM route (alternative route for lidocaine), give it in the deltoid area.
- Remember that IM injections increase creatine kinase (CK) levels. The CK-MM isoenzyme (which originates in skeletal muscle, not cardiac muscle) level increases significantly in patients who receive an IM injection.
- Don't crush sustained-release tablets.
- Be aware that sustained-release and extended-release medications aren't interchangeable.
- Take safety precautions if adverse CNS reactions occur.
- Notify the prescriber about adverse reactions. If signs of lidocaine toxicity occur, stop the drug at once and notify the prescriber. Continued infusion could lead to seizures, cardiovascular collapse, coma, and respiratory arrest.
- Use IV forms of these drugs to treat acute arrhythmias. Discontinue the drug and notify the prescriber if arrhythmias worsen or if ECG changes, such as widening QRS complex or substantially prolonged PR interval, are evident.

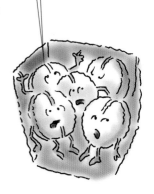

Keep in mind that you shouldn't crush sustained-release tablets—and we're all feeling a bit crushed in here!

Postadministration
(Evaluate outcomes)
- Observe the patient for signs of adequate tissue perfusion demonstrated by normal vital signs.
- Monitor the patient's health status including potential for adverse reactions throughout therapy.
- Evaluate the patient's and family's understanding of drug therapy.

Class IC antiarrhythmics

Class IC antiarrhythmics are used to treat certain severe, refractory (resistant) ventricular arrhythmias. Class IC antiarrhythmics include:
- flecainide acetate
- propafenone hydrochloride.

Pharmacokinetics

After oral administration, class IC antiarrhythmics are absorbed well, distributed in varying degrees, and probably metabolized by the liver. They are excreted primarily by the kidneys, except for propafenone which is excreted primarily in feces. (See *Class IC antiarrhythmics: Propafenone.*)

Pharmacodynamics

Class IC antiarrhythmics primarily slow conduction along the heart's conduction system. Moricizine decreases the fast inward current of sodium ions of the action potential, depressing the depolarization rate and effective refractory period.

Pharmacotherapeutics

Like class IB antiarrhythmics, class IC antiarrhythmic drugs are used to treat life-threatening ventricular arrhythmias. They are also used to treat supraventricular arrhythmias (abnormal heart rhythms that originate above the bundle branches of the heart's conduction system).

Treating troublesome tachycardia

Flecainide and propafenone may also be used to prevent PSVT in patients without structural heart disease.

Drug interactions

Class IC antiarrhythmics may exhibit additive effects when administered with other antiarrhythmics. Here are some other interactions:

- When used with digoxin (Lanoxin), flecainide and propafenone increase the risk of digoxin toxicity.
- Quinidine increases the effects of propafenone.
- Cimetidine (Tagamet) may increase the plasma level and the risk of toxicity of moricizine.
- Propafenone increases the serum concentration and effects of metoprolol (Lopressor) and propranolol (Inderal).
- Warfarin (Coumadin) may increase the level of propafenone.

Side effects/Adverse reactions

Class IC antiarrhythmics can produce serious adverse reactions, including the development of new arrhythmias and aggravation of existing arrhythmias. These drugs aren't given to patients with structural heart defects because of a high incidence of resulting mortality. Other cardiovascular adverse reactions include palpitations, shortness of breath, chest pain, heart failure, and cardiac arrest.

Because propafenone has beta-adrenergic blocking properties, it may also cause bronchospasm.

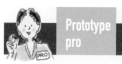

Prototype pro

Class IC antiarrhythmics: Propafenone, flecainide

Black Box Warning: Increased mortality. Avoid use in asymptomatic and symptomatic non-life-threatening ventricular arrhythmias. ■

Actions
- Reduces inward sodium current in Purkinje and myocardial cells
- Decreases excitability, conduction velocity, and automaticity in AV nodal, His-Purkinje, and intraventricular tissue
- Prolongs refractory period in AV nodal tissue

Indications
- Life-threatening ventricular arrhythmias

Nursing considerations
- Administer with food to minimize adverse GI reactions.
- Notify the prescriber if the QRS complex increases by more than 25%.
- During use with digoxin, monitor the ECG and digoxin levels frequently.

Can't stomach it

GI adverse reactions include abdominal pain, heartburn, nausea, and vomiting.

The Three-Step Approach

Nursing management for patients needing class IC antiarrhythmics includes these three steps.

Preadministration

(Recognize and analyze cues)
- Assess the patient's arrhythmia before therapy and regularly thereafter.
- Measure the apical pulse rate and blood pressure before giving the drug.
- Monitor serum drug levels as indicated.
- Monitor blood studies, such as liver function tests, as indicated.
- Assess for adverse reactions and drug interactions.
- Assess the patient's and family's knowledge of drug therapy.

(Prioritize hypothesis—priority patient problems)
- Altered tissue perfusion
- Injury risk
- Knowledge deficiency

(Generate solutions)
- The patient's tissue perfusion will improve as demonstrated by stable blood pressure, cardiac monitoring, and adequate urine output.
- The patient will remain free of injury from adverse reactions.
- The patient will verbalize an understanding of drug therapy.

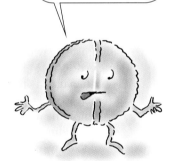

Be safe… notify the prescriber about adverse reactions— even if they appear to be unrelated.

Medication administration

(Take action)
- Monitor the ECG continuously when therapy starts and when the dosage is adjusted.
- Monitor the patient's vital signs frequently and assess for signs of toxicity and adverse reactions.
- Do not crush sustained-release tablets.
- Take safety precautions if adverse CNS reactions occur.
- Notify the prescriber about adverse reactions, even if they seem unrelated.
- Use IV forms of these drugs to treat acute arrhythmias.
- Administer the drug with food to minimize adverse reactions as indicated.

- Notify the prescriber if the PR interval or QRS complex increases by more than 25%. A reduction in dosage may be necessary.
- Monitor the ECG and digoxin levels frequently if used with digoxin.

Postadministration

(Evaluate outcomes)

- Observe the patient for signs of adequate tissue perfusion demonstrated by normal vital signs.
- Monitor the patient's health status including potential for adverse reactions throughout therapy.
- Evaluate the patient's and family's understanding of drug therapy.

Class II antiarrhythmics

Class II antiarrhythmics are composed of beta-adrenergic antagonists, which are also known as *beta-adrenergic blockers* or *beta blockers*. Beta-adrenergic blockers used as antiarrhythmics include:

- metoprolol succinate (Toprol XL) and metoprolol tartrate (Lopressor)
- esmolol (Brevibloc)
- propranolol (Inderal)

Pharmacokinetics

Metoprolol (Lopressor) and propranolol (Inderal) are absorbed almost entirely from the GI tract after an oral dose. Esmolol (Brevibloc) which can only be given IV is immediately available throughout the body. Metoprolol tartrate is available in IV form.

WARNING: Do not confuse metoprolol succinate, which is extended release and metoprolol tartrate, which is immediate release. They are considerably different.

No breaking and entering

Esmolol (Brevibloc) has low lipid solubility. That means that it cannot penetrate the blood-brain barrier (highly fatty cells that act as barriers between the blood and brain). Propranolol (Inderal) has high lipid solubility and readily crosses the blood-brain barrier, which accounts for its side effect of vivid dreams.

Just a little gets the job done

Propranolol undergoes significant first-pass effect, leaving only a small portion of this drug available to be distributed to the body.

Esmolol is metabolized exclusively by red blood cells (RBCs), with only 1% excreted in the urine. Approximately 50% of acebutolol is excreted in feces. Propranolol's metabolites are excreted in urine as well.

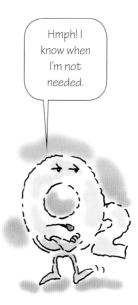

Hmph! I know when I'm not needed.

Pharmacodynamics

Class II antiarrhythmics block beta-adrenergic receptor sites in the conduction system of the heart. As a result, the ability of the SA node to fire spontaneously (automaticity) is slowed. The ability of the AV node and other cells to receive and conduct an electrical impulse to nearby cells (conductivity) is also reduced.

Cutting back on contractions

Class II antiarrhythmics also reduce the strength of the heart's contractions. When the heart beats less forcefully, it doesn't require as much oxygen to do its work.

Pharmacotherapeutics

Class II antiarrhythmics slow ventricular rates in patients with atrial flutter, atrial fibrillation, and paroxysmal atrial tachycardia.

Drug interactions

Class II antiarrhythmics can cause a variety of drug interactions:
- Administering class II antiarrhythmics with phenothiazines and other antihypertensive drugs increases the antihypertensive effect.
- Administration with nonsteroidal anti-inflammatory drugs (NSAIDs) can cause fluid and water retention, decreasing the antihypertensive effects of the drug.
- The effects of sympathomimetics may be reduced when taken with class II antiarrhythmics.

Depressing news

- Beta-adrenergic blockers given with verapamil or other antiarrhythmic or antihypertensive drugs can depress the heart, causing hypotension, bradycardia, AV block, and asystole.
- Beta-adrenergic blockers reduce the effects of sulfonylureas.
- The risk of digoxin toxicity increases when digoxin is taken with esmolol.

Side effects/Adverse reactions

Common adverse reactions to class II antiarrhythmics include:
- arrhythmias
- bradycardia
- heart failure
- hypotension
- GI reactions, such as nausea, vomiting, and diarrhea
- bronchoconstriction
- fatigue.

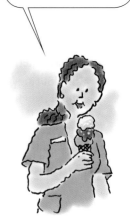

Monitor the patient's intake and output and daily weight. I may go a little overboard on the intake here if I'm not careful!

The Three-Step Approach

Nursing management for patients needing class II antiarrhythmics includes these three steps.

Preadministration

(Recognize and analyze cues)

- Assess the patient's arrhythmia before therapy and regularly thereafter.
- Measure the apical pulse rate and blood pressure before giving the drug.
- Monitor serum drug levels as indicated.
- Monitor blood studies, such as liver function tests, as indicated.
- Be alert for adverse reactions and drug interactions.
- Evaluate the patient's and family's knowledge of drug therapy.
- Monitor the patient's intake and output and daily weight.

(Prioritize hypothesis—priority patient problems)

- Altered tissue perfusion
- Injury risk
- Knowledge deficiency

(Generate solutions)

- The patient's tissue perfusion will improve as demonstrated by stable blood pressure, cardiac monitoring, and adequate urine output.
- The patient will remain free of injury from adverse reactions.
- The patient will verbalize an understanding of drug therapy.
- The patient will demonstrate correct drug administration.

Medication administration

(Take action)

- Monitor the ECG continuously when therapy starts, when the dosage is adjusted, and especially during IV therapy.
- Monitor the patient's vital signs frequently and assess for signs of toxicity and adverse reactions.
- Don't crush sustained-release tablets.
- Take safety precautions if adverse CNS reactions occur.
- Notify the prescriber about adverse reactions.
- Use IV forms of these drugs for treating acute arrhythmias; they may be given as a loading dose IV or diluted with normal saline solution and given by intermittent infusion.
- Check the apical pulse before giving the drug. If you detect extremes in pulse rate, withhold the drug and call the prescriber immediately.
- Administer the drug with meals as indicated.
- Before any surgical procedure, notify the anesthesiologist that the patient is receiving this drug.

- Don't discontinue the IV form of the drug abruptly; symptoms may worsen with increased tachycardia, arrhythmias, or hypertension.

Postadministration
(Evaluate outcomes)
- Observe the patient for signs of adequate tissue perfusion demonstrated by normal vital signs.
- Monitor the patient's health status including potential for adverse reactions throughout therapy.
- Evaluate the patient's and family's understanding of drug therapy.

> Check the patient's apical pulse before giving a beta-adrenergic blocker. If you detect a too fast or too slow pulse, withhold the drug and call the prescriber.

Class III antiarrhythmics

Class III antiarrhythmics are used to treat ventricular arrhythmias. Drugs in this class include amiodarone (Pacerone), dofetilide (Tikosyn), ibutilide (Corvert), and sotalol (Betapace).

Class distinctions

Sotalol is a nonselective (not having a specific affinity for a receptor) beta-adrenergic blocker (class II) that also has class III properties. The class III antiarrhythmic effects are more predominant, especially at higher doses, so sotalol is usually listed as a class III antiarrhythmic.

Pharmacokinetics

The absorption of class III antiarrhythmics varies widely.

Slow but sure

After oral administration, amiodarone is absorbed slowly at widely varying rates. This drug is distributed extensively and accumulates in many sites, especially in organs with a rich blood supply and fatty tissue. It is highly protein bound in plasma, mainly to albumin. Sotalol is also slowly absorbed, with the amount varying between 60% and 100% with minimal protein binding.

Absolute absorption

Dofetilide is very well absorbed from the GI tract, with almost 100% overall absorption and with approximately 70% being bound to plasma proteins. Ibutilide is administered IV only, with absorption of 100%.

Pharmacodynamics

Although the exact mechanism of action isn't known, class III antiarrhythmics are thought to suppress arrhythmias by converting a unidirectional block to a bidirectional block. They have little or no effect on depolarization. These drugs delay repolarization and lengthen the refractory period and duration of the action potential.

Pharmacotherapeutics

Class III antiarrhythmics are used for ventricular arrhythmias. Dofetilide and ibutilide are used for symptomatic atrial fibrillation and flutter. Amiodarone is the first-line drug of choice for ventricular tachycardia and ventricular fibrillation. (See *Class III antiarrhythmics: Amiodarone.*)

Drug interactions

These drug interactions can occur with class III antiarrhythmics:
- Amiodarone increases quinidine, procainamide, and phenytoin levels.
- Amiodarone increases the risk of digoxin toxicity.
- Cimetidine (Tagamet) may increase the level of amiodarone.
- The effects of warfarin (Coumadin) are enhanced when taken with amiodarone.

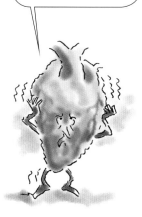

All this talk about "life-threatening arrhythmias" and other drug interactions is really stressing me out!

Prototype pro

Class III antiarrhythmics: Amiodarone (Pacerone)

Black Box Warning: Potential pulmonary toxicity, hepatotoxicity, proarrhythmic effects; hospitalization for the administration of the loading dose and highly recommended for dosage changes ■

Actions
• Thought to prolong the refractory period and duration of action potential and to decrease repolarization

Indications
• Life-threatening ventricular tachycardia and ventricular fibrillation not responding to any other drug
• Suppression of supraventricular tachycardias

Nursing considerations
• Be aware that the drug poses major and potentially life-threatening management problems in patients at risk for sudden death and should be used only in patients with documented, life-threatening, recurrent ventricular arrhythmias who are nonresponsive to adequate doses of other antiarrhythmics or when alternative drugs can't be tolerated.
• Know that amiodarone can cause fatal toxicities, including hepatic and pulmonary toxicity.
• Be aware that the drug causes vision impairment; most adults taking amiodarone develop corneal microdeposits, and cases of optic neuritis have been reported.
• Administer an oral loading dose in three equal doses; give with meals to decrease GI intolerance.
• Only give the drug IV if the patient is closely monitored for cardiac function and resuscitation equipment is available.
• Oral forms of the drug shouldn't be taken with grapefruit juice because it interferes with drug metabolism.

- Ibutilide should not be administered within 4 hours of other class I or class III antiarrhythmics because of the potential for prolonged refractory state.
- Dofetilide should not be administered with cimetidine, ketoconazole, megestrol, prochlorperazine, trimethoprim, sulfamethoxazole, or verapamil because the combination may induce life-threatening arrhythmias.
- Sotalol should not be administered with droperidol because of an increased risk of life-threatening arrhythmias.
- Severe hypotension may develop when IV amiodarone is administered too rapidly.

Side effects/Adverse reactions

Side effects/adverse reactions to class III antiarrhythmics, especially amiodarone, vary widely and commonly lead to drug discontinuation. A common adverse effect is aggravation of arrhythmias.

Other adverse reactions vary by drug:

- Amiodarone may also produce hypotension, bradycardia, nausea, and anorexia. Severe pulmonary toxicity occurs in 15% of patients and can be fatal. Vision disturbances and corneal microdeposits may also occur.
- Ibutilide may cause sustained ventricular tachycardia, QT interval prolongation, hypotension, nausea, and headache.
- Sotalol may cause AV block, bradycardia, ventricular arrhythmias, bronchospasm, and hypotension.

The Three-Step Approach

Nursing management for patients needing class III antiarrhythmics includes these three steps.

Preadministration

(Recognize and analyze cues)
- Assess the patient's arrhythmia before therapy and regularly thereafter.
- Assess potassium and magnesium prior to starting therapy. Correct hypokalemia and hypomagnesemia before therapy to reduce the risk of arrhythmias.
- Measure the patient's apical pulse rate and blood pressure before giving the drug.
- Monitor serum drug levels as indicated.
- Monitor blood studies, such as liver function tests, as indicated.
- Assess the patient's and family's knowledge of drug therapy.

(Prioritize hypothesis—priority patient problems)
- Altered tissue perfusion
- Injury risk
- Knowledge deficiency

(Generate solutions)

- The patient's tissue perfusion will improve as demonstrated by stable blood pressure, cardiac monitoring, and adequate urine output.
- The patient will remain free of injury from adverse reactions.
- The patient will verbalize an understanding of drug therapy.

Medication administration

(Take action)

- Monitor the ECG continuously when therapy starts and when the dosage is adjusted.
- Monitor the patient's vital signs frequently and assess for signs of toxicity and adverse reactions.
- During and after administration, make sure proper equipment and facilities, such as cardiac monitoring, intracardiac pacing, a cardioverter-defibrillator, and medication for treatment of sustained ventricular tachycardia, are available.
- Be alert for adverse reactions and drug interactions.

A stable situation

- Remember that admixtures and approved diluents are chemically and physically stable for 24 hours at room temperature or 48 hours if refrigerated.
- Don't crush sustained-release tablets.
- Be aware that sustained-release and extended-release medications aren't interchangeable.
- Take safety precautions if adverse CNS reactions occur.
- Notify the prescriber about adverse reactions.
- Use IV forms of the drug to treat acute arrhythmias.

Postadministration

(Evaluate outcomes)

- Observe the patient for signs of adequate tissue perfusion demonstrated by normal vital signs.
- Monitor the patient's health status including potential for adverse reactions throughout therapy.
- Evaluate the patient's and family's understanding of drug therapy

Class IV antiarrhythmics

Class IV antiarrhythmics are composed of calcium channel blockers. Calcium channel blockers used to treat arrhythmias include verapamil and diltiazem.

One mission

Verapamil and diltiazem (Cardizem) are used to treat supraventricular arrhythmias with rapid ventricular response rates (rapid heart rate in which the rhythm originates above the ventricles).

Pharmacokinetics

Class IV antiarrhythmics are rapidly and completely absorbed from the GI tract after PO administration; only about 20% to 35% reaches systemic circulation. About 90% of the circulating drug is bound to plasma proteins. Class IV antiarrhythmics are metabolized in the liver and excreted in the urine as unchanged drug and active metabolites.

Pharmacodynamics

Class IV antiarrhythmics inhibit calcium ion influx across cardiac and smooth muscle cells, thus decreasing myocardial contractility and oxygen demand. They also dilate coronary arteries and arterioles.

Pharmacotherapeutics

This class of drugs is used to relieve angina, lower blood pressure, and restore normal sinus rhythm.

Drug interactions

These drug interactions may occur with class IV antiarrhythmics:
- Furosemide (Lasix) forms a precipitate when mixed with diltiazem injection. Give through separate IV lines.
- Anesthetics may potentiate the effects of class IV antiarrhythmics.
- Cyclosporine levels may be increased by diltiazem, resulting in toxicity; avoid using these drugs together.
- Diltiazem (Cardizem) may increase levels of digoxin. Monitor the patient and drug levels.
- Cimetidine (Tagamet) may inhibit diltiazem metabolism, resulting in toxicity.
- Propranolol (Inderal) and other beta-adrenergic blockers may precipitate heart failure or prolong cardiac conduction time with diltiazem and, therefore, should be used together cautiously.
- Antihypertensives and quinidine may cause hypotension when used with verapamil; monitor blood pressure.
- Disopyramide, flecainide, and propranolol and other beta-adrenergic blockers may cause heart failure when used with verapamil.
- Verapamil may decrease lithium levels.
- Rifampin may decrease the effects of verapamil.
- Black catechu may cause additive effects when used with verapamil.

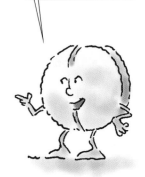

Class IV antiarrhythmics are used to relieve angina, lower blood pressure, and restore normal sinus rhythm.

Don't drink and…

- Grapefruit juice may increase verapamil levels.
- Verapamil enhances the effects of alcohol; discourage concurrent use.

Side effects/Adverse reactions

The following adverse effects can occur when taking class IV antiarrhythmics.

Mild effects

- Dizziness
- Headache
- Hypotension
- Constipation
- Nausea
- Rash

Serious effects

- Heart failure
- Bradycardia
- AV block
- Ventricular asystole
- Ventricular fibrillation
- Pulmonary edema

The Three-Step Approach

Nursing management for patients needing class IV antiarrhythmics includes these three steps.

Preadministration

(Recognize and analyze cues)
- Obtain a history of the patient's underlying condition before therapy and reassess regularly thereafter.
- Assess the patient's arrhythmia before therapy and regularly thereafter.
- Measure the patient's apical pulse rate and blood pressure before giving the drug.
- Monitor the patient's intake and output.
- Monitor serum drug levels as indicated.
- Monitor blood studies, such as liver function tests, as indicated.
- Be alert for adverse reactions and drug interactions.
- Evaluate the patient's and family's knowledge of drug therapy.

(Prioritize hypothesis—priority patient problems)
- Altered tissue perfusion
- Injury risk

- Knowledge deficiency

(Generate solutions)
- The patient's tissue perfusion will improve as demonstrated by stable blood pressure, cardiac monitoring, and adequate urine output.
- The patient will remain free of injury from adverse reactions.
- The patient will verbalize an understanding of drug therapy.

Medication administration

(Take action)
- Monitor the ECG continuously when therapy starts and when the dosage is adjusted.
- Monitor the patient's vital signs frequently and assess for signs of toxicity and adverse reactions.
- Don't crush sustained-release tablets.
- Know that sustained-release and extended-release drug forms aren't interchangeable.

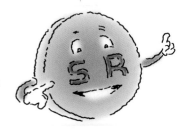

Don't confuse me with an extended-release form of the drug. I'm sustained release. We're not the same.

Forget the fluids

- Fluid and sodium intake may need to be restricted to minimize edema.
- Take safety precautions if adverse CNS reactions occur.
- Notify the prescriber about adverse reactions.
- Use IV forms of the drug for treating acute arrhythmias; cardiac monitoring is required during administrations.
- Withhold the dose and notify the prescriber if the patient's systolic pressure drops below 90 mm Hg or the heart rate drops to less than 60 beats/minute or follow the prescriber's ordered parameters for withholding the medication.
- Help the patient walk because dizziness can occur.
- If the drugs are being used to terminate supraventricular tachycardia, the prescriber may have the patient perform vagal maneuvers after receiving the drug.

Postadministration

(Evaluate outcomes)
- Observe the patient for signs of adequate tissue perfusion demonstrated by normal vital signs.
- Monitor the patient's health status including potential for adverse reactions throughout therapy.
- Evaluate the patient's and family's understanding of drug therapy.

Adenosine

Adenosine is an injectable antiarrhythmic drug indicated for acute treatment of PSVT.

Pharmacokinetics

After IV administration, adenosine probably is distributed rapidly throughout the body and metabolized inside RBCs as well as in vascular endothelial cells.

Pharmacodynamics

Adenosine depresses the pacemaker activity of the SA node, reducing heart rate and the ability of the AV node to conduct impulses from the atria to the ventricles.

Pharmacotherapeutics

Adenosine is especially effective against reentry tachycardias (when an impulse depolarizes an area of heart muscle and returns and repolarizes it) that involve the AV node.

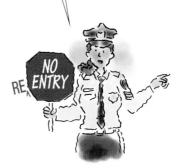

Adenosine is especially effective against reentry tachycardias that involve the AV node.

Packs a punch against PSVT (paroxysmal supraventricular tachycardia)

Adenosine is also effective in more than 90% of PSVT cases. It's predominantly used to treat arrhythmias associated with accessory bypass tracts (brief periods of rapid heart rate in which the rhythm's origin is above the ventricle), as in Wolff-Parkinson-White syndrome, a condition in which strands of heart tissue formed during fetal development abnormally connect structures such as the atria and ventricles, bypassing normal conduction. This condition is also known as a *preexcitation syndrome*.

Drug interactions

Adenosine has various drug interactions:
- Methylxanthines antagonize the effects of adenosine so that the patient may need larger doses of adenosine.
- Dipyridamole and carbamazepine potentiate the effects of adenosine, which may call for smaller doses of adenosine.
- When adenosine is administered with carbamazepine, the risk of heart block increases.
- Caffeine and theophylline may decrease adenosine's effects.

Side effects/Adverse reactions

Adenosine may cause facial flushing, shortness of breath, dizziness, dyspnea, and chest discomfort.

The Three-Step Approach

Nursing management for patients needing adenosine therapy include these three steps.

Preadministration

(Recognize and analyze cues)

- Assess the patient's arrhythmia before therapy and regularly thereafter.
- Measure the apical pulse rate and blood pressure before giving the drug.
- Be alert for adverse reactions and drug interactions.
- Assess the patient's and family's knowledge of drug therapy.

(Prioritize hypothesis—priority patient problems)

- Altered tissue perfusion
- Injury risk
- Knowledge deficiency

(Generate solutions)

- The patient's tissue perfusion will improve as demonstrated by stable blood pressure, cardiac monitoring, and adequate urine output.
- The patient will remain free of injury from adverse reactions.
- The patient will verbalize an understanding of drug therapy.

Medication administration

(Take action)

- Monitor the ECG continuously when therapy starts and when the dosage is adjusted.
- Monitor the patient's vital signs frequently and assess for signs of toxicity and adverse reactions.
- If the solution is cold, check for crystals that may form. If crystals are visible, gently warm the solution to room temperature. Don't use unclear solutions.

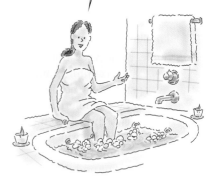

If crystals form in a cold solution, gently warm the solution to room temperature. This is my favorite way to warm up!

Speed is key

- Give rapidly for effective drug action. Give directly into the vein if possible. If an IV line is used, inject the drug into the most proximal port and follow with a rapid saline flush to ensure that the drug reaches systemic circulation quickly.
- If ECG disturbances occur, withhold the drug, obtain a rhythm strip, and notify the prescriber immediately.
- Tell the patient that flushing or chest pain that lasts for 1 to 2 minutes after the drug is injected may occur.
- Take safety precautions before administration because the patient may experience a brief loss of consciousness as the heart block increases.
- Notify the prescriber about adverse reactions.

Postadministration

(Evaluate outcomes)

- Observe the patient for signs of adequate tissue perfusion demonstrated by normal vital signs.

- Monitor the patient's health status including potential for adverse reactions throughout therapy.
- Evaluate the patient's and family's understanding of drug therapy.

Antianginal drugs

Although angina's cardinal symptom is chest pain, the drugs used to treat angina aren't typically analgesics. Rather, antianginal drugs treat angina by reducing myocardial oxygen demand (reducing the amount of oxygen the heart needs to do its work), by increasing the supply of oxygen to the heart, or both. (See *How antianginal drugs work*, page 264.)

The three classes of antianginal drugs discussed in this section include:
- nitrates (for treating acute angina)
- beta-adrenergic blockers (for long-term prevention of angina)
- calcium channel blockers (used when other drugs fail to prevent angina).

Nitrates

Nitrates are the drugs of choice for relieving acute angina. Nitrates commonly prescribed to treat angina include:
- isosorbide dinitrate (Isordil)
- isosorbide mononitrate (Imdur)
- nitroglycerin.

Pharmacokinetics

Nitrates can be administered in a variety of ways.

All absorbed...

Nitrates given sublingually (under the tongue), buccally (in the pocket of the cheek), as chewable tablets, or as lingual aerosols (sprayed onto or under the tongue) are absorbed almost completely because of the rich blood supply of the mucous membranes of the mouth.

... half-absorbed...

Swallowed nitrate capsules are absorbed through the mucous membranes of the GI tract, and only about half the dose enters circulation.

Transdermal nitrates (a patch or ointment placed on the skin) are absorbed slowly and in varying amounts, depending on the quantity of drug applied, the location where the patch is applied, the surface area of skin used, and the circulation to the skin.

Pharm function

How antianginal drugs work

Angina occurs when the coronary arteries, the heart's primary source of oxygen, supply insufficient oxygen to the myocardium. This increases the heart's workload, increasing heart rate, preload (blood volume in the ventricles at the end of diastole), afterload (pressure in the arteries leading from the ventricles), and force of myocardial contractility. The antianginal drugs relieve angina by decreasing one or more of these four factors. This illustration summarizes how antianginal drugs affect the cardiovascular system.

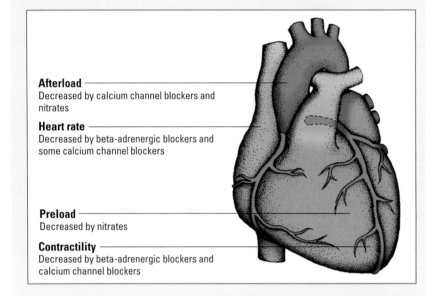

Afterload
Decreased by calcium channel blockers and nitrates

Heart rate
Decreased by beta-adrenergic blockers and some calcium channel blockers

Preload
Decreased by nitrates

Contractility
Decreased by beta-adrenergic blockers and calcium channel blockers

... or not absorbed at all

IV nitroglycerin, which doesn't need to be absorbed, goes directly into circulation. (See *Nitrates: Nitroglycerin.*)

Pharmacodynamics

Nitrates cause the smooth muscle of the veins and, to a lesser extent, the arteries to relax and dilate. Nitrates work in the following ways:
- When the veins dilate, less blood returns to the heart.
- This, in turn, reduces the amount of blood in the ventricles at the end of diastole, when the ventricles are full. (This blood volume in the ventricles just before contraction is called *preload.*)

- By reducing preload, nitrates reduce ventricular size and ventricular wall tension (the left ventricle doesn't have to stretch as much to pump blood). This, in turn, reduces the oxygen requirements of the heart.

Lighten the load

The arterioles provide the most resistance to the blood pumped by the left ventricle (called *peripheral vascular resistance*). Nitrates decrease afterload by dilating the arterioles, reducing resistance, easing the heart's workload, and easing the demand for oxygen.

Pharmacotherapeutics

- Nitrates are used to relieve and prevent angina.

The short story...

Rapidly absorbed nitrates, such as nitroglycerin, are the drugs of choice for relief of acute angina because they have a rapid onset of action, are easy to take, and are inexpensive

... or the long one

Longer acting nitrates, such as the daily nitroglycerin transdermal patch, are convenient and can be used to prevent chronic angina. Oral nitrates are also used because they seldom produce serious adverse reactions.

Drug interactions

These drug interactions may occur with nitrates:
- Severe hypotension can result when nitrates interact with alcohol.
- Sildenafil should not be taken within 24 hours of nitrates because of possible enhanced hypotensive effects.
- Absorption of sublingual nitrates may be delayed when taken with an anticholinergic drug.
- Marked orthostatic hypotension (a drop in blood pressure when a person stands up) with light-headedness, fainting, or blurred vision may occur when calcium channel blockers and nitrates are used together.

Side effects/Adverse reactions

Most adverse reactions to nitrates are caused by changes in the cardiovascular system. The reactions usually disappear when the dosage is reduced.

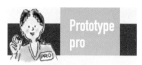

Prototype pro

Nitrates: Nitroglycerin

Actions
- Relaxes vascular smooth muscle
- Causes general vasodilation

Indications
- Acute or chronic anginal attacks

Nursing considerations
- Monitor for adverse effects, such as headache, dizziness, orthostatic hypotension, tachycardia, flushing, palpitations, and hypersensitivity reactions.
- Monitor vital signs closely.
- Treat headaches with acetaminophen or aspirin.

Nitrates are used to treat acute angina because of their rapid onset of action.

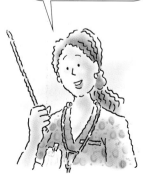

My aching head...

Headache is the most common adverse reaction. Hypotension may occur, accompanied by dizziness and increased heart rate.

The Three-Step Approach

Nursing management for patients needing nitrate therapy include these three steps.

Preadministration

(Recognize and analyze cues)

- Assess the patient's pain level and blood pressure prior to administration.
- Assess if the patient has received nitrate therapy before.
- Be sure to review current medications.
- If administering nitroglycerin intravenously, be sure to secure tubing that is specific to infusion of nitroglycerin.
- If using the pump spray for translingual administration, prime the pump with 5 sprays into the air away from people, prior to initiation, pump may need to be reprimed with 1 pump if not used within 6 weeks, and 5 pumps if not used within 3 months. Do not shake the spray prior to administration.
- Assess expiration date of sublingual tablets prior to administration.

(Prioritize hypothesis—priority patient problems)

- Altered tissue perfusion
- Hypotension risk
- Knowledge deficiency

(Generate solutions)

- The patient will maintain adequate tissue perfusion demonstrated by a reduction in chest pain and stable blood pressure and urine output.
- The patient will maintain a normal blood pressure.
- The patient will verbalize the purpose of nitrates as well as discuss steps for proper administration.

Medication administration

(Take action)

- Monitor vital signs.
- Monitor the effectiveness of the prescribed drug.
- Observe for adverse reactions.
- Be aware that the drug may initially cause headache until tolerance develops or the dosage is minimized.

  Sublingual nitrates:
  - Administer sublingual nitrate tablets at the first sign of anginal pain, placing the tablet under the tongue until it's completely

absorbed. The dose can be repeated every 5 minutes until three doses have been administered.

- Advise the patient to avoid eating or drinking anything for 10 minutes after administration of nitroglycerin

Translingual nitrates:

- Administer translingual nitrate spray (1 to 2 sprays) at the first sign of anginal pain, spraying onto or under the tongue. Do not inhale the medication. Repeat the dose if angina persists every 5 minutes with a maximum of 3 sprays in 15 minutes (Amsterdam et al., 2014).

Oral nitrates:

- Tablets may be given on an empty stomach, either 30 minutes before or 1 to 2 hours after meals. Teach the patient to swallow tablets whole, not chew them.
- Have the patient sit or lie down when receiving the first nitrate dose. Take the patient's pulse and blood pressure before giving the dose and when the drug action starts.
- Don't give a beta-adrenergic blocker or calcium channel blocker to relieve acute angina.
- Withhold the dose and notify the prescriber if the patient's heart rate is less than 60 beats/minute or the systolic blood pressure drops below 90 mm Hg, or follow the prescriber's ordered parameters for withholding the medication.

Intravenous nitroglycerin:

- Dilute IV nitroglycerin with D_5W or normal saline solution for injection, using a glass bottle or specialized polymer IV bag.
- Avoid the use of IV filters because the drug binds to plastic.
- Special nonabsorbent polyvinyl chloride tubing is available from the manufacturer.
- Titrate the drug and administer with an infusion control device.
- With IV nitroglycerin, monitor blood pressure and pulse rate every 5 to 15 minutes while adjusting the dosage and every hour thereafter.

Transdermal nitrates:

- Place topical ointments on paper as prescribed and then place the paper on a nonhairy area and secure the patch with paper tape. Remove excess ointment from the previous site when applying the next dose.
- Remember to rotate application sites and wear gloves with application to avoid getting any ointment on your fingers.
- Make sure there are no other older patches, or ointments on the skin before applying a new dose to avoid overdose.

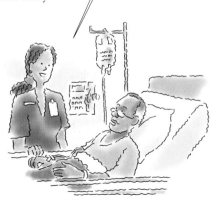

Have the patient sit or lie down when receiving the first nitrate dose.

- Remove a transdermal patch before defibrillation. The aluminum backing on the patch may ignite or cause burns with electric current.

Postadministration

(Evaluate outcomes)

- Observe the patient for signs of adequate tissue perfusion demonstrated by normal vital signs.
- Observe the patient for adverse reactions such as hypotension.
- Evaluate the patient's and family's understanding of drug therapy. (See *Teaching about nitrates*)

Teaching about nitrates

If nitrates are prescribed, review these points with the patient and caregivers:

- It's essential to understand how to use the prescribed form of the drug.
- Take the drug regularly, as prescribed, and make sure the drug is accessible at all times.
- Don't discontinue the drug abruptly without your prescriber's approval. Coronary vasospasm can occur.
- If taking nitrates, you may need an additional dose before anticipated stress or at bedtime if angina is nocturnal. Check with your prescriber.
- Remove patches if undergoing MRI to avoid the patch from heating up and possibly causing a burn.
- Avoid alcohol during drug therapy.
- Remove a used transdermal patch before applying a new one.
- Change to an upright position slowly. Go up and down stairs carefully and lie down at the first sign of dizziness.
- Store nitrates in a cool, dark place in a tightly closed container. To ensure freshness, replace sublingual tablets every 3 months and remove the cotton because it absorbs the drug.
- Store sublingual tablets in their original container or another container specifically approved for this use and carry the container in a jacket pocket or purse, not in a pocket close to the body.
- As indicated, take your pulse before taking the medication, such as with beta-adrenergic blockers and calcium channel blockers. Withhold the dose and alert your prescriber if your pulse rate is below 60 beats/ minute.
- If taking nitroglycerin sublingually, contact emergency services if three tablets taken 5 minutes apart don't relieve anginal pain.
- Report serious or persistent adverse reactions to your prescriber.
- Place the buccal tablet between your lip and gum above the incisors or between your cheek and gum. Don't swallow or chew the tablet.
- Nitroglycerin tablets do have a shelf-life and lose effectiveness over time.
- If using the pump spray for translingual administration, prime the pump with 5 sprays prior to initiation, pump may need to be reprimed with 1 pump if not used within 6 weeks, and 5 pumps if not used within 3 months. Spray onto or under the tongue. Do not inhale the medication. Do not shake the medication prior to use.

Beta-adrenergic antagonists

Beta-adrenergic antagonists (also called *beta-adrenergic blockers*) are used for long-term prevention of angina and are one of the main types of drugs used to treat hypertension. Beta-adrenergic blockers include:
- atenolol (Tenormin)
- carvedilol (Coreg)
- metoprolol tartrate (Lopressor)
- nadolol (Corgard)
- propranolol hydrochloride (Inderal).

Pharmacokinetics

Metoprolol (Lopressor) and propranolol (Inderal) are absorbed almost entirely from the GI tract, whereas less than half the dose of atenolol (Tenormin) or nadolol (Corgard) is absorbed. These beta-adrenergic blockers are distributed widely. Propranolol is highly protein-bound; the other beta-adrenergic blockers are poorly protein-bound. (See *Beta$_1$- and beta$_2$-adrenergic blockers: Propranolol* and *Beta$_1$-adrenergic blockers: Metoprolol*, page 269 and 271.)

Propranolol and metoprolol are metabolized in the liver, and their metabolites are excreted in urine. Carvedilol is metabolized in the liver and excreted in the bile and feces. Atenolol and nadolol are not metabolized and are excreted unchanged in urine and feces.

Prototype pro

Beta$_1$- and beta$_2$-adrenergic blockers: Propranolol (Inderal)

Black Box Warning: Do not suddenly stop taking this medication. Decrease dosage gradually over 1 to 2 weeks. ∎

Actions
- Reduces cardiac oxygen demand by blocking catecholamine-induced increases in heart rate, blood pressure, and force of myocardial contraction
- Depresses renin secretion and prevents vasodilation of cerebral arteries
- Relieves anginal and migraine pain, lowers blood pressure, restores normal sinus rhythm, and helps limit myocardial infarction (MI) damage

Indications
- Angina pectoris
- Mortality reduction after MI
- Supraventricular, ventricular, and atrial arrhythmias
- Tachyarrhythmias caused by excessive catecholamine action during anesthesia, hyperthyroidism, or pheochromocytoma
- Hypertension
- Prevention of frequent, severe, uncontrollable, or disabling migraine or vascular headache
- Essential tremor
- Hypertrophic cardiomyopathy

Pharmacodynamics

Beta-adrenergic blockers decrease blood pressure and block beta-adrenergic receptor sites in the heart muscle and conduction system. This decreases heart rate and reduces the force of the heart's contractions, resulting in a lower demand for oxygen.

Pharmacotherapeutics

Beta-adrenergic blockers are indicated for the long-term prevention of angina. Metoprolol may be given IV in acute coronary syndrome, followed by an oral dose. Carvedilol and metoprolol are indicated for heart failure. Beta-adrenergic blockers are also first-line therapy for treating hypertension.

Drug interactions

Several drugs interact with beta-adrenergic blockers:
• Antacids delay absorption of beta-adrenergic blockers.
• NSAIDs can decrease the hypotensive effects of beta-adrenergic blockers.
• Lidocaine toxicity may occur when the drug is taken with beta-adrenergic blockers.
• The requirements for insulin and oral antidiabetic drugs can be altered by beta-adrenergic blockers.
• The ability of theophylline to produce bronchodilation is impaired by nonselective beta-adrenergic blockers.

Side effects/Adverse reactions

Side effects/adverse reactions to beta-adrenergic blockers include:
• bradycardia, angina, heart failure, and arrhythmias, especially AV block
• fainting
• fluid retention
• peripheral edema

Prototype pro

Beta₁-adrenergic blockers: Metoprolol (Lopressor)

Black Box Warning: Do not suddenly stop taking this medication. Decrease dosage gradually over 1 to 2 weeks. ■

Actions
• Competes with beta-adrenergic agonists for available beta-adrenergic receptor sites

Indications
• Hypertension

• Angina pectoris

Nursing considerations
• Monitor for adverse reactions, such as fatigue, dizziness, bradycardia, hypotension, heart failure, and AV block.
• Withhold the drug as ordered if the apical pulse is less than 60 beats/minute.
• Monitor blood pressure frequently.

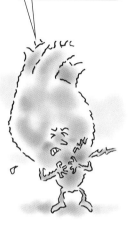

Don't stop a beta-adrenergic blocker suddenly. That could trigger angina, hypertension, arrhythmias, and MI. That's not good!

• shock
• nausea and vomiting
• diarrhea
• significant constriction of the bronchioles.

Not so fast...

Suddenly stopping a beta-adrenergic blocker may trigger angina, hypertension, arrhythmias, and acute MI.

The Three-Step Approach

Nursing management for patients needing beta-adrenergic blockers includes these three steps.

Preadministration

(Recognize and analyze cues)
• Assess the patient's arrhythmia before therapy and regularly thereafter.
• Measure the apical pulse rate and blood pressure before giving the drug.
• Monitor serum drug levels as indicated.
• Monitor blood studies, such as liver function tests, as indicated.
• Be alert for adverse reactions and drug interactions.
• Assess the patient's and family's knowledge of drug therapy.

(Prioritize hypothesis—priority patient problems)
• Altered tissue perfusion
• Hypotension risk
• Nonadherence

(Generate solutions)
- The patient will maintain adequate tissue perfusion demonstrated by a reduction in chest pain and stable blood pressure and urine output.
- The patient will maintain a normal blood pressure.
- The patient will verbalize the purpose of the drug as well as discuss steps for proper administration.

Medication administration

(Take action)
- Monitor the ECG continuously when therapy starts, when the dosage is adjusted, and particularly during IV therapy.
- Monitor the patient's vital signs frequently; assess for signs of toxicity and adverse reactions
- Don't crush sustained-release tablets.
- Be aware that sustained-released and extended-release medications aren't interchangeable.
- Take safety precautions if adverse CNS reactions occur.
- Notify the prescriber about adverse reactions.
- Use IV forms of the drug for treating acute arrhythmias. IV forms may be given as a loading dose IV or may be diluted with normal saline solution and given by intermittent infusion.
- Know that the drug may be given with meals as indicated.
- Before any surgical procedure, notify the anesthesiologist that the patient is receiving this drug.
- Don't discontinue the drug abruptly as the patient may experience chest pain.
- Provide patient teaching.

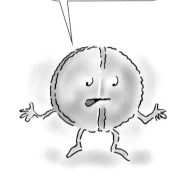

Watch your patient closely for drug interactions. You know, I don't always get along with just any old drug.

Postadministration

(Evaluate outcomes)
- Observe the patient for signs of adequate tissue perfusion demonstrated by normal vital signs.
- Observe the patient for adverse reactions such as hypotension.
- Evaluate the patient's and family's understanding of drug therapy

Calcium channel blockers

Calcium channel blockers are commonly used to prevent angina that does not respond to drugs in either of the other antianginal classes. Several of the calcium channel blockers are also used as antiarrhythmics and in the treatment of hypertension.

Calcium channel blockers used to treat angina include:
- amlodipine besylate (Norvasc)
- diltiazem (Cardizem)
- nicardipine (Cardene)
- nifedipine (Procardia)
- verapamil.

How calcium channel blockers work

Calcium channel blockers increase myocardial oxygen supply and slow cardiac impulse formation. Apparently, the drugs produce these effects by blocking the slow calcium channel. This action inhibits the influx of extracellular calcium ions across both myocardial and vascular smooth muscle cell membranes. Calcium channel blockers achieve this blockade without changing serum calcium concentrations.

No calcium = dilation

This calcium blockade causes the coronary arteries (and, to a lesser extent, the peripheral arteries and arterioles) to dilate, decreasing afterload and increasing myocardial oxygen supply.

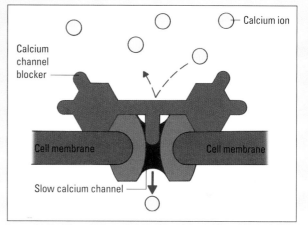

Pharmacokinetics

When administered orally, calcium channel blockers are absorbed quickly and almost completely. Because of the first-pass effect, however, the bioavailability of these drugs is much lower. Calcium channel blockers are highly bound to plasma proteins.

Speedy through the liver

All calcium channel blockers are metabolized rapidly and almost completely in the liver.

Pharmacodynamics

Calcium channel blockers prevent the passage of calcium ions across the myocardial cell membrane and vascular smooth muscle cells. This causes dilation of the coronary and peripheral arteries, which decreases the force of the heart's contractions and reduces the workload of the heart. (See *How calcium channel blockers work*, page 273.)

Putting on the brakes

By preventing arterioles from constricting, calcium channel blockers also reduce afterload, resulting in a decreased oxygen demand of the heart.

Some calcium channel blockers (diltiazem and verapamil) also reduce the heart rate by slowing conduction through the SA and AV nodes. A slower heart rate reduces the heart's need for additional oxygen.

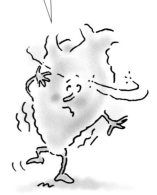

Such adverse reactions! Headache, flushing, weakness, dizziness… Ohhh…

Prototype pro

Calcium channel blockers: Verapamil

Actions
- Inhibits calcium ion influx across the cardiac and smooth muscle cells
- Reduces myocardial contractility and oxygen demand
- Dilates coronary arteries and arterioles

Indications
- Angina relief
- Decreased blood pressure
- Abnormal sinus rhythm

Nursing considerations
- A patient with severely compromised cardiac function or one taking beta-adrenergic blockers should receive lower doses of verapamil.
- Monitor cardiac rhythm and blood pressure during the start of therapy and with dose adjustments.
- Notify the prescriber if signs and symptoms of heart failure occur, such as swelling of the hands and feet and shortness of breath.

Pharmacotherapeutics

Calcium channel blockers are used only for long-term prevention of angina, not for short-term relief of chest pain. Calcium channel blockers are particularly effective for preventing Prinzmetal angina. (See *Calcium channel blockers: Verapamil.*)

Drug interactions

These drug interactions can occur with calcium channel blockers:
- Calcium salts and vitamin D reduce the effectiveness of calcium channel blockers.
- Nondepolarizing blocking drugs may enhance the muscle relaxant effect when taken with calcium channel blockers.
- Verapamil and diltiazem increase the risk of digoxin toxicity and enhance the action of carbamazepine.

Side effects/Adverse reactions

As with other antianginal drugs, cardiovascular reactions are the most common and serious adverse reactions to calcium channel blockers. Possible adverse reactions include orthostatic hypotension, heart failure, hypotension, and arrhythmias, such as bradycardia and AV block. Other possible adverse reactions include dizziness, headache, flushing, weakness, and persistent peripheral edema.

The Three-Step Approach

Nursing management for patients needing calcium channel blocker therapy includes these three steps.

Preadministration

(Recognize and analyze cues)
- Obtain a history of the patient's underlying condition before therapy and reassess regularly thereafter.

- Assess the patient's arrhythmia before therapy and regularly thereafter.
- Measure the apical pulse rate and blood pressure before giving the drug.
- Monitor serum drug levels as indicated.
- Monitor blood studies, such as liver function tests, as indicated.
- Be alert for adverse reactions and drug interactions.
- Assess the patient's and family's knowledge of drug therapy.

(Prioritize hypothesis—priority patient problems)
- Altered tissue perfusion
- Hypotension risk
- Knowledge deficiency

(Generate solutions)
- The patient will maintain adequate tissue perfusion demonstrated by stable blood pressure, cardiac monitoring, and adequate urine output.
- The patient will maintain a normal blood pressure.
- The patient will verbalize the purpose of the drug as well as discuss steps for proper administration.

Medication administration

(Take action)
- Monitor the ECG continuously when therapy starts and when the dosage is adjusted.
- Monitor the patient's vital signs frequently and assess for signs of toxicity and adverse reactions.
- Don't crush sustained release tablets.
- Be aware that sustained released and extended release medications aren't interchangeable.
- Take safety precautions if adverse CNS reactions occur.
- Notify the prescriber about adverse reactions.
- Know that IV forms are used for treating acute arrhythmias; cardiac monitoring is required during administration.
- If the patient's systolic pressure is below 90 mm Hg or the heart rate drops below 60 beats/minute, withhold the dose and notify the prescriber, or follow the prescriber's ordered parameters for withholding the medication.

Help your patient walk the walk

- Assist the patient with ambulation during the start of therapy because dizziness can occur.
- If the drug is being used to terminate supraventricular tachycardia, the prescriber may have the patient perform vagal maneuvers after receiving the drug.
- Advise the patient that fluid and sodium intake may need to be restricted to minimize edema.
- Provide patient teaching.

Postadministration

(Evaluate outcomes)

- Evaluate the patient for signs of adequate tissue perfusion demonstrated by normal vital signs and adequate rhythm.
- Observe the patient for adverse reactions such as hypotension.
- Evaluate the patient's and family's understanding of drug therapy.

Antihypertensive drugs

Antihypertensive drugs are used to treat hypertension, a disorder characterized by elevation in systolic blood pressure, diastolic blood pressure, or both.

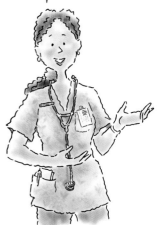

Antihypertensive drugs are used to treat hypertension. That makes sense!

A word to the wise

According to the Eighth Report of the Joint National Committee on Prevention, Detection, Evaluation, and Treatment of High Blood Pressure, several classes of drugs have been shown in clinical trials to be effective in treating hypertension (James et al., 2014). Diuretics, primarily thiazide diuretics, may be used as initial therapy in treating most patients with hypertension. (These drugs are discussed in Chapter 11, Genitourinary drugs.) Other classes of drugs used to treat hypertension include:

- angiotensin-converting enzyme (ACE) inhibitors
- angiotensin-receptor blockers (ARBs)
- beta-adrenergic antagonists
- calcium channel blockers.

If these drugs are ineffective, treatment continues with sympatholytic drugs (other than beta-adrenergic blockers), direct vasodilators, selective aldosterone-receptor antagonists, or a combination of drugs. For black patients, it is recommended to start on two agents depending on the severity of the hypertension and/or evidence of organ damage such as kidney or eye damage (James et al., 2014).

Angiotensin-converting enzyme inhibitors

ACE inhibitors reduce blood pressure by interrupting the renin-angiotensin activating system (RAAS). Commonly prescribed ACE inhibitors include:

- benazepril (Lotensin)
- captopril
- enalapril (Vasotec)
- fosinopril sodium

ACE inhibitors: Captopril

Black Box Warning: This medication may cause fetal/neonatal morbidity/mortality if used in pregnancy. ■

Actions
- Thought to inhibit ACE, preventing conversion of angiotensin I to angiotensin II (Reduced formation of angiotensin II decreases peripheral arterial resistance, thus decreasing aldosterone secretion.)

Indications
- Sodium and water retention
- High blood pressure
- Impaired renal function in patients with diabetes

Nursing considerations
- Monitor white blood cell (WBC) and differential counts before therapy, every 2 weeks for the first 3 months of therapy, and periodically thereafter.
- Give the drug 1 hour before meals because food may reduce drug absorption.
- Withhold the dose and notify the prescriber if the patient develops fever, sore throat, leukopenia, hypotension, or tachycardia.
- Keep in mind that light-headedness and syncope can develop in hot weather, with inadequate fluid intake, vomiting, diarrhea, and excessive perspiration.

- lisinopril (Zestril)
- moexipril
- quinapril hydrochloride, Accupril
- ramipril (Altace)
- trandolapril.

Pharmacokinetics

ACE inhibitors are absorbed from the GI tract, distributed to most body tissues, metabolized somewhat in the liver, and excreted by the kidneys. Ramipril also is excreted in feces. Enalaprilat is the only intravenous ACE inhibitor available.

Pharmacodynamics

ACE inhibitors work by preventing the conversion of angiotensin I to angiotensin II. Angiotensin II is a potent vasoconstrictor that increases peripheral resistance and promotes the excretion of aldosterone (which promotes sodium and water retention). As angiotensin II is reduced, arterioles dilate, reducing peripheral vascular resistance.

By reducing aldosterone secretion, ACE inhibitors promote the excretion of sodium and water, reducing the amount of blood the heart needs to pump and reducing blood pressure.

Pharmacotherapeutics

ACE inhibitors may be used alone or in combination with other agents, such as a thiazide diuretic, to treat hypertension. They are commonly used when beta-adrenergic blockers or diuretics are ineffective.

All ACE inhibitors are indicated for use in heart failure for the following situations:

- left ventricular systolic failure (unless contraindicated or intolerant)
- left ventricular systolic dysfunction without symptoms of heart failure
- after acute MI (especially in patients with prior myocardial injury) to reduce mortality
- left ventricular dysfunction (recent or remote) to prevent or delay the development of left ventricular dilation and overt heart failure
- combined use with beta-adrenergic blockers to produce complementary effects
- combined use with diuretics if fluid retention persists.

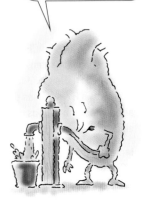

ACE inhibitors reduce the amount of blood I need to pump. Thank goodness! Pumping can be hard work!

Multiple uses

Lisinopril, ramipril, and trandolapril are also indicated for use in patients who have had an MI to improve survival and to reduce morbidity and mortality in patients with left ventricular dysfunction.

Historically speaking…

Ramipril is also indicated to prevent major cardiovascular events in patients with a history of vascular disease or diabetes. It is also used to reduce overall cardiovascular risk, including death, nonfatal MI, nonfatal stroke, and complications of diabetes.

Drug interactions

ACE inhibitors can cause several different types of interactions with other cardiovascular drugs:

- All ACE inhibitors enhance the hypotensive effects of diuretics and other antihypertensives such as beta-adrenergic blockers. They can also increase serum lithium levels, possibly resulting in lithium toxicity.
- When ACE inhibitors are used with potassium-sparing diuretics, potassium supplements, or potassium-containing salt substitutes, hyperkalemia may occur.
- ACE inhibitors may interact with other medications, both prescribed and over the counter. For example, patients taking ACE inhibitors should avoid taking NSAIDs. In addition to decreasing the antihypertensive effects of ACE inhibitors, NSAIDs may alter renal function.
- Food decreases the absorption of ACE inhibitors.

On their own

Captopril, enalapril, and lisinopril may become less effective when administered with NSAIDs. Antacids may impair the absorption of fosinopril and quinapril.

Side effects/Adverse reactions

ACE inhibitors can cause these adverse reactions:
- headache
- fatigue
- dry, nonproductive, persistent cough
- angioedema
- GI reactions
- increased serum potassium concentrations
- tickling in the throat
- transient elevations of BUN and serum creatinine levels (indicators of kidney function).

They can cause problems with fetal circulation and shouldn't be administered during the second or third trimester of pregnancy.

Captopril cautions

Captopril may cause protein in the urine, reduced neutrophils and granulocytes (types of WBCs), rash, loss of taste, hypotension, or a severe allergic reaction.

The Three-Step Approach

Nursing management for patients needing ACE inhibitors includes these three steps.

Preadministration

(Recognize and analyze cues)
- Obtain a baseline blood pressure and pulse rate and rhythm; recheck regularly.
- Monitor the patient for adverse reactions and drug interactions.
- Monitor the patient's weight and fluid and electrolyte status.
- Assess the patient's underlying condition before therapy and regularly thereafter.
- Monitor laboratory results, including WBC and differential counts, potassium level, and renal function (BUN and creatinine clearance levels and urinalysis).

(Prioritize hypothesis—priority patient problems)
- Hypotension risk
- Hypertension
- Knowledge deficiency

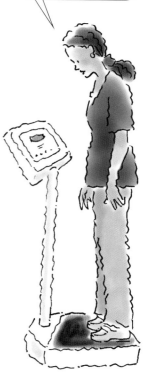

Be sure to monitor the weight of a patient taking ACE inhibitors.

(Generate solutions)
- The patient will not develop hypotension and will verbalize understanding of the risk associated with orthostatic hypotension.
- The patient will maintain a normal blood pressure.
- The patient will verbalize the purpose of the drug as well as discuss steps for proper administration.

Medication administration

(Take action)
- Observe the patient's tolerance of the drug's therapeutic effects. The dosage may need to be increased.

Potential patch problems

- Monitor a patient using a transdermal patch for dermatitis and ask about pruritus. Keep in mind that the patch can require several days to take effect and that interim oral therapy may be needed.
- If giving orally, administer the drug before meals as indicated.
- Follow the manufacturer's guidelines when mixing and administering parenteral drugs (enalaprilat (Vasotec IV)).
- Prevent or minimize orthostatic hypotension by helping the patient to get up slowly and by teaching the patient to avoid sudden changes in position.
- Maintain the patient's nonpharmacologic therapies, such as sodium restriction, calorie reduction, stress management, and exercise program.
- Keep in mind that drug therapy may be given to lower blood pressure rapidly in some hypertensive emergency situations.
- Know that the dosage is usually adjusted to the patient's blood pressure and tolerance.
- To improve adherence of a transdermal patch, apply an adhesive overlay. Place the patch at a different site each week and remove the old patch before applying the new one.

Avoiding an electrifying experience

- Remove a transdermal patch before defibrillation to prevent arcing.
- Periodic eye examinations are recommended.

Postadministration

(Evaluate outcomes)
- Evaluate the patient's blood pressure and observe for adverse reactions such as hypotension.
- Evaluate the patient's and family's understanding of drug therapy.

Angiotensin II receptor blocking agents

ARBs lower blood pressure by blocking the vasoconstrictive effects of angiotensin II. Available ARBs include:

- candesartan cilexetil (Atacand)
- irbesartan (Avapro)
- losartan (Cozaar)
- olmesartan (Benicar)
- telmisartan (Micardis)
- valsartan (Diovan).

Pharmacokinetics

ARBs have varying pharmacokinetic properties, and all are highly bound to plasma proteins.

Pharmacodynamics

ARBs act by interfering with the RAAS. They selectively block the binding of angiotensin II to the angiotensin II receptor. This prevents the vasoconstricting and aldosterone-secreting effects of angiotensin II (a potent vasoconstrictor), resulting in a blood pressure decrease.

No inhibitions

ARBs do not inhibit the production of ACE that's responsible for the conversion of angiotensin I to angiotensin II, nor do they cause a breakdown in bradykinin (a vasodilator). (See *Angiotensin II receptor blockers: Losartan.*)

Pharmacotherapeutics

ARBs may be used alone or in combination with other agents, such as a diuretic, for the treatment of hypertension. Valsartan may also be used as an alternative to ACE inhibitors or for the management of heart failure. Irbesartan and losartan are indicated for patients with type 2 diabetes because of their inherent renal protective effect.

Drug interactions

These drug interactions may occur with ARBs:

- Losartan taken with fluconazole may increase levels of losartan, leading to increased hypotensive effects.
- NSAIDs reduce the antihypertensive effects of ARBs.
- Rifampin may increase metabolism of losartan, leading to decreased antihypertensive effect.
- Potassium supplements can increase the risk of hyperkalemia when used with ARBs.
- Losartan taken with lithium may increase lithium levels.

Prototype pro

Angiotensin II receptor blockers: Losartan (Cozaar)

Actions

- Inhibits vasoconstricting and aldosterone-secreting effects of angiotensin II by selectively blocking binding of angiotensin II to receptor sites in many tissues, including vascular smooth muscle and adrenal glands

Indications

- High blood pressure

Nursing considerations

- Monitor blood pressure before therapy and regularly thereafter.
- Regularly assess kidney function (creatinine and BUN levels).

Side effects/Adverse reactions

Side effects/adverse effects of ARBs include:

- headache
- fatigue
- cough and tickling in the throat
- angioedema
- GI reactions
- increased serum potassium
- transient elevations of BUN and serum creatinine levels.
  ARBs shouldn't be used during the second and third trimesters
of pregnancy; this can result in injury to or death of the fetus.

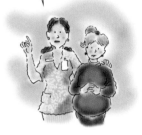

ARBs shouldn't be used during the second and third trimesters because of the risk of injury or death to the fetus.

The Three-Step Approach

Nursing management for patients needing ARB therapy includes these three steps.

Preadministration

(Recognize and analyze cues)

- Obtain a baseline blood pressure and pulse rate and rhythm; recheck regularly.
- Monitor the patient for adverse reactions.
- Monitor the patient's weight and fluid and electrolyte status.

(Prioritize hypothesis—priority patient problems)

- Injury risk
- Hypertension risk
- Knowledge deficiency

(Generate solutions)

- The patient's blood pressure will be maintained within acceptable limits, minimizing the risk for injury.
- The patient will verbalize the purpose of the drug as well as discuss steps for proper administration.

Medication administration

(Take action)

- If giving orally, administer the drug with food or at bedtime as indicated.
- Follow the manufacturer's guidelines when mixing and administering parenteral drugs.
- Prevent or minimize orthostatic hypotension by helping the patient to get up slowly and teaching the patient to avoid sudden changes in position.
- Maintain the patient's nonpharmacologic therapies, such as sodium restriction, calorie reduction, stress management, and exercise program.
- Keep in mind that drug therapy may be given to lower blood pressure rapidly in some hypertensive emergency situations.

- Observe the patient's tolerance of the drug and monitor the drug's therapeutic effects. The dosage may need to be adjusted.
- Monitor a patient with a transdermal patch for dermatitis; ask about pruritus. The patch can require several days to take effect and that the patient may need interim oral therapy.
- Know that the dosage is usually adjusted to the patient's blood pressure and tolerance.
- To improve adherence of a transdermal patch, apply an adhesive overlay. Place the patch at a different site each week and completely remove the old patch before applying the new one to prevent overdose.
- Remove a transdermal patch before defibrillation to prevent arcing.
- Periodic eye examinations are recommended.

Postadministration
(Evaluate outcomes)
- Evaluate the patient's blood pressure and observe for adverse reactions such as hypotension.
- Evaluate the patient's and family's understanding of drug therapy.

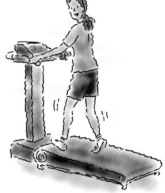

The patient on ARBs should maintain nonpharmacologic therapies, including an exercise program. Let's keep up the pace!

SOMETHING NEW....A new class of drugs

Prototype pro

Angiotensin receptor neprilysin inhibitor (ARNI): Sacubitril and valsartan (Entresto)

- Only drug in its class, shown to improve mortality and morbidity in heart failure patients with reduced cardiac function of less than 35% when compared to ACE inhibitors or solitary ARB (McMurray et al., 2014).

Actions
- Inhibits neprilysin, causing vasodilation and a reduction in fluid volume. Additionally, has the benefit of an ARB. By blocking the angiotensin receptor, it inhibits vasoconstriction and the water retaining effects of aldosterone

Indications
- Indicated to reduce the risk of cardiovascular death and hospitalization in chronic heart failure patients with reduced ejection fraction.

Nursing considerations
- Upon initiating Entresto if the patient is on an ACE inhibitor such as lisinopril, they must stop taking other ACE inhibitors for 36 hours (referred to as a washout period) before changing the medication.
- Verify the patient is not receiving an ARB simultaneously.
- For severe renal failure, dose reduction is required.
- May increase lithium levels.
- DO NOT use in hepatic failure.
Adverse reactions:
- Similar to ARB, cough, angioedema (rare), hypotension, renal impairment, hyperkalemia

Beta-adrenergic antagonists

Beta-adrenergic antagonists, or beta-adrenergic blockers, are one of the main types of drugs used to treat hypertension, including ocular hypertension. They're also used for long-term prevention of angina. Beta-adrenergic blockers used for hypertension include:

- acebutolol
- atenolol (Tenormin)
- betaxolol
- bisoprolol
- carteolol
- metoprolol tartrate (Lopressor)
- nadolol (Corgard)
- pindolol
- propranolol hydrochloride (Inderal)
- timolol.

Pharmacokinetics

The pharmacokinetics of beta-adrenergic blockers varies by drug. Acebutolol, betaxolol, carteolol, metoprolol (Lopressor) pindolol, propranolol (Inderal), and timolol are absorbed almost entirely from the GI tract, whereas less than half of atenolol or nadolol is absorbed. GI tract absorption of bisoprolol is approximately 80%.

Acebutolol, carteolol, propranolol, metoprolol, and timolol are metabolized in the liver, and their metabolites are excreted in urine. Atenolol and nadolol aren't metabolized and are excreted unchanged in urine and feces. Betaxolol is metabolized in the liver and is primarily excreted in urine. Bisoprolol is partially eliminated by renal pathways. Approximately 50% of the drug is excreted in the urine and about 2% in feces. Pindolol is metabolized in the liver (about 65% of the dose), and 35% to 50% of the dose is excreted unchanged in urine.

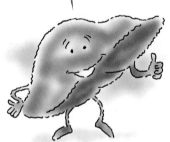

Pharmacokinetics varies by drug, but many beta-adrenergic antagonists are metabolized by me and their metabolites are excreted in urine.

Pharmacodynamics

Beta-adrenergic blockers decrease blood pressure and block beta-adrenergic receptor sites in the heart muscle and conduction system. This decreases heart rate and reduces the force of the heart's contractions, resulting in a lower demand for oxygen.

Pharmacotherapeutics

Beta-adrenergic blockers are used as first-line therapy for treating hypertension and are also indicated for the long-term prevention of angina.

The "eyes" have it

Betaxolol, carteolol, and timolol are also used for ocular hypertension. Ophthalmic agents may still have some systemic effects depending on dosage.

Drug interactions

Several drugs interact with beta-adrenergic blockers:
- Antacids delay absorption of beta-adrenergic blockers.
- NSAIDs can decrease the hypotensive effects of beta-adrenergic blockers.
- Lidocaine toxicity may occur when the drug is taken with beta-adrenergic blockers.
- The requirements for insulin and oral antidiabetic drugs can be altered by beta-adrenergic blockers.
- The ability of theophylline to produce bronchodilation is impaired by nonselective beta-adrenergic blockers.
- Hypotensive effects may be increased when beta-adrenergic blockers are administered with diuretics.

Side effects/aAdverse reactions

Side effects/adverse reactions to beta-adrenergic blockers include:
- bradycardia, angina, heart failure, and arrhythmias, especially AV block
- fainting
- fluid retention
- peripheral edema
- dizziness
- shock
- nausea and vomiting
- diarrhea
- significant constriction of the bronchioles.

Slow to a halt

Suddenly stopping a beta-adrenergic blocker may trigger angina, hypertension, arrhythmias, and acute MI.

The Three-Step Approach

Nursing management for patients needing beta-adrenergic blocker therapy includes these three steps.

Preadministration

(Recognize and analyze cues)
- Obtain a baseline blood pressure and pulse rate and rhythm; recheck regularly.
- Monitor the ECG when therapy starts, when the dosage is adjusted, and particularly during IV therapy.

- Monitor the patient's vital signs frequently; assess for signs of toxicity and adverse reactions.
- Measure the apical pulse rate and blood pressure before giving the drug.
- Monitor blood studies, such as liver function tests, as indicated.
- Evaluate the patient's and family's knowledge of drug therapy.

(Prioritize hypothesis—priority patient problems)
- Hypotension risk
- Injury risk
- Knowledge deficiency

(Generate solutions)
- Blood pressure will be maintained within acceptable limits.
- Risk for injury will be minimized.
- The patient will verbalize an understanding of drug therapy.

Medication administration
(Take action)
- Don't crush sustained-release tablets.
- Be aware that sustained-release and extended-release medications aren't interchangeable.
- Take safety precautions if adverse CNS reactions occur.
- Notify the prescriber about adverse reactions.
- Know that the dosage is usually adjusted to the patient's blood pressure and tolerance.
- Be alert for adverse reactions and drug interactions.
- Prevent or minimize orthostatic hypotension by helping the patient to get up slowly and by telling the patient not to make sudden movements.
- Use IV forms of the drug for treating severe hypertension. IV forms may be given as a loading dose IV or may be diluted with normal saline solution and given by intermittent infusion.
- If systolic blood pressure is below 90 mm Hg or heart rate is below 60 beats/minute, withhold the dose and notify the prescriber, or follow the prescriber's ordered parameters for withholding the medication.
- Know that the drug may be given with meals as indicated.
- Before any surgical procedure, notify the anesthesiologist that the patient is receiving this drug.
- Don't discontinue IV administration abruptly.

Postadministration
(Evaluate outcomes)
- Blood pressure is maintained within acceptable limits.
- Patient sustains no injury from orthostatic hypotension.
- Patient and family demonstrate an understanding of drug therapy.

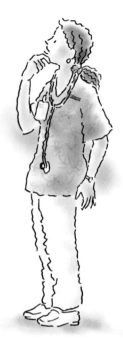

Calcium channel blockers

Calcium channel blockers are commonly used to treat hypertension. Several are also used to treat arrhythmias and to prevent angina that doesn't respond to other antianginal drugs.

Calcium channel blockers used to treat hypertension include:
- amlodipine besylate (Norvasc)
- diltiazem (Cardizem)
- isradipine
- nicardipine (Cardene)
- nifedipine (Procardia)
- nisoldipine (Sular)
- verapamil.

Pharmacokinetics

When administered orally, calcium channel blockers are absorbed quickly and almost completely. Because of the first-pass effect, however, the bioavailability of these drugs is much lower. Food decreases amlodipine absorption by 30%, and high-fat foods increase the peak concentration of nisoldipine. Calcium channel blockers are highly bound to plasma proteins.

All calcium channel blockers are metabolized rapidly and almost completely in the liver and are primarily excreted in urine.

Pharmacodynamics

Calcium channel blockers prevent the passage of calcium ions across the myocardial cell membrane and vascular smooth muscle cells. This causes dilation of the coronary and peripheral arteries, which decreases the force of the heart's contractions and reduces the workload of the heart and decreases blood pressure. By preventing arterioles from constricting, calcium channel blockers also reduce afterload, resulting in a decreased oxygen demand of the heart.

No need for extra O_2

Some calcium channel blockers (diltiazem and verapamil) also reduce the heart rate by slowing conduction through the SA and AV nodes. A slower heart rate reduces the heart's need for additional oxygen.

Pharmacotherapeutics

Calcium channel blockers are used to treat hypertension and for long-term prevention of angina. They shouldn't be used for short-term relief of chest pain. Calcium channel blockers are particularly effective for preventing Prinzmetal's angina.

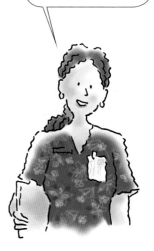

Calcium channel blockers are particularly effective for preventing Prinzmetal's angina.

Drug interactions

These drug interactions can occur with calcium channel blockers:

- Calcium salts and vitamin D reduce the effectiveness of calcium channel blockers.
- The muscle relaxant effect of calcium channel blockers may be enhanced when taken with nondepolarizing blocking drugs.
- Verapamil and diltiazem increase the risk of digoxin toxicity, enhance the action of carbamazepine, and can produce myocardial depression.

Side effects/Adverse reactions

Possible adverse reactions include headache, dizziness, weakness, orthostatic hypotension, heart failure, hypotension, peripheral edema, palpitations, and arrhythmias such as tachycardia. Bradycardia and AV block also occur with diltiazem and verapamil.

The Three-Step Approach

Nursing management for patients needing calcium channel blocker therapy includes these three steps.

Preadministration

(Recognize and analyze cues)

- Obtain a history of the patient's underlying condition before therapy and reassess regularly thereafter.
- Obtain a baseline blood pressure and pulse rate and rhythm; recheck regularly.
- Monitor the ECG when therapy starts and when the dosage is adjusted.
- Measure the apical pulse rate and blood pressure before giving the drug.
- Monitor serum drug levels as indicated.
- Monitor blood studies, such as liver function tests, as indicated.
- Be alert for adverse reactions and drug interactions.
- Evaluate the patient's and family's knowledge of drug therapy.

(Prioritize hypothesis—priority patient problems)

- Hypotension risk
- Injury risk
- Knowledge deficiency

(Generate solutions)

- Blood pressure will be maintained within acceptable limits.
- Risk for injury will be minimized.
- The patient will verbalize an understanding of drug therapy.

Medication administration

- Don't crush sustained-release tablets.
- Be aware that sustained-release and extended-release medications aren't interchangeable.
- Monitor the patient's vital signs frequently and assess for signs of toxicity and adverse reactions.
- Take safety precautions if adverse CNS reactions occur.
- Notify the prescriber about adverse reactions.
- If the patient's systolic pressure is below 90 mm Hg or the heart rate drops below 60 beats/minute, withhold the dose and notify the prescriber, or follow the prescriber's ordered parameters for withholding the medication.
- Assist the patient with ambulation during the start of therapy because dizziness can occur.
- Advise the patient that fluid and sodium intake may need to be restricted to minimize edema.

Postadministration

(Evaluate outcomes)
- Evaluate the patient's blood pressure and observe for adverse reactions such as hypotension.
- Evaluate the patient's and family's understanding of drug therapy.

Diuretic drugs

Diuretic drugs include several classes of diuretics that reduce blood pressure by increasing urine output and decreasing edema, circulating blood volume, and cardiac output. See Chapter 11, Genitourinary drugs, for specific information on the various types of diuretics.

Sympatholytic drugs

Sympatholytic drugs include several different types of drugs that reduce blood pressure by inhibiting or blocking the sympathetic nervous system. They're classified by their site or mechanism of action and include:
- central-acting sympathetic nervous system inhibitors (clonidine hydrochloride and methyldopa) (See *Centrally acting sympatholytics: Clonidine*, Page 290)
- alpha-adrenergic blockers (doxazosin, phentolamine, prazosin, and terazosin) (See *Alpha-adrenergic blockers: Doxazosin*, Page 290)
- mixed alpha- and beta-adrenergic blockers (carvedilol and labetalol)

Centrally acting sympatholytic: Clonidine (Catapres)

Actions
- Inhibits central vasomotor centers, decreasing sympathetic outflow to the heart, kidneys, and peripheral vasculature
- Decreases peripheral vascular resistance
- Decreases systolic and diastolic blood pressure
- Decreases heart rate

Indications
- High blood pressure

Nursing considerations
- The drug is adjusted to the patient's blood pressure and tolerance.
- When stopping therapy in a patient receiving both clonidine and a beta-adrenergic blocker, gradually withdraw the beta-adrenergic blocker first to minimize adverse reactions.
- Discontinuing clonidine for surgery isn't recommended.

Alpha-adrenergic blockers: Doxazosin (Cardura)

Actions
- Acts on peripheral vasculature to produce vasodilation

Indications
- High blood pressure

Nursing considerations
- The dosage must be increased gradually, with adjustments every 2 weeks for hypertension.
- Monitor blood pressure.
- Monitor the ECG for arrhythmias.

Pharmacokinetics

Most sympatholytic drugs are absorbed well from the GI tract, distributed widely, metabolized in the liver, and excreted primarily in urine.

Pharmacodynamics

All sympatholytic drugs inhibit stimulation of the sympathetic nervous system. This causes dilation of the peripheral blood vessels or decreased cardiac output, thereby reducing blood pressure.

Pharmacotherapeutics

If blood pressure can't be controlled by beta-adrenergic blockers and diuretics, an alpha-adrenergic blocker (such as prazosin) or a mixed alpha- and beta-adrenergic blocker (such as labetalol) may be used.

Try and try again

If the patient still fails to achieve the desired blood pressure, the prescriber may add a drug from a different class, substitute a drug in the same class, or increase the drug dosage.

Drug interactions

Sympatholytic drugs can create the following drug interactions:
- Clonidine plus tricyclic antidepressants may increase blood pressure.

- Clonidine taken with CNS depressants may worsen CNS depression.
- Carvedilol taken with antidiabetic agents may result in an increased hypoglycemic effect.
- Carvedilol taken with calcium channel blockers and digoxin may result in increased digoxin levels.
- Carvedilol taken with rifampin decreases levels of carvedilol.

Side effects/Adverse reactions

Sympatholytic drugs can also produce significant adverse reactions. Possible adverse reactions to sympatholytic drugs vary by type. For example, alpha-adrenergic blockers may cause hypotension.

Central problems

Side effects/adverse reactions to central-acting drugs include:
- depression
- drowsiness
- edema
- liver dysfunction
- numbness and tingling
- vertigo.

"G" whiz

Side effects/adverse reactions to guanadrel include:
- difficulty breathing
- excessive urination
- fainting or dizziness
- orthostatic hypotension
- drowsiness
- diarrhea
- headache.

Side effects/adverse reactions to guanethidine include:
- decreased heart contractility
- diarrhea
- fluid retention
- orthostatic hypotension.

Reserpine results

Side effects/adverse reactions to reserpine include:
- abdominal cramps
- diarrhea
- angina
- blurred vision
- bradycardia

- bronchoconstriction
- decreased libido
- depression
- drowsiness
- edema
- nasal congestion
- weight gain.

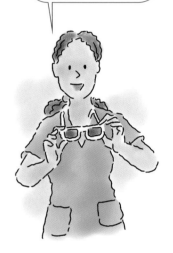

Look sharp! Adverse reactions to reserpine include abdominal cramps, diarrhea, angina, and blurred vision.

The Three-Step Approach

Nursing management for patients needing sympatholytic drug therapy includes these three steps.

Preadministration

(Recognize and analyze cues)
- Obtain a baseline blood pressure and pulse rate and rhythm; recheck regularly.
- Follow the manufacturer's guidelines when mixing and administering parenteral drugs.
- Monitor a patient with a transdermal patch for dermatitis and ask about pruritus. Keep in mind that the patch can require several days to take effect and that interim oral therapy may be needed.

(Prioritize hypothesis—priority patient problems)
- Hypotension risk
- Injury risk
- Knowledge deficiency

(Generate solutions)
- The patient will maintain blood pressure within acceptable limits.
- The patient will not experience injury associated with drug therapy.
- The patient will verbalize understanding of drug therapy.

Medication administration

(Take action)
- If giving orally, administer the drug with food or at bedtime as indicated.
- Monitor the patient for adverse reactions.
- Monitor the patient's weight and fluid and electrolyte status.
- Monitor the patient's adherence with treatment.
- Observe the patient's tolerance of the drug and monitor for the drug's therapeutic effects. The patient may require a dosage adjustment.

- Prevent or minimize orthostatic hypotension by helping the patient to get up slowly and by telling the patient not to make sudden movements.
- Maintain the patient's nonpharmacologic therapies, such as sodium restriction, calorie reduction, stress management, and exercise program.
- Keep in mind that drug therapy may be given to lower blood pressure rapidly in some hypertensive emergency situations.
- Keep in mind that the dosage is usually adjusted to the patient's blood pressure and tolerance.
- To improve adherence of a transdermal patch, apply an adhesive overlay. Place the patch at a different site each week.
- Remove a transdermal patch before defibrillation to prevent arcing.
- Periodic eye examinations are recommended.

Postadministration

(Evaluate outcomes)
- Evaluate the patient's blood pressure and observe for adverse reactions such as hypotension.
- Evaluate the patient's and family's understanding of drug therapy. (See *Teaching about antihypertensives.*)

Education edge

Teaching about antihypertensives

If antihypertensives are prescribed, review these points with the patient and caregivers:
- Take the drug exactly as prescribed. Don't stop the drug abruptly. Abrupt discontinuation may cause severe rebound hypertension.
- The last oral dose is usually administered at bedtime.
- The transdermal patch usually adheres despite showering and other routine daily activities. Use an adhesive overlay to improve skin adherence if necessary. Place the patch at a different site each week.
- The drug can cause drowsiness, but tolerance to this adverse effect will develop.
- Be aware of the adverse reactions caused by this drug and notify your prescriber of serious or persistent reactions (dizziness, coughing, light-headedness, hypotension).
- Avoid sudden changes in position to prevent dizziness, light-headedness, or fainting, which are signs of orthostatic hypotension.
- Avoid hazardous activities until the full effects of the drug are known. Also avoid physical exertion, especially in hot weather.
- Consult with your prescriber before taking any OTC medications or herbal remedies; serious drug interactions can occur.
- Comply with therapy.

Direct vasodilators

Direct vasodilators decrease systolic and diastolic blood pressure. They act on arteries, veins, or both. Examples of these drugs include:
- hydralazine
- minoxidil
- nitroprusside.

Hypertension that hangs on tight

Hydralazine and minoxidil are usually used to treat resistant or refractory hypertension. Nitroprusside are reserved for use in hypertensive crisis. (See *Vasodilators: Nitroprusside.*)

Pharmacokinetics

Most vasodilating drugs are absorbed rapidly and distributed well. They're all metabolized in the liver, and most are excreted by the kidneys.

Pharmacodynamics

The direct vasodilators relax peripheral vascular smooth muscles, causing the blood vessels to dilate. This lowers blood pressure by increasing the diameter of the blood vessels, reducing total peripheral resistance.

Pharmacotherapeutics

Vasodilating drugs are rarely used alone to treat hypertension. Rather, they're usually used in combination with other drugs to treat the patient with moderate to severe hypertension (hypertensive crisis).

Drug interactions

Few drug interactions occur with vasodilating drugs. Some that may occur, however, include the following:
- The antihypertensive effects of hydralazine and minoxidil are increased when they're given with other antihypertensive drugs, such as methyldopa.
- Vasodilating drugs may produce additive effects when given with nitrates, such as isosorbide dinitrate or nitroglycerin.

Side effects/Adverse reactions

Direct vasodilators commonly produce adverse reactions related to reflex activation of the sympathetic nervous system. As blood pressure falls, the sympathetic nervous system is stimulated, producing such compensatory measures as vasoconstriction and tachycardia.

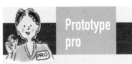

Prototype pro

Vasodilators: Nitroprusside

Actions
- Relaxes arteriolar and venous smooth muscle

Indications
- High blood pressure
- Increased preload and afterload

Nursing considerations
- Monitor thiocyanate levels every 72 hours; excessive doses or rapid infusion may cause cyanide toxicity.
- Monitor for adverse effects and signs of cyanide toxicity, including profound hypotension, metabolic acidosis, dyspnea, headache, loss of consciousness, ataxia, and vomiting.
- Monitor blood pressure every 5 minutes at the start of infusion and every 15 minutes thereafter.
- An IV solution must be wrapped in foil because it's sensitive to light.

Other reactions to sympathetic stimulation include:
- palpitations
- angina
- edema
- breast tenderness
- fatigue
- headache
- rash
- severe pericardial effusion.

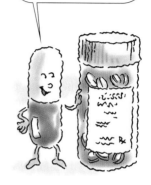

Successful treatment of hypertension usually requires a team approach.

The Three-Step Approach

Nursing management for patients needing vasodilator therapy includes these three steps.

Preadministration

(Recognize and analyze cues)
- Obtain a baseline blood pressure and pulse rate and rhythm; recheck regularly.
- Assess for patent IV site for infusion.

(Prioritize hypothesis—priority patient problems)
- Hypotension risk
- Injury risk
- Knowledge deficiency

(Generate solutions)
- The patient will maintain blood pressure within acceptable limits.
- The patient will not experience injury associated with vasodilator drug therapy.
- The patient will demonstrate an understanding of vasodilator drug therapy.

Medication administration

(Take action)
- If giving orally, administer the drug with food or at bedtime as indicated.
- Follow the manufacturer's guidelines when mixing and administering parenteral drugs.
- Prevent or minimize orthostatic hypotension by helping the patient to get up slowly and by telling the patient not to make sudden movements.
- Because excessive doses or rapid infusion of nitroprusside can cause cyanide toxicity, check thiocyanate levels every 72 hours. Levels above 100 mcg/mL may cause toxicity. Signs of toxicity include profound hypotension, metabolic acidosis, dyspnea, headache, loss of consciousness, ataxia, and vomiting.
- Monitor the patient for adverse reactions and drug interactions.

- Monitor the patient's weight and fluid and electrolyte status.
- Observe the patient's tolerance of the drug and monitor the drug's therapeutic effects. The dosage may need to be adjusted.

Curses! Foiled again

- Keep in mind that nitroprusside is sensitive to light; wrap IV solutions of this drug in foil. A fresh solution should have a faint brownish tint. Discard the drug after 24 hours.
- Infuse IV forms with an infusion pump, usually piggybacked through a peripheral line with no other medications.
- If administering IV, check blood pressure every 5 minutes at the start of the infusion and every 15 minutes thereafter with nitroprusside; titrate the dosage according to blood pressure parameters ordered by the prescriber. If severe hypotension occurs, stop the infusion, and notify the prescriber. Effects of the drug quickly reverse due to its short half-life.
- If cyanide toxicity occurs, stop the drug immediately and notify the prescriber.
- Maintain the patient's nonpharmacologic therapies, such as sodium restriction, calorie reduction, stress management, and exercise program.
- Keep in mind that drug therapy may be given to lower blood pressure rapidly in some hypertensive emergency situations.
- Know that the dosage is usually adjusted to the patient's blood pressure and tolerance.

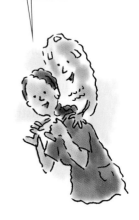

IV infusions of the drug are usually piggybacked through a peripheral line with no other medications.

Postadministration

(Evaluate outcomes)
- Evaluate blood pressure to assess for and respond to hypotension.
- Evaluate patient's and family's understanding of drug therapy.

Selective aldosterone-receptor antagonist

Eplerenone (Inspra), the only selective aldosterone receptor antagonist, produces sustained increases in plasma renin and serum aldosterone. This inhibits the negative feedback mechanism of aldosterone on renin secretion. It selectively binds to mineralocorticoid receptors. The result is an antihypertensive effect.

Pharmacokinetics

Eplerenone has a plasma protein binding of 50% and is primarily bound to alpha-1-acid glycoproteins after oral administration. Its metabolism is controlled by the cytochrome P450 isoform 3A4 (CYP3A4), and less than 5% of the dose is excreted unchanged in urine and feces.

Pharmacodynamics

Eplerenone blocks the binding of aldosterone, an important part of the RAAS. Aldosterone causes increases in blood pressure through sodium reabsorption.

Pharmacotherapeutics

Eplerenone is used to lower blood pressure.

Drug interactions

Eplerenone levels may be increased when the drug is taken with inhibitors of CYP3A4 (erythromycin, saquinavir, verapamil, and fluconazole).

Side effects/Adverse reactions

Eplerenone may cause hyperkalemia (resulting in arrhythmias), cough, diarrhea, fatigue, vaginal bleeding, and breast swelling.

The Three-Step Approach

Preadministration
(Recognize and analyze cues)
- Obtain a baseline blood pressure and pulse rate and rhythm; recheck regularly.
- Monitor the patient for adverse reactions.
- Monitor the patient's weight and fluid and electrolyte status, including potassium levels.
- Monitor the patient's compliance with treatment.

Prioritize hypothesis—priority patient problems
- Electrolyte imbalance risk
- Knowledge deficiency

(Generate solutions)
- The patient will maintain electrolyte balance.
- The patient will verbalize an understanding of drug therapy.

Medication administration
(Take action)
- If giving orally, administer the drug with food or at bedtime as indicated.
- Prevent or minimize orthostatic hypotension by helping the patient to get up slowly and by telling the patient not to make sudden movements.
- Don't give the patient potassium supplements or salt substitutes that contain potassium because eplerenone may cause hyperkalemia.
- Maintain the patient's nonpharmacologic therapies, such as sodium restriction, calorie reduction, stress management, and exercise program.

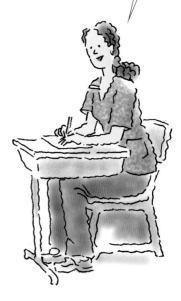

Eplerenone is in a class by itself!

- Know that the dosage is usually adjusted to the patient's blood pressure and tolerance.
- Periodic eye examinations are recommended.

Postadministration
(Evaluate outcomes)
- Patient sustains no trauma from orthostatic hypotension.
- Patient sustains no injury.
- Patient and family demonstrate an understanding of drug therapy.

Antilipemic drugs

Antilipemic drugs are used to lower abnormally high blood levels of lipids, such as cholesterol, triglycerides, and phospholipids. The risk of developing coronary artery disease increases when serum lipid levels are elevated. These drugs are used in combination with lifestyle changes, such as proper diet, weight loss, and exercise, and treatment of any underlying disorder.

Antilipemic drug classes include:
- bile-sequestering drugs
- fibric acid derivatives
- 3-hydroxy-3-methylglutaryl coenzyme A (HMG-CoA) reductase inhibitors
- nicotinic acid
- cholesterol absorption inhibitors.

Bile-sequestering drugs

The bile-sequestering drugs are cholestyramine, colesevelam, and colestipol hydrochloride. These drugs are resins that remove excess bile acids from the fat deposits under the skin.

Pharmacokinetics
Bile-sequestering drugs aren't absorbed from the GI tract. Instead, they remain in the intestine, where they combine with bile acids for about 5 hours and are eventually excreted in feces.

Pharmacodynamics
The bile-sequestering drugs lower blood levels of low-density lipoproteins (LDLs). These drugs combine with bile acids in the intestines to form an insoluble compound that's then excreted in feces. The decreasing level of bile acid in the gallbladder triggers the liver to synthesize more bile acids from their precursor, cholesterol.

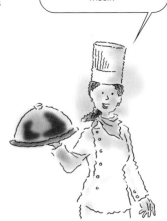

Would you care for a side of bile-sequestering drugs with your low-fat meal?

Calling all cholesterol!

As cholesterol leaves the bloodstream and other storage areas to replace the lost bile acids, blood cholesterol levels decrease. Because the small intestine needs bile acids to emulsify lipids and form chylomicrons, absorption of all lipids and lipid-soluble drugs decreases until the bile acids are replaced.

Pharmacotherapeutics

Bile-sequestering drugs are the drugs of choice for treating type IIa hyperlipoproteinemia (familial hypercholesterolemia) in a patient who isn't able to lower LDL levels through dietary changes. A patient whose blood cholesterol levels indicate a severe risk of coronary artery disease is most likely to require one of these drugs as a supplement to his diet.

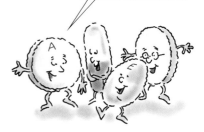

Ha! Let those bile-sequestering drugs just *try* and reduce our absorption!

Drug interactions

Bile-sequestering drugs produce the following drug interactions:
- Bile acid–binding resins of bile-sequestering drugs may interfere with the absorption of digoxin, oral phosphate supplements, and hydrocortisone.
- Bile-sequestering drugs may decrease absorption of propranolol, tetracycline, furosemide, penicillin G, hydrochlorothiazide, and gemfibrozil.
- Bile-sequestering drugs may reduce absorption of lipid-soluble vitamins, such as A, D, E, and K. Poor absorption of vitamin K can affect prothrombin time significantly, increasing the risk of bleeding.

Side effects/Adverse reactions

Short-term adverse reactions to bile-sequestering drugs are relatively mild. More severe reactions can result from long-term use. Adverse GI effects with long-term therapy include severe fecal impaction, vomiting, diarrhea, and hemorrhoid irritation.

Less likely

Rarely, peptic ulcers and bleeding, gallstones, and inflammation of the gallbladder may occur.

The Three–Step Approach

Nursing management for patients needing bile-sequestering drugs includes these three steps.

Preadministration
(Recognize and analyze cues)
- Assess the patient's cholesterol level and pruritus before therapy as appropriate.

- Monitor blood cholesterol and lipid levels before and periodically during therapy. Monitor the drug's effectiveness by checking cholesterol and triglyceride levels every 4 weeks or by asking the patient whether pruritus has diminished or abated as appropriate.
- Monitor CK levels when therapy begins and every 6 months thereafter. Also check CK levels if a patient who takes a cholesterol synthesis inhibitor complains of muscle pain.
- Monitor the patient for adverse reactions and drug interactions.
- Monitor the patient for fat-soluble vitamin deficiency because long-term use may be linked to deficiency of vitamins A, D, E, and K and folic acid.
- Evaluate the patient's and family's knowledge of drug therapy.

(Prioritize hypothesis—priority patient problems)
- Injury risk
- Knowledge deficiency

(Generate solutions)
- The patient will demonstrate lower cholesterol levels.
- Adverse drug effects will be minimized decreasing the risk of injury to the patient.
- The patient will verbalize an understanding of drug therapy.

Medication administration
(Take action)
- If severe constipation develops, decrease the dosage, add a stool softener, or discontinue the drug.
- Give all other drugs at least 1 hour before or 4 to 6 hours after cholestyramine to avoid blocking their absorption.

Mixing it up
- Mix powder forms of bile-sequestering drugs with 120 to 180 mL of liquid. Never administer dry powder alone because the patient may accidentally inhale it.
- To mix the powder, sprinkle it on the surface of a preferred beverage or wet food (soup, applesauce, crushed pineapple). Let it stand for a few minutes, and then stir it to obtain uniform suspension. Know that mixing with carbonated beverages may result in excess foaming. Use a large glass and mix slowly.

Postadministration
(Evaluate outcomes)
- Evaluate the patient's cholesterol levels.
- Evaluate for and promptly address adverse drug effects.
- Evaluate patient's and family's understanding of drug therapy. (See *Teaching about antilipemics*, Page 301.)

Education edge

Teaching about antilipemics

If antilipemics are prescribed, review these points with the patient and caregivers:

• Take the drug exactly as prescribed. If you take a bile-sequestering drug, never take the dry form. Esophageal irritation or severe constipation may result.

• Use a large glass and sprinkle the powder on the surface of a preferred beverage. Let the mixture stand a few minutes; then stir thoroughly. The best diluents are water, milk, and juice (especially pulpy fruit juice). Mixing with carbonated beverages may result in excess foaming. After drinking this preparation, swirl a small additional amount of liquid in the same glass and then drink it to ensure ingestion of the entire dose.

• Diet is very important in controlling serum lipid levels. Maintain proper dietary management of serum lipids (restricting total fat and cholesterol intake) as well as control of other cardiac disease risk factors.

• Drink 2 to 3 qt (2 to 3 L) of fluid daily and report persistent or severe constipation.

• Weight control, exercise, and smoking cessation programs may be appropriate.

• If you also take bile acid resin, take fenofibrate 1 hour before or 4 to 6 hours after bile acid resin.

• When taking fenofibrate promptly report symptoms of unexplained muscle weakness, pain, or tenderness, especially if accompanied by malaise or fever.

• Have periodic eye examinations.

• Don't crush or chew extended-release tablets.

Fibric acid derivatives

Fibric acid is produced by several fungi. Two derivatives of this acid are fenofibrate and gemfibrozil. These drugs are used to reduce high triglyceride levels and, to a lesser extent, high LDL levels.

Pharmacokinetics

Fenofibrate and gemfibrozil are absorbed readily from the GI tract and are highly protein-bound. Fenofibrate undergoes rapid hydrolysis, and gemfibrozil undergoes extensive metabolism in the liver. Both drugs are excreted in urine.

Pharmacodynamics

Although the exact mechanism of action for these drugs isn't known, researchers believe that fibric acid derivatives may:

• reduce cholesterol production early in its formation
• mobilize cholesterol from the tissues
• increase cholesterol excretion
• decrease synthesis and secretion of lipoproteins
• decrease synthesis of triglycerides.

A silver lining

Gemfibrozil produces two other effects:

- It increases high-density lipoprotein (HDL) levels in the blood (remember, this is "good" cholesterol).
- It increases the serum's capacity to dissolve additional cholesterol.

Pharmacotherapeutics

Fibric acid derivatives are used primarily to reduce triglyceride levels, especially very-low-density triglycerides, and secondarily to reduce blood cholesterol levels.

Because of their ability to reduce triglyceride levels, fibric acid derivatives are useful in treating patients with types II, III, IV, and mild type V hyperlipoproteinemia.

Drug interactions

These drug interactions may occur:

- Fibric acid drugs may displace acidic drugs, such as barbiturates, phenytoin, thyroid derivatives, and cardiac glycosides.
- The risk of bleeding increases when fibric acid derivatives are taken with oral anticoagulants.
- Fibric acid derivatives can lead to adverse GI effects.

Side effects/Adverse reactions

Side effects/adverse reactions to fibric acid derivatives include headache, dizziness, blurred vision, arrhythmias, thrombocytopenia, and rash. GI effects include epigastric pain, dyspepsia, nausea, vomiting, and diarrhea or constipation.

The Three-Step Approach

These nursing process steps are appropriate for patients undergoing treatment with fibric acid derivatives.

Preadministration

(Recognize and analyze cues)

- Assess the patient's cholesterol level before therapy as appropriate.
- Assess liver function tests before starting therapy.
- Monitor CK levels when therapy begins.
- Monitor the patient for fat-soluble vitamin deficiency because long-term use may be linked to deficiency of vitamins A, D, E, and K and folic acid.
- If the patient is taking fenofibrate, monitor for muscle pain, tenderness, or weakness, especially if malaise or fever is present.
- Evaluate the patient's and family's knowledge of drug therapy.

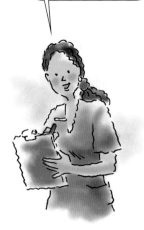

Here's a checklist for you: Fibric acid derivatives can cause headache, dizziness, blurred vision, arrhythmias, thrombocytopenia, rash, and GI effects.

(Prioritize hypothesis—priority patient problems)
- Injury risk
- Knowledge deficiency

(Generate solutions)
- The nurse will monitor closely for potential injury risks associated with complications from adverse reactions.
- The patient will demonstrate lower cholesterol levels.
- The patient and family will demonstrate understanding of drug therapy.

Medication administration

(Take action)
- Monitor blood cholesterol and lipid levels periodically during therapy. Monitor the drug's effectiveness by checking cholesterol and triglyceride levels every 4 weeks or by asking the patient whether pruritus has diminished or abated as appropriate.
- Monitor CK levels every 6 months after initiation. Also check CK levels if a patient who takes a cholesterol synthesis inhibitor complains of muscle pain.
- Monitor the patient for adverse reactions and drug interactions.
- If severe constipation develops, decrease the dosage, add a stool softener, or discontinue the drug.
- Administer a daily fibric acid derivative at prescribed times.
- Withdraw therapy in a patient who doesn't have an adequate response after 2 months of treatment with the maximum dosage.
- Give fenofibrate with meals to increase bioavailability.
- Give gemfibrozil 30 minutes before breakfast and dinner.
- Evaluate renal function and triglyceride levels of a patient with severe renal impairment before dosage increases.
- Reinforce the importance of adhering to a triglyceride-lowering diet.
- Instruct the patient who also takes bile acid resin to take fenofibrate 1 hour before or 4 to 6 hours after bile acid resin.

Postadministration

(Evaluate outcomes)
- Evaluate the patient's cholesterol levels.
- Evaluate for and promptly address adverse drug effects.
- Evaluate patient's and family's understanding of drug therapy.

HMG-CoA reductase inhibitors

As their name implies, HMG-CoA reductase inhibitors (also known as the *statins*) lower lipid levels by interfering with cholesterol synthesis. These drugs include atorvastatin calcium (Lipitor), fluvastatin sodium, lovastatin, pitavastatin, pravastatin sodium, rosuvastatin (Crestor), and simvastatin (Zocor). (See *Antilipemics: Atorvastatin* (Lipitor).)

Pharmacokinetics

With the exception of pravastatin, HMG-CoA reductase inhibitors are highly bound to plasma proteins. All undergo extensive first-pass metabolism. Their specific pharmacokinetic properties vary slightly.

Pharmacodynamics

HMG-CoA reductase inhibitors inhibit the enzyme that's responsible for the conversion of HMG-CoA to mevalonate, an early rate-limiting step in the biosynthesis of cholesterol.

Pharmacotherapeutics

Statin drugs are used primarily to reduce LDL cholesterol levels and to reduce total blood cholesterol levels. These agents also produce a mild increase in HDL cholesterol levels.

Because of their ability to lower cholesterol levels, statins are indicated for the treatment of primary hypercholesterolemia (types IIa and IIb).

Event preventer

As a result of their effect on LDL and total cholesterol, these drugs are indicated for primary and secondary prevention of cardiovascular events.

Drug interactions

These drug interactions may occur:
- Atorvastatin (Lipitor), simvastatin (Zocor), or lovastatin, when combined with niacin, erythromycin, clarithromycin, immunosuppressant drugs (especially cyclosporine), gemfibrozil, itraconazole, ketoconazole, or fluconazole, may increase the risk of myopathy (muscle wasting and weakness) or rhabdomyolysis (potentially fatal breakdown of skeletal muscle, causing renal failure).
- All HMG-CoA reductase inhibitors should be administered 1 hour before or 4 hours after bile-sequestering drugs (cholestyramine, colestipol, colesevelam).
- Lovastatin and simvastatin may increase the risk of bleeding when administered with warfarin.

Side effects/Adverse reactions

HMG-CoA reductase inhibitors may alter liver function studies, increasing aspartate aminotransferase, alanine aminotransferase, alkaline phosphatase, and bilirubin levels. Other hepatic effects may include pancreatitis, hepatitis, and cirrhosis.

Prototype pro

Antilipemics: Atorvastatin (Lipitor)

Actions
- Inhibits HMG-CoA reductase

Indications
- High plasma cholesterol and lipoprotein levels

Nursing considerations
- Use the drug only after diet and other, nonpharmacologic treatments prove ineffective.
- Restrict the patient to a standard low-cholesterol diet before and during therapy.
- Before starting treatment, perform a baseline lipid profile to exclude secondary causes of hypercholesterolemia. Liver function test results and lipid levels should be obtained before therapy, after 6 and 12 weeks, following a dosage increase, and periodically thereafter.
- Before starting treatment, a baseline CK may be obtained and the patient should be routinely monitored for myopathy, which may be an indication of rhabdomyolysis.

Oh, the pain of it all…

Myalgia is the most common musculoskeletal effect, although arthralgia and muscle cramps may also occur. Myopathy and rhabdomyolysis are rare but potentially severe reactions that may occur with these drugs.

Possible adverse GI reactions include nausea, vomiting, diarrhea, abdominal pain, flatulence, and constipation.

The Three-Step Approach

Nursing management for patients needing HMG-CoA reductase inhibitors (also known as the *statins*) includes these three steps.

Preadministration

(Recognize and analyze cues)
- Assess the patient's cholesterol level before therapy as appropriate.
- Monitor blood cholesterol and lipid levels before and periodically during therapy. Monitor the drug's effectiveness by checking cholesterol and triglyceride levels every 4 weeks or by asking the patient whether pruritus has diminished or abated as appropriate.
- Monitor CK levels when therapy begins and every 6 months thereafter. Also check CK levels if a patient who takes a cholesterol synthesis inhibitor complains of muscle pain.
- Liver function tests should be performed at the start of therapy and periodically thereafter. A liver biopsy may be performed if enzyme level elevations persist.
- Monitor the patient for fat-soluble vitamin deficiency because long-term use may be linked to deficiency of vitamins A, D, E, and K and folic acid.
- Evaluate the patient's and family's knowledge of drug therapy.

(Prioritize hypothesis—priority patient problems)
- Injury risk
- Knowledge deficiency

(Generate solutions)
- The patient will demonstrate lower cholesterol levels.
- The nurse will monitor for potential injury risks associated with complications from adverse reactions.
- The patient and family will demonstrate understanding of drug therapy.

Medication administration

(Take action)
- Monitor the patient for adverse reactions and drug interactions.
- If severe constipation develops, decrease the dosage, add a stool softener, or discontinue the drug.

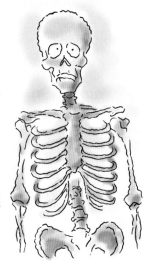

I know statins help reduce LDL levels, but I'm not too crazy about the joint pain they can cause.

- Give the drug before meals and at bedtime as applicable. Give lovastatin with an evening meal, simvastatin in the evening, and fluvastatin and pravastatin at bedtime.

Postadministration
(Evaluate outcomes)
- Evaluate the patient's cholesterol levels.
- Evaluate for and promptly address adverse drug effects.
- Evaluate patient's and family's understanding of drug therapy.

Nicotinic acid

Also known as *niacin*, nicotinic acid is a water-soluble vitamin that decreases triglyceride and apolipoprotein B-100 levels and increases HDL levels. The drug is available in immediate-release and extended-release tablets.

Pharmacokinetics

Nicotinic acid is moderately bound to plasma proteins; its overall binding ranges from 60% to 70%. The drug undergoes rapid metabolism by the liver to active and inactive metabolites. About 75% of the drug is excreted in urine.

Pharmacodynamics

The way that nicotinic acid lowers triglyceride and apolipoprotein levels is unknown. However, it may work by inhibiting hepatic synthesis of lipoproteins that contain apolipoprotein B-100, promoting lipoprotein lipase activity, reducing free fatty acid mobilization from adipose tissue, and increasing fecal elimination of sterols.

Pharmacotherapeutics

Nicotinic acid is used primarily as an adjunct to lower triglyceride levels in patients with type IV or V hyperlipidemia who are at high risk for pancreatitis. The drug also may be used to lower cholesterol and LDL levels in patients with hypercholesterolemia. It's commonly used with other antilipemics to meet LDL goals and to increase the HDL level for patients who have a lower-than-desired HDL level.

Just say no

This antilipemic is contraindicated in patients who are hypersensitive to nicotinic acid and in those with hepatic or renal dysfunction, active peptic ulcer disease, gout, heart disease, muscle disorder, or arterial bleeding. Also, because nicotinic acid can cause hyperglycemia, it's not prescribed for patients with diabetes.

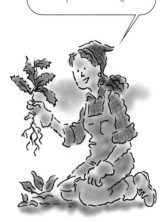

Giving kava with nicotinic acid may increase the risk of hepatotoxicity.

Drug interactions

These drug interactions can occur with nicotinic acid:

- Together, nicotinic acid and an HMG-CoA reductase inhibitor may increase the risk of muscle wasting and weakness, myopathy, or life-threatening breakdown of skeletal muscle, causing renal failure or rhabdomyolysis.
- A bile-sequestering drug, such as cholestyramine can bind with nicotinic acid and decrease its effectiveness.
- When given with nicotinic acid, kava may increase the risk of hepatotoxicity.

Side effects/Adverse reactions

High doses of nicotinic acid may produce vasodilation and cause flushing. Extended-release forms tend to produce less severe vasodilation than immediate-release forms. To help minimize flushing, aspirin may be given 30 minutes before nicotinic acid, or the extended-release form may be given at night.

Nicotinic acid can cause hepatotoxicity; the risk of this adverse reaction is greater with extended-release forms. Other adverse effects include nausea, vomiting, diarrhea, and epigastric or substernal pain.

The Three–Step Approach

Nursing management for patients needing nicotinic acid drug therapy includes these three steps.

Preadministration

(Recognize and analyze cues)

- Assess the patient's cholesterol level and pruritus before therapy, as appropriate.
- Monitor blood cholesterol and lipid levels before and periodically during therapy. Monitor the drug's effectiveness by checking cholesterol and triglyceride levels every 4 weeks or by asking the patient whether pruritus has diminished or abated as appropriate.
- Monitor CK levels when therapy begins and every 6 months thereafter. Also check CK levels if a patient who takes a cholesterol synthesis inhibitor complains of muscle pain.
- Monitor the patient for adverse reactions and drug interactions.
- Monitor the patient for fat-soluble vitamin deficiency because long-term use may be linked to deficiency of vitamins A, D, E, and K and folic acid.
- Evaluate the patient's and family's knowledge of drug therapy.

(Prioritize hypothesis—priority patient problems)

- Injury risk
- Knowledge deficiency

(Generate solutions)

- The patient will demonstrate lower cholesterol levels.
- The nurse will monitor for potential injury risks associated with complications from adverse reactions.
- The patient and family will demonstrate understanding of drug therapy.

Medication administration

(Take action)

- If severe constipation develops, decrease the dosage, add a stool softener, or discontinue the drug.
- Administer aspirin as appropriate to help reduce flushing.
- Know that timed-release niacin or niacinamide may prevent excessive flushing that occurs with large dosages. However, timed-release niacin has been linked to hepatic dysfunction, even at low dosages.
- Give the drug with meals to minimize GI adverse effects.
- To decrease flushing, advise the patient to take the drug with a low-fat snack and to avoid taking it after alcohol, hot beverages, hot or spicy foods, a hot shower, or exercise.

Postadministration

(Evaluate outcomes)

- Evaluate the patient's cholesterol levels.
- Evaluate for and promptly address adverse drug effects.
- Evaluate patient's and family's understanding of drug therapy.

Cholesterol absorption inhibitors

As their name implies, cholesterol absorption inhibitors inhibit the absorption of cholesterol and related phytosterols from the intestine. Ezetimibe is the drug that falls under this class.

Pharmacokinetics

Ezetimibe (Zetia) is absorbed and extensively conjugated to an active form and is highly bound to plasma proteins. The drug is primarily metabolized in the small intestine and is excreted by the biliary and renal routes.

Pharmacodynamics

Ezetimibe reduces blood cholesterol levels by inhibiting the absorption of cholesterol by the small intestine.

Ezetimibe reduces blood cholesterol levels by inhibiting the absorption of cholesterol by the small intestine.

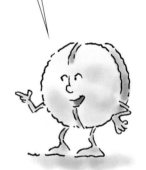

On the edge

The drug works at the brush border of the small intestine to inhibit cholesterol absorption. This leads to a decrease in delivery of intestinal cholesterol to the liver, causing a reduction in hepatic cholesterol stores and an increase in clearance from the blood.

Pharmacotherapeutics

Ezetimibe may be administered alone as adjunctive therapy to diet for treatment of primary hypercholesterolemia and homozygous sitosterolemia. The drug is also indicated as adjunctive therapy, administered in addition to HMG-CoA reductase inhibitors, for the treatment of primary hypercholesterolemia and homozygous familial hypercholesterolemia.

Helping things along

Ezetimibe helps to further lower total cholesterol and LDL and further increase HDL cholesterol in patients who can't achieve their desired goals with maximum-dose HMG-CoA reductase inhibitor therapy.

Drug interactions

Cholestyramine may decrease the effectiveness of ezetimibe. Fenofibrate, gemfibrozil, and cyclosporine lead to an increased level of ezetimibe.

Side effects/Adverse reactions

The most common adverse reactions to ezetimibe include:
- fatigue
- abdominal pain
- diarrhea
- pharyngitis
- sinusitis
- arthralgia and back pain
- cough.

When ezetimibe is given with an HMG-CoA reductase inhibitor, the most common adverse reactions are:
- chest or abdominal pain
- dizziness
- headache
- diarrhea
- pharyngitis
- sinusitis
- upper respiratory tract infection
- arthralgia, myalgia, and back pain.

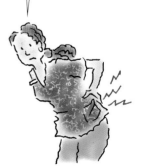

Whether you take ezetimibe alone or with HMG-CoA, it can sometimes cause back pain. Ouch!

The Three-Step Approach

Nursing management for patients needing cholesterol absorption inhibitor therapy includes these three steps.

Preadministration

(Recognize and analyze cues)
- Assess the patient's cholesterol level and pruritus before therapy as appropriate.
- Monitor blood cholesterol and lipid levels before and periodically during therapy.
- Assess the patient's and family's knowledge of drug therapy.

(Prioritize hypothesis—priority patient problems)
- Injury risk
- Knowledge deficiency

(Generate solutions)
- The patient will demonstrate lower cholesterol levels.
- The nurse will monitor for potential injury risks associated with complications from adverse reactions.
- The patient and family will demonstrate understanding of drug therapy.

Medication administration

(Take action)
- Monitor the drug's effectiveness by checking cholesterol and triglyceride levels every 4 weeks or by asking the patient whether pruritus has diminished or abated as appropriate.
- Monitor the patient for fat-soluble vitamin deficiency because long-term use may be linked to deficiency of vitamins A, D, E, and K and folic acid.
- Monitor CK levels when therapy begins and every 6 months thereafter. Also check CK levels if a patient who takes a cholesterol synthesis inhibitor or reports muscle pain.
- Be alert for adverse reactions and drug interactions.
- If severe constipation develops, decrease the dosage, add a stool softener, or discontinue the drug.
- Teach the patient how to follow a cholesterol-lowering diet as appropriate.

Postadministration

(Evaluate outcomes)
- Evaluate the patient's cholesterol levels.
- Evaluate for and promptly address adverse drug effects.
- Evaluate patient's and family's understanding of drug therapy

Quick quiz

1. A patient is being discharged with a new prescription for translingual nitroglycerin. Which patient statement indicates additional teaching is required?

    A. "I will shake the medication before I spray it in my mouth."
    B. "I can use this medication if I have chest pain."
    C. "If I still have chest pain after 3 sprays within 15 minutes, I should call 911."
    D. "I can spray this medicine on my tongue or under it."

Answer: A. Translingual nitroglycerin should not be shaken prior to administration. This patient statement requires further education from the nurse. All other statements are accurate.

2. A patient taking nitroglycerin intravenously for the treatment of chest pain reports a headache. What nursing action is appropriate?

    A. Titrate to decrease the nitroglycerin drip
    B. Assess the heart rate
    C. Notify the provider
    D. Administer PRN Tylenol

Answer: D. The most common adverse reaction to nitrates is headache. Nitrates dilate the blood vessels in the meningeal layers between the brain and cranium. The most appropriate nursing action is to administer PRN Tylenol to treat the headache pain. If the patient continues to have chest pain, it is not appropriate to decrease the nitroglycerin drip. While the nurse can assess the heart rate, the report of a headache is not likely to be related to the heart rate, rather it is a known adverse effect of nitroglycerin. The nurse would not need to notify the provider unless the ordered Tylenol does not treat the patient's headache pain.

3. Which life-threatening reaction is associated with ACE inhibitors?

    A. Seizure
    B. Sexual dysfunction
    C. Dizziness
    D. Angioedema

Answer: D. Angioedema is life-threatening reaction that may occur with ACE inhibitor agents. It is life-threatening because the swelling can occlude the airway. Dizziness can occur with ACE inhibitors and can be a sign of hypotension. Dizziness is not life threatening. Sexual dysfunction can occur with ACE inhibitors; however, this is not a life-threatening reaction. Seizure is unlikely with ACE inhibitors.

4. The charge nurse is teaching a group of new nurses about digoxin. Which teaching will the nurse include? Select all that apply.
  A. This drug has a wide therapeutic index.
  B. Digoxin is often used to control the heart rate with atrial fibrillation.
  C. Brands of digoxin are interchangeable.
  D. Vision changes are a sign of digoxin toxicity.
  E. There is no antidote for digoxin overdose or toxicity.

Answer: B, D. When teaching about digoxin, the nurse will include that digoxin has a narrow therapeutic index of safety (not wide). If the patient receives too much, it can create digoxin toxicity or become fatal. Digoxin can be used to control the heart rate. Brands and forms of digoxin are different and are not interchangeable. Vision changes are a sign of digoxin toxicity, and there is an antidote that can be used for digoxin toxicity.

Scoring

☆☆☆ If you answered all four questions correctly, A+! You're aces with ACE inhibitors and all of the other cardiovascular drugs.

 ☆☆ If you answered three questions correctly, cool! Cardiovascular drugs aren't causing you any complications.

  ☆ If you answered fewer than three questions correctly, stay mellow! This is a complex chapter, and it might just require another dose.

Suggested References

Amsterdam, E. A., Wenger, N. K., Brindis, R. G., et al.; American College of Cardiology; American Heart Association Task Force on Practice Guidelines; Society for Cardiovascular Angiography and Interventions; Society of Thoracic Surgeons; American Association for Clinical Chemistry. (2014). 2014 AHA/ACC guideline for the management of patients with non-ST-elevation acute coronary syndromes: A report of the American College of Cardiology/American Heart Association Task Force on Practice Guidelines. *J Am Coll Cardiol, 64*(24), e139–e228. doi: 10.1016/j.jacc.2014.09.017.

Elliot, W. J., & Varon, J. (2020). Evaluation and treatment of hypertensive emergencies in adults. In *UpToDate*.

Flesher, L. A., Fleischmann, K. E., Auerbach, A. D., Barnason, S. A., Beckman, J. A., Bozkurt, B., …Wijeysundera, D. N. (2014). 2014 ACC/AHA guideline on perioperative cardiovascular evaluation and management of patients undergoing noncardiac surgery: a report of the American College of Cardiology/American Heart Association Task Force on Practice Guidelines. *J Am Coll Cardiol, 64*, e77–e137.

James, P. A., Ortiz, E., et al. (2014). 2014 evidence-based guideline for the management of high blood pressure in adults: (JNC8). *JAMA, 311*(5), 507–520.

McMurray, J., Packer, M., Desai, A., et al. (2014). Angiotensin-neprilysin inhibition versus enalapril in heart failure. *The New England Journal of Medicine, 371*, 993–1004. doi: 10.1056/NEJMoa1409077.

Overgaard, C. B., & Džavík, V. (2008). Inotropes and vasopressors: Review of physiology and clinical use in cardiovascular disease. *Circulation, 118*, 1047–1056. https://doi.org/10.1161/CIRCULATIONAHA.107.728840

Ponikowski, P., Voors, A. A., Anker, S. D., Bueno, H., Cleland, J. G. F., Coats A. J. S., … van der Meer, P.; ESC Scientific Document Group. (2016). 2016 ESC guidelines for the diagnosis and treatment of acute and chronic heart failure: The Task Force for the diagnosis and treatment of acute and chronic heart failure of the European Society of Cardiology (ESC) Developed with the special contribution of the Heart Failure Association (HFA) of the ESC. European Heart Journal, 37(27), 2129–2200. https://doi.org/10.1093/eurheartj/ehw128

Yancy, C. W., Jessup, M., Bozkurt, B., Butler, J., Casey, D. E. Jr, Colvin, M. M., … Westlake, C. (2017). 2017 ACC/AHA/HFSA focused update of the 2013 ACCF/AHA guideline for the management of heart failure: A report of the American College of Cardiology/American Heart Association Task Force on Clinical Practice Guidelines and the Heart Failure Society of America. *Circulation, 136*, e137–e161. doi: 10.1161/CIR.0000000000000509.

Chapter 9

Respiratory drugs

Just the facts

In this chapter, you'll learn:

◆ classes of drugs that affect the respiratory system

◆ uses and varying actions of these drugs

◆ absorption, distribution, metabolization, and excretion of these drugs

◆ drug interactions, side effects, and adverse reactions to these drugs.

Drugs and the respiratory system

The respiratory system, which extends from the nose to the pulmonary capillaries, performs the essential function of gas exchange (oxygen and carbon dioxide) between the body and its environment.

Drugs used to improve respiratory symptoms are available in inhalation and systemic formulations. These include:

- beta$_2$-adrenergic agonists
- anticholinergics
- corticosteroids
- leukotriene modifiers
- mast cell stabilizers
- methylxanthines
- expectorants
- antitussives
- decongestants.

Antihistamines also improve respiratory function and are discussed in the Anti-inflammatory, antiallergy, and immunosuppressant, pages 645.

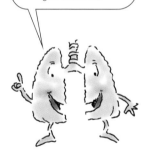

Are you ready to learn about respiratory system drugs? Then take a deep breath and let's get started.

Beta$_2$-adrenergic agonists

Beta$_2$-adrenergic agonists, or beta agonists, are used for the treatment of symptoms associated with asthma and chronic obstructive pulmonary disease (COPD) (Lemanske, 2019). Agents in this class can be divided into two categories:

- short-acting
- long-acting.

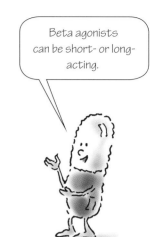

Beta agonists can be short- or long-acting.

The short...

Short-acting beta agonists (SABAs) are used for acute therapy and include:

- albuterol (systemic, inhalation)
- levalbuterol (inhalation)
- terbutaline (systemic).

... and long of it

Long-acting beta agonists (LABAs) are used for long-term control and include:

- albuterol (oral, systemic)
- formoterol (inhalation)
- salmeterol (inhalation).

Better together

Combination agents that contain inhaled beta agonists, anticholinergics, and or corticosteroids may be used for better control and include:

- albuterol and ipratropium (inhalation)
- budesonide and formoterol (inhalation)
- formoterol and mometasone (inhalation)
- salmeterol and fluticasone (inhalation).

Pharmacokinetics

Beta agonists are minimally absorbed from the GI tract. Inhaled formulations generally exert their effects locally. After inhalation, beta agonists appear to be absorbed in the respiratory tract. These drugs do not cross the blood-brain barrier. They are extensively metabolized in the liver to inactive compounds and are rapidly excreted in urine (Karch, 2020).

Pharmacodynamics

Beta agonists relax smooth muscle in the airways and allow increased airflow to the lungs. They increase levels of cyclic adenosine monophosphate through the stimulation of beta₂-adrenergic receptors in the smooth muscle, resulting in bronchodilation. Beta agonists may lose their selectivity at higher doses, which can increase the risk of toxicity (Karch, 2020). Inhaled agents are preferred because they act locally in the lungs, resulting in fewer adverse effects than systemically absorbed formulations.

Pharmacotherapeutics

Short-acting inhaled beta agonists are the drugs of choice for fast relief of symptoms in asthmatic patients. They are primarily used on an as-needed basis for asthma and COPD and are also effective for prevention of exercise-induced asthma.

From morning till night

Some patients with COPD use short-acting inhaled beta agonists around the clock on a specified schedule. However, excessive use of these agents may indicate poor asthma control, requiring reassessment of the therapeutic regimen (Lemanske, 2019).

Strictly regimented

Long-acting agents are more appropriately used with anti-inflammatory agents, specifically inhaled corticosteroids, to help control asthma. They must be administered on schedule to be most effective. These drugs are especially useful when a patient exhibits nocturnal asthmatic symptoms. Because of their delayed onset, long-acting beta agonists aren't used for acute symptoms. They are also ineffective against the chronic inflammation associated with asthma. When used daily, long-acting agents prevent asthma attacks but will not relieve asthma attacks already under way and should not be used as rescue inhalers.

Drug interactions

Interactions with beta agonists aren't as common when using inhaled formulations. Beta-adrenergic blockers decrease the bronchodilation effects of the beta agonists; therefore, these drugs should be used together cautiously.

Side effects/adverse reactions

Side effects and adverse reactions to SABAs include:
- paradoxical bronchospasm
- tachycardia
- palpitations
- tremors
- dry mouth.

Side effects and adverse reactions to LABAs include:
- bronchospasm
- tachycardia
- palpitation
- hypertension
- tremors.

The Three-Step Approach

Nursing management for the patient receiving treatment with beta agonists include these three steps.

Preadministration

(Recognize and analyze cues)

- Assess the patient's respiratory condition before therapy and regularly thereafter.
- Assess peak flow readings before starting treatment and periodically thereafter.
- Be alert for adverse reactions and drug interactions.
- Assess the patient's and family's knowledge of drug therapy.

(Prioritize hypothesis—priority patient problems)

- Altered breathing pattern
- Impaired gas exchange
- Knowledge deficiency

(Generate solutions)

- Breathing patterns will improve as evidenced by regular and even respiratory rate and rhythm.
- Gas exchange will be adequate as evidenced by improved peak flow rates, oxygen saturation, and arterial blood gas (ABG) levels.
- The patient and family members will demonstrate correct drug understanding, administration, and use.

Medication administration

(Take action)

- Report insufficient relief or a worsening condition.
- Obtain an order for a mild analgesic if a drug-induced headache occurs.
- Teach the patient and family not to use long-acting beta agonists for reversing bronchospasm during an acute asthma attack.
- For the inhalation formulation, teach the patient to hold their breath for several seconds after inhalation and wait at least 2 minutes before taking another inhalation of the drug.

Postadministration

(Evaluate outcomes)

- The patient exhibits a normal breathing pattern.
- The patient exhibits improved gas exchange.
- The patient and family understand drug therapy. (See *Teaching about bronchodilators*, page 318.)

Teaching about bronchodilators

See Education edge: Teaching template in Chapter 3, page 38 for general teaching for all medications. Specific points to review with patients and family for bronchodilator therapy:

• Note that some medications should be taken every 12 hours, even if you're feeling better, and other drugs, such as albuterol, should only be used in an acute attack.

• Take the prescribed drug 30 to 60 minutes before exercise as directed to prevent exercise-induced bronchospasm.

• Contact your prescriber if the medication no longer provides sufficient relief or if you need more than four inhalations per day. This may be a sign that asthma symptoms are worsening. Don't increase the dosage of the drug.

• Don't take bronchodilators with other drugs, over-the-counter preparations, or herbal remedies without your prescriber's consent.

• Follow these instructions for using a metered-dose inhaler as appropriate:

  – Clear your nasal passages and throat.

  – Breathe out, expelling as much air from your lungs as possible.

  – Place the mouthpiece well into your mouth and inhale deeply as you release the dose from the inhaler.

  – Hold your breath for several seconds, remove the mouthpiece, and exhale slowly.

  – Avoid accidentally spraying the medication into your eyes. Temporary blurring of vision may result.

• If more than one inhalation is ordered, wait at least 2 minutes between each subsequent inhalation.

• If you use a corticosteroid inhaler, use the bronchodilator first, and then wait about 5 minutes before using the corticosteroid. This process allows the bronchodilator to open air passages for maximum effectiveness of the corticosteroid.

• Take a missed dose as soon as you remember, unless it's almost time for the next dose; in that case, skip the missed dose. Don't double the dose.

• Whenever possible, use a spacer device with your metered-dose inhaler to achieve more effect from the medication. Remember to wash and dry the device after each use.

Anticholinergics

Anticholinergics competitively antagonize the actions of acetylcholine and other cholinergic agonists at receptors. Although oral anticholinergics generally aren't used to treat asthma and COPD because of their tendency to thicken secretions and form mucus plugs in the airways, one anticholinergic—ipratropium—is used for COPD.

Ipratropium

Inhaled ipratropium bromide is a bronchodilator used primarily in patients suffering from COPD to prevent wheezing, difficulty breathing, chest tightness, and coughing. It may also be used as an adjunct to beta agonists (Dweik, 2021).

Pharmacokinetics

Ipratropium is minimally absorbed from the GI tract. It exerts its effects locally through inhalation.

Pharmacodynamics

Ipratropium blocks the parasympathetic nervous system rather than stimulating the sympathetic nervous system. To exert its anticholinergic effects, this drug inhibits muscarinic receptors, which results in bronchodilation (Dweik, 2021).

Pharmacotherapeutics

Ipratropium is used in patients with COPD. It may also be used as an adjunctive therapy for the treatment of asthma; however, it is less effective as a form of long-term management. It's commonly used in combination with a SABA on a scheduled basis. It is also used to treat rhinorrhea and is available as a nasal spray.

Drug interactions

Drug interactions aren't as likely when using an inhaled formulation of ipratropium. Use antimuscarinic and anticholinergic agents cautiously with ipratropium.

Side effects/adverse reactions

The most common side effects and adverse reactions to anticholinergics include:
- nervousness
- tachycardia
- nausea and vomiting
- dizziness
- headache
- paradoxical bronchospasm with excessive use
- difficulty urinating
- constipation
- dry mouth.

The Three-Step Approach

Nursing management for patients receiving treatment with anticholinergics include these three steps.

Preadministration
(Recognize and analyze cues)
- Assess the patient's respiratory condition before therapy and regularly thereafter.
- Assess peak flow readings before starting treatment and periodically thereafter.
- Be alert for side effects, adverse reactions, and drug interactions.

- Assess the patient's and family's knowledge of drug therapy.

(Prioritize hypothesis—priority patient problems)

- Altered breathing pattern
- Impaired gas exchange
- Knowledge deficiency

(Generate solutions)

- Breathing patterns will improve as evidenced by regular and even respiratory rate and rhythm.
- Gas exchange will be adequate as evidenced by improved peak flow rates, oxygen saturation, and ABG levels.
- The patient and family members will demonstrate correct drug understanding, administration, and use.

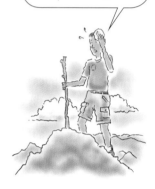

Assess... whew! ... peak flow readings before starting treatment and then periodically.

Medication administration

(Take action)

- Report insufficient relief or a worsening condition.
- Obtain an order for a mild analgesic if a drug-induced headache occurs.

Acutely ineffective

- Be aware that the drug isn't effective for treating acute episodes of bronchospasm when rapid response is needed.
- Monitor the medication regimen. Total inhalations shouldn't exceed 12 in 24 hours, and total nasal sprays shouldn't exceed 8 in each nostril in 24 hours.
- If more than one inhalation is ordered, 2 minutes should elapse between inhalations. If more than one type of inhalant is ordered, always give the bronchodilator first and wait 5 minutes before administering the other inhalant.
- Give the drug on time to ensure maximal effect.
- Notify the prescriber if the drug fails to relieve bronchospasms.
- Provide patient teaching.

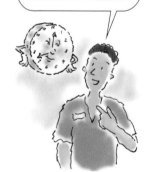

Watch that clock! Keep in mind that total inhalations shouldn't exceed 12 in 24 hours, and total nasal sprays shouldn't exceed 8 in each nostril in 24 hours.

Close your eyes

- Warn the patient to keep eyes closed when using ipratropium because it can cause acute narrow-angle glaucoma if it gets in the eyes. Instruct the patient to call the prescriber immediately if the drug gets in the eyes.

Postadministration

(Evaluate outcomes)

- The patient exhibits normal breathing pattern.
- The patient exhibits improved gas exchange.
- The patient and family understand drug therapy and demonstrate correct use and administration.

Corticosteroids

Corticosteroids are anti-inflammatory agents available in both inhaled and systemic formulations for the short- and long-term control of asthma symptoms. This class consists of many drugs with differing potencies.

The nose knows

Inhaled corticosteroids include:
- beclomethasone dipropionate
- budesonide
- ciclesonide
- fluticasone propionate
- triamcinolone acetonide
- mometasone.

Over the lips, past the gums

Oral corticosteroids include:
- prednisolone
- prednisone.

A vein attempt

IV corticosteroids include:
- dexamethasone
- hydrocortisone
- methylprednisolone.

Pharmacokinetics

Inhaled corticosteroids are minimally absorbed, although absorption increases as the dose is increased. Oral prednisone is readily absorbed and extensively metabolized in the liver to the active metabolite, prednisolone. IV forms have a rapid onset but offer no more advantage over oral forms.

Pharmacodynamics

Corticosteroids inhibit the production of cytokines, leukotrienes, and prostaglandins; the recruitment of eosinophils; and the release of other inflammatory mediators. They also have various effects elsewhere in the body that cause many of the long-term adverse effects associated with these agents. (See *Corticosteroid warning,* page 322.)

> Make sure the patient knows to close his eyes when using ipratropium. Serious eye problems, including acute narrow-angle glaucoma, can occur if solution gets in the eyes.

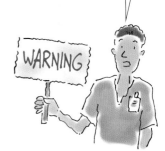

Corticosteroid Warning

Consider these points about special populations before administering corticosteroids:
• Growth should be monitored in children, especially when taking systemic agents or higher doses of inhaled agents.
• Older adults may benefit from specific medications, diet, and exercise intended to prevent osteoporosis while on these agents, especially when receiving higher doses of inhaled steroids or systemic agents.
• Patients with diabetes may require closer monitoring of blood glucose while on steroids.

• Corticosteroid levels are negligible in the breast milk of mothers who are receiving less than 20 mg/day of oral prednisone. The amount found in breast milk can be minimized if the mother waits at least 4 hours after taking prednisone to breast-feed the infant.
• To reduce the risk of side effects and adverse reactions occurring with the inhaled agents, use the lowest possible doses to maintain control. Spacers should be used to administer doses, and patients should rinse their mouths out following administration.

Pharmacotherapeutics

Corticosteroids are the most effective agents available for the long-term treatment and prevention of asthma exacerbations. Systemic formulations are commonly reserved for moderate to severe acute exacerbations but are also used in those with severe asthma that's refractory to other measures. Systemic corticosteroids should be used at the lowest effective dosage and for the shortest possible period to avoid adverse effects (Fanta, 2021).

Inhaled corticosteroids remain the mainstay of therapy to prevent future exacerbations for most asthmatics with mild to severe disease. Use of inhaled corticosteroids reduces the need for systemic steroids in many patients, thus reducing the risk of serious long-term adverse effects. Inhaled corticosteroids should not be used for acute symptoms; rather, short-acting inhaled beta agonists should be used (Fanta, 2021).

Drug interactions

Interactions aren't likely when using inhaled formulations. Hormonal contraceptives, ketoconazole, and macrolide antibiotics can increase the activity of corticosteroids in general and may require a dosage decrease of the steroid. Barbiturates, cholestyramine, and phenytoin can decrease the effectiveness of corticosteroids and may require a dosage increase of the steroid.

Side effects/adverse reactions

Possible side effects and adverse reactions to inhaled corticosteroids include:
• mouth irritation
• oral candidiasis

- upper respiratory tract infection
- cough and hoarseness.

Possible side effects and adverse reactions to oral corticosteroids include:
- hyperglycemia
- nausea and vomiting
- headache
- insomnia
- growth suppression in children.

The Three-Step Approach

Nursing management for patients undergoing treatment with corticosteroids include these three steps.

Preadministration

(Recognize and analyze cues)
- Assess the patient's respiratory condition before therapy and regularly thereafter.
- Assess peak flow readings before starting treatment and periodically thereafter.
- Be alert for adverse reactions and drug interactions.
- Evaluate the patient's and family's knowledge of drug therapy.

(Prioritize hypothesis—priority patient problems)
- Altered breathing pattern
- Impaired gas exchange
- Knowledge deficiency

(Generate solutions)
- Breathing pattern will improve as evidenced by regular and even respiratory rate and rhythm.
- Gas exchange will be adequate as evidenced by improved peak flow rates, oxygen saturation, and ABG levels.
- The patient and family members will demonstrate understanding, administration, and correct drug use.

Medication administration

(Take action)
- Report insufficient relief or worsening of condition.
- Give oral doses with food to prevent GI irritation.
- Take precautions to avoid exposing the patient to infection.
- Don't stop the drug abruptly.
- Notify the prescriber of severe or persistent adverse reactions.
- Avoid prolonged use of corticosteroids, especially in children.

Postadministration

(Evaluate outcomes)
- The patient exhibits normal breathing pattern.
- The patient exhibits improved gas exchange.

- The patient and family members understand the drug therapy and demonstrate administration and correct use.

Leukotriene modifiers

Although inhaled corticosteroids are the preferred option for treatment of mild asthma, leukotriene modifiers can be also used for the prevention and long-term control of mild asthma (Fanta, 2021). There are two types of leukotriene modifiers:

- *Leukotriene receptor antagonists* (LTRAs) include zafirlukast and montelukast. (See *Leukotriene modifiers: Zafirlukast.*)
- *Leukotriene formation inhibitors* include zileuton. Zileuton is used for more severe asthma (Fanta, 2021).

Pharmacokinetics

All leukotriene modifiers are extensively metabolized, have a rapid absorption, and are highly protein-bound (more than 90%).

Factoring in food

Zafirlukast's absorption is decreased by food. Montelukast has a rapid absorption from the GI tract and may be given with food. Administration of zileuton with food doesn't affect the rate of absorption. Patients with hepatic impairment may require a dosage adjustment.

Pharmacodynamics

Leukotrienes are substances that are released from mast cells, eosinophils, and basophils. They can result in smooth muscle contraction of the airways, increased permeability of the vasculature, increased secretions, and activation of other inflammatory mediators. Leukotrienes are inhibited by two different mechanisms:

1. The leukotriene receptor antagonists (zafirlukast and montelukast) are competitive inhibitors of the leukotriene D4 and E4 receptors that inhibit leukotriene from interacting with its receptor and blocking its action (Fanta, 2021).
2. The leukotriene formation inhibitor (zileuton) inhibits the production of 5-lipoxygenase, an enzyme that inhibits the formation of leukotrienes, which are known to contribute to swelling, bronchoconstriction, and mucus secretion seen in patients with asthma (Fanta, 2021).

Pharmacotherapeutics

Leukotriene modifiers are primarily used to prevent and control asthma exacerbations in patients with mild to moderate disease. They aren't effective in an acute asthma attack. They may also be used as steroid-sparing agents in some patients.

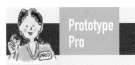

Prototype Pro

Leukotriene modifiers: Zafirlukast

Actions
- Selectively competes for leukotriene receptor sites, blocking inflammatory action

Indications
- Prophylaxis and long-term management of mild, persistent asthma

Nursing considerations
- This drug isn't indicated for reversing bronchospasm in acute asthma attacks.
- Give cautiously to older adults and those with hepatic impairment.
- Drug absorption is decreased by food; give the drug 1 hour before or 2 hours after meals.
- Monitor liver function studies in patients with suspected hepatic dysfunction. The drug may need to be discontinued if hepatic dysfunction is confirmed.

Drug interactions

Many drug interactions may occur with leukotriene modifiers that results in toxicity including:

- Zafirlukast use with phenytoin or warfarin.
- Zafirlukast and zileuton use with amlodipine, atorvastatin, carbamazepine, clarithromycin, cyclosporine, erythromycin, hormonal contraceptives, itraconazole, ketoconazole, lovastatin, nelfinavir, nifedipine, ritonavir, sertraline, simvastatin, or warfarin.
- Zafirlukast, zileuton, and montelukast use with amiodarone, cimetidine, fluconazole, fluoxetine, fluvoxamine, isoniazid, metronidazole, or voriconazole.

Leukotriene modifiers have a decreased effectiveness when given with carbamazepine, phenobarbital, phenytoin, primidone, or rifampin.

- If the patient is a smoker, nicotine can result in decreased effectiveness of zileuton.

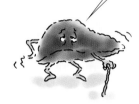

Zileuton is contraindicated in patients with active liver disease—which actually makes me feel more inactive.

Side effects/adverse reactions

Side effects and adverse reactions to leukotriene modifiers include:

- headache
- dizziness
- nausea and vomiting
- myalgia
- cough.

Zileuton is contraindicated in patients with active liver disease and in children under the age of 12 due to risk of hepatotoxicity.

Black Box Warning

Preparing for practice: Leukotriene modifier: Montelukast

- **Black Box Warning:** Montelukast has been linked to psychological reactions, such as agitation, aggression, hallucinations, depression, and suicidal thinking.
- ***Changes in practice…***Because of this new warning, the FDA is now recommending that montelukast only be used to treat patients with allergic rhinitis and asthma that does not respond to alternative medications.
- Educate patient to seek medical advice right away if they experience any of these reactions.

Source: Boyce, J. (2021). Antileukotriene agents in the management of asthma. In R. A. Wood & B. S. Bochner (Eds.), *UpToDate*.

The Three-Step Approach

Nursing management for patients undergoing treatment with leukotriene modifiers include these three steps.

Preadministration

(Recognize and analyze cues)
- Assess the patient's respiratory condition before therapy and regularly thereafter.
- Assess peak flow readings before starting treatment and periodically thereafter.
- Use cautiously in patients with hepatic impairment.
- Be alert for adverse reactions and drug interactions.
- Evaluate the patient's and family's knowledge of drug therapy.

(Prioritize hypothesis—priority patient problems)
- Altered breathing pattern
- Impaired gas exchange
- Knowledge deficiency

(Generate solutions)
- Breathing pattern will improve as evidenced by regular and even respiratory rate and rhythm.
- Gas exchange will be adequate as evidenced by improved peak flow rates, oxygen saturation, and ABG levels.
- The patient will demonstrate correct drug administration.

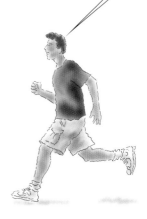

With the proper medication, exercise-induced asthma doesn't have to stop you in your tracks.

Medication administration

(Take action)
- Report insufficient relief or worsening of condition.
- Do not use these drugs for reversing bronchospasm during an acute asthma attack.
- Administer zafirlukast 1 hour before or 2 hours after meals.

Postadministration

(Evaluate outcomes)
- The patient exhibits normal breathing pattern.
- The patient exhibits improved gas exchange.
- The patient and family understand drug therapy.

Mast cell stabilizers

Mast cell stabilizers are used for the prevention and long-term control of asthma in children five and older and those with mild disease. These drugs are ineffective in the management of an acute asthma attack. The main medication in this class is cromolyn sodium.

Pharmacokinetics

Mast cell stabilizers are minimally absorbed from the GI tract. Inhaled formulations exert effects locally.

Pharmacodynamics

The mechanism of action of mast cell stabilizers involves inhibiting the release of inflammatory mediators by stabilizing the mast cell membrane through the inhibition of chloride channels (Parada, 2021).

Pharmacotherapeutics

Mast cell stabilizers control the inflammatory process and are used for the prevention and long-term control of asthma symptoms. Cromolyn is an option for children and patients with exercise-induced asthma when inhaled glucocorticoids are contraindicated or result in side effects and adverse reactions (Parada, 2021).

Handling hay fever

The intranasal form of cromolyn (Canada) and the ophthalmic form of nedocromil (Canada) are used to treat seasonal allergies.

Drug interactions

There are no known drug interactions for nedocromil or cromolyn sodium.

Side effects/adverse reactions

Side effects and adverse reactions to inhaled mast cell stabilizers may include:
- pharyngeal and tracheal irritation
- cough.

The Three-Step Approach

Nursing management for patients undergoing treatment with mast cell stabilizers include these three steps.

Preadministration

(Recognize and analyze cues)
- Assess the patient's respiratory condition before therapy and regularly thereafter.
- Assess peak flow readings before starting treatment and periodically thereafter.
- Be alert for adverse reactions and drug interactions.
- Evaluate the patient's and family's knowledge of drug therapy.

(Prioritize hypothesis—priority patient problems)
- Altered breathing pattern
- Impaired gas exchange
- Knowledge deficiency

(Generate solutions)
- Breathing pattern will improve as evidenced by regular and even respiratory rate and rhythm.
- Gas exchange will be adequate as evidenced by improved peak flow rates, oxygen saturation, and ABG levels.
- The patient and family members will demonstrate understanding, administration, and correct drug use.

Medication administration

(Take action)
- Report insufficient relief or worsening of condition.
- Do not use these drugs for reversing bronchospasm during an acute asthma attack.
- Monitor for side effects or adverse reactions of therapy.

Postadministration

(Evaluate outcomes)
- The patient exhibits normal breathing pattern.
- The patient exhibits improved gas exchange.
- The patient and family understand drug therapy and demonstrate correct administration and use.

Methylxanthines

Methylxanthines, also called *xanthines*, are used to treat breathing disorders. Examples of methylxanthines include:
- aminophylline
- anhydrous theophylline.

Aminophylline is a theophylline derivative. Theophylline is the most used oral methylxanthine. Aminophylline is preferred when IV methylxanthine treatment is required.

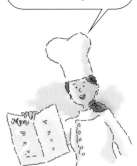

High-fat meals can increase theophylline concentrations and increase the risk of toxicity.

Pharmacokinetics

When methylxanthines are given as an oral solution or a rapid-release tablet, they're absorbed rapidly and completely. They're converted in the body to an active form, which is principally theophylline. High-fat meals can increase theophylline concentrations and increase the risk of toxicity.

pH scale weighs in

Absorption of slow-release forms of theophylline depends on the patient's gastric pH. Food can also alter absorption. When converting patient dosages from IV aminophylline to theophylline by mouth (PO), the dosage is decreased by 20%.

Theophylline is approximately 56% protein bound in adults and 36% protein bound in neonates. It readily crosses the placental barrier and is secreted in breast milk. Smokers and patients on dialysis may need higher doses.

Theophylline is metabolized primarily in the liver by the CYP1A2 enzyme, and, in adults and children, about 10% of a dose is excreted unchanged in urine. Therefore, no dosage adjustment is required in a patient with renal insufficiency. Older adult patients and patients with liver dysfunction may require lower doses. Because infants have immature livers with reduced metabolic functioning, as much as one half of a dose may be excreted unchanged in their urine. Theophylline levels need to be collected to evaluate and avoid toxicity. The therapeutic serum concentration is 10 to 20 mcg/mL (SI, 44 to 111 µmol/L) (Hendeles & Weinberger, 2021). Levels need to be assessed when a dose is initiated or changed, and when drugs are added or removed from a patient's medication regimen.

Pharmacodynamics

Methylxanthines work in several ways.

Taking it easy

Methylxanthines decrease airway reactivity and relieve bronchospasm by relaxing bronchial smooth muscle. Theophylline inhibits phosphodiesterase, resulting in smooth-muscle relaxation as well as bronchodilation and a decrease in inflammatory mediators (namely, mast cells, T cells, and eosinophils). Much of theophylline's toxicity may be due to increased catecholamine release.

Driven to breathe

In obstructive airway disease (chronic bronchitis, emphysema, and apnea), methylxanthines appear to increase the sensitivity of the brain's respiratory center to carbon dioxide and stimulate the respiratory drive. Methylxanthines help to improve exercise tolerance in patients with COPD (Aboussouan, 2021).

Pumped up

In chronic bronchitis and emphysema, these drugs reduce fatigue of the diaphragm, the respiratory muscle that separates the abdomen from the thoracic cavity. They also improve ventricular function and, therefore, the heart's pumping action.

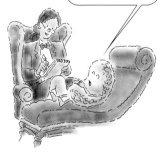

"So you're telling me methylxanthines increase your sensitivity to carbon dioxide?"

"Yes, and it always ends up stimulating my respiratory drive!"

Pharmacotherapeutics

Methylxanthines are used as second- or third-line agents for the long-term control of and prevention of symptoms related to:
- asthma
- chronic bronchitis
- emphysema.

Oh baby

Theophylline has been used to treat neonatal apnea (periods of not breathing in a neonate) and has been effective in reducing severe bronchospasm in infants with cystic fibrosis.

Drug interactions

Theophylline drug interactions occur with those substances that inhibit or induce the CYP1A2 enzyme system:

- Inhibitors of CYP1A2 decrease the metabolism of theophylline, thus increasing the serum concentration. This results in increased adverse reactions or toxicity. The dose of theophylline may need to be reduced. Examples of CYP1A2 inhibitors include ketoconazole, erythromycin, clarithromycin, cimetidine, isoniazid, fluvoxamine, hormonal contraceptives, ciprofloxacin, ticlopidine, and zileuton.
- Inducers of CYP1A2 increase the metabolism of theophylline, decreasing the serum concentration. This results in possible therapeutic failure. The dose of theophylline may need to be increased. Examples of CYP1A2 inducers include rifampin, carbamazepine, phenobarbital, phenytoin, and St. John's wort.
- Smoking cigarettes or marijuana increases theophylline elimination, decreasing its serum concentration and effectiveness. Alcohol misuse can increase theophylline effects.
- Taking adrenergic stimulants or drinking beverages that contain caffeine or caffeine-like substances may result in additive adverse reactions to theophylline or signs and symptoms of methylxanthine toxicity.
- Activated charcoal may decrease theophylline levels.
- Receiving isoflurane with theophylline and theophylline derivatives increases the risk of cardiac toxicity.
- Theophylline and its derivatives may reduce the effects of lithium by increasing its rate of excretion.
- Thyroid hormones may reduce theophylline levels; antithyroid drugs may increase theophylline levels.

Side effects/adverse reactions

Side effects and adverse reactions to methylxanthines may be transient or symptomatic of toxicity.

Gut reactions

Side effects and adverse GI system reactions include:

- nausea and vomiting
- abdominal cramping
- epigastric pain
- anorexia
- diarrhea.

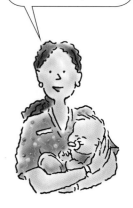

Sleep tight, little one. Theophylline is used to treat neonatal apnea.

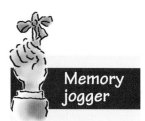

Memory jogger

How can you remember what theophylline and its salts are used to treat? Simple: Just remember that you really need to "ACE" this one! It's used for long-term control and prevention of symptoms related to:

- **A**sthma
- **C**hronic bronchitis
- **E**mphysema.

Nerve racking

Side effects and adverse central nervous system (CNS) reactions include:

- headache
- irritability, restlessness, and anxiety
- insomnia
- dizziness.

Heart of the matter

Side effects and adverse cardiovascular reactions include:

- hypotension
- tachycardia
- palpitations
- arrhythmias.

The Three-Step Approach

Nursing management for patients undergoing treatment with methylxanthines include these three steps.

Preadministration

(Recognize and analyze cues)

- Assess the patient's respiratory condition before therapy and regularly thereafter.
- Assess peak flow readings before starting treatment and periodically thereafter.
- Be alert for adverse reactions and drug interactions.
- Monitor vital signs and measure fluid intake and output. Expected clinical effects include improvement in the quality of pulse and respirations.
- The xanthine metabolism rate varies among individuals; the dosage is determined by weight and by monitoring the patient's response, tolerance, pulmonary function, and serum theophylline level.
- Evaluate the patient's and family's knowledge of drug therapy.

(Prioritize hypothesis—priority patient problems)

- Altered breathing pattern
- Impaired gas exchange
- Knowledge deficiency

(Generate solutions)

- Breathing pattern will improve as evidenced by regular and even respiratory rate and rhythm.
- Gas exchange will be adequate as evidenced by improved peak flow rates, oxygen saturation, and ABG levels.
- The patient will verbalize an understanding of drug therapy.

Medication administration

(Take action)

- Report insufficient relief or worsening of condition.
- Give PO doses around the clock, using a sustained-release product at bedtime.
- Use a commercially available infusion solution for IV use or mix the drug in dextrose 5% in water (D_5W). Use an infusion pump for a continuous infusion.

Smoked out

- The dosage may need to be increased in cigarette smokers and in habitual marijuana smokers because smoking causes the drug to be metabolized faster.
- The daily dose may need to be decreased in patients with heart failure or hepatic disease and in older patients because metabolism and excretion may be decreased.
- Monitor the patient's vital signs.
- Measure and record the patient's intake and output.
- Tell the patient to avoid caffeine.

Postadministration

(Evaluate outcomes)

- The patient exhibits normal breathing pattern.
- The patient exhibits improved gas exchange.
- The patient and family members understand drug therapy. (See *Teaching about methylxanthines.*)

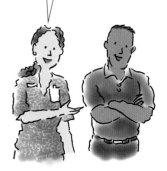

"Did you know that smoking causes xanthines to be metabolized faster?"

Education edge

Teaching about methylxanthines

See Education edge: Teaching template in Chapter 3, page 38 for general teaching for all medications. Specific points to review with patients and family for methylxanthine therapy:

- For a child who can't swallow capsules, sprinkle the contents of capsules over soft food and instruct the child to swallow without chewing.
- Relieve GI symptoms by taking the oral form of the drug with a full glass of water after meals.
- Dizziness may occur at the start of therapy, especially in an older adult.
- Change position slowly and avoid hazardous activities during drug therapy.
- If you're a smoker while on drug therapy and then you quit, notify your prescriber; your dosage may need to be reduced.
- Report signs and symptoms of toxicity to your prescriber, including tachycardia, anorexia, nausea, vomiting, diarrhea, restlessness, irritability, and headache.
- Have blood levels monitored periodically.
- Avoid foods with caffeine.

Expectorants

Expectorants reduce the thickness, adhesiveness, and surface tension of mucus, making it easier to clear the airways.

Guaifenesin

The most commonly used expectorant is guaifenesin, a common component of over the counter (OTC) cold and flu medications.

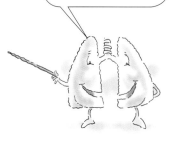

Expect to see this expectorant listed as a component in many OTC cold and flu medications.

Pharmacokinetics

Guaifenesin is absorbed through the GI tract, metabolized by the liver, and excreted primarily by the kidneys.

Pharmacodynamics

By increasing the production of respiratory tract fluids, guaifenesin reduces the thickness, adhesiveness, and surface tension of mucus, making it easier to clear it from the airways. It also provides a soothing effect on mucous membranes of the respiratory tract. The result is a more productive cough.

Pharmacotherapeutics

Guaifenesin helps make mucus easier to cough up and is used for the relief of symptoms caused by productive coughs from many disorders, such as:

* colds
* minor bronchial irritation
* bronchitis
* influenza
* sinusitis
* bronchial asthma
* emphysema.

Drug interactions

Guaifenesin isn't known to have specific drug interactions.

Side effects/adverse reactions

Side effects and adverse reactions to guaifenesin include those associated with an allergic reaction and:

* vomiting (if taken in large doses)
* diarrhea
* drowsiness
* nausea
* abdominal pain
* headache
* hives or skin rash.

The Three-Step Approach

Nursing management for patients undergoing treatment with an expectorant include these three steps.

Preadministration

(Recognize and analyze cues)
- Assess the patient's sputum production before and after giving the drug.
- Monitor the patient for worsening condition or other symptoms indicating respiratory complications.
- Evaluate the patient's and family's knowledge of drug therapy.

(Prioritize hypothesis—priority patient problems)
- Ineffective airway clearance
- Infection risk
- Knowledge deficiency

(Generate solutions)
- The patient will have a patent airway.
- The patient will not exhibit symptoms of respiratory complications such as infection.
- The patient will verbalize an understanding of drug therapy.

Medication administration

(Take action)
- Administer the medication as directed; give with a full glass of water as appropriate.

The acid test

- Be aware that the drug may interfere with laboratory tests for 5-hydroxyindoleacetic acid and vanillylmandelic acid.
- Report ineffectiveness of the drug to the prescriber; also report if the patient's cough persists or if signs and symptoms worsen.
- Encourage the patient to perform deep-breathing exercises.
- Advise the patient not to take other medications, OTC products, or herbal remedies unless approved by the prescriber or a pharmacist.

Postadministration

(Evaluate outcomes)
- The patient's lungs are clear, and respiratory secretions are normal.
- The patient is free from respiratory complications.
- The patient and family understand drug therapy.

Antitussives

Antitussive drugs suppress or inhibit coughing. They're typically used to treat dry, nonproductive coughs. The major antitussives include:
- benzonatate
- codeine

- dextromethorphan hydrobromide
- hydrocodone bitartrate.

Pharmacokinetics

Antitussives are absorbed well through the GI tract, metabolized in the liver, and excreted in urine. Opioid antitussives are excreted in breast milk and should be used during pregnancy only if the benefits outweigh the risks.

Pharmacodynamics

Antitussives act in slightly different ways:
- Benzonatate acts by anesthetizing stretch receptors throughout the bronchi, alveoli, and pleura.
- Codeine, dextromethorphan, and hydrocodone suppress the cough reflex by direct action on the cough center in the medulla of the brain, thus lowering the cough threshold.

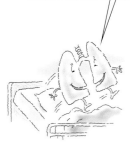

Antitussives are used to relieve a dry, nonproductive cough, allowing for a good night's sleep.

Pharmacotherapeutics

The uses of these drugs vary slightly, but each treats a serious, nonproductive cough that interferes with a patient's ability to rest or carry out activities of daily living.

Testing 1, 2, 3

Benzonatate relieves cough caused by pneumonia, bronchitis, the common cold, and chronic pulmonary diseases such as emphysema. It can also be used during bronchial diagnostic tests, such as bronchoscopy, when the patient must avoid coughing.

And the winner is…

Dextromethorphan is the most widely used cough suppressant in the United States and may provide better antitussive activity than codeine. Its popularity may stem from the fact that it isn't associated with sedation, respiratory depression, or addiction at usual dosages. However, dextromethorphan should not be used by those taking selective serotonin reuptake inhibitors (SSRIs).

When the going gets tough

The opioid antitussives (typically codeine and hydrocodone) are usually reserved for treating intractable cough but can be used for less serious coughs. Opioids should be used cautiously in older adults and are listed in the Beers Criteria for Inappropriate Use of Medications.

IN THE KNOW! Changes in practice…

Although codeine is still used as a cough suppressant, evidence varies on its effectiveness. Providers are using other options to reduce coughing (Weinberger & Silvestri, 2021).

Drug interactions

Antitussives may interact with other drugs in the following ways:
- Codeine and hydrocodone may cause excitation, an extremely elevated temperature, hypertension or hypotension, and coma when taken with monoamine oxidase (MAO) inhibitors.
- Dextromethorphan use with MAO inhibitors may produce excitation, an elevated body temperature, hypotension, and coma.

Dangerous depression
- Codeine may cause increased CNS depression—including drowsiness, lethargy, stupor, respiratory depression, coma, and death—when taken with other CNS depressants, including alcohol, barbiturates, sedative-hypnotics, and phenothiazines.

Side effects/Adverse reactions

Benzonatate can cause different kinds of adverse reactions than the opioid antitussives codeine, dextromethorphan, and hydrocodone.

Benzonatate

Benzonatate needs to be swallowed whole; chewing or crushing can produce a local anesthetic effect in the mouth and throat, which can compromise the airway. The following side effects and adverse reactions can also occur when taking benzonatate:
- dizziness
- sedation
- headache
- nasal congestion
- burning in the eyes
- GI upset or nausea
- constipation
- skin rash, eruptions, or itching
- chills
- chest numbness.

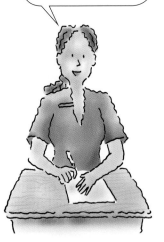

Different types of antitussives can cause different kinds of adverse reactions.

Opioid antitussives

Common side effects and adverse reactions to the opioid antitussives include nausea, vomiting, sedation, dizziness, and constipation. Other reactions include:
- pupil constriction
- bradycardia or tachycardia
- hypotension
- stupor
- seizures
- circulatory collapse
- respiratory arrest.

The Three-Step Approach

Nursing management for patients undergoing treatment with antitussives include these three steps.

Preadministration

(Recognize and analyze cues)
- Obtain a history of the patient's cough.
- Be alert for adverse reactions and drug interactions.
- Monitor the patient's hydration level if adverse GI reactions occur.
- Evaluate the patient and family members' knowledge of drug therapy.

(Prioritize hypothesis—priority patient problems)
- Altered airway clearance
- Fatigue
- Knowledge deficiency

(Generate solutions)
- The patient will have a patent airway.
- The patient will state that fatigue is lessened.
- The patient and family will verbalize an understanding of drug therapy.

Medication administration

(Take action)
- Report ineffectiveness of the drug to the prescriber; also report if the patient's cough persists or if signs and symptoms worsen.
- Encourage the patient to perform deep-breathing exercises.
- Advise the patient not to take other medications, OTC products, or herbal remedies until talking with the prescriber or a pharmacist.
- Tell the patient taking an opioid antitussive to avoid driving and drinking alcohol.

Postadministration

(Evaluate outcomes)
- The patient's lungs are clear, and respiratory secretions are normal.
- The patient's cough is relieved.
- The patient and family members understand drug therapy.

Decongestants

Decongestants may be classified as systemic or topical, depending on how they are administered.

How swell!

As sympathomimetic drugs, systemic decongestants stimulate the sympathetic nervous system to reduce swelling of the respiratory tract's vascular network. Systemic decongestants include:
- ephedrine
- phenylephrine
- pseudoephedrine.

In the clear

Topical decongestants are also powerful vasoconstrictors. When applied directly to swollen mucous membranes of the nose, they provide immediate relief from nasal congestion. Topical decongestants include:

- ephedrine, epinephrine, and phenylephrine (sympathomimetic amines)
- naphazoline, oxymetazoline, and tetrahydrozoline.

Pharmacokinetics

The pharmacokinetic properties of decongestants vary. When taken orally, the systemic decongestants are absorbed readily from the GI tract and widely distributed throughout the body into various tissues and fluids, including cerebrospinal fluid, the placenta, and breast milk.

All in a day's work

Systemic decongestants are slowly and incompletely metabolized by the liver and excreted largely unchanged in the urine within 24 hours of oral administration.

In the neighborhood

Topical decongestants act locally on the alpha-adrenergic receptors of the vascular smooth muscle in the nose, causing the arterioles to constrict. As a result of this local action, absorption of the drug becomes negligible.

Pharmacodynamics

The properties of systemic and topical decongestants vary slightly.

Direct and to the point

The systemic decongestants cause vasoconstriction by directly stimulating alpha-adrenergic receptors in the blood vessels of the body. They also cause contraction of urinary and GI sphincters, pupil dilation, and decreased secretion of insulin.

Indirect hit

These drugs may also act indirectly, resulting in the release of norepinephrine from storage sites in the body, which leads to peripheral vasoconstriction.

On a clear day...

Like systemic decongestants, topical decongestants stimulate alpha-adrenergic receptors in the smooth muscle of the blood vessels in the nose, resulting in vasoconstriction. The combination of reduced blood flow to the nasal mucous membranes and decreased capillary permeability reduces swelling. This action improves respiration by helping to drain sinuses, clear nasal passages, and open eustachian tubes.

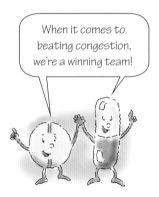

When it comes to beating congestion, we're a winning team!

Pharmacotherapeutics

Systemic and topical decongestants are used to relieve the symptoms of swollen nasal membranes resulting from:
- allergic rhinitis (hay fever)
- vasomotor rhinitis
- acute coryza (profuse discharge from the nose)
- sinusitis
- the common cold.

It's a group effort

Systemic decongestants are usually given with other drugs, such as antihistamines, antimuscarinics, antipyretic-analgesics, and antitussives.

Advantage, topical

Topical decongestants provide two major advantages over systemics: minimal side effects and adverse reactions and rapid symptom relief.

Drug interactions

Because they produce vasoconstriction, which reduces drug absorption, drug interactions involving topical decongestants seldom occur. However, systemic decongestants may interact with other drugs:
- Increased CNS stimulation may occur when systemic decongestants are taken with other sympathomimetic drugs, including epinephrine, norepinephrine, dopamine, dobutamine, isoproterenol, metaproterenol, and terbutaline.
- When taken with MAO inhibitors, systemic decongestants may cause severe hypertension or a hypertensive crisis, which can be life-threatening. These drugs should not be used together.
- Alkalinizing drugs may increase the effects of pseudoephedrine by reducing its urinary excretion.

Side effects/adverse reactions

Most side effects and adverse reactions to decongestants result from CNS stimulation and include:
- nervousness
- restlessness and insomnia
- nausea
- palpitations and tachycardia
- difficulty urinating
- elevated blood pressure.

Systemic decongestants

Systemic decongestants also exacerbate hypertension, hyperthyroidism, diabetes, benign prostatic hyperplasia, glaucoma, and heart disease.

Taking MAO inhibitors with systemic decongestants may cause severe hypertension, even a hypertensive crisis.

Topical decongestants

The most common side effects and adverse reactions associated with prolonged use (more than 5 days) of topical decongestants is rebound nasal congestion. Other reactions include burning and stinging of the nasal mucosa, sneezing, and mucosal dryness or ulceration.

The Three-Step Approach

Nursing management for patients undergoing treatment with decongestants include these three steps.

Preadministration

(Recognize and analyze cues)
- Assess the patient's condition before and after giving the drug.
- Assess the patient's nares for signs of bleeding.
- Be alert for side effects, adverse reactions, and drug interactions.
- Evaluate the patient and family members' knowledge of drug therapy.

(Prioritize hypothesis—priority patient problems)
- Ineffective airway clearance
- Knowledge deficiency

(Generate solutions)
- The patient will have a patent airway.
- The patient and family members will understand drug therapy and demonstrate correct drug administration.

Medication administration

(Take action)
- Report ineffectiveness of the drug to the prescriber; also report if the patient's symptoms persists or if signs and symptoms worsen.
- Encourage the patient to perform deep-breathing exercises.
- Advise the patient not to take other medications, OTC products, or herbal remedies until talking with the prescriber or a pharmacist.
- Identify and correct hypoxia, hypercapnia, and acidosis, which may reduce drug effectiveness or increase adverse reactions, before or during ephedrine administration.
- Give the last dose at least 2 hours before bedtime to minimize insomnia.
- Instruct the patient to limit use of intranasal forms to 3 to 5 days to prevent rebound congestion.

Postadministration

(Evaluate outcomes)
- Patient's lungs are clear, and respiratory secretions are normal.
- Patient and family members understand drug therapy and demonstrates correct administration.

Quick quiz

1. A nurse is educating a patient who just received a bronchodilator prescription. Which statement requires further teaching?
    A. "I need to wash and dry the device after each use."
    B. "I will take the drug 30 to 60 minutes before exercising."
    C. "If I miss a dose, I need to take it as soon as I remember even if it is almost time for the next dose."
    D. "A spacer device should be used with my metered-dose inhaler to achieve more effect from the medication."

Answer: C. Take a missed dose as soon as you remember, unless it's almost time for the next dose; in that case, skip the missed dose. Do not double the dose. Further teaching is not needed for A, B, and D as these are correct statements.

2. A nurse is caring for a patient with uncontrolled hypertension who is experiencing severe nasal congestion. Which form of nasal decongestant would the nurse anticipate being ordered?
    A. IM
    B. Oral
    C. Topical
    D. Sublingual

Answer: C. Topical decongestants, such as a topical nasal spray, act locally with minimal adverse reactions and rapid symptom relief. Systemic decongestants can exacerbate hypertension.

3. A nurse is caring for a patient with asthma. Which medication would the nurse anticipate being prescribed for long-term treatment and prevention of asthma exacerbation?
    A. Beta agonists
    B. Corticosteroids
    C. Anticholinergics
    D. Leukotriene modifiers

Answer: B. Inhaled corticosteroids remain the mainstay of therapy to prevent future exacerbations for most asthmatics. Use of inhaled corticosteroids reduces the need for systemic steroids in many patients, thus reducing the risk of serious long-term adverse effects.

4. A nurse is caring for a patient who is experiencing an acute asthma attack. Which medication does the nurse anticipate administering?
    A. Albuterol
    B. Benzonatate
    C. Guaifenesin
    D. Pseudoephedrine

Answer: A. Short-acting inhaled beta agonists, such as albuterol, should be used for treating acute episodes of bronchospasm when rapid response is needed. Benzonatate, guaifenesin, and pseudoephedrine are not effective in terminating an acute asthma attack.

5. A nurse is administering aminophylline IV to a patient experiencing an exacerbation of bronchitis. Which side effects would the nurse report to the provider immediately?
- A. Nausea and vomiting
- B. Headache and dizziness
- C. Abdominal cramping and diarrhea
- D. Palpitations and cardiac arrhythmias

Answer: D. Palpitations and cardiac arrhythmias due to aminophylline indicates that the electrical impulses of the heart are irregular. This side effect/adverse reaction may be harmful to the patient and should be reported to the provider immediately. Although the other side effects/adverse reactions may result from aminophylline, they are not as potentially dangerous as the cardiac arrhythmias.

Scoring

☆☆☆ If you answered all five questions correctly, good job! You can take a deep breath and move on to the next chapter.

☆☆ If you answered three or four questions correctly, you're as relaxed as bronchial smooth muscle on xanthines.

☆ If you answered fewer than three questions correctly, you may need another dose of the chapter to clear your head about respiratory drugs.

Suggested References

Aboussouan, L. (2021). Role of mucoactive agents and secretion clearance techniques in COPD. In U. Hatipoglu & H. Hollingsworth (Eds.), *UpToDate*.

Boyce, J. (2021). Antileukotriene agents in the management of asthma. In R. A. Wood & B. S. Bochner (Eds.), *UpToDate*.

Dweik, R. (2021). Role of anticholinergic therapy in COPD. In J. Stoller (Ed.), *UpToDate*.

Fanta, C. (2021). Treatment of intermittent and mild persistent asthma in adolescents and adults. In B. S. Bochner (Ed.), *UpToDate*.

Hendeles, L., & Weinberger, M. (2021). Theophylline use in asthma. In B. S. Bochner & R. A. Wood (Eds.), *UpToDate*.

Karch, A. (2020). *Focus on nursing pharmacology* (8th ed.). Philadelphia, PA: Lippincott Williams & Wilkins

Lemanske, R. (2019). Beta agonists in asthma: Acute administration and prophylactic use. In B. S. Bochner (Ed.), *UpToDate*.

Parada, N. (2021). The use of chromones (cromoglycates) in the treatment of asthma. In B. S. Bochner (Ed.), *UpToDate*.

Weinberger, S., & Silvestri, R. (2021). Treatment of subacute and chronic cough in adults. In P. J. Barnes & T. E. King (Eds.), *UpToDate*.

Chapter 10

Gastrointestinal drugs

Just the facts

In this chapter, you'll learn:

◆ classes of drugs used to improve GI function

◆ uses and varying actions of these drugs

◆ absorption, distribution, metabolization, and excretion of these drugs

◆ drug interactions, side effects, and adverse reactions to these drugs.

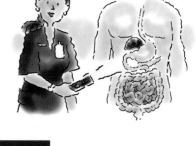

Let's shed some light on the subject. The drugs in this chapter are used to improve function in the GI tract—the pharynx, esophagus, stomach, and intestines.

Drugs and the gastrointestinal system

The GI tract is basically a hollow, muscular tube that begins at the mouth and ends at the anus; it encompasses the pharynx, esophagus, stomach, and the small and large intestines. Its primary functions are to digest and absorb foods and fluids and excrete metabolic waste.

Role call

Classes of drugs used to improve GI function include:

• antiulcer drugs
• tumor necrosis factor-alpha (TNF-alpha) blocker drugs
• adsorbent, antiflatulent, and digestive drugs
• antidiarrheal and laxative drugs
• obesity drugs
• antiemetic drugs.

Antiulcer drugs

Antiulcer drugs are used to treat gastroesophageal reflux disease (GERD) and peptic ulcers. GERD is the reflux of gastric contents into the esophagus causing symptoms that may be associated with mucosal tissue injury (Kahrilas, 2021). A peptic ulcer is a circumscribed lesion in the mucosal membrane, developing in the lower esophagus, stomach, duodenum, or jejunum (Drini, 2017).

Common culprits

The major causes of peptic ulcers include:
- bacterial infection with *Helicobacter pylori*
- the use of nonsteroidal anti-inflammatory drugs (NSAIDs)
- Risk factors include:
  - cigarette smoking, which causes hypersecretion and impairs ulcer healing
  - heavy alcohol use, which causes hypersecretion of gastric acid
  - a genetic predisposition, which accounts for 20% to 50% of patients with peptic ulcers (Vakil, 2021a).

Busting bacteria or bolstering balance

Antiulcer drugs are formulated to eradicate *H. pylori* or restore the balance between acid and pepsin secretions and the GI mucosal defense. (See *Where drugs affect GI secretions*, page 346.) These drugs include:
- systemic antibiotics
- antacids
- histamine-2 (H_2) receptor antagonists
- proton pump inhibitors
- other antiulcer drugs, such as misoprostol and sucralfate.

Systemic antibiotics

H. pylori is a Gram-negative bacteria that's thought to be a major causative factor in peptic ulcer formation and gastritis (inflammation of the stomach lining) (Vakil, 2021a). Eradicating the bacteria promotes ulcer healing and decreases recurrence.

It takes two

Successful treatment involves a combination of drugs that include systemic antibiotics and antisecretory agents (Vakil, 2021a). One common combination used for ulcers caused by *H. pylori* includes two systemic antibiotics (tetracycline and metronidazole), and bismuth subsalicylate.

Systemic antibiotics used to treat *H. pylori* include:
- amoxicillin
- clarithromycin
- metronidazole
- tetracycline.

Pharmacokinetics

Systemic antibiotics are variably absorbed from the GI tract.

Where drugs affect GI secretions

Antiulcer drugs and digestive drugs that affect GI secretions can decrease secretory activity, block the action of secretions, form a protective coating on the lining, or replace missing enzymes. The illustration below depicts where these types of GI drugs act.

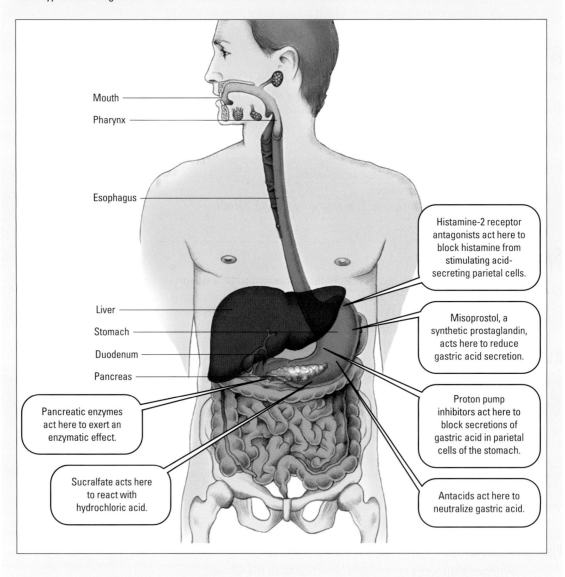

Mouth

Pharynx

Esophagus

Liver

Stomach

Duodenum

Pancreas

Histamine-2 receptor antagonists act here to block histamine from stimulating acid-secreting parietal cells.

Misoprostol, a synthetic prostaglandin, acts here to reduce gastric acid secretion.

Pancreatic enzymes act here to exert an enzymatic effect.

Proton pump inhibitors act here to block secretions of gastric acid in parietal cells of the stomach.

Sucralfate acts here to react with hydrochloric acid.

Antacids act here to neutralize gastric acid.

Got milk?

Food, especially dairy products, decreases the absorption of tetracycline but doesn't significantly delay the absorption of the other antibiotics.

All of these antibiotics are distributed widely and are excreted primarily in urine.

Pharmacodynamics

Antibiotics act by treating the *H. pylori* infection. They're usually combined with a proton pump inhibitor or H_2-receptor antagonist to decrease stomach acid and further promote healing (Vakil, 2021a).

Pharmacotherapeutics

Systemic antibiotics are indicated for *H. pylori* eradication to reduce the risk of an ulcer.

Sounds like a plan

Treatment plans include the use of an antibiotic and a proton pump inhibitor for 14 days and then continue the proton pump inhibitor for 6 more weeks to reduce acid in patients with peptic ulcers. Additional antibiotics or antisecretory agents may be used for more complex ulcers and treatment may last longer.

Drug interactions

Tetracycline and metronidazole can interact with many other drugs. For example, tetracycline increases digoxin levels and, when combined with methoxyflurane, increases the risk of nephrotoxicity. Metronidazole and tetracycline increase the risk of bleeding when taken with oral anticoagulants.

Side effects/adverse reactions

Antibiotics used to improve GI tract function may lead to side effects and adverse reactions, such as:

- Metronidazole, clarithromycin, and tetracycline commonly cause mild GI disturbances.
- Clarithromycin and metronidazole may produce abnormal tastes.
- Metronidazole may cause a disulfiram-like reaction (nausea, vomiting, headache, cramps, flushing) when combined with alcohol. Discourage concomitant use.
- Amoxicillin may cause diarrhea.

The Three-Step Approach

Nursing management for patients undergoing treatment with systemic antibiotics includes these three steps.

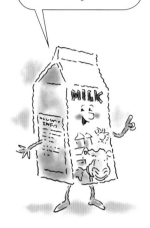

Dairy products and other foods decrease the absorption of the antibiotic tetracycline.

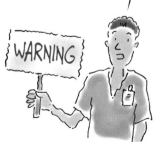

Avoid drinking alcohol while taking metronidazole as a severe reaction may occur.

Preadministration

(Recognize and analyze cues)
- Assess the patient's infection before therapy and regularly thereafter.
- Assess for signs and symptoms of the patient's ulcer.
- Watch for edema, especially in the patient who is also receiving antibiotics, such as metronidazole, that may cause sodium retention.
- Assess for side effects, adverse reactions, and drug interactions.
- Identify risk factors for peptic ulcer disease, such as cigarette smoking, stress, and drug therapy with irritating medications (aspirin, other NSAIDs, corticosteroids, or antineoplastics).
- Assess the patient's and family's understanding of drug therapy.

(Prioritize hypothesis—priority patient problems)
- Altered health maintenance
- Hypovolemia
- Knowledge deficiency

(Generate solutions)
- The patient's overall health status will improve.
- Stable vital signs and the patient's urine output will indicate improved fluid volume status.
- The patient and family or caregiver will demonstrate an understanding of drug therapy.

Medication administration

(Take action)
- Administer drugs as prescribed for the patient's condition and diagnosis.
- Use measures to prevent or minimize peptic ulcer disease and gastric acid–induced esophageal disorders such as GERD.
- Observe the patient for improvement in signs and symptoms.
- Instruct the patient to take the full course of antibiotics.

Postadministration

(Evaluate outcomes)
- Patient is free from infection.
- Patient maintains adequate hydration throughout antibiotic therapy.
- Patient and family members demonstrate an understanding of drug therapy. (See *Teaching about antiulcer drugs*, page 349.)

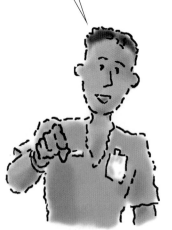

Make sure to evaluate for adequate hydration in the patient taking systemic antibiotics.

Education edge

Teaching about antiulcer drugs

See Education Edge: Teaching template in Chapter 3, page 38 for general teaching for all medications. Specific points to review with patients and family for antiulcer drugs:

- Elevate the head of the bed.
- Avoid abdominal distention by eating small meals.
- Don't lie down for 1 to 2 hours after eating.
- Decrease intake of fats, chocolate, citric juices, coffee, and alcohol.
- Avoid smoking.
- As possible, take steps to avoid obesity, constipation, and other conditions that increase intra-abdominal pressure.
- Take medications with enough water to avoid irritating the esophagus.
- Take antiulcer drugs as directed; underuse decreases their effectiveness and overuse increases adverse effects.

- Swallow capsules whole unless otherwise instructed; some medications can be sprinkled on applesauce if they're difficult to swallow.
- Take medications with or without food as prescribed, when applicable.
- Eat a well-balanced diet.
- Get adequate rest.
- Exercise regularly.
- Avoid gastric irritants such as NSAIDs.
- Reduce psychological stress; employ stress management techniques as needed.
- Don't take other medications, over-the-counter (OTC) preparations, or herbal remedies without first consulting with the prescriber.

Antacids

Antacids are OTC medications used in combination with other drugs to treat peptic ulcers. Antacids are usually a combination of the following:
- aluminum hydroxide
- calcium carbonate
- magnesium hydroxide (Vakil, 2021b).

In addition, the medication simethicone, a miscellaneous GI agent, can be used as an antacid.

Pharmacokinetics

Antacids work locally in the stomach by neutralizing gastric acid. They don't need to be absorbed to treat peptic ulcers. Antacids are distributed throughout the GI tract and are eliminated primarily in feces.

Pharmacodynamics

The acid-neutralizing action of antacids reduces the total amount of acid in the GI tract, allowing peptic ulcers time to heal.

> By reducing the amount of acid in the GI tract, antacids allow peptic ulcers time to heal. Which gives me some time to relax …

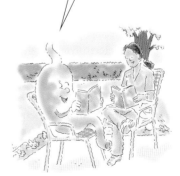

Pepsin, a digestive enzyme needed for protein breakdown, acts more effectively when the stomach is highly acidic; therefore, as acidity drops, pepsin action is also reduced. An acidic gastric environment with pepsin is associated with higher risks of peptic ulcers. Reducing gastric pH allows healing to occur (Vakil, 2021c).

Myth buster

Contrary to popular belief, antacids don't work by coating peptic ulcers or the lining of the GI tract.

Pharmacotherapeutics

Antacids are primarily prescribed to relieve pain and are used adjunctively in peptic ulcer disease.

Churn, churn, churn

Antacids also relieve symptoms of acid indigestion, heartburn, dyspepsia (burning or indigestion), and GERD.

Foiling phosphate absorption

Antacids may be used to control hyperphosphatemia (elevated blood phosphate levels) in kidney failure. Because calcium binds with phosphate in the GI tract, calcium carbonate antacids prevent phosphate absorption (Berkoben, 2021). (See *Antacids: Aluminum hydroxide*.)

Drug interactions

All antacids can interfere with the absorption of oral drugs if given at the same time. Absorption of digoxin, phenytoin, ketoconazole, iron salts, isoniazid, quinolones, and tetracycline may be reduced if taken within 2 hours of antacids. If a patient is taking an antacid in addition to other drugs, separate the drugs' administration times.

Side effects/adverse reactions

All side effects and adverse reactions to antacids are dose related and include:
- diarrhea (magnesium-based antacids)
- constipation (calcium- and aluminum-based antacids)
- electrolyte imbalances
- aluminum accumulation in serum.

The Three–Step Approach

Nursing management for patients undergoing treatment with antacids includes these three steps.

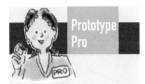

Prototype Pro

Antacids: Aluminum hydroxide

Actions
- Reduces total acid load in the GI tract
- Elevates gastric pH to reduce pepsin activity
- Strengthens the gastric mucosal barrier
- Increases esophageal sphincter tone

Indications
- GI discomfort

Nursing considerations
- Shake suspensions well.
- When administering through a nasogastric (NG) tube, make sure that the tube is patent and placed correctly; after instilling, flush the tube with water to ensure passage to the stomach and to clear the tube.
- Don't give other oral drugs within 2 hours of antacid administration. This may cause premature release of enteric coated drugs in the stomach.

Preadministration

(Recognize and analyze cues)
- Assess the patient's condition before therapy and regularly thereafter.
- Record the number and consistency of stools.
- Assess the patient for side effects and adverse reactions.
- Monitor the patient receiving long-term, high-dose aluminum hydroxide for fluid and electrolyte imbalance, especially if the patient is on a sodium-restricted diet.
- Monitor phosphate levels in the patient receiving aluminum hydroxide.
- Watch for signs of hypercalcemia in the patient receiving calcium carbonate.

(Prioritize hypothesis—priority patient problems)
- Constipation
- Electrolyte imbalance risk
- Knowledge deficiency

(Generate solutions)
- The patient's underlying symptoms will improve.
- Laboratory studies will show normal electrolyte balance.
- The patient and family or caregiver will demonstrate an understanding of antacid therapy.

Medication administration

(Take action)
- Manage constipation with laxatives or stool softeners or ask the prescriber about switching the patient to a magnesium preparation.
- If the patient suffers from diarrhea, obtain an order for an antidiarrheal as needed and ask the prescriber about switching the patient to an antacid containing aluminum.
- Shake the container of a liquid form well.
- When giving the drug through an NG tube, make sure that the tube is patent and placed correctly. After instilling the drug, flush the tube with water to ensure passage to the stomach and to clear the tube.

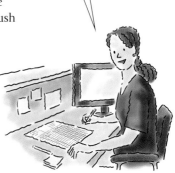

Laxatives, stool softeners, or antidiarrheals may be ordered to counteract the effects of antacids.

Postadministration

(Evaluate outcomes)
- Patient verbalizes relief of symptoms (pain, heartburn, etc.).
- Patient maintains a normal electrolyte balance.
- Patient and family or caregiver demonstrate an understanding of drug therapy. (See *Teaching about antacids*, page 352.)

Teaching about antacids

See Education Edge: Teaching template in Chapter 3, page 38 for general teaching for all medications. Specific points to review with patients and family for antacids:

• Don't take antacids indiscriminately or switch antacids without the prescriber's consent.

• Don't take calcium carbonate with milk or other foods high in vitamin D.

• Shake the suspension form well before taking it.

• Some antacids, such as aluminum hydroxide, may color stools white or cause white streaks.

• To prevent constipation, increase fluid and roughage intake and increase activity level.

H₂-receptor antagonists

H_2-receptor antagonists are commonly prescribed antiulcer drugs in the United States. Drugs in this category include:

• cimetidine
• famotidine
• nizatidine.

Pharmacokinetics

Cimetidine and nizatidine are absorbed rapidly and completely from the GI tract. Famotidine isn't completely absorbed. Food and antacids may reduce the absorption of H_2-receptor antagonists.

H_2-receptor antagonists are distributed widely throughout the body, metabolized by the liver, and excreted primarily in urine.

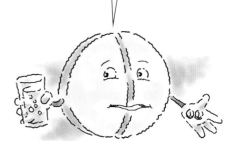

Food and antacids may reduce my absorption, making it more difficult for me to achieve my peak performance.

Pharmacodynamics

H_2-receptor antagonists block histamine from stimulating the acid-secreting parietal cells of the stomach (Vakil, 2021b).

Really in a bind

Acid secretion in the stomach depends on the binding of gastrin, acetylcholine, and histamine to receptors on the parietal cells. If the binding of any one of these substances is blocked, acid secretion is reduced. By binding with H_2 receptors, H_2-receptor antagonists block the action of histamine in the stomach and reduce acid secretion. (See *H₂-receptor antagonists: Famotidine*, page 353.)

Pharmacotherapeutics

H$_2$-receptor antagonists are used therapeutically to:
- promote healing of duodenal and gastric ulcers
- provide long-term treatment of pathologic GI hypersecretory conditions such as Zollinger-Ellison syndrome
- reduce gastric acid production and prevent stress ulcers in severely ill patients and in those with reflux esophagitis or upper GI bleeding.

Drug interactions

H$_2$-receptor antagonists may interact with antacids and other drugs:
- Antacids reduce the absorption of cimetidine, nizatidine, and famotidine.
- Cimetidine may increase the blood levels of oral anticoagulants, propranolol (and possibly other beta-adrenergic blockers), benzodiazepines, tricyclic antidepressants, theophylline, procainamide, quinidine, lidocaine, phenytoin, calcium channel blockers, cyclosporine, carbamazepine, and opioid analgesics by reducing their metabolism in the liver and their subsequent excretion.
- Cimetidine taken with carmustine increases the risk of bone marrow toxicity.
- Cimetidine inhibits ethyl alcohol metabolism in the stomach, resulting in higher blood alcohol levels.

Side effects/adverse reactions

Using H$_2$-receptor antagonists may lead to side effects and adverse reactions, especially in older adults or in patients with altered hepatic or renal function.

A rash of reactions
- Cimetidine may produce headache, dizziness, malaise, muscle pain, nausea, diarrhea or constipation, rashes, itching, loss of sexual desire, gynecomastia, and impotence.
- Famotidine and nizatidine produce few adverse reactions, with headaches being the most common, followed by constipation or diarrhea and rash.

The Three-Step Approach

Nursing management for patients undergoing treatment with H$_2$-receptor antagonists includes these three steps.

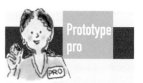

Prototype
pro

H$_2$-receptor antagonists: Famotidine

Actions
- Inhibits histamine's action at H$_2$ receptors in gastric parietal cells
- Reduces gastric acid output and concentration regardless of the stimulating agent (histamine, food, insulin, caffeine, betazole, or pentagastrin) or basal conditions

Indications
- GERD
- Zollinger-Ellison syndrome
- Duodenal ulcer
- Gastric ulcer
- Heartburn

Nursing considerations
- Monitor for side effects or adverse effects such as headache.
- Monitor for signs of GI bleeding such as blood in the patient's feces.

Preadministration

(Recognize and analyze cues)
- Assess for adverse reactions, especially hypotension and arrhythmias.
- Periodically monitor laboratory tests, such as complete blood count and renal and hepatic studies.

(Prioritize hypothesis—priority patient problems)
- Altered tissue integrity risk (GI mucosa)
- Hypotension risk (cimetidine)
- Knowledge deficiency

(Generate solutions)
- The patient's tissue integrity will improve as evidenced by a reduction in underlying symptoms.
- The patient will maintain adequate cardiac output as evidenced by stable vital signs and adequate urine output.
- The patient and family or caregiver will demonstrate an understanding of drug therapy.

Medication administration

(Take action)
- Administer a once-daily dose at bedtime to promote compliance. Twice-daily doses should be administered in the morning and evening; multiple doses, with meals and at bedtime.
- Don't exceed the recommended infusion rates when administering H_2-receptor antagonists IV; doing so increases the risk of adverse cardiovascular effects. Continuous IV infusion may suppress acid secretion more effectively.
- Administer antacids at least 1 hour before or after H_2-receptor antagonists. Antacids can decrease drug absorption.
- Anticipate dosage adjustments for the patient with renal disease.
- Avoid stopping the drug abruptly.

Postadministration

(Evaluate outcomes)
- Patient experiences decrease in or relief from upper GI symptoms with drug therapy.
- Patient maintains a normal heart rhythm.
- Patient and family or caregiver demonstrate an understanding of drug therapy. (See *Teaching about H_2-receptor antagonists*, page 355.)

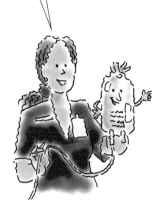

Be aware! Exceeding the recommended infusion rates when administering H_2-receptor antagonists IV increases the risk of adverse cardiovascular effects.

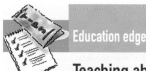

Teaching about H$_2$-receptor antagonists

See Education Edge: Teaching template in Chapter 3, page 38 for general teaching for all medications. Specific points to review with patients and family for H$_2$-receptor antagonist:

- Take the drug with a snack if desired.
- Take the drug as prescribed; don't stop taking the drug suddenly.
- If taking the drug once daily, take it at bedtime for best results.
- Continue to take the drug even after pain subsides to allow for adequate healing.
- If the prescriber approves, you may also take antacids, especially at the beginning of therapy when pain is severe.
- Don't take antacids within 1 hour of taking an H$_2$-receptor antagonist.

- Don't take the drug for more than 8 weeks unless specifically ordered to do so by the prescriber.
- Don't self-medicate for heartburn longer than 2 weeks without consulting the prescriber.
- Be aware of possible side effects and adverse reactions and report unusual effects.
- Avoid smoking during therapy; smoking stimulates gastric acid secretion and worsens the disease.
- Immediately report black tarry stools, diarrhea, confusion, or rash.
- Don't take other drugs, OTC products, or herbal remedies without first consulting with the prescriber or a pharmacist.

Proton pump inhibitors

Proton pump inhibitors (PPIs) disrupt chemical binding in stomach cells to reduce acid production, lessening irritation and allowing peptic ulcers to better heal. PPIs are more effective in healing ulcers than other antiulcer agents especially for NSAID-induced ulcers when NSAID therapy must continue (Vakil, 2021b). They include:
- dexlansoprazole
- esomeprazole
- lansoprazole
- omeprazole
- pantoprazole
- rabeprazole.

Pharmacokinetics

Proton pump inhibitors are given orally in enteric coated formulas to bypass the stomach because they're highly unstable in acid. They dissolve in the small intestine and are rapidly absorbed. Esomeprazole, lansoprazole, and pantoprazole can also be given IV (Karch, 2020).

Bound and determined

These drugs are highly protein bound and extensively metabolized by the liver to inactive compounds and then eliminated in urine.

Pharmacodynamics

Proton pump inhibitors block the last step in gastric acid secretion by combining with hydrogen, potassium, and adenosine triphosphate in the parietal cells of the stomach (Drini, 2017). (See *Proton pump inhibitors: Omeprazole.*)

Pharmacotherapeutics

Proton pump inhibitors are indicated for:
- short-term treatment of active gastric ulcers
- active duodenal ulcers
- erosive esophagitis
- symptomatic GERD that isn't responsive to other therapies
- active peptic ulcers associated with *H. pylori* infection (in combination with antibiotics)
- long-term treatment of hypersecretory states such as Zollinger-Ellison syndrome.

Drug interactions

Proton pump inhibitors may interfere with the metabolism of diazepam, phenytoin, and warfarin, causing increased half-lives and elevated plasma concentrations of these drugs.

Proton pump interference

Proton pump inhibitors may also interfere with the absorption of drugs that depend on gastric pH for absorption, such as ketoconazole, digoxin, ampicillin, magnesium, vitamin B_{12}, calcium, and iron salts.

Side effects/adverse reactions

Side effects and adverse reactions to proton pump inhibitors include:
- abdominal pain
- flatulence
- diarrhea
- nausea and vomiting
- malabsorption of vitamins and minerals (magnesium, calcium, iron, and vitamin B_{12}) (Wolfe, 2021).

Too much of a good thing!

Prolonged use of proton pump inhibitors has been associated with higher risk of osteoporosis, *Clostridiodes* infection, hypomagnesemia, and community-acquired pneumonia.

The Three-Step Approach

Nursing management for patients undergoing treatment with proton pump inhibitors includes these three steps.

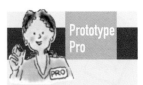

Prototype Pro

Proton pump inhibitors: Omeprazole

Actions
- Inhibits activity of acid (proton) pump and binds to hydrogen, potassium, and adenosine triphosphate, located at the secretory surface of the gastric parietal cells, to block gastric acid formation

Indications
- GERD
- Zollinger-Ellison syndrome
- Duodenal ulcer
- Gastric ulcer
- *H. pylori* infection

Nursing considerations
- Monitor the patient for adverse effects, such as headache, dizziness, and nausea.
- Administer the drug 30 minutes before meals.

Preadministration

(Recognize and analyze cues)
- Assess the patient's condition before therapy and regularly thereafter.
- Assess the patient for side effects, adverse reactions, and drug interactions.
- Monitor the patient's hydration status if adverse GI reactions occur.
- Assess the patient and family or caregiver's knowledge of drug therapy.

(Prioritize hypothesis—priority patient problems)
- Altered tissue integrity (GI mucosa)
- Hypovolemia
- Knowledge deficiency

(Generate solutions)
- The patient's tissue integrity will improve as evidenced by a reduction in presenting symptoms.
- The patient will maintain adequate fluid volume as evidenced by stable vital signs and urine output.
- The patient and family or caregivers will demonstrate an understanding of drug therapy.

Medication administration

(Take action)
- Administer the drug 30 minutes before meals.
- Dosage adjustments aren't needed for patients with renal or hepatic impairment.
- Tell the patient to swallow capsules whole and not to open or crush them.
- When giving IV esomeprazole, lansoprazole, or pantoprazole, check the package insert and your facility's policy for reconstitution, compatibility, and infusion time information.

Postadministration

(Evaluate outcomes)
- Patient responds well to therapy.
- Patient maintains adequate hydration throughout therapy.
- Patient and family or caregivers demonstrate an understanding of drug therapy. (See *Teaching about proton pump inhibitors*, page 358.)

> Remember:
> Give proton pump inhibitors 30 minutes before meals.

Teaching about proton pump inhibitors

See Education Edge: Teaching template in Chapter 3, page 38 for general teaching for all medications. Specific points to review with patients and family for proton pump inhibitors:

• Take the drug before eating; however, oral pantoprazole may be taken with or without food.

• Swallow the tablets or capsules whole; don't crush or chew them. These formulations are delayed release and long acting; opening, crushing, or chewing them destroys the drug's effects.

• If swallowing capsules is difficult, lansoprazole capsules can be opened and mixed with 60 mL of apple, orange, vegetable, or tomato juice. Capsule contents can also be sprinkled on 1 tablespoon of applesauce, pudding, cottage cheese, or yogurt. Swallow the mixture immediately without chewing the granules.

• Observe for the drug's effects; if symptoms persist or side effects or adverse reactions (such as headache, diarrhea, abdominal pain, and nausea or vomiting) occur, notify the prescriber.

Other antiulcer drugs

Research on the usefulness of other drugs in treating peptic ulcer disease continues. Two other antiulcer drugs currently in use are:
• misoprostol (a synthetic prostaglandin E_1)
• sucralfate (a gastrointestinal protectant).

Pharmacokinetics

Each of these drugs has slightly different pharmacokinetic properties.

An active acid

After an oral dose, misoprostol is absorbed extensively and rapidly. It's metabolized to misoprostol acid, which is clinically active, meaning it can produce a pharmacologic effect. Misoprostol acid is highly protein bound and is excreted primarily in urine.

Goes on by the GI

Sucralfate is minimally absorbed from the GI tract. It's excreted in feces.

Pharmacodynamics

The actions of these drugs vary.

Reduce and boost

Misoprostol protects against peptic ulcers caused by NSAIDs by reducing the secretion of gastric acid and by boosting the production of gastric mucus, a natural defense against peptic ulcers.

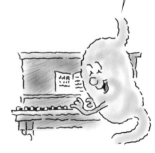

Misoprostol reduces gastric acid and boosts production of gastric mucus—a natural defense against peptic ulcers. That's music to my ears!

A sticky situation

Sucralfate works locally in the stomach, rapidly reacting with hydrochloric acid to form a thick, pastelike substance that adheres to the gastric mucosa and especially to ulcers. By binding to the ulcer site, sucralfate actually protects the ulcer from the damaging effects of acid and pepsin to promote healing. This binding usually lasts for 6 hours. Sucralfate is considered safe for women who are pregnant or breast-feeding as the drug is not well absorbed in the GI tract (Kahrilas, 2021).

Pharmacotherapeutics

Each of these drugs has its own therapeutic uses.

Attention to prevention

Misoprostol prevents peptic ulcers caused by NSAIDs in patients at high risk for complications resulting from gastric ulcers.

To treat and prevent

Sucralfate is used for short-term treatment (up to 8 weeks) of duodenal or gastric ulcers and prevention of recurrent ulcers or stress ulcers.

Drug interactions

Misoprostol and sucralfate may interact with other drugs:
- Antacids may bind with misoprostol or decrease its absorption. However, this effect doesn't appear to be clinically significant.
- Cimetidine, digoxin, norfloxacin, phenytoin, fluoroquinolones, tetracycline, and theophylline decrease the absorption of sucralfate.
- Antacids may reduce the binding of sucralfate to the gastric and duodenal mucosa, reducing its effectiveness.

Side effects/adverse reactions

Side effects and adverse reactions to misoprostol include:
- diarrhea (common and usually dose related)
- abdominal pain
- gas
- indigestion
- nausea and vomiting
- spontaneous abortion (women of childbearing age shouldn't become pregnant while taking misoprostol).
  Side effects and adverse reactions to sucralfate include:
- constipation
- nausea and vomiting
- dry mouth
- metallic taste.

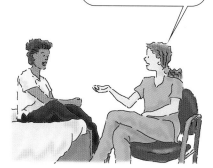

Since you are taking misoprostol, let's talk about contraceptive methods and possible alternative treatments. This drug can harm the fetus if pregnancy occurs.

The Three-Step Approach

Nursing management for patients undergoing treatment with the antiulcer drugs misoprostol and sucralfate includes these three steps.

Preadministration

(Recognize and analyze cues)

- Assess the patient's condition before therapy and regularly thereafter.
- Assess for adverse reactions and drug interactions.
- Assess women for pregnancy or breast-feeding (misoprostol).

Pregnancy precaution

- If a female patient is taking misoprostol, the drug can cause danger to the fetus if pregnancy occurs; discuss contraceptive methods or alternative treatment.
- Monitor the patient's hydration status if adverse GI reactions occur.
- Assess the patient and family or caregiver's understanding of drug therapy.

(Prioritize hypothesis—priority patient problems)

- Altered tissue integrity (GI mucosa)
- Hypovolemia
- Knowledge deficiency

(Generate solutions)

- The patient's tissue integrity will improve as evidenced by a reduction in presenting symptoms.
- The patient will maintain adequate fluid volume as evidenced by stable vital signs and urine output.
- The patient and family or caregivers will demonstrate an understanding of drug therapy.

Medication administration

(Take action)

- Administer sucralfate 1 hour before meals and at bedtime.
- Administer misoprostol with food.
- Tell the patient to continue the prescribed regimen at home to ensure complete healing. Explain that pain and ulcerative symptoms may subside within the first few weeks of therapy.
- Urge the patient to avoid cigarette smoking because it may increase gastric acid secretion and worsen the disease.

The spice of life

- Tell the patient to avoid alcohol, chocolate, spicy foods, or anything that irritates the stomach.

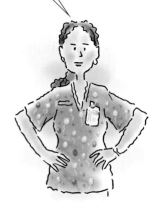

No butts about it! Cigarette smoking may increase gastric acid secretions and worsen ulcers.

- Elevate the head of the bed for comfort.
- Tell the patient to avoid large meals within 2 hours before bedtime.
- In women, start misoprostol therapy on the second or third day of the next normal menses to ensure that the patient isn't pregnant and that she is using effective contraception.

Postadministration
(Evaluate outcomes)
- Patient responds well to therapy.
- Patient maintains adequate hydration throughout therapy.
- Patient and family or caregivers demonstrate an understanding of drug therapy.

Tumor necrosis factor–alpha (TNF–alpha) blockers

Infliximab is an anti-TNF biologic medication used for treatment of Crohn's disease and ulcerative colitis. Crohn's disease is a chronic inflammation, most commonly associated with the small intestine, causing thickened mucosal walls and deep ulcers. Ulcerative colitis is a chronic inflammation, most commonly associated with the rectum and large intestine, causing small ulcers and abscess formation. The anti-TNF medication infliximab binds to TNF-alpha and inhibits its activity thus reducing the inflammation in the digestive tract (Lichtenstein, 2021).

Not for drive-through or carryout

This drug must be administered in a health care setting, frequently a physician's office, as it is administered via IV. Patients should be monitored for reactions during the infusion and for 2 hours after the infusion has completed. Patients typically receive a dose every 1 to 2 months.

Pharmacokinetics

Infliximab is administered intravenously and distributed within the vascular compartment, and it is thought to be excreted through the renal system. Terminal half-life of infliximab is approximately 14 days.

Pharmacodynamics

Infliximab is a monoclonal antibody that acts by binding to TNF-alpha to defuse its activity and inhibit its binding with receptors. This mechanism of action causes a reduction in the infiltration of inflammatory cells. This decrease in inflammation reduces the occurrence of common inflammatory bowel disease symptoms such as abdominal pain, chronic diarrhea, and weight loss.

Pharmacotherapeutics

Infliximab is prescribed for patients age six and older with moderate to severe Crohn's disease or ulcerative colitis whose condition has not improved with conventional medications. Infliximab is administered on a maintenance schedule after an initial introduction dosing and has proven effective in reducing symptoms, promoting clinical remission, and reducing or eliminating the need for long-term corticosteroid use.

Drug interactions

Studies have shown that infliximab may impact cytochrome P450 enzymes, resulting in unanticipated adverse reactions. Drugs with common interactions with cytochrome P450 enzymes include warfarin, antidepressants, antiepileptic drugs, and statins. Infliximab may influence a normal immune response to a live-virus vaccine, so patients who are taking infliximab should postpone immunizations until treatment is complete.

Side effects/adverse reactions

Infliximab increases the risk of serious infection, including tuberculosis (TB). Caution should be used when prescribed for patients with long-term or current infection. Patients should know that they will be tested for TB prior to initiation of therapy with infliximab, and they should immediately report any signs or symptoms of developing infection (Adegbola et al., 2018).

The Three–Step Approach

Nursing management for patients undergoing treatment with an anti-TNF medication includes these three steps.

Preadministration
(Recognize and analyze cues)
- Obtain a baseline assessment of the patient's bowel patterns and GI history before starting therapy.
- Assess the patient for side effects, adverse reactions, and drug interactions.
- Assess the patient for new or recurrent infection prior to administration including WBC, temperature, and other signs of infection.
- Obtain medication history.
- Assess the patient's fluid and electrolyte status during administration.

- Determine whether the patient maintains adequate fluid intake and diet and exercise.
- Assess patient for contraindications to the drug including older adults (higher risk of infection), patients with hematologic conditions, and those with hepatitis B.
- Assess the patient and family or caregiver's knowledge of drug therapy.
- Monitor the patient's CBC and liver enzymes throughout therapy and report abnormalities.

(Prioritize hypothesis—priority patient problems)
- Diarrhea
- Acute pain
- Infection risk
- Knowledge deficiency

(Generate solutions)
- The patient will experience fewer flares of symptoms.
- The patient's pain will decrease.
- The patient will remain infection free and be free from side effects or adverse reactions.
- The patient and family or caregiver will demonstrate an understanding of drug therapy.

Medication administration
(Take action)
- Administer the drug exactly as prescribed.
- Avoid infusing infliximab with other drugs or through plasticized polyvinyl IV tubing.
- Monitor the patient for signs of infusion reaction including fever, chills, pruritus, dyspnea, or chest pain during and for 2 hours postadministration.
- Notify the prescriber immediately of serious adverse reactions.
- Teach the patient to report any signs or symptoms of infection or enlarged lymph nodes immediately.
- Teach the patient to avoid live vaccines during treatment.

Postadministration
(Evaluate outcomes)
- Patient response is a reduction in symptoms.
- Patient regains normal bowel elimination pattern and consistency and is free from pain.
- Patient is infection free and is free from side effects and adverse reactions.
- Patient and family or caregiver demonstrate an understanding of drug therapy.

Adsorbent, antiflatulent, and digestive drugs

Adsorbent, antiflatulent, and digestive drugs aid healthy GI functions. They're used to fight undesirable toxins, acids, and gases in the GI tract.

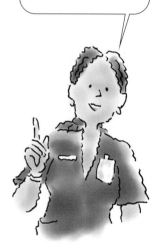

Adsorbent drugs are used as antidotes to toxins.

Adsorbent drugs

Natural and synthetic adsorbent drugs, or adsorbents, are prescribed as antidotes for the ingestion of toxins, substances that can lead to poisoning or overdose (Hendrickson & Kusin, 2021).

It's no picnic

The most commonly used clinical adsorbent is activated charcoal, a black powder residue obtained from the distillation of various organic materials.

Pharmacokinetics

Quick action required

Activated charcoal must be administered soon after toxic ingestion because it can only bind with drugs or poisons that haven't yet been absorbed from the GI tract. Activated charcoal, which isn't absorbed or metabolized by the body, is excreted unchanged in feces (Hendrickson & Kusin, 2021).

Pharmacodynamics

Because adsorbent drugs attract and bind toxins in the intestine, they inhibit toxins from being absorbed from the GI tract. However, this binding doesn't change toxic effects caused by earlier absorption of the poison.

Pharmacotherapeutics

Activated charcoal is a general-purpose antidote used for many types of acute oral poisoning.

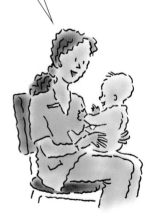

Children younger than age 1 shouldn't be given activated charcoal.

Contraindications

Activated charcoal or multidose activated charcoal should be avoided in acute poisoning from mineral acids, alkalines, cyanide, ethanol, methanol, iron, sodium chloride alkali, inorganic acids, or organic solvents. It should also be avoided in children younger than age 1 or if the patient has a risk of GI obstruction, perforation, or hemorrhage; decreased or absent bowel sounds; a history of recent GI surgery; or depressed mental state (Hendrickson & Kusin, 2021).

Drug interactions

Activated charcoal can decrease the absorption of oral medications; therefore, these medications (other than those used to treat the ingested toxin) should not be administered orally within 2 hours of taking activated charcoal.

Side effect/adverse reactions

Activated charcoal turns stool black and may cause constipation. A laxative such as sorbitol may be given with activated charcoal to prevent constipation and improve taste. Aspiration is a major concern with activated charcoal administration (Hendrickson & Kusin, 2021).

The Three-Step Approach

Nursing management for patients undergoing treatment with adsorbent drugs includes these three steps.

Preadministration

(Recognize and analyze cues)
- Obtain a history of the substance reportedly ingested, including time of ingestion, if possible. Activated charcoal isn't effective for all drugs and toxic substances.
- Assess for side effects, adverse reactions, and drug interactions.
- Assess the patient and family or caregiver's knowledge of drug therapy.

(Prioritize hypothesis—priority patient problems)
- Injury risk
- Aspiration risk
- Knowledge deficiency

(Generate solutions)
- The patient's risk of injury from poisoning will be minimized.
- The patient will be free from aspiration.
- The patient and the family or caregivers will demonstrate an understanding of drug therapy.

Medication administration

(Take action)
- Don't give the drug to a semiconscious or unconscious patient unless the airway is protected and an NG tube is in place for installation.
- Mix the powdered form with tap water to form the consistency of thick syrup. Add a small amount of fruit juice or flavoring to make it more palatable.
- Give by NG tube after lavage if needed.
- Take precautions to prevent aspiration.

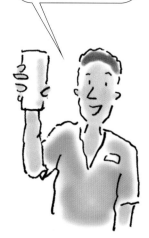

Here's a tip: Once you've mixed the powdered form of the adsorbent with tap water, add a small amount of fruit juice to make it more palatable.

Down with dairy

- Don't give the drug in ice cream, milk, or sherbet; these may reduce absorption.
- Repeat the dose if the patient vomits shortly after administration if prescribed.
- Keep airway, oxygen, and suction equipment nearby.
- Follow treatment with a stool softener or laxative to prevent constipation.
- Tell the patient that stools will be black.

Postadministration

(Evaluate outcomes)

- Patient doesn't experience injury from ingesting toxic substances or from overdose.
- Patient is free from aspiration and other side effects and adverse reactions.
- Patient exhibits no signs of deficient fluid volume.
- Patient and family or caregivers demonstrate an understanding of drug therapy.

Antiflatulent drugs

Antiflatulent drugs, or antiflatulents, disperse gas pockets in the GI tract. They're available alone or in combination with antacids. The major antiflatulent drug currently in use is simethicone.

Pharmacokinetics

Simethicone isn't absorbed from the GI tract. It's distributed only in the intestinal lumen and is eliminated intact in feces.

Pharmacodynamics

Simethicone creates foaming action in the GI tract. It produces a film in the intestines that disperses mucus-enclosed gas pockets.

Pharmacotherapeutics

Simethicone may be prescribed to treat conditions in which excess gas is a problem, such as:
- functional gastric bloating
- postoperative gaseous bloating
- diverticular disease
- spastic or irritable colon
- the swallowing of air.

Drug interactions

Simethicone doesn't interact significantly with other drugs.

Side effects/adverse reactions

Simethicone doesn't cause any known adverse reactions. It has, however, been associated with excessive belching or flatus.

The Three-Step Approach

Nursing management for patients undergoing treatment with antiflatulent drugs includes these three steps.

Preadministration

(Recognize and analyze cues)
- Assess the patient's condition before therapy and regularly thereafter.
- Assess for underlying cause of gas
- Assess the patient and family or caregiver's knowledge of drug therapy.

(Prioritize hypothesis—priority patient problems)
- Acute pain
- Knowledge deficiency

(Generate solutions)
- The patient's pain will decrease.
- The patient and family or caregivers will demonstrate an understanding of drug therapy.

Medication administration

(Take action)
- Make sure that the patient chews the tablet form before swallowing.
- Teach patient to avoid gas forming foods and carbonated drinks.

A shaky situation

- If giving the suspension form, make sure to shake the bottle or container thoroughly to distribute the solution.
- Inform the patient that the drug doesn't prevent gas formation.
- Encourage the patient to change position frequently and to ambulate to help pass flatus.

Postadministration

(Evaluate outcomes)
- Patient's gas pain is relieved.
- Patient and family or caregivers demonstrate an understanding of drug therapy.

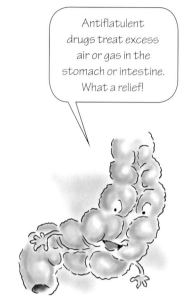

Antiflatulent drugs treat excess air or gas in the stomach or intestine. What a relief!

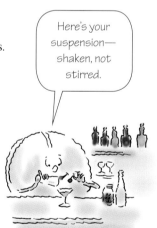

Here's your suspension—shaken, not stirred.

Digestive drugs

Digestive drugs (also called *digestants*) aid digestion in patients who are missing enzymes or other substances needed to digest food. A digestive drug that functions in the GI tract, liver, and pancreas is the pancreatic enzyme drug pancrelipase, which contains lipase, protease, and amylase (Freedman, 2021). Different forms of pancrelipase are available such as enteric and nonenteric formulas.

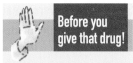

Pharmacokinetics

Digestive drugs aren't absorbed; they act locally in the GI tract and are excreted in feces.

Pharmacodynamics

The action of pancrelipase resembles the action of the body substances it replaces. Pancreatic enzyme replacement therapy (PERT) replaces missing pancreatic enzymes. Pancreatic enzyme supplementation provides additional enzymes to ensure adequate levels of enzymes are available for use in digestion (Freedman, 2021). They exert their effect in the duodenum and upper jejunum of the upper GI tract.

Pharmacotherapeutics

Pancrelipase contains enzymes to digest proteins, carbohydrates, and fat.

For the enzyme impaired

Pancreatic enzymes are administered to patients with insufficient levels of pancreatic enzymes, such as those with pancreatitis, pancreatic cancer, cystic fibrosis, and sometimes following gastric resection and/or bypass. They may also be used to treat steatorrhea (a disorder of fat metabolism characterized by fatty, foul-smelling stools). (See *Pancreatic enzymes warning*.)

Drug interactions

Antacids, calcium and magnesium supplements, and dairy products reduce the effects of pancreatic enzymes and shouldn't be given at the same time. Pancreatic enzymes may also decrease the absorption of folic acid and iron and reduce effectiveness of the oral diabetic drugs acarbose and miglitol.

Side effects/adverse reactions

Adverse reactions to pancreatic enzymes include:
- diarrhea
- nausea
- abdominal cramping.

Before you give that drug!

Pancreatic enzymes warning

Pancreatic enzymes should be given before meals. This ensures that the drug is available in the small intestine to help digestion. Giving pancreatic enzymes at another time, such as 1 hour or more after eating or during a meal, decreases the drug's effectiveness.

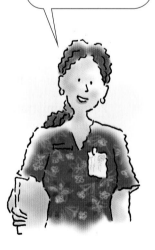

Patients with pancreatitis or cystic fibrosis may require pancreatic enzyme administration because their bodies may not produce enough on their own.

The Three-Step Approach

Nursing management for patients undergoing treatment with digestive drugs includes these three steps.

Preadministration

(Recognize and analyze cues)

- Assess the patient's condition before therapy and regularly thereafter. A decrease in the number of bowel movements and improved stool consistency indicate effective therapy.
- Obtain results of fecal elastase or fecal fat testing.
- Monitor the patient's diet to ensure a proper balance of fat, protein, and starch intake. This helps avoid indigestion. The dosage varies according to the degree of maldigestion and malabsorption, the amount of fat in the diet, and the enzyme activity of the drug.
- Assess the patient and family or caregiver's knowledge of drug therapy.
- Assess the patient's and family's knowledge and attitudes about nutrition.

(Prioritize hypothesis—priority patient problems)

- Malnutrition
- Nonadherence
- Knowledge deficiency

(Generate solutions)

- The patient's nutritional status will improve as evidenced by laboratory tests and weight.
- The patient will adhere with the prescribed drug regimen.
- The patient and family or caregivers will demonstrate an understanding of drug therapy.

Medication administration

(Take action)

- Administer the drug before or with each meal as applicable. If dairy products are consumed, take enzymes 15 minutes prior to the meal.
- For older infants, the powdered form may be mixed with applesauce and given before meals.
- Avoid contact with or inhalation of the powder form; it may be irritating.
- Older children may take capsules with food.
- Tell the patient not to crush or chew enteric-coated dosage forms. Capsules containing enteric-coated microspheres may be opened and their contents sprinkled on a small amount of soft food, such as applesauce. Follow administration with a glass of water or juice.
- Review food preferences and diet orders with the patient and family or caregivers.
- Provide food and fluids that the patient enjoys at times of preference, if possible.

Teaching about digestive drugs

See Education Edge: Teaching template in Chapter 3, page 38 for general teaching for all medications. Specific points to review with patients and family for digestive drugs:

• Exercise and stay active to aid the digestion and improve appetite.
• Minimize the use of strong pain medications and sedatives because these drugs may cause drowsiness and deter eating and drinking.

• Have routine checkups to monitor weight, fluid intake, urine output, and laboratory studies and to assess nutritional outcomes.

- Treat signs and symptoms or disorders that may interfere with nutrition, such as pain, nausea, vomiting, or diarrhea.
- Consult with a dietitian if special diets are ordered. Provide foods the patient likes, selecting nutritionally better choices that fall within the prescribed diet.

Postadministration

(Evaluate outcomes)
- Patient maintains normal digestion of fats, carbohydrates, and proteins.
- Patient complies with the prescribed drug regimen.
- Patient and family or caregivers demonstrate an understanding of drug therapy. (See *Teaching about digestive drugs*.)

Antidiarrheal and laxative drugs

Diarrhea and constipation represent the two major symptoms related to disturbances of the large intestine.

Antidiarrheals act systemically or locally and include:
- opioid-related drugs
- kaolin and pectin (a combination drug and the only one that acts locally).

Laxatives stimulate defecation and include:
- hyperosmolar drugs
- dietary fiber and related bulk-forming substances
- emollients
- stimulants
- lubricants
- 5-HT$_3$-receptor antagonists
- probiotics.

Opioid-related drugs

Opioid-related drugs decrease peristalsis (involuntary, progressive wavelike intestinal movement that pushes fecal matter along) in the intestines and include:

- diphenoxylate with atropine
- difenoxin with atropine
- loperamide.

> Opioid-related drugs decrease the wavelike movement of peristalsis.

Pharmacokinetics

Diphenoxylate with atropine and difenoxin with atropine is readily absorbed from the GI tract. Loperamide is slowly absorbed after oral administration.

These drugs are distributed in serum, metabolized in the liver, and excreted primarily in feces (Karch, 2020). Diphenoxylate with atropine is metabolized to difenoxin, its biologically active major metabolite.

Pharmacodynamics

These opium derivatives slow GI motility by depressing the circular and longitudinal muscle action (peristalsis) in the large and small intestines. These drugs also decrease expulsive contractions throughout the colon.

Pharmacotherapeutics

Diphenoxylate with atropine, difenoxin with atropine, and loperamide are used to treat short-term diarrhea. (See *Antidiarrheals: Loperamide.*)

Drug interactions

These opium derivatives may enhance the depressant effects of barbiturates, alcohol, opioids, tranquilizers, and sedatives.

Contraindications

Avoid use of antidiarrheal agents in patients with diarrhea due to poisoning or with hepatic dysfunction (Karch, 2020).

Side effects/adverse reactions

Side effects and adverse reactions to diphenoxylate with atropine and loperamide include:

- constipation
- nausea and vomiting
- abdominal discomfort or distention
- drowsiness
- fatigue

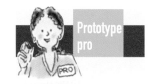

Prototype pro

Antidiarrheals: Loperamide

Actions
- Inhibits peristaltic activity, prolonging transit of intestinal contents

Indications
- Diarrhea

Nursing considerations
- Monitor the drug's effect on bowel movements.
- If giving by NG tube, flush the tube to clear it and to ensure the drug's passage to the stomach.
- Oral liquids are available in different concentrations. Check the dosage carefully.
- For children, an oral liquid that doesn't contain alcohol should be considered.

- central nervous system (CNS) depression
- tachycardia
- paralytic ileus (reduced or absent peristalsis in the intestines).

The Three-Step Approach

Nursing management for patients undergoing treatment with antidiarrheal drugs includes these three steps.

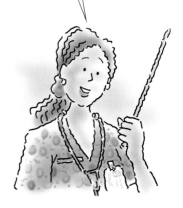

Before giving antidiarrheals, make sure you correct fluid and electrolyte disturbances, which may cause dehydration.

Preadministration

(Recognize and analyze cues)
- Assess the patient's condition and diarrhea before therapy and regularly thereafter.
- Monitor the patient's fluid and electrolyte balance.
- Monitor the patient's hydration status if adverse GI reactions occur.
- Evaluate the patient for side effects and adverse reactions.
- Assess the patient and family or caregiver's knowledge of drug therapy.

(Prioritize hypothesis—priority patient problems)
- Diarrhea
- Hypovolemia
- Injury risk
- Knowledge deficiency

(Generate solutions)
- The patient will have normal bowel movements.
- The patient will maintain adequate fluid and electrolyte balance as evidenced by intake and output.
- The patient will be free from injury associated with fluid and electrolyte imbalances or central nervous system depression.
- The patient and family or caregivers will demonstrate an understanding of drug therapy.

Medication administration

(Take action)
- Correct fluid and electrolyte disturbances before starting the drug; dehydration may increase the risk of delayed toxicity in some cases.
- Use naloxone to treat respiratory depression caused by overdose for opium derivative antidiarrheals.
- Take safety precautions if the patient experiences adverse CNS reactions.
- Notify the prescriber about serious or persistent side effects or adverse reactions occur.

Postadministration

(Evaluate outcomes)

- Patient's diarrhea is relieved.
- Patient maintains adequate hydration and electrolyte balance.
- Patient is free from injury.
- Patient and family or caregivers demonstrate an understanding of drug therapy. (See *Teaching about antidiarrheals*, page 374.)

Other antidiarrheals

Other antidiarrheal drugs include kaolin and pectin, usually in combination with bismuth subsalicylate.

Kaolin and pectin

Kaolin and pectin mixtures are locally acting OTC antidiarrheals. They work by adsorbing irritants and soothing the intestinal mucosa. The combination of kaolin and pectin relieves mild to moderate acute diarrhea or may be used to temporarily relieve chronic diarrhea until the cause is determined and definitive treatment starts. These antidiarrheals can interfere with the absorption of digoxin or other drugs from the intestinal mucosa if administered at the same time.

Kaolin and pectin mixtures cause few adverse reactions. However, constipation may occur, especially in older adults, patients who are debilitated, and in cases of overdose or prolonged use.

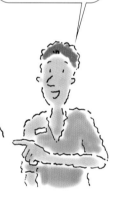

> Kaolin and pectin may cause constipation, especially for patients who are older or are debilitated.

Bismuth subsalicylate

Bismuth subsalicylate relieves diarrhea, nausea, and dyspepsia. This gastrointestinal agent is absorbed from the GI tract, is metabolized in the liver, and is excreted in urine (Karch, 2020). Side effects and adverse reactions are similar to other salicylate products such as GI bleeding, hearing loss or tinnitus, and Reye's syndrome in children and adolescents.

Selective 5-HT₃-receptor antagonists

Alosetron, a selective antagonist of serotonin 5-HT$_3$ receptors, is used to treat irritable bowel syndrome (IBS) in women who have severe diarrhea (Wald, 2021). IBS is a disorder of the colon that's characterized by constipation or diarrhea.

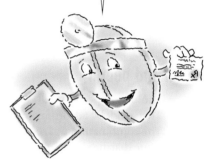

Because of the potential for serious adverse effects, alosetron is prescribed only by doctors enrolled in the drug's prescribing program.

Pharmacokinetics

Alosetron is rapidly absorbed after oral administration. It's metabolized by the cytochrome P450 pathway.

Pharmacodynamics

Alosetron selectively inhibits 5-HT$_3$ receptors on enteric neurons in the GI tract. By inhibiting activation of these cation channels, neuronal depolarization is blocked, resulting in decreased visceral pain, colonic transit, and GI secretions—factors that usually contribute to the symptoms of IBS.

Pharmacotherapeutics

Alosetron is used for the short-term treatment of women with IBS whose primary symptom is diarrhea that has lasted longer than 6 months and has not responded to conventional treatment. Don't give this drug if the patient is constipated. Stop the drug if constipation develops. This drug is not indicated for men.

Education edge

Teaching about antidiarrheals

See Education Edge: Teaching template in Chapter 3, page 38 for general teaching for all medications. Specific points to review with patients and family for antidiarrheals:

- Take the drug exactly as prescribed; be aware that excessive use of opium preparations can lead to dependence.
- Notify your prescriber if diarrhea lasts for more than 2 days, if acute abdominal signs and symptoms or bleeding occur, or if the drug is ineffective.
- Avoid hazardous activities that require alertness if CNS depression occurs.
- Maintain intake of fluids and electrolytes, about 2 to 3 L/day.

- Avoid food and fluids that can irritate the GI tract while diarrhea is present.
- Schedule rest periods and decrease activity while diarrhea persists to reduce peristalsis.
- Avoid bismuth subsalicylate if GI bleeding occurs, in children or adolescents with fever, or in patients with bleeding disorders as the medication is related to salicylates.

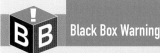

Black Box Warning

Preparing for Practice: Alosetron

Monitor patient for GI adverse reactions including ischemic colitis and constipation. Report symptoms of ischemic colitis and constipation immediately as they have resulted in serious illness and death.

Lexicomp. (2019). Alosetron: Drug information. In *UpToDate*. Retrieved from www.uptodate.com

Drug interactions

Avoid using alosetron if the patient is taking CYP1A2 inhibitors (abametapir); 5-HT3 antagonist (apomorphine or tramadol); serotonergic agents; eluxadoline, fluvoxamine, or viloxazine; or if the patient smokes tobacco. In addition, avoid using alosetron with other drugs that decrease GI motility to prevent the risk of constipation. (*See Preparing for Practice: Alosetron.*)

Side effects/adverse reactions

Alosetron has produced serious, and sometimes fatal, adverse reactions, including:
- ischemic colitis
- serious complications of constipation, including obstruction, perforation, and toxic megacolon.

The Three-Step Approach

Nursing management for patients undergoing treatment with a selective 5-HT$_3$-receptor antagonist include these three steps.

Preadministration
(Recognize and analyze cues)
- Obtain a baseline assessment of the patient's bowel patterns and GI history before starting therapy.
- Assess the patient for adverse reactions and drug interactions.
- Monitor the patient's bowel pattern throughout therapy. Assess bowel sounds and color and consistency of stools.
- Assess the patient's fluid and electrolyte status during administration.
- Determine whether the patient maintains adequate fluid intake, diet, and exercise.
- Determine if the patient smokes tobacco.
- Assess the patient's and family's knowledge of drug therapy.

A collection of contraindications

- Assess the patient for contraindications to alosetron, such as constipation, intestinal obstruction, stricture, toxic megacolon, GI perforation, GI adhesions, ischemic colitis, impaired intestinal circulation, thrombophlebitis, hypercoagulable state, Crohn's disease, ulcerative colitis, or diverticulitis (Lexicomp, 2019).

Key nursing diagnoses (prioritize hypothesis—priority patient problems)
- Diarrhea
- Constipation risk
- Injury risk
- Knowledge deficiency

Planning outcome goals (generate solutions)
- The patient will maintain regular bowel movements without diarrhea or constipation.
- The patient will be free from side effects/adverse reactions of alosetron.
- The patient's pain will decrease.
- The patient and family or caregiver will demonstrate an understanding of drug therapy.

Medication administration

(Take action)
- Time drug administration so that bowel evacuation doesn't interfere with scheduled activities or sleep.
- Make sure that the patient has easy access to a bedpan or bathroom.
- Institute measures to prevent constipation including adequate fluid intake, diet, and exercise.
- Determine patient's understanding of the risks and benefits of the drug.
- Teach patient to take alosetron with or without food. However, taking with food may decrease absorption.
- Teach patient to follow up with their health care provider in 4 weeks after treatment begins.
- Teach patient to report any symptoms of ischemic colitis or constipation immediately.
- Teach patient if they miss a dose, skip that dose. Do not take 2 doses close together.
- Teach patient to store medication away from light and moisture.

Postadministration

(Evaluate outcomes)
- Patient regains normal bowel elimination pattern.
- Patient is free from side effects/adverse reactions.
- Patient states that pain is relieved with stool evacuation.
- Patient and family or caregiver demonstrate an understanding of drug therapy.

Laxatives

Laxative, or cathartic, drugs are used for a variety of situations including:
- relief of constipation
- preparing for colon or rectal procedures or surgery
- prevent straining after a vaginal birth, myocardial infarction, and other conditions where straining causes injury
- rid the lower intestine of poisons or the GI tracts of helminths (Karch, 2020).

Laxatives are classified according to how they work in the body.

Osmolar laxatives

Osmolar laxatives work by drawing water into the intestine, thereby promoting bowel distention and peristalsis. They include:
- glycerin
- lactulose
- saline compounds, such as magnesium salts, sodium biphosphate, sodium phosphate, polyethylene glycol (PEG), and electrolytes
- sorbitol.

Pharmacokinetics

The pharmacokinetic properties of osmolar laxatives vary. Glycerin is placed directly into the colon by enema or suppository and isn't absorbed systemically.

Intestine marks the spot

Lactulose enters the GI tract orally and is minimally absorbed. As a result, the drug is distributed only in the intestine. It's metabolized by bacteria in the colon and excreted in feces.

Saline away

After saline compounds are introduced into the GI tract orally or as an enema, some of their ions are absorbed. Absorbed ions are excreted in urine, the unabsorbed drug in feces.

And then there's PEG

PEG is a nonabsorbable solution that acts as an osmotic drug but doesn't alter electrolyte balance.

Pharmacodynamics

Hyperosmolar laxatives produce a bowel movement by drawing water into the intestine. Fluid accumulation distends the bowel and promotes peristalsis and a bowel movement. (See *Osmolar laxatives: Magnesium hydroxide*, page 378.)

Osmolar laxatives: Magnesium hydroxide

Actions
- Reduces total acid in the GI tract
- Elevates gastric pH to reduce pepsin activity
- Strengthens the gastric mucosal barrier
- Increases esophageal sphincter tone

Indications
- Upset stomach
- Constipation
- Inadequate magnesium level

Nursing considerations
- Monitor the drug's effect on bowel movements.
- Shake the suspension well. Give the drug with a large amount of water when used as a laxative.
- When used with an NG tube, make sure the tube is placed properly and is patent. After instilling the drug, flush the tube with water to ensure passage to the stomach and to maintain tube patency.

Pharmacotherapeutics

The uses of hyperosmolar laxatives vary:
- Glycerin is helpful in bowel retraining.
- Lactulose is used to treat constipation and helps promote ammonia excretion from the intestines in patients with liver disease.
- Saline compounds are used when prompt and complete bowel evacuation is required.

Drug interactions

Osmolar laxatives don't interact significantly with other drugs. However, the absorption of oral drugs administered 1 hour before PEG is significantly decreased.

Side effects/adverse reactions

Side effects and adverse reactions to osmolar laxatives involve fluid and electrolyte imbalances.
- Side effects and adverse reactions to glycerin include weakness and fatigue.
- Lactulose may cause abdominal distention, gas, and abdominal cramps; nausea and vomiting; diarrhea; hypokalemia; hypovolemia; and increased blood glucose level.
- Saline compounds may cause:
  - weakness
  - lethargy
  - dehydration
  - hypernatremia
  - hypermagnesemia

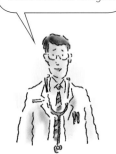

Adverse reactions to glycerin include weakness and fatigue.

○ hyperphosphatemia
○ hypocalcemia
○ cardiac arrhythmias
○ shock.
- These side effects and adverse reactions may occur with PEG: nausea, abdominal fullness, explosive diarrhea, and bloating.

> A high-fiber diet is the most natural way to prevent or treat constipation. Dietary fiber is the part of plants not digested in the small intestine.

Dietary fiber and related bulk-forming laxatives

Close resemblance

Bulk-forming laxatives, which resemble dietary fiber, contain natural and semisynthetic polysaccharides and cellulose. These laxatives include:
- methylcellulose
- polycarbophil
- psyllium hydrophilic mucilloid.

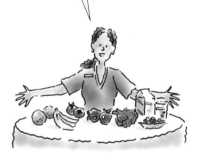

Pharmacokinetics

Dietary fiber and bulk-forming laxatives aren't absorbed systemically. The polysaccharides in these drugs are converted by intestinal bacterial flora into osmotically active metabolites that draw water into the intestine. Dietary fiber and bulk-forming laxatives are excreted in feces.

Pharmacodynamics

Dietary fiber and bulk-forming laxatives increase stool mass and water content, promoting peristalsis. (See *Bulk-forming laxatives: Psyllium*)

Prototype pro

Bulk-forming laxatives: Psyllium

Actions
- Absorbs water and expands to increase bulk and moisture content of stool, thus encouraging peristalsis and bowel movements

Indications
- Constipation

Nursing considerations
- Mix the drug with at least 8 oz (240 mL) of cold, pleasant-tasting liquid such as orange juice to mask grittiness. Stir only a few seconds. Have the patient drink the mixture immediately, before it congeals. Follow administration with another glass of liquid.
- Psyllium may reduce the patient's appetite if taken before meals.
- This drug isn't absorbed systemically and is nontoxic.
- Psyllium is useful in patients who are deliberated and in patients with postpartum constipation, IBS, or diverticular disease. It's also used to treat chronic laxative abuse and combined with other laxatives to empty the colon before barium enema examination.
- Advise patients with diabetes to check the drug's label and to use a brand that doesn't contain sugar.

Pharmacotherapeutics

Bulk-forming laxatives are used to:
- treat simple cases of constipation, especially constipation resulting from a low-fiber or low-fluid diet
- aid patients recovering from acute myocardial infarction (MI) or cerebral aneurysms who need to avoid Valsalva's maneuver (forced expiration against a closed airway) and maintain soft stool
- manage patients with IBS and diverticulosis.

Drug interactions

Decreased absorption of digoxin, warfarin, and salicylates occurs if these drugs are taken within 2 hours of fiber or bulk-forming laxatives.

Side effects/adverse reactions

Side effects and adverse reactions to dietary fiber and related bulk-forming laxatives include:
- flatulence
- a sensation of abdominal fullness
- intestinal obstruction
- fecal impaction (hard feces that can't be removed from the rectum)
- esophageal obstruction (if sufficient liquid hasn't been administered with the drug)
- severe diarrhea.

Emollient laxatives

Emollient laxatives—also known as *stool softeners*—include the calcium and sodium salts of docusate.

Pharmacokinetics

Administered orally, emollient laxatives are absorbed and excreted through bile in feces.

Pharmacodynamics

Emollient laxatives emulsify the fat and water components of feces in the small and large intestines. This detergent action allows water and fats to penetrate the stool, making it softer and easier to eliminate. Emollients also stimulate electrolyte and fluid secretion from intestinal mucosal cells. (See *Emollient laxatives: Docusate*, Page 381.)

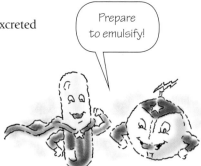

Prepare to emulsify!

Prototype pro

Emollient laxatives: Docusate

Actions
• Reduces surface tension of interfacing liquid contents of the bowel, promoting incorporation of additional liquid into stool, thus forming a softer mass

Indications
• Stool softening for patients who should avoid straining during a bowel movement

Nursing considerations
• Monitor the drug's effect on bowel movements.

• Be alert for side effects, adverse reactions, and drug interactions.
• This drug is the laxative of choice for patients who shouldn't strain during defecation (including those recovering from MI or rectal surgery), for patients with rectal or anal disease that makes passage of firm stool difficult, and for patients with postpartum constipation.
• Discontinue the drug if abdominal cramping occurs and notify the prescriber.
• Docusate doesn't stimulate intestinal peristaltic movements.

Pharmacotherapeutics

Emollient laxatives are the drugs of choice for softening stools in patients who should avoid straining during a bowel movement, including those with:
• recent MI or surgery
• disease of the anus or rectum
• increased intracranial pressure (ICP)
• hernias.

Drug interactions

Taking oral doses of mineral oil with oral emollient laxatives increases the systemic absorption of mineral oil. This increased absorption may result in tissue deposits of the oil.

Proceed with caution

Because emollient laxatives may enhance the absorption of many oral drugs, drugs with low margins of safety (narrow therapeutic index) should be administered cautiously.

Side effects/adverse reactions

Although side effects and adverse reactions to emollient laxatives seldom occur, they may include:
• a bitter taste
• diarrhea
• throat irritation
• mild, transient abdominal cramping.

Determine whether the patient maintains adequate fluid intake, diet, and exercise.

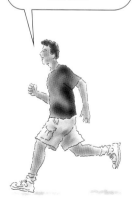

Stimulant laxatives

Stimulant laxatives, also known as *irritant cathartics*, include:

- bisacodyl
- cascara sagrada
- castor oil
- phenolphthalein
- senna
- sodium picosulfate.

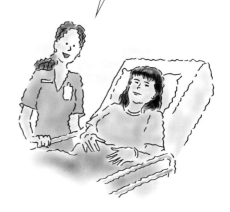

Stimulant laxatives are used to empty the bowel before general surgery, sigmoidoscopic or proctoscopic procedures, and radiologic procedures.

Pharmacokinetics

Stimulant laxatives are minimally absorbed and are metabolized in the liver. The metabolites are excreted in urine and feces.

Pharmacodynamics

Stimulant laxatives stimulate peristalsis and produce a bowel movement by irritating the intestinal mucosa or stimulating nerve endings of the intestinal smooth muscle.

Powering up peristalsis

Castor oil also increases peristalsis in the small intestine.

Pharmacotherapeutics

Stimulant laxatives are the preferred drugs for emptying the bowel before general surgery, sigmoidoscopic or proctoscopic procedures, and radiologic procedures such as barium studies of the GI tract.

Conquering constipation

Besides their use before surgery and procedures, stimulant laxatives are used to treat constipation caused by prolonged bed rest, neurologic dysfunction of the colon, and constipating drugs such as opioids.

Package deal

Combining three ingredients to form one package (packet) of two types of laxatives is used to prepare a patient for proctoscopy or colonoscopy procedures. The three ingredients in the packet include sodium picosulfate, magnesium oxide, and anhydrous citric acid. Magnesium oxide and anhydrous citric acid combine to form magnesium citrate, an osmotic diuretic. Sodium picosulfate is a stimulant laxative.

Drug interactions

No significant drug interactions occur with stimulant laxatives. However, because stimulant laxatives produce increased intestinal motility, they reduce the absorption of other oral drugs administered at the same time, especially sustained-release forms.

Side effects/adverse reactions

Side effects and adverse reactions to stimulant laxatives include:
- weakness
- nausea
- abdominal cramps
- mild inflammation of the rectum and anus
- urine discoloration (with cascara sagrada or senna use).

Lubricant laxatives

Mineral oil is the main lubricant laxative in current clinical use.

Pharmacokinetics

In its nonemulsified form, mineral oil is minimally absorbed; the emulsified form is about half absorbed.

Mineral oil on the move

Absorbed mineral oil is distributed to the mesenteric lymph nodes, intestinal mucosa, liver, and spleen. Mineral oil is metabolized by the liver and excreted in feces. (See *Lubricant laxatives: Mineral oil.*)

Prototype pro

Lubricant laxatives: Mineral oil

Actions
- Increases water retention in stool by creating a barrier between the colon wall and feces that prevents colonic reabsorption of fecal water

Indications
- Constipation

Nursing considerations
- Monitor the drug's effect on bowel movements.
- Be alert for adverse reactions and drug interactions.
- Give the drug on an empty stomach.
- Give the drug with fruit juice or a carbonated drink to disguise its taste, or may be given by enema.

Pharmacodynamics

Mineral oil lubricates the stool and the intestinal mucosa and prevents water reabsorption from the bowel lumen. The increased fluid content of feces increases peristalsis. Rectal administration by enema also produces distention.

Pharmacotherapeutics

Mineral oil is used to treat constipation and maintain soft stools when straining is contraindicated, such as after a recent MI (to avoid Valsalva maneuver), eye surgery (to prevent increased pressure in the eye), or cerebral aneurysm repair (to avoid increased ICP). Administered orally or by enema, mineral oil is also used to treat patients with fecal impaction.

Drug interactions

To minimize drug interactions, administer mineral oil at least 2 hours before other drugs. These drug interactions may occur:

- Mineral oil may impair the absorption of many oral drugs, including fat-soluble vitamins, hormonal contraceptives, and anticoagulants.
- Mineral oil may interfere with the antibacterial activity of nonabsorbable sulfonamides.

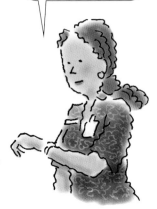

You can minimize drug interactions by giving mineral oil at least 2 hours before other drugs.

Side effects/adverse reactions

Side effects and adverse reactions to mineral oil include:

- nausea
- vomiting
- diarrhea
- abdominal cramping.

Drugs for chronic constipation

Chronic constipation is defined as persistent constipation over a period of 3 months or more. Chronic constipation occurs in patients with IBS with constipation (IBS-C) and patients taking long-term opioids for chronic pain.

Chloride channel activator

Lubiprostone (Amitiza) is a bicyclic fatty acid derived from prostaglandin E_1 analog approved for use of chronic constipation and IBS-C in women over the age of 18.

Guanylate cyclase-C agonist

Linaclotide (Linzess) is indicated in the treatment of IBS-C.

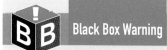

Black Box Warning

Preparing for practice: Lubiprostone and linaclotide

Caution: Use is approved for those over age 18. These drugs are contraindicated in known or suspected mechanical GI obstruction or pregnancy.

Pharmacokinetics

Lubiprostone and linaclotide are minimally absorbed in the systemic circulation.

Pharmacodynamics

Lubiprostone activates chloride channels in the small intestine to increase intestinal fluid secretion and motility.

Linaclotide acts locally on intestinal epithelium, increasing chloride and bicarbonate secretion into intestines and inhibiting sodium ion absorption. Water absorption into the lumen improves defecation.

Pharmacotherapeutics

Lubiprostone and linaclotide are indicated for chronic idiopathic and opioid-induced constipation and IBS-C in patients who have not responded to fiber and osmotic laxatives. They help to reduce abdominal pain associated with chronic constipation.

Drug interactions

None identified

Side effects/adverse reactions

- Diarrhea, if severe is associated with fluid and electrolyte imbalances
- Abdominal pain
- Flatulence
- Abdominal distention

A word about probiotics

Probiotics are microorganisms primarily derived from food, most notably, from cultured milk products. One microorganism commonly used is Lactobacillus although others are available. Probiotics are used to colonize the intestine with beneficial bacteria in conditions such as *Clostridioides difficile*, infectious diarrhea colitis, IBS, and Crohn's disease (Sartor, 2021).

Commercially prepared probiotics are available and their efficacy is under investigation. Although benefits from probiotic include growth suppression of "unwanted" bacteria in the colon and modulation of the immune systems, some probiotics from cultured milk products may create problems for those who are lactose intolerant or they may not colonize in the intestine (Sartor, 2021).

The Three-Step Approach

These nursing process steps are appropriate for patients undergoing treatment with laxatives include these three steps.

Preadministration

(Recognize and analyze cues)
- Obtain a baseline assessment of the patient's bowel patterns and GI history before giving a laxative.
- For linaclotide—assess the patient's medication list. Dosages may need to be decreased if the patient is taking antihypertensives or methadone. Determine if the patient is pregnant—patients need to have a negative pregnancy test to begin therapy.
- Determine whether the patient maintains adequate fluid intake, diet, and exercise.
- Assess the patient's bowel pattern throughout therapy. Assess bowel sounds and color and consistency of stools.
- Monitor the patient's fluid and electrolyte status during administration.
- Assess for side effects, adverse reactions, and drug interactions.
- Assess the patient and family or caregiver's knowledge of drug therapy.

(Prioritize hypothesis—priority patient problems)
- Diarrhea
- Constipation
- Acute pain
- Knowledge deficiency

(Generate solutions)
- The patient will maintain regular bowel movements without diarrhea or constipation.
- The patient's pain will decrease.
- The patient and family or caregivers will demonstrate an understanding of drug therapy.

Medication administration

(Take action)
- Time drug administration so that bowel evacuation doesn't interfere with scheduled activities or sleep.
- Shake suspensions well; give with a large amount of water as applicable.
- If administering the drug through an NG tube, make sure that the tube is placed properly and is patent. After instilling the drug, flush the tube with water to ensure passage to the stomach and to maintain tube patency.

- Don't crush enteric coated tablets.
- Make sure that the patient has easy access to a bedpan or bathroom.
- Institute measures to prevent constipation such as adequate fluid and dietary fiber intake.
- Administer on an empty stomach at least 30 minutes before the first meal of the day (lubiprostone and linaclotide).
- When giving mineral oil by mouth, give it on an empty stomach.
- Perform rectal administration according to facility protocol (lubricant laxatives).
- Mix drugs as directed and give with a large amount of water, as applicable (dietary fiber and bulk forming laxatives).
- Keep in mind that the laxative effect usually occurs in 12 to 24 hours but may be delayed for up to 3 days (dietary fiber and bulk forming laxatives).
- Teach patient to use birth control measures/methods to prevent pregnancy while on lubiprostone.

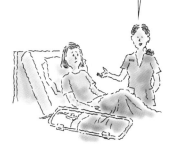

Schedule laxative administration so that the drug's effects don't interfere with the patient's activities or sleep.

Postadministration

(Evaluate outcomes)

- Patient regains a normal bowel elimination pattern without constipation or diarrhea.
- Patient states that pain is relieved with stool evacuation.
- Patient and family or caregivers demonstrate an understanding of drug therapy. (See *Teaching about laxatives*.)

Education edge

Teaching about laxatives

If laxatives are prescribed, review these points with the patient and family or caregivers:

- Therapy should be short term. Misuse or prolonged use can result in nutritional imbalances.
- Diet, exercise, and fluid intake are important in maintaining normal bowel function and preventing or treating constipation.
- Drink at least 6 to 10 glasses (8 oz each) of fluid daily, unless contraindicated.
- Exercise regularly to help with bowel elimination.
- Stool softeners and bulk-forming laxatives may take several days to achieve results.

- If using a bulk-forming laxative, remain active and drink plenty of fluids.
- Stimulant laxatives may cause harmless urine discoloration.
- Include foods high in fiber, such as bran and other cereals, fresh fruit, and vegetables, in your diet.
- Frequent or prolonged use of some laxatives can result in dependence.
- Never take laxatives when experiencing acute abdominal pain, nausea, or vomiting. A ruptured appendix or other serious complications may result.
- Notify the prescriber if signs and symptoms persist or if the laxative doesn't work.

Obesity drugs

Obesity drugs can help patients who are morbidly obese and have health problems that will likely improve with weight loss. These drugs are used in combination with a weight management program that includes diet, physical activity, and behavior modification. They should be used only for improving health, not for cosmetic weight loss (Perreault, 2021).

Obesity drugs include:
- appetite suppressant or anorectic or sympathomimetic agents (phentermine, diethylpropion, benzphetamine, and phendimetrazine)
- lipase inhibitors (orlistat)
- glucagon-like peptide 1 (GLP-1) receptor agonists or antidiabetics (liraglutide and semaglutide)
- combination agents (phentermine-topiramate and bupropion-naltrexone)

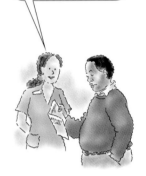

Drugs for obesity should be used in combination with a weight management program that includes diet, physical activity, and behavior modification.

Appetite suppressant or anorectic or sympathomimetic agents

Phentermine, diethylpropion, benzphetamine, and phendimetrazine are used for 12 weeks or less, for weight management in patients who are obese, due to side effects, adverse reactions, potential for misuse, and need for regulatory surveillance (Perreault, 2021).

Pharmacokinetics

Phentermine is rapidly absorbed from the intestine and distributed throughout the body. It's excreted in urine.

Pharmacodynamics

These sympathomimetic agents increase the amount of norepinephrine and dopamine in the brain, which suppresses appetite and causes early satiety (Perreault, 2021).

Pharmacotherapeutics

Appetite suppressants or sympathomimetic agents are used primarily in morbidly obese patients for whom weight loss will improve health and prevent death. Phentermine is the primary first line drug for weight management in patients who are obese (Perreault, 2021).

Drug interactions

Obesity drugs have the following interactions:
- Appetite suppressants taken with cardiovascular stimulants may increase risk of hypertension and arrhythmias.
- When taken with CNS stimulants, appetite suppressants can result in anxiety and insomnia.

- Appetite suppressants taken with serotonergic drugs (including selective serotonin reuptake inhibitors such as fluoxetine and triptan, antimigraine drugs such as sumatriptan, lithium, and dextromethorphan, which is commonly found in cough syrup) can cause agitation, confusion, hypomania, impaired coordination, loss of consciousness, nausea, and tachycardia.

Side effects/adverse reactions

Side effects and adverse reactions include:
- elevated heart rate
- hypertension
- insomnia
- dry mouth
- constipation
- nervousness (Perreault, 2021).

Lipase inhibitors

Lipase inhibitors, such as orlistat, are used to manage weight in patients who are obese.

Pharmacokinetics

Orlistat isn't absorbed systemically; its action occurs in the GI tract, and it's excreted in the feces.

Pharmacodynamics

Orlistat binds to gastric and pancreatic lipases in the GI tract, making them unavailable to break down fats. This prevents absorption of 30% of the fat ingested in a meal. Stools have an increased fat content.

Pharmacotherapeutics

Lipase inhibitors, sometimes called fat blockers, inhibit lipase enzymes in breaking down fats in the GI tract. The patient does not absorb fat or calories associated with fats, which results in weight loss. Evidence indicates orlistat improves blood pressure and serum lipid levels, although this may be due to the actual weight loss versus the medication (Perreault, 2021).

Drug interactions

Patients taking warfarin may need dosage adjustments due to the decrease in vitamin K absorption.

Side effects/adverse reactions

Orlistat may cause side effects and adverse reactions listed below:
- Gastrointestinal: abdominal pain, oily spotting, fecal urgency, flatulence with discharge, fatty stools, fecal incontinence, and increased defecation, although these effects usually subside after a few weeks.

- Fat soluble vitamins A, D, E, and K are not absorbed.
- Acute renal injury.

Proceed with caution

Patients who are pregnant, have a history of renal stones caused by calcium oxalate, or who have chronic malabsorption conditions should not take lipase inhibitors.

Glucagon-like peptide 1 (GLP-1) receptor agonists

The two drugs under this classification, liraglutide and semaglutide, are also classified as antidiabetics.

Pharmacokinetics

Liraglutide is administered via subcutaneous injection while semaglutide can be administered orally or via subcutaneous injection. The GLP-1 receptor antagonists are highly protein bound and are excreted in both urine and feces. These drugs slow gastric emptying, altering other medications ability to absorb (Lexicomp, 2021).

Pharmacodynamics

These drugs work by increasing insulin secretion and decreasing glucagon secretion.

Pharmacotherapeutics

Liraglutide and semaglutide are used as antidiabetic agents in patients with type 2 diabetes along with diet and exercise regimen. They both are used as weight management treatments for patients who are obese. Liraglutide is used for chronic weight management in patients who have a comorbid condition such as type 2 diabetes, hypertension, or hyperlipidemia.

Drug interactions

Taking GLP-1 receptor antagonists with other drugs may enhance hypoglycemic effect:
- androgens
- hypoglycemic agents
- MAO inhibitors
- quinolones
- salicylates
- SSRIs
- sulfonylureas.
  Taking GLP-1 receptor antagonists with other drugs may increase the effect of the other drugs:
- furosemide
- levothyroxine.

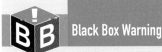

Black Box Warning

Preparing for practice: GLP-1 receptor antagonists

Liraglutide and semaglutide may cause thyroid C-cell tumors. Monitor the patient and teach the patient to report symptoms of thyroid tumors including hoarseness, a mass in the neck, dysphagia, and dyspnea (Lexicomp, 2021).

Side effects/adverse reactions

Side effects and adverse reactions to GLP-1 receptor antagonist liraglutide include:

- acute renal injury
- gallbladder disease
- gastrointestinal: diarrhea, nausea, vomiting, dyspepsia, abdominal pain
- pancreatitis
- increased heart rate
- medullary thyroid carcinoma
- liraglutide: local injection site irritation.

Side effects and adverse reactions to GLP-1 receptor antagonist semaglutide include:

- the above side effects and adverse reactions
- diabetic retinopathy.

(*See Preparing for practice: GLP-1 receptor antagonists.*)

Proceed with caution

GLP-1 receptor antagonists should be discontinued at least 2 months before pregnancy occurs (Perreault, 2021).

Combination agents

There are two combination drugs under this classification, phentermine-topiramate and bupropion-naltrexone that are used to manage weight in patients who are obese.

Naltrexone has been used to treat alcohol and drug addiction, and bupropion is indicated for smoking cessation and treatment of depression. The drug is intended to work on impulse, reward, and/or hunger centers in the brain to reduce appetite and decrease the urge to consume food for emotional comfort.

The Three–Step Approach

Nursing management for patients undergoing treatment with obesity drugs include these three steps.

Preadministration

(Recognize and analyze cues)

- Assess the patient for factors and health risks related to excess weight, such as cardiovascular disease, diabetes, and sleep apnea.
- Determine the patient's blood pressure and pulse rate before starting therapy with sympathomimetic and lipase inhibitor agents.
- Assess the patient for side effects and adverse reactions during treatment.
- Assess such laboratory values as cholesterol, triglycerides, HbA1C, glucose, and renal function.
- Assess the patient's caloric intake before starting therapy.
- Measure the patient's weight, waist circumference, and body mass index before, during, and after treatment.
- Assess the patient's motivation to adhere to a weight management program.
- Assess patient and family or caregiver's knowledge of drug therapy.

(Prioritize hypothesis—priority patient problems)

- Overweight
- Altered body image perception
- Altered health maintenance
- Knowledge deficiency

(Generate solutions)

- The patient will lose weight appropriately.
- The patient will experience a positive body image with weight loss.
- The patient will maintain or enhance health.
- The patient will verbalize an understanding of drug therapy.

Medication administration

(Take action)

- Promote exercise and healthy eating as part of an overall strategy to lose weight.
- Specific actions for patients taking phentermine
  - Explain to the patient that phentermine is for short-term use only. Don't give this drug to a patient with hypertension, cardiovascular disease, or a history of drug misuse.
  - Assess the patient taking phentermine for agitation and anxiety.
  - Monitor blood pressure at regular intervals throughout therapy.

- Specific actions for patients taking orlistat
  - ○ Because orlistat prevents absorption of fat-soluble vitamins—including A, D, E, and K—make sure the patient takes a multivitamin daily 2 hours before or after taking orlistat.
- Specific actions for patients taking GLP-1 receptor antagonists
  - ○ Teach patient that if they miss a dose, skip the dose, and restart the regimen as prescribed at the next dose time.
  - ○ Teach patient not to mix insulin and liraglutide or semaglutide in the same syringe. Use two separate syringes.
  - ○ Liraglutide: Teach patient they can take the drug without regard to meals but to take at the same time each day.
  - ○ Semaglutide: Teach patient to take oral medication 30 to 60 minutes before first food/drink intake of the day with 4 oz or less of plain water only.
  - ○ Semaglutide: Monitor therapeutic index for medications taken with semaglutide because the index may show an increase or a decrease in response.

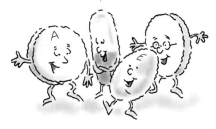

Orlistat prevents the absorption of fat-soluble vitamins, so make sure you administer us daily 2 hours before or after orlistat.

Postadministration

(Evaluate outcomes)
- Patient decreases caloric intake and loses weight.
- Patient regains a positive body image.
- Patient verbalizes an understanding of drug therapy. (See *Teaching about obesity drugs.*)

Education edge

Teaching about obesity drugs

If obesity drugs are prescribed, review these points with the patient and family or caregivers:

- Take an appetite suppressant in the morning to decrease your appetite during the day and to prevent the drug from interfering with sleep at night.
- If you're taking phentermine, take it 30 minutes before meals or as a single dose in the morning. Avoid caffeine.
- Keep in mind that the drug may lose its effectiveness over time; you should not use it for more than 3 months.

- If you're taking orlistat, take one capsule with each main meal (or up to 1 hour after a meal) three times a day. If you miss a meal, skip that dose. Take a multivitamin that contains fat-soluble vitamins A, D, E, and K daily, at least 2 hours before or after taking orlistat.

Antiemetic drugs

Antiemetic drugs decrease nausea, vomiting, and are used to prevent motion sickness.

Antiemetics

The major antiemetics include:
- antihistamines, including dimenhydrinate, diphenhydramine hydrochloride, hydroxyzine hydrochloride, hydroxyzine pamoate, meclizine hydrochloride, and trimethobenzamide hydrochloride
- phenothiazines, including chlorpromazine hydrochloride, perphenazine, prochlorperazine maleate, and promethazine hydrochloride
- serotonin receptor ($5-HT_3$) antagonists, including ondansetron, dolasetron, granisetron, and palonosetron
- cannabinoids, including dronabinol and nabilone
- neurokinin receptor antagonists, including aprepitant and fosaprepitant
- anticholinergic, including scopolamine
- glucocorticoids, including dexamethasone.

Pharmacokinetics

The pharmacokinetic properties of antiemetics may vary slightly. Most antiemetics are absorbed well from the GI tract, are metabolized primarily by the liver, and excreted in urine or feces. Inactive metabolites are excreted in urine.

Pharmacodynamics

Five major receptive sites, when activated, stimulate the vomiting reflex. These receptors sites are muscarinic (M1), dopamine (D2), histamine (H1), serotonin (5-HT3), and neurokinin 1 (substance P) (Longstreth & Hasketh, 2021). The role of antiemetics is to block or antagonize the receptor so the vomiting reflex is inhibited. The action of antiemetics may vary depending on the site of action.

Blocking action
Antihistamines block H_1 receptors, which prevents acetylcholine from binding to receptors in the vestibular nuclei.

The trigger zone
Phenothiazines produce their antiemetic effect by blocking the dopaminergic receptors in the chemoreceptor trigger

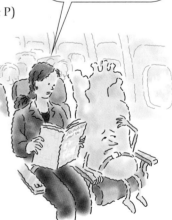

Did you take your antihistamine before boarding the plane?

zone in the brain. (This area of the brain, near the medulla, stimulates the vomiting center in the medulla, causing vomiting.) These drugs may also directly depress the vomiting center.

Two spots to block

Serotonin receptor antagonists block serotonin stimulation centrally in the chemoreceptor trigger zone and peripherally in the vagal nerve terminals, both of which stimulate vomiting.

How?

How glucocorticoids, such as dexamethasone, work is unknown (Longstreth & Hasketh, 2021). Cannabinoids block serotonin receptors and neurokinin agents block substance P.

Pharmacotherapeutics

The uses of antiemetics include relief of nausea and vomiting that result from underlying conditions, prevention of motion sickness, and side effects of medication including chemotherapy. Examples of underlying conditions include:

- postoperative nausea and vomiting
- pregnancy
- gastroenteritis
- gastric outlet obstruction.

Motion potion

With the exception of trimethobenzamide, the antihistamines and anticholinergics are specifically used for nausea and vomiting caused by inner ear stimulation. As a consequence, these drugs prevent or treat motion sickness. They usually prove most effective when given before activities that produce motion sickness and are much less effective when nausea or vomiting has already begun.

Much more severe

Phenothiazines and serotonin receptor antagonists control severe nausea and vomiting from various causes. They're used when vomiting becomes severe and potentially hazardous, such as postsurgical or viral nausea and vomiting.

Chemotherapy

Phenothiazines, serotonin receptor antagonists, cannabinoids, neurokinin receptor antagonists, and glucocorticoids may be prescribed to control nausea and vomiting resulting from cancer chemotherapy and radiotherapy. (See *Other antiemetics*, Page 396.)

Other antiemetics

Here are other antiemetics currently in use.

Cannabinoid: Dronabinol

Dronabinol, a purified derivative of cannabis, is a schedule II drug (meaning it has a high potential for misuse) used to treat the nausea and vomiting resulting from cancer chemotherapy in patients who don't respond adequately to conventional antiemetics. It's also been used to stimulate the appetite in patients with acquired immunodeficiency syndrome. However, dronabinol can accumulate in the body, and the patient can develop tolerance or physical and psychological dependence. Side effects and adverse reactions, especially for older adults, result in limited use for the treatment of nausea and vomiting (Longstreth & Hasketh, 2021).

Neurokinin receptor antagonists: Aprepitant and fosaprepitant

Aprepitant is used to prevent chemotherapy-induced nausea and vomiting. It works by blocking neurokinin receptors in the brain. It's given orally 1 hour before chemotherapy for the first 3 days of treatment.

Fosaprepitant is administered IV only. Commonly prescribed with glucocorticoid and a serotonin receptor antagonist. However, the doses must be reduced when given with glucocorticoids (Longstreth & Hasketh, 2021).

Anticholinergic: Scopolamine

Scopolamine (M1 receptor antagonist) prevents motion sickness, but its use is limited because of its sedative and anticholinergic effects. The drug is delivered via transdermal patches (Longstreth & Hasketh, 2021).

D2 antagonist: Metoclopramide

Metoclopramide hydrochloride is principally used to treat GI motility disorders, including gastroparesis in diabetic patients. It's also used to prevent chemotherapy-induced nausea and vomiting.

Glucocorticoids: Dexamethasone

Dexamethasone is commonly prescribed in combination with other antiemetic, including neurokinin and serotonin receptor antagonists to prevent chemotherapy induced nausea and vomiting (Longstreth & Hasketh, 2021).

Drug interactions

Antiemetics may have many significant interactions:

- Antihistamines and phenothiazines can produce additive CNS depression and sedation when taken with CNS depressants, such as barbiturates, tranquilizers, antidepressants, alcohol, and opioids.
- Antihistamines can cause additive anticholinergic effects, such as constipation, dry mouth, vision problems, and urine retention, when taken with anticholinergic drugs, including tricyclic antidepressants, phenothiazines, and antiparkinsonian drugs.
- Phenothiazine antiemetics taken with anticholinergic drugs increase the anticholinergic effect and decrease antiemetic effects.
- Droperidol plus phenothiazine antiemetics increase the risk of extrapyramidal effects (abnormal involuntary movements).

Side effects/adverse reactions

The use of these antiemetic drugs may lead to adverse reactions:

- Antihistamine antiemetics produce drowsiness; paradoxical CNS stimulation may also occur.

- Phenothiazines can produce extrapyramidal symptoms such as dystonia and tardive dyskinesia. Hypotension and orthostatic hypotension with an increased heart rate, fainting, and dizziness are common adverse reactions to phenothiazines.
- CNS effects associated with phenothiazine and serotonin receptor antagonist antiemetics include confusion, anxiety, euphoria, agitation, depression, headache, insomnia, restlessness, and weakness.
- The anticholinergic effect of antiemetics may cause constipation, dry mouth and throat, painful or difficult urination, urine retention, impotence, and visual and auditory disturbances.
- Neurokinin receptor antagonists may cause fatigue, neutropenia, hypotension, and bradycardia.
- Glucocorticoids side effects and adverse reactions include insomnia, mood changes, and a feeling of increased energy.
- Cannabinoid side effects and adverse reactions include vertigo, dysphoria, and hypotension.

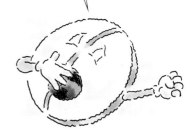

Antihistamines and phenothiazines can produce additive CNS depression and sedation when taken with CNS depressants.

The Three-Step Approach

Nursing management for patients undergoing treatment with antiemetics includes these three steps.

Preadministration

(Recognize and analyze cues)

- Assess the patient's condition before therapy and regularly thereafter.
- Assess for side effects, adverse reactions, and drug interactions.
- Assess the patient and family or caregiver's knowledge of drug therapy.

(Prioritize hypothesis—priority patient problems)

- Nausea
- Vomiting
- Hypovolemia
- Knowledge deficiency

(Generate solutions)

- The patient will exhibit improved health as evidenced by decreased nausea and vomiting.
- The patient will maintain adequate fluid volume balance as evidenced by intake and output, vital signs, and electrolyte evaluations.
- The patient and family or caregivers will demonstrate an understanding of drug therapy.

Medication administration

(Take action)

- Monitor the patient for the drug's effect.
- Administer the drug as directed to promote GI effectiveness and relieve distress.

- Give IM injections deeply into a large muscle mass. Rotate injection sites.
- Do not give antiemetics subcutaneously.
- For prevention of motion sickness, tell the patient to take the drug 30 to 60 minutes before travel.
- Warn the patient to avoid alcohol and hazardous activities until the drug's CNS effects are known.
- Stop the drug 4 days before allergy skin tests.

Postadministration

(Evaluate outcomes)

- Patient reports relief of nausea and vomiting.
- Patient maintains fluid volume.
- Patient and family or caregivers demonstrate an understanding of drug therapy.

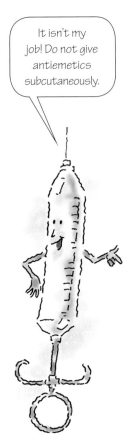

It isn't my job! Do not give antiemetics subcutaneously.

Quick quiz

1. The nurse is educating a patient about when to take dimenhydrinate (antihistamine). When would the nurse teach the patient to take the medication?
    A. After meals
    B. During the acute nausea and vomiting stage
    C. Prior to activities that may produce motion sickness
    D. After completing activities that may produce motion sickness

Answer: C. Antihistamines such as dimenhydrinate are most effective as antiemetics when taken prior to activities that may produce motion sickness.

2. A nurse is following up with a patient who is being treated for obesity. The patient states, "I have to take fat-soluble vitamins 2 hours before taking my medication." Which medication would the nurse anticipate the patient is taking?
    A. Orlistat
    B. Linaclotide
    C. Omeprazole
    D. Simethicone

Answer: A. Orlistat prevents absorption of fat-soluble vitamins so they should be taken 2 hours before or after orlistat. Linaclotide is a medication used to treat constipation. Omeprazole is commonly prescribed for acid reflux, and simethicone is used to treat flatulence and bloating.

3. Which drug or drug type, if prescribed, would the nurse monitor therapeutic levels of diazepam, phenytoin, and warfarin?

    A. Antacids
    B. Proton pump inhibitors
    C. Sucralfate
    D. Simethicone

Answer: B. Proton pump inhibitors can cause increased half-lives and elevated plasma concentration of diazepam, phenytoin, and warfarin.

4. A patient is admitted to the medical surgical floor and is scheduled for a sigmoidoscopy. Which drug would the nurse anticipate giving the patient for bowel preparation?

    A. Glucocorticoid
    B. Stimulant laxative
    C. Proton pump inhibitor
    D. Selective 5-HT-receptor antagonist

Answer: B. Stimulant laxatives are preferred in bowel emptying prior to procedures related to the lower GI tract.

5. The nurse is caring for a patient with pancreatic cancer. Which drug does the nurse anticipate giving?

    A. Lactulose
    B. Pancrelipase
    C. Scopolamine
    D. Methylcellulose

Answer: B. Pancreatic enzymes, such as pancrelipase, are administered to patients with insufficient levels of pancreatic enzymes, such as patients with pancreatic cancer.

Scoring

✮✮✮   If you answered all five questions correctly, thumbs up! Your knowledge of GI drugs is gastronomical.

✮✮   If you answered three or four questions correctly, nice work! You are doing well!

✮   If you answered fewer than three questions correctly, don't panic. You may need some more time to digest the material.

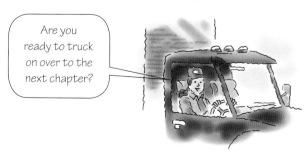

Are you ready to truck on over to the next chapter?

Suggested References

Adegbola, S. O., Sahnan, K., Warusavitarne, J., Hart, A., & Tozer, P. (2018). Anti-TNF therapy in Crohn's disease. *International Journal of Molecular Sciences, 19*(8), 2244, 1–21. https://doi.org/10.3390/ijms19082244

Bello, N. T. (2019). Update on drug safety evaluation of naltrexone/bupropion for the treatment of obesity. *Expert Opinion on Drug Safety, 18*(7), 549–552. doi: 10.1080/14740338.2019.1618268

Berkoben, M. (2021). Management of hyperphosphatemia in adults with chronic kidney disease. In J. S. Berns (Ed.), *UpTodate.* Waltham, MA: UpToDate.

Drini, M. (2017). Peptic ulcer disease and non-steroidal anti-inflammatory drugs. *Australian Prescriber, 40*(3), 91–93. https://doi.org/10.18773/austprescr.2017.037

Freedman, S. (2021). Treatment of chronic pancreatitis. In D. C. Whitcomb (Ed.), *UpToDate.* Waltham, MA: UpToDate.

Hendrickson, R., & Kusin, S. (2021). Gastrointestinal decontamination of the poisoned patient. In S. J. Traub, & M. M. Burns (Eds.), *UpToDate.* Waltham, MA: UpToDate.

Kahrilas, P. (2021). Clinical manifestations and diagnosis of gastroesophageal reflux in adults. In N. J. Talley (Ed.), *UpToDate.* Waltham, MA: UpToDate.

Karch, A. (2020). *Focus on nursing pharmacology* (8th ed.). Philadelphia, PA: Wolters Kluwer.

Lexicomp. (2019). Alosetron: Drug information. In *UpToDate.* Waltham, MA: UpToDate.

Lexicomp. (2021). Semaglutide: Drug information. In *UpToDate.* Waltham, MA: UpToDate.

Lichtenstein, G. (2021). Treatment of Crohn disease in adults: Dosing and monitoring of tumor necrosis inhibitors. In J. T. Lamont (Ed.), *UpToDate.* Waltham, MA: UpToDate.

Longstreth, G., & Hasketh, P. (2021). Characteristics of antiemetics. In N. J. Talley (Ed.), *UpToDate.* Waltham, MA: UpToDate.

Perreault, L. (2021). Obesity in adults: Drug therapy. In F. X. Pi-Sunyer (Ed.), *UpToDate.* Waltham, MA: UpToDate.

Sartor, R. (2021). Probiotics for gastrointestinal diseases. In J. T. Lamont (Ed.), *UpToDate.* Waltham, MA: UpToDate.

Vakil, N. (2021a). Peptic ulcer disease: Epidemiology, etiology, and pathogenesis. In M. Feldman (Ed.), *UpToDate.* Waltham, MA: UpToDate.

Vakil, N. (2021b). Antiulcer medications: Mechanisms of action, pharmacology, and side effects. In M. Feldman (Ed.), *UpToDate.* Waltham, MA: UpToDate.

Vakil, N. (2021c). Physiology of gastric acid secretion. In M. Feldman (Ed.), *UptoDate.* Waltham, MA: UpToDate.

Wald, A. (2021). Treatment of irritable bowel syndrome. In N. J. Talley (Ed.), *UpToDate.* Waltham, MA: UpToDate.

Wolfe, M. M. (2021). Proton pump inhibitors: Overview of use and adverse effects in the treatment of acid related disorders. In M. Feldman (Ed.), *UpToDate.* Waltham, MA: UpToDate.

Chapter 11

Genitourinary drugs

Just the facts

In this chapter, you'll learn:

♦ classes of drugs used to treat genitourinary (GU) disorders

♦ uses and varying actions of these drugs

♦ absorption, distribution, metabolization, and excretion of these drugs

♦ drug interactions and adverse reactions to these drugs.

Drugs and the genitourinary system

The genitourinary (GU) system consists of the reproductive system (the sex organs) and the urinary system, which includes the kidneys, ureters, bladder, and urethra. The kidneys perform most of the work of the urinary system.

Multitalented

The kidneys perform several vital tasks, including:
- disposing of wastes and excess ions in the form of urine
- filtering blood, which regulates its volume and chemical makeup
- helping to maintain fluid and electrolytes and acid-base balance
- producing and regulating several hormones and enzymes
- converting vitamin D to a more active form
- helping to regulate blood pressure and volume by secreting renin.

Helping hands

The main types of drugs used to treat GU disorders include:
- diuretics
- urinary tract antispasmodics
- benign prostatic hyperplasia therapy drugs
- erectile dysfunction therapy drugs
- hormonal contraceptives.

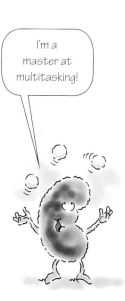

I'm a master at multitasking!

Diuretics

Diuretics trigger the excretion of water and electrolytes from the kidneys, making these drugs a primary choice in the treatment of renal disease, edema, hypertension, and heart failure.

Thiazide and thiazidelike diuretics

Derived from sulfonamides, thiazide and thiazidelike diuretics are used to treat edema and to prevent the development and recurrence of renal calculi. They're also used for disorders such as hypertension and heart failure.

Thiazide diuretics include:
- chlorothiazide (Diuril)
- hydrochlorothiazide (Microzide).
  Thiazidelike diuretics include:
- indapamide
- chlorthalidone
- metolazone (Zaroxolyn).

Pharmacokinetics

Thiazide diuretics are absorbed rapidly but incompletely from the GI tract after oral administration. They cross the placenta and are secreted in breast milk. These drugs differ in how well they're metabolized, but all are excreted primarily in urine. (See *Thiazide diuretics: Hydrochlorothiazide [Microzide]*.) Thiazidelike diuretics are absorbed from the GI tract. All of these drugs are primarily excreted in urine.

Prototype pro

Thiazide diuretics: Hydrochlorothiazide (Microzide)

Actions
- Increases water elimination from the body

Indications
- Edema
- Hypertension

Nursing considerations
- Monitor for adverse effects, especially hypokalemia

(symptoms include leg cramps and muscle aches).
- Frequently monitor weight and blood pressure.
- Assess for signs of orthostatic blood pressure changes, which could lead to falls and injuries.

Pharmacodynamics

Thiazide and thiazide-like diuretics promote the excretion of water by preventing the reabsorption of sodium in the kidneys. As the kidneys excrete the excess sodium, water is excreted with it. These drugs also increase the excretion of chloride, potassium, and bicarbonate, which can result in electrolyte imbalances. Thiazide diuretics also lower blood pressure by causing arteriolar vasodilation.

Turning down the volume

Initially, diuretic drugs decrease circulating blood volume, leading to reduced cardiac output. However, if therapy is maintained, cardiac output stabilizes but plasma fluid volume decreases.

Pharmacotherapeutics

Thiazides are used for long-term treatment of hypertension; they are also used most commonly to treat edema caused by kidney or liver disease, and mild or moderate heart failure. Because these drugs decrease the level of calcium in urine, they may be used alone or with other drugs to prevent the development and recurrence of renal calculi.

Pointing out a paradox

In patients with diabetes insipidus (a disorder characterized by excessive urine production and excessive thirst resulting from reduced secretion of antidiuretic hormone), thiazides paradoxically decrease urine volume, possibly through sodium depletion and plasma volume reduction.

Drug interactions

Drug interactions related to thiazide and thiazidelike diuretics result in altered fluid volume, blood pressure, and serum electrolyte levels:

- These drugs may decrease excretion of lithium, causing lithium toxicity.
- Nonsteroidal anti-inflammatory drugs (NSAIDs), including cyclooxygenase-2 (COX-2) inhibitors, may reduce the antihypertensive effect of these diuretics.
- Use of these drugs with other potassium-depleting drugs and digoxin may cause an additive effect, increasing the risk of digoxin toxicity.
- These diuretics may increase the response to skeletal muscle relaxants.
- Use of these drugs may increase blood glucose levels, requiring higher doses of insulin or oral antidiabetic drugs.
- These drugs may produce additive hypotension when used with antihypertensives.

Side effects/adverse reactions

The most common side effects and adverse reactions to thiazide and thiazidelike diuretics include:

- reduced blood volume
- orthostatic hypotension
- hypokalemia

Administering thiazide diuretics along with antihypertensives can result in additive hypotension.

Prototype pro

Thiazide-like diuretics: Indapamide (no trade name at the time of production)

Actions
• Diuretic effect at the kidney's distal tubule level

Indications
• Mild to moderate hypertension
• Edema in heart failure

Nursing considerations
• Administer in the morning to prevent nocturia.
• May be used with a potassium-sparing diuretic to prevent potassium loss.

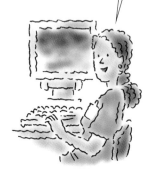

• hyperglycemia
• hyponatremia.

Each of these can be detrimental if not discovered and corrected early in the process, which constitutes an adverse effect.

Education edge

Teaching about diuretics

See Common teaching points in Chapter 3, page 38 for general education regarding all medications. Specific points to review with patients and family for diuretic therapy:
• Take the drug at the same time each day to prevent nocturia.
• You may take the drug with food if you experience gastrointestinal irritation.
• Seek your health care provider's approval before taking any other drug, including over-the-counter medications and herbal remedies.
• Record weight each morning after voiding and before breakfast, in the same type of clothing, and using the same scale.
• Report chest, back, or leg pain; shortness of breath; increased fluid accumulation or weight gain (more than 2 lb [0.9 kg]) daily; or excess water loss (as evidenced by a weight loss of more than 2 lb daily) to your health care provider immediately.

• Photosensitivity reactions can occur 10 to 14 days after initial sun exposure.
• Avoid high-sodium foods (such as lunch meat, smoked meats, and processed cheeses); don't add table salt to foods.
• Clarify with your health care provider whether you are taking a potassium-depleting or potassium-sparing diuretic. If you're taking a potassium-depleting diuretic, include potassium-rich foods (such as bananas, oranges, and potatoes) in your diet. If you're taking a potassium-sparing diuretic, you do not need to eat additional foods that are rich in potassium.
• Avoid hot beverages, excessive sweating, and the use of hot tubs or saunas.
• If taking a loop diuretic, report any hearing loss immediately to the health care provider. These drugs can induce transient deafness. (Permanent deafness is associated with administration of high dose IV furosemide or in low dose furosemide when given to patients with impaired kidney function (Brater & Ellison, 2021).)

Loop diuretics

Loop diuretics are highly potent drugs. They include bumetanide (Bumex), ethacrynic acid (Edecrin), furosemide (Lasix), and torsemide (no trade name at the time of publication).

Pharmacokinetics

Loop diuretics are absorbed well in the GI tract and are rapidly distributed. These diuretics are highly protein bound. They undergo partial or complete metabolism in the liver, except for furosemide, which is excreted primarily unchanged. Loop diuretics are excreted primarily by the kidneys.

Pharmacodynamics

Loop diuretics are the most potent diuretics available, producing the greatest volume of diuresis (urine production). Loop diuretics have a high potential for causing severe adverse reactions. (See *Pharm Fact Alert*.)

The scoop on the loop

Loop diuretics received their name because they act primarily on the thick ascending loop of Henle (the part of the nephron responsible for concentrating urine) to increase the excretion of sodium, chloride, and water. These drugs also inhibit sodium, chloride, and water reabsorption in the proximal tubule. They also activate renal prostaglandins, which result in dilation of the blood vessels of the kidneys, lungs, and the rest of the body.

Pharmacotherapeutics

Loop diuretics are used to treat edema associated with renal disease (including nephrotic syndrome), hepatic cirrhosis, and heart failure (Huxel et al., 2021) as well as to treat hypertension (usually with a potassium-sparing diuretic or potassium supplement to prevent hypokalemia). (See *Loop diuretics: Furosemide*, page 406.)

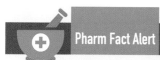

Pharm Fact Alert

Loop diuretics such as bumetanide, furosemide, and torsemide are considered to be nonantimicrobial sulfonamides. Evidence shows that these are generally tolerated in patients with sulfonamide antibiotic allergy (Montanaro, 2020); however, it is important to document the specific sulfa drug to which the patient experienced a reaction, and what the reaction was. Communicate this information to the health care provider to determine if one of these diuretics is still recommended.

Prototype Pro

Loop diuretics: Furosemide

Actions
- Inhibits sodium and chloride reabsorption from proximal and distal tubules, and in the loop of Henle, thus increasing renal excretion of sodium, chloride, and water
- Increases excretion of potassium (like thiazide diuretics)
- Produces greater maximum diuresis and electrolyte loss than a thiazide diuretic

Indications
- Edema related to heart failure, liver failure, or renal failure
- Hypertension (although thiazide diuretics are preferred over loop diuretics as first-line treatment (Whelton et al., 2017))

Nursing considerations
- Monitor for serious adverse effects, such as pancreatitis, hematologic disorders, and electrolyte imbalances (especially hypokalemia, signs of which include leg cramps and muscle aches).
- Monitor weight and blood pressure frequently.

Drug interactions

Loop diuretics produce a variety of drug interactions:

- The risk of ototoxicity (damage to the organs of hearing) increases when aminoglycosides or platinum-based antineoplastic agents are taken with loop diuretics (especially with high doses of furosemide).
- They reduce the hypoglycemic effects of oral antidiabetic drugs, which can result in hyperglycemia.
- They have been shown to interfere with the serum concentration of lithium; therapy should be closely monitored if a loop diuretic is used in conjunction with lithium therapy.
- The risk of electrolyte imbalances that can trigger arrhythmias increases when cardiac glycosides and loop diuretics are taken together.
- Use with digoxin may cause additive toxicity, increasing the risk of digoxin toxicity and arrhythmias. It is recommended that health care providers avoid this combination of drugs (Huxel et al., 2021).

Side effects/adverse reactions

The most common side effects are dizziness, headache, gastrointestinal upset, dehydration, hypernatremia, and hypokalemia.

Black Box Warning

Preparing for practice: Bumetanide and furosemide

Prior to administration of bumetanide or furosemide the nurse must recognize that these drugs carry a black box warning about the possibility for extreme diuresis and subsequent fluid and electrolyte depletion. Symptoms included in the box below may indicate hypovolemia, hypokalemia, and/or hyponatremia and should be reported immediately to the health care provider.

Hypovolemia	Hypokalemia	Hyponatremia
Neuro: headache, fatigue, dizziness, and increased thirst Musculoskeletal: weakness Cardiovascular: cool, clammy skin Genitourinary: low urine output	Musculoskeletal: weakness, muscle cramps Gastrointestinal: constipation Cardiovascular: arrhythmia	Neuro: headache, confusion, loss of energy, drowsiness/fatigue, restlessness/irritability, and coma Musculoskeletal: muscle weakness, spasms or cramps, seizures Gastrointestinal: nausea/vomiting

Source: Lippincott Williams & Wilkins. (2020). *Nursing2021 drug handbook (nursing drug handbook)* (41st ed.). LWW.

Potassium-sparing diuretics

Potassium-sparing diuretics have weaker diuretic and antihypertensive effects than other diuretics but provide the advantage of conserving potassium. These drugs include amiloride hydrochloride (Midamor), eplerenone (Inspra), spironolactone (Aldactone), and triamterene (Dyrenium).

Pharmacokinetics

Potassium-sparing diuretics are only available orally and are absorbed in the GI tract. They're metabolized by the liver and excreted primarily in urine.

Pharmacodynamics

The direct action of potassium-sparing diuretics on the collecting ducts and distal tubule of the kidneys results in urinary excretion of sodium, water, bicarbonate, and calcium. The drug also decreases the excretion of potassium and hydrogen ions. These effects lead to reduced blood pressure and increased serum potassium levels.

Compare and contrast

Structurally similar to aldosterone, spironolactone acts as an aldosterone antagonist. Aldosterone promotes the retention of sodium and water and the loss of potassium, whereas spironolactone counteracts these effects by competing with aldosterone for receptor sites. As a result, sodium, chloride, and water are excreted and potassium is retained.

Pharmacotherapeutics

Potassium-sparing diuretics are used to treat:
- edema
- ascites due to cirrhosis
- heart failure
- hypertension
- primary hyperaldosteronism.

Drug interactions

Giving potassium-sparing diuretics with potassium supplements or angiotensin-converting enzyme inhibitors increases the risk of hyperkalemia. Concurrent use of spironolactone and digoxin increases the risk of digoxin toxicity. When given with lithium, lithium toxicity can occur. NSAIDs cause a decrease in action of the potassium-sparing diuretic.

Adverse reactions

Potassium-sparing effects can lead to hyperkalemia, especially if given with a potassium supplement or high-potassium diet. Spironolactone may lead to gynecomastia or erectile dysfunction. Additionally, it may cause irregular periods or postmenopausal bleeding in females.

Drop that banana!

- Instruct the patient to avoid salt substitutes and potassium-rich foods, except with practitioner approval. Consult a dietitian.
- Because potassium-sparing diuretics may cause dizziness, headache, or vision disturbances, advise the patient to avoid driving or performing activities requiring mental alertness or physical dexterity until the response to the diuretic is known.

Don't forget to remind your patients taking thiazide or thiazidelike diuretics to consume plenty of potassium-rich foods.

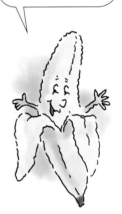

Osmotic diuretics

Osmotic diuretics cause diuresis through osmosis, moving fluid into the extracellular spaces. They include mannitol (Osmitrol).

Pharmacokinetics

Administered IV for rapid distribution, osmotic diuretics are freely filtered by the glomeruli of the kidney—except for mannitol, which is only slightly metabolized. Osmotic diuretics are excreted primarily in urine.

Pharmacodynamics

Osmotic diuretics receive their name because they increase the osmotic pressure of the glomerular filtrate, which inhibits the reabsorption of sodium and water. They create an osmotic gradient in the glomerular filtrate and the blood. In the glomerular filtrate, the gradient prevents sodium and water reabsorption. In the blood, the gradient allows fluid to be drawn from the intracellular to the intravascular spaces.

Pharmacotherapeutics

Osmotic diuretics are used to treat acute renal failure and cerebral edema and to reduce intracranial and intraocular pressure. Mannitol is used to promote diuresis in acute renal failure and to promote urinary excretion of toxic substances.

Drug interactions

No significant drug interactions are known to be associated with mannitol.

Adverse reactions

Osmotic diuretics can cause seizures, thrombophlebitis, and pulmonary congestion. Other significant effects are headaches, chest pains, tachycardia, blurred vision, chills, and fever.

The pressure's building…

Mannitol may cause rebound increased intracranial pressure (ICP) 8 to 12 hours after diuresis. It also may cause rhinitis, thirst, and urine retention.

An irritating problem

Take steps to avoid infiltration because osmotic diuretics may cause mild irritation or even necrosis.

The Three-Step Approach

Nursing management for patients receiving diuretic therapy includes these three steps. Be certain to pay particular attention to the type of diuretic being given, and personalize care accordingly.

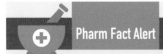

Preadministration

(Recognize and analyze cues)

- Establish baseline values before therapy begins and watch for significant changes.
- Observe a baseline complete blood count (CBC) (including a white blood cell [WBC] count); liver function tests; and levels of serum electrolytes, carbon dioxide, magnesium, BUN, and creatinine. Review periodically and report abnormalities.
- Observe for edema and ascites. Pay particular attention to the legs of ambulatory patients and the sacral area of patients on bed rest.
- Record weight (taken at the same time each morning in similar clothing), intake, and output carefully every 24 hours. Continue doing so after medication administration.
- Recognize that dosage for a patient with hepatic dysfunction may be reduced and that a dosage for a patient with renal impairment or oliguria may be increased.

(Prioritize hypothesis—priority patient problems)

- Potential for fluid and electrolyte imbalance

(Generate solutions)

- Excess fluid will be excreted while the patient maintains a normal fluid volume.
- Electrolyte imbalance will not occur.
- The patient and family will express an understanding of diuretic therapy.

Medication administration

(Take action)

- Administer in the morning to ensure that major diuresis occurs before bedtime. To prevent nocturia, don't administer later than 6 p.m.

- Administer most IV doses slowly over 1 to 2 minutes to prevent hypotension (follow current drug guidelines). Mannitol should be given over 3 minutes to several hours, based on provider order, depending on the reason for administration of this drug and the solution concentration.
- Administer with food or milk to prevent GI upset.
- Collaborate with the health care provider and dietician about the possible need for a high-potassium diet and/or supplementation for patients who are taking diuretics that are **not** potassium sparing.
- Ensure that a urinal or bedpan is within reach or that the bathroom is easily accessible to prevent falls.
- Teach to use sunscreen and wear protective clothing to prevent photosensitivity reactions.
- Teach how to avoid postural hypotension by getting up slowly.

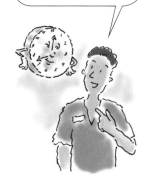

To prevent nocturia, don't administer diuretics after 6 p.m.

Postadministration

(Evaluate outcomes)

- If the patient has diabetes or is at risk for diabetes mellitus (DM), monitor the blood glucose levels because diuretics may cause hyperglycemia.
- Monitor serum creatinine and blood urea nitrogen (BUN) levels and blood uric acid levels.
- Monitor and document intake and output carefully.
- Monitor for changes in the sodium and potassium levels; signs of hyperkalemia include confusion, hyperexcitability, muscle weakness, flaccid paralysis, arrhythmias, abdominal distention, and diarrhea.
- Monitor for vital sign changes, especially during quick diuresis.
- Monitor serum digoxin levels if digoxin and loop diuretics are given concurrently.
- Monitor for evidence of excessive diuresis, which can culminate in dehydration; symptoms include hypotension, tachycardia, poor skin turgor, excessive thirst, and dry or cracked mucous membranes.
- Monitor for signs and symptoms of hyperkalemia, such as confusion, hyperexcitability, muscle weakness, flaccid paralysis, arrhythmias, abdominal distention, and diarrhea.
- Monitor for signs of increased intracranial pressure and circulatory overload for patients taking osmotic diuretics.
- Evaluate the patient's and family's knowledge of diuretic therapy. (See *Teaching about diuretics*, page 404.)

Urinary tract antispasmodics

Urinary tract antispasmodics help decrease urinary tract muscle spasms. They include darifenacin (Enablex), fesoterodine (Toviaz), mirabegron (Myrbetriq), oxybutynin (Ditropan XL), solifenacin (VESIcare), tolterodine (Detrol), and trospium (no trade name at the time of publication).

Pharmacokinetics

Urinary tract antispasmodics are most often administered orally and are rapidly absorbed. Trospium is administered orally but is poorly absorbed. These drugs are all widely distributed, metabolized in the liver, and excreted in urine. Urinary tract antispasmodics also cross the placenta and are excreted in breast milk.

Pharmacodynamics

Urinary tract antispasmodics relieve smooth muscle spasms by inhibiting parasympathetic activity, which causes the detrusor and urinary muscles to relax. Urinary antispasmodics, with the exception of mirabegron, exhibit anticholinergic effects.

Pharmacotherapeutics

Urinary tract antispasmodics are used for patients with overactive bladders who have symptoms of urinary frequency, urgency, or incontinence.

Urgent symptoms

Mirabegron (Myrbetriq) and trospium (no trade name at the time of publication) are also indicated for patients with overactive bladders who have symptoms of urge urinary incontinence, and oxybutynin acts as an antispasmodic for uninhibited or reflex neurogenic bladder. (See *How oxybutynin works*.)

Drug interactions

Urinary tract antispasmodics have few drug interactions:
- Use with anticholinergic agents may increase dry mouth, constipation, and other anticholinergic effects.
- Urinary tract antispasmodics may decrease the effectiveness of phenothiazines (that is, chlorpromazine and prochlorperazine [Procomp]) and haloperidol (Haldol).
- Trospium (no trade name at the time of publication) may interfere with the elimination of certain drugs excreted through the kidneys (such as digoxin, metformin, and vancomycin), resulting in increased blood levels of these drugs.

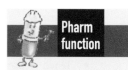
Pharm function

How oxybutynin works

When acetylcholine is released within the bladder, it attaches to receptors on the surface of smooth muscle in the bladder, stimulating bladder contractions. Oxybutynin suppresses these involuntary contractions by blocking the release of acetylcholine. This anticholinergic effect is what makes oxybutynin useful in the treatment of overactive bladder.

Adverse reactions

Possible adverse reactions to urinary tract antispasmodics include:
- blurred vision
- headache
- somnolence
- urinary retention
- dry mouth
- dyspepsia
- constipation
- nausea
- vomiting
- weight gain
- pain
- acute and secondary angle-closure glaucoma.

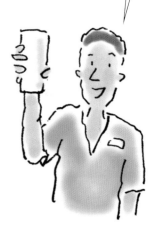

It may sound counterintuitive, but it's often best to encourage your patient to increase fluid intake when taking an antispasmodic to relieve urinary incontinence.

The Three-Step Approach

Nursing management for patients receiving urinary tract antispasmodics includes these three steps.

Preadministration

(Recognize and analyze cues)
- Assess signs and symptoms before beginning therapy.

(Prioritize hypothesis—priority patient problems)
- Potential for infection due to reflex urinary incontinence
- Discomfort or pain

(Generate solutions)
- Comfort will increase.
- Incontinence will decrease.

Medication administration

(Take action)
- Administer trospium at least 1 hour before meals or on an empty stomach.

Postadministration

(Evaluate outcomes)
- Encourage ongoing small, frequent meals to help prevent nausea.
- Unless contraindicated, encourage the patient to increase fluid intake to 2 to 3 L/day.
- Monitor intake and output, and discomfort or pain level.
- Regularly reassess for episodes of incontinence.
- Teach according to the information in *"Teaching about urinary tract antispasmodics,"* page 414.

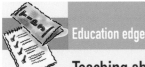

Teaching about urinary tract antispasmodics

If urinary tract antispasmodics are prescribed, review these points with the patient and family:

• Take the drug with meals to decrease GI upset.

• This drug may decrease your ability to sweat; do not engage in activities that may cause you to overheat.

• Take the drug whole; do not chew, crush, or cut the tablet.

• Suck on hard candy or ice chips to relieve dry mouth if this symptom develops.

• Drink adequate fluids to prevent constipation.

• Notify the health care provider if you cannot urinate, develop a fever or severe constipation, or experience blurring of your vision.

• Follow up by undergoing periodic cystometry as recommended by your health care provider.

Benign prostatic hyperplasia therapy drugs

The medications used to treat benign prostatic hyperplasia (BPH) belong to two drug classes, alpha-blockers and 5a-reductase inhibitors. Both groups of medications improve urinary flow.

Alpha-blockers and 5a-reductase inhibitors

Alpha-blockers have an end effect of relaxing muscles, which facilitates the flow of urine. As a drug class, their primary use is for treatment of hypertension. The 5a-reductase inhibitors work differently, as they prevent growth of the prostate by blocking development of dihydrotestosterone (DHT).

Alpha-blockers used to treat BPH include:

• alfuzosin (Uroxatral)
• doxazosin (Cardura)
• tamsulosin (Flomax)
• terazosin (no trade name at the time of publication).

5a-Reductrase inhibitors used to treat BPH include:

• dutasteride (Avodart)
• finasteride (Proscar).

Pharmacokinetics

BPH-related medications are administered orally and are rapidly absorbed. These drugs are all widely distributed and metabolized in the liver. Alpha-blockers are excreted in both the urine and feces, while 5a-reductase inhibitors are almost primarily excreted in the feces. Although doxazosin (Cardura), an alpha-blocker, can be found in human milk, these alpha-blockers have not been tested in pregnant women, and benefit must outweigh risk to the fetus for use to be considered. Make note that 5a-reductase inhibitors are **prohibited** for use in pregnant woman due to potential to cause birth defects.

Pharmacodynamics

Alpha-blockers decrease smooth muscle tone in the prostate and bladder neck to facilitate flow of urine. Drugs in the 5a-reductase inhibitor class stop the conversion of testosterone to dihydrotestosterone (DHT), the hormone that causes prostate growth. Their action reduces the size of the prostate, reducing urethral constriction and facilitating urinary flow.

Pharmacotherapeutics

Alfuzosin, doxazosin, dutasteride, finasteride, and tamsulosin are all used in the treatment of benign prostatic hyperplasia. Doxazosin and terazosin are also used to treat hypertension. Tamsulosin can be used as an additive treatment with ureteral stones, and dutasteride may be used in the treatment of male pattern baldness.

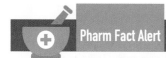

Pharm Fact Alert

5a-Reductase inhibitors are not intended for use with women and are specifically contraindicated in use with women of childbearing age and pregnancy. Due to potential for absorption, women should not handle these drugs or engage in sex with those taking the drug, since it is present in semen. The presence of erectile dysfunction medications in breast milk has not been studied; therefore, use with breast-feeding is contraindicated.

Source: Lippincott Williams & Wilkins. (2020). *Nursing2021 drug handbook (nursing drug handbook)* (41st ed.). LWW.

Drug interactions

Alpha-blockers used in the treatment of BPH may interact with other drugs in the following ways:

- Use with other alpha-blockers should be avoided due to expected interactions.
- Combination with medications that reduce blood pressure such as antihypertensives and diuretics have the potential to cause hypotension.
- Erectile dysfunction medications that are PDE5 inhibitors may cause symptomatic hypotension.
- CYP3A4 medications and select anti-infectives can increase serum levels of the alpha-blocker and attribute to hypotension.
- Dutasteride levels may be increased when combined with CYP3A4 medications. No significant drug interactions are known to be associated with finasteride.

Adverse reactions

Alpha-blockers carry a severe risk of orthostatic hypotension and syncope especially during administration of the first few doses. This is called the first-dose effect. Additional cardiovascular symptoms associated with alpha-blockers include tachycardia, palpitations, and fluid retention.

Drugs in the 5a-reductase inhibitor group are associated with genitourinary complications such as ejaculation disorders, erectile dysfunction, decreased libido, and gynecomastia.

The Three–Step Approach

Nursing management for patients receiving urinary tract antispasmodics includes these three steps.

Preadministration

(Recognize and analyze cues)

- Assess for signs of prostate cancer, which can mimic BPH.
- Assess for symptoms of obstruction such as urinary retention and/ or decreased urinary flow.
- Review baseline prostate-specific antigen (PSA) level.
- Obtain baseline vital signs.
- Recognize that if doxazosin or tamsulosin dosing has been interrupted even briefly, it should be restarted at a lower initial dose before titrating upward.

(Prioritize hypothesis—priority patient problems)

- Potential for injury due to orthostatic hypotension

(Generate solutions)

- Cardiac output will be maintained.
- Symptoms of BPH will be reduced.

Medication administration

(Take action)

- Practice safe handling as 5a-reductase inhibitors are potential teratogens.
- If giving tamsulosin, administer 30 minutes after the same meal daily.
- Administer medication whole, do not crush, chew, divide or open medications.

Postadministration

(Evaluate outcomes)

- If priapism occurs, report this immediately, as it is a medical emergency that must be treated immediately.
- Monitor for orthostatic hypotension because of the first-dose effect with initial dosing and dosing changes.
- Monitor cardiac output.
- Teach according to the information in *"Teaching about benign prostatic hyperplasia medications."*

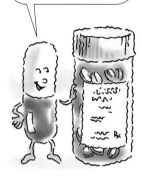

I'm a 5a-reductase inhibitor. Pregnant women and those of childbearing age should not touch me.

Education edge

Teaching about benign prostatic hyperplasia medications

If medications to treat benign prostatic hyperplasia are prescribed, review these points with the patient and caregivers:
- Take the drug as prescribed. Do not crush, open, divide, or chew.
- Do not stop taking medication abruptly.
- Caution about the first-dose effect of low blood pressure.
- Explain signs of orthostatic hypotension and how to perform slow position changes.
- Avoid driving or dangerous activities until effects are known.
- Teach that priapism is a medical emergency that must be reported.

- Pregnant women and those of childbearing age should not handle 5a-reductase inhibitors. Since the medication is found in semen, contact with semen must also be avoided by this population.
- Teach patients taking finasteride to report changes in breast tissue to their provider.
- Teach patients taking dutasteride (or a combination drug in which dutasteride is one of the ingredients) to avoid blood donation while taking the drug and for 6 months after the last dose.

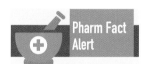

Pharm Fact Alert

Patients taking dutasteride (or a combination drug in which dutasteride is one of the ingredients) should not donate blood while taking this medication, and for at least 6 months after the last dose, as this drug is teratogenic.

Erectile dysfunction therapy drugs

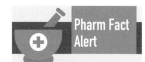

Erectile dysfunction therapy drugs treat penile erectile dysfunction that results from a lack of blood flowing through the corpus cavernosum. This type of erectile dysfunction usually stems from vascular and neurologic conditions. Drugs used for erectile dysfunction include alprostadil (Caverject, Edex, Muse, Prostin VR), avanafil (Stendra), sildenafil (Revatio, Viagra), tadalafil (Cialis), and vardenafil (Levitra).

Pharm Fact Alert

Alprostadil is not indicated for use in women.

Pharmacokinetics

Erectile dysfunction drugs are well absorbed in the GI tract. Distribution of these drugs isn't known. The majority of these drugs—including avanafil, sildenafil, tadalafil, and vardenafil—are given orally, metabolized in the liver, and excreted in feces.

An exceptional drug

Alprostadil is the exception: it's administered directly into the corpus cavernosum, metabolized in the lungs, and excreted in urine.

Pharmacodynamics

Avanafil, sildenafil, tadalafil, and vardenafil selectively inhibit the phosphodiesterase type 5 receptors, which causes an increase in blood levels of nitric oxide. This increase in nitric oxide levels activates the cGMP enzyme, which relaxes smooth muscles and allows blood to flow into the corpus cavernosum, causing an erection.

Alprostadil acts locally, promoting smooth muscle relaxation, which causes an increase in blood flow to the corpus cavernosum and produces an erection.

Pharmacotherapeutics

Avanafil, alprostadil, sildenafil, tadalafil, and vardenafil are all used in the treatment of erectile dysfunction. Sildenafil is also indicated for the treatment of pulmonary arterial hypertension.

Drug interactions

Erectile dysfunction drugs may interact with other drugs in the following ways:
- Nitrates and alpha-adrenergic blockers used in combination with erectile dysfunction drugs may cause severe hypotension and potentially serious cardiac events.
- Ketoconazole, itraconazole, and erythromycin may result in increased levels of vardenafil or tadalafil.
- Protease inhibitors, such as atazanavir or ritonavir, may cause increased tadalafil or vardenafil levels.

Watch out! Nitrates and alpha-adrenergic blockers used with erectile dysfunction drugs can cause severe hypotension and potentially serious cardiac events.

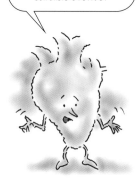

Adverse reactions

Sildenafil increases the risk of cardiovascular events by decreasing supine blood pressure and cardiac output. Patients with known cardiovascular disease have an increased risk of cardiovascular events, including myocardial infarction (MI), sudden cardiac death, ventricular arrhythmias, cerebrovascular hemorrhage, transient ischemic attack, and hypertension.

Other reactions to these drugs include headache, dizziness, flushing, dyspepsia, and vision changes. Prolonged erections (more than 4 hours) can result in irreversible damage to erectile tissue. Alprostadil can cause penile pain.

The Three-Step Approach

Nursing management for patients receiving urinary tract antispasmodics includes these three steps.

Preadministration

(Recognize and analyze cues)
- Assess for signs of cardiovascular risk.
- Obtain baseline vital signs, giving particular attention to blood pressure and heart rate.
- Collaborate with the health care provider to assure that a baseline electrocardiogram has been ordered.

(Prioritize hypothesis—Priority patient problems)
- Potential for injury

(Generate solutions)
- Cardiac output will be maintained.
- Patient will verbalize satisfaction with the drug's intended action.

Medication administration

(Take action)
- Explain that the drug will not protect against pregnancy or the transmission of sexually transmitted infections.
- If the patient is also taking medication to manage human immunodeficiency virus (HIV), caution about the risk of adverse reactions, including hypotension and priapism.
- If the patient is taking alprostadil, teach proper preparation and administration of the drug. Review aseptic technique, warn them that bleeding at the injection site can increase the risk of transmitting blood-borne diseases to any partners, and explain that they should only use the drug as directed.

Pharm Fact Alert

Patients taking the brand name drug Muse should be taught to refrain from sexual intercourse with a pregnant woman unless a condom barrier is used.

Teaching about erectile dysfunction drugs

If an erectile dysfunction drug is prescribed, review these points with the patient:

• This drug won't work without the presence of sexual stimulation.

• Take this drug as directed before anticipated sexual activity; timing will be specific to the individual drug prescribed. Some drugs can be taken up to 4 hours prior to intercourse, whereas others must be taken within 30 minutes of intercourse.

• If you have an erection that lasts longer than 4 hours, seek medical attention; this is considered a medical emergency.

• Tell all health care providers that you are taking this drug.

• Do not take this drug if you are taking nitrates or alpha-adrenergic blockers for high blood pressure or angina.

• Do not take this drug with alcohol.

Postadministration

(Evaluate outcomes)

• If priapism occurs, report this immediately, as it is a medical emergency that must be treated immediately.

• Monitor for signs of orthostatic hypotension.

• Monitor cardiac output.

• Evaluate patient's satisfaction with the drug's action.

• Teach according to the information in *"Teaching about erectile dysfunction drugs."*

Hormonal contraceptives

Hormonal contraceptives inhibit ovulation. Contraceptives typically contain a combination of hormones. For example, ethinyl estradiol is an estrogen hormone that may be combined with desogestrel, drospirenone, levonorgestrel, norethindrone, norgestimate, or norgestrel, which are progesterone hormones. However, many of the progesterones mentioned are used independently of estrogen for progesterone-only contraception.

Pharmacokinetics

Hormonal contraceptives are absorbed from the GI tract and are widely distributed. They're metabolized in the liver and excreted in urine and feces.

Patch power

Some forms of hormonal contraceptives are available in a transdermal patch form. These contraceptives are absorbed through the skin but have similar distribution, metabolism, and excretion as orally administered contraceptives.

Insertable contraception

Some forms of hormonal contraception are available by insertable methods. One form is a silicone ring that contains combination hormones. Another method is an intrauterine device (IUD), placed by a women's health care provider, that contain progesterone-only hormones. The contraceptive devices have similar distribution, metabolism, and excretion as orally administered contraceptives. However, they are absorbed either through the vaginal mucosa when using the ring or through the uterus when using an IUD.

Pharmacodynamics

The primary mechanism of action of combination hormonal contraceptives (estrogen and progestin) is the suppression of gonadotropins, which inhibits ovulation. Estrogen suppresses secretion of follicle-stimulating hormone, which blocks follicular development and ovulation. Progestin suppresses the secretion of luteinizing hormone, which prevents ovulation, even if the follicle develops. Progestin also thickens the cervical mucus; this interferes with sperm migration and causes endometrial changes that prevent implantation of a fertilized ovum.

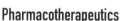

It looks like we're not welcome here, guys!

DO NOT ENTER

Pharmacotherapeutics

The primary purpose for taking hormonal contraceptives is the prevention of pregnancy in women. Certain hormonal contraceptives are used to treat moderate acne, and others may be used to alleviate menstrual cramping.

Drug interactions

Hormonal contraceptives can interact with other medications in various ways:
- Antibiotics, oxcarbazepine, phenytoin, topiramate, and modafinil are known to decrease the effectiveness of oral contraceptives. A patient taking these drugs with a hormonal contraceptive must be taught to additionally use a barrier contraceptive if pregnancy is not desired.
- Atorvastatin may increase serum estrogen levels.
- Cyclosporine and theophylline have an increased risk of toxicity when taken with hormonal contraceptives.

- Prednisone increases the therapeutic and possibly toxic effects of hormonal contraceptives.
- Several herbal medications can affect serum levels of hormonal contraceptives.

Adverse reactions

Potentially serious adverse reactions to hormonal contraceptives include arterial thrombosis, thrombophlebitis, pulmonary embolism, myocardial infarction, cerebral hemorrhage or thrombosis, hypertension, gallbladder disease, and hepatic adenomas.

Other adverse reactions include:
- acne
- bleeding or spotting between menstrual periods
- bloating
- breast tenderness or enlargement
- changes in libido
- diarrhea
- difficulty wearing contact lenses
- unusual hair growth
- weight fluctuations
- upset stomach
- vomiting.

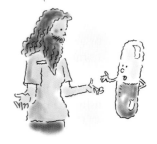

I know hormonal contraceptives can cause unusual hair growth, but this is ridiculous!

The Three-Step Approach

Nursing management for patients receiving urinary tract antispasmodics includes these three steps.

Preadministration

(Recognize and analyze cues)
- Collect a full history, as hormonal contraceptives are contraindicated in patients with a history of thrombophlebitis or thromboembolic disorders, deep vein thrombosis, cerebrovascular accidents, coronary artery disease, known carcinoma of the breast, any estrogen-dependent neoplasm, abnormal genital bleeding, or cholestatic jaundice with pregnancy. Caution must be used in patients with fibrocystic breast disease, migraines, hypertension, and diabetes, and in patients who smoke (which increases the cardiovascular risk).
- Obtain baseline vital signs, giving particular attention to blood pressure.
- Collaborate with the health care provider to assure that a baseline electrocardiogram has been ordered.

(Prioritize hypothesis—Priority patient problems)
- Potential for injury

(Generate solutions)
- Pregnancy will be avoided.

Medication administration

(Take action)

- Teach how to take pills (21-, 28-, or 91-day packets), how to apply the patch, or insert the ring.
- Explain that hormonal contraceptives do not decrease the risk of transmission of sexually transmitted infections and that a barrier method should be used for that purpose.

Postadministration

(Evaluate outcomes)

- Teach about possible drug interactions and when to use an additional form of contraception.
- Teach according to the information in *"Teaching about hormonal contraceptives."*

Quick quiz

1. Which teaching will the nurse provide to a patient prescribed a 5a-reductase inhibitor for benign prostatic hyperplasia?

    A. Hypotension and syncope may occur.
    B. Antibiotics reduce efficacy of this drug.
    C. Report priapism immediately.
    D. Avoid unprotected sex with women of childbearing age.

Answer: D. Women of childbearing age should not handle 5a-reductase inhibitors nor should they come into contact with the semen of men who take these medications. Hypotension and syncope are associated with alpha-blockers. Antibiotics reduce the efficacy of hormonal contraceptives. Decreased libido—not priapism—is associated with 5a-reductase inhibitors.

2. Which condition is most likely to benefit from treatment with a thiazide diuretic?

    A. Benign prostatic hyperplasia
    B. Fluid retention
    C. Erectile dysfunction
    D. Desire for contraception

Answer: B. Thiazide diuretics are used primarily to treat hypertension and edema, so fluid retention is the condition that will best benefit from this type of drug. Thiazide diuretics are not used to treat BPH, erectile dysfunction, or to minimize the chance for contraception.

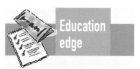

Teaching about hormonal contraceptives

If a hormonal contraceptive is prescribed, review these points with the patient (or caregiver, as needed):

- Take this medication at the same time each day and as directed by your health care provider.
- If you miss a period, contact your health care provider; you may be pregnant.
- Report to the nearest emergency department if you have chest pain, difficulty breathing, leg pain, or severe abdominal pain or headache. These symptoms could indicate a serious adverse reaction.
- Do not take this drug if you think you're pregnant.
- Do not smoke while taking hormonal contraceptives.

3. When teaching a patient how to take erectile dysfunction medication, which information will the nurse provide?
   A.   Take as prescribed 30 minutes to 4 hours before sex.
   B.   Take in combination with a nitrate.
   C.   High blood pressure may occur when taking.
   D.   Alcohol will enhance the effect of this drug.

Answer: A. The patient should take the medication between 30 minutes and 4 hours before intercourse. The exact timing is dependent upon the specific drug prescribed. Erectile dysfunction drugs should not be taken with a nitrate. Hypotension—not hypertension—is likely to occur when taking this type of drug. Alcohol should not be used when taking a drug for erectile dysfunction.

4. When caring for a patient taking oral hormonal contraceptives, which teaching will be emphasized by the nurse?
   A.   Take daily at any time.
   B.   Take 30 minutes before sex.
   C.   Avoid smoking.
   D.   Continue taking if pregnant.

Answer: C. Smoking significantly increases the risk of cardiovascular complications when combined with hormonal contraceptives and should be avoided. Oral hormonal contraceptives should be taken at the same time daily. They are not taken 30 minutes before sex. Oral hormonal contraceptives should be discontinued if the patient becomes pregnant.

Scoring

☆☆☆   If you answered all four questions correctly, terrific! Everything's flowing smoothly for you when it comes to GU drugs.

☆☆   If you answered three questions correctly, super! Your stream of knowledge about GU drugs is impressive.

☆   If you answered fewer than three questions correctly, don't panic! Relax, review the chapter, and try again.

Suggested References

Akbari, P., & Khorasani-Zadeh, A. (2021). Thiazide diuretics. [Updated 2020 July 10]. In *StatPearls [Internet]*. Treasure Island, FL: StatPearls Publishing. Retrieved from https://www.ncbi.nlm.nih.gov/books/NBK532918/

Brater, D., & Ellison, D. (2021). Loop diuretics: Dosing and major side effects. In R. Sterns & M. Emmett (Eds.), *UpToDate*. Waltham, MA.

Epocrates online. (2021). *Avanafil*. Retrieved from https://online.epocrates.com/drugs/685710/Stendra/Monograph

Huxel, C., Raja, A., & Ollivierre-Lawrence, M. (2021). Loop diuretics. In *StatPearls [Internet]*. Treasure Island, FL: StatPearls Publishing. Retrieved from https://www.ncbi.nlm.nih.gov/books/NBK546656/

Montanaro, A. (2020). Sulfonamide allergy in HIV-uninfected patients. In N. Adkinson (Ed.), *UpToDate*. Waltham, MA.

National Center for Biotechnology Information. (n.d.). *Avanafil*. PubChem. Retrieved from https://pubchem.ncbi.nlm.nih.gov/compound/9869929#section=Absorption-Distribution-and-Excretion

Prescriber's Digital Reference. (2021a). *Hydrochlorothiazide–Drug summary*. Retrieved from https://www.pdr.net/drug-summary/Microzide-hydrochlorothiazide-2130#14

Prescriber's Digital Reference. (2021b). *Indapamide—Drug summary*. Retrieved from https://www.pdr.net/drug-summary/Indapamide-indapamide-2292

Salisbury, B., & Tadi, P. (2021 January). 5 Alpha reductase inhibitors. [Updated 2021 January 31]. In *StatPearls [Internet]*. Treasure Island, FL: StatPearls Publishing. Retrieved from https://www.ncbi.nlm.nih.gov/books/NBK555930/

U.S. Food & Drug Administration. (n.d.a). *Drugs@FDA: FDA-approved drugs*. https://www.accessdata.fda.gov/scripts/cder/daf/index.cfm

U.S. Food & Drug Administration. (n.d.b). *Ethacrynic acid*. https://www.accessdata.fda.gov/drugsatfda_docs/label/2016/205609Orig1s000lbl.pdf

U.S. Food & Drug Administration. (n.d.c). *Hydrochlorothiazide tablets*. Accessdata.Fda.Gov. https://www.accessdata.fda.gov/drugsatfda_docs/label/2011/040735s004,040770s003lbl.pdf

U.S. Food & Drug Administration. (n.d.d). *Lasix*. https://www.accessdata.fda.gov/drugsatfda_docs/label/2010/016273s061lbl.pdf

U.S. Food & Drug Administration. (n.d.e). *Spironolactone*. https://www.accessdata.fda.gov/drugsatfda_docs/label/2018/012151s075lbl.pdf

Whelton, P., et al. (2017). 2017 ACC/AHA/AAPA/ABC/ACPM/AGS/APhA/ASH/ASPC/NMA/PCNA: Guideline for the prevention, detection, evaluation, and management of high blood pressure in adults: A report of the American College of Cardiology/American Heart Association Task Force on Clinical Practice Guidelines. *Hypertension, 71*(6), e13–e115.

Chapter 12

Hematologic drugs

Just the facts

In this chapter, you'll learn:

◆ classes of drugs used to treat hematologic disorders

◆ uses and varying actions of these drugs

◆ absorption, distribution, metabolization, and excretion of these drugs

◆ drug interactions and adverse reactions to these drugs.

Drugs and the hematologic system

The hematologic system includes plasma (the liquid component of blood) and blood cells, such as red blood cells (RBCs), white blood cells (WBCs), and platelets. Types of drugs used to treat disorders of the hematologic system include:

- hematinic drugs
- anticoagulant drugs
- thrombolytic drugs.

Hematinic drugs

Hematinic drugs provide essential building blocks for RBC production. They do so by increasing hemoglobin, the necessary element for oxygen transportation.

Taking aim at anemia

Drugs used to treat microcytic and macrocytic anemias are hematinic drugs. These drugs include iron, vitamin B_{12}, and folic acid. Some normocytic anemias are treated with epoetin alfa and darbepoetin alfa.

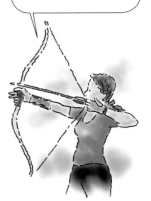

Hematinic drugs give me the tools I need to take aim at anemia.

Iron

Iron preparations are used to treat the most common form of anemia—iron deficiency anemia. Iron preparations discussed in this section include ferrous fumarate, ferrous gluconate, ferrous sulfate, iron dextran (INFeD), iron sucrose (Venofer), and sodium ferric gluconate complex.

Pharmacokinetics

Iron is absorbed primarily from the duodenum and upper jejunum of the intestine. The formulations do not vary in their rate of absorption, but they do vary in the amount of elemental iron supplied.

What's in store?

The amount of iron absorbed depends partially on the body's stores of iron. When body stores are low or RBC production is accelerated, iron absorption may increase by 20% to 30%. On the other hand, when total iron stores are large, only about 5% to 10% of iron is absorbed.

Form and function

Enteric coated preparations decrease iron absorption because, in that form, iron is not released until after it leaves the duodenum. The lymphatic system absorbs the parenteral form after IM injections.

Iron is transported by the blood and bound to transferrin, its carrier plasma protein. About 30% of the iron is stored primarily as hemosiderin or ferritin in the reticuloendothelial cells of the liver, spleen, and bone marrow. About 66% of the total body iron is contained in hemoglobin. Excess iron is excreted in urine, stool, and sweat and through intestinal cell sloughing. Excess iron is also secreted in breast milk.

Pharmacodynamics

Although iron has other roles, its most important role is the production of hemoglobin. About 80% of the iron in the plasma goes to the bone marrow, where it is used for erythropoiesis (production of RBCs).

Pharmacotherapeutics

Oral iron therapy is used to prevent or treat iron deficiency anemia. It is also used to prevent anemia in children ages 6 months to 2 years because this is a period of rapid growth and development.

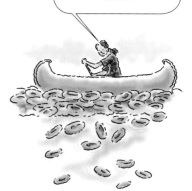

Iron is transported by the blood. It's an interesting way to travel!

Baby makes two

A woman who is pregnant may need iron supplements to replace the iron used by the developing fetus. She should take oral iron therapy in the form of prenatal vitamins unless she is unable to take iron. Women who are pregnant with iron deficiency anemia can show symptoms of:

- pallor
- shortness of breath
- palpitations
- hair loss
- headaches
- dizziness
- leg cramps
- irritability
- fatigue
- decreased breast milk production.

Women with iron deficiency are at an increased risk of complications such as susceptibility to infection, eclampsia, hemorrhage, and need for blood transfusion in the peripartum time frame due to blood loss. Iron deficiency anemia can also lead to problems with placental development, fetal demise, infection, and decreased iron stores in the newborn (Garzon et al., 2020).

Babies who are strictly breast-fed may require additional iron supplementation at about 4 months of age until able to routinely consume foods with iron. Infants who are formula fed will likely have iron needs met, as most formulas sold in the United States are fortified with iron. Infants who are fed with a combination of breast milk and formula will have different iron needs. Visits to the pediatrician and monitoring laboratory values can detect iron deficiency anemia in children and be treated as recommended by the physician (Centers for Disease Control and Prevention, 2020).

An alternate route

Parenteral iron therapy is used for patients who cannot absorb oral preparations, are not compliant with oral therapy, or have bowel disorders (such as ulcerative colitis or Crohn's disease). Patients with end-stage renal disease who receive hemodialysis may also receive parenteral iron therapy at the end of their dialysis session. Parenteral iron therapy corrects the iron store deficiency quickly; however, the anemia is not corrected any faster than it would be with oral preparations.

Two of a kind

There are two parenteral iron products available. Iron dextran (INFeD) is given by either IM injection or slow continuous IV infusion. Iron sucrose (Venofer), indicated for use in the hemodialysis patient, is administered by IV infusion.

Drug interactions

Iron absorption is reduced by antacids as well as by such foods as spinach, whole-grain breads and cereals, coffee, tea, eggs, and milk products. Other drug interactions involving iron include the following:

- Tetracycline, demeclocycline, minocycline (Minocin), doxycycline (Vibramycin), methyldopa, quinolones, levofloxacin (Levaquin), norfloxacin, ofloxacin, gatifloxacin, lomefloxacin, moxifloxacin, sparfloxacin, ciprofloxacin (Cipro), levothyroxine (Synthroid), and penicillamine (Cuprimine) absorption may be reduced when taken with oral iron preparations.
- Cholestyramine (Questran), cimetidine (Tagamet), magnesium trisilicate (Gaviscon), and colestipol (Colestid) may reduce iron absorption in the GI tract.
- Cimetidine (Tagamet) and other histamine-2 receptor antagonists may decrease GI absorption of iron.

Side effects/Adverse reactions

The most common adverse reaction to iron therapy is gastric irritation and constipation. Iron preparations also darken the stool. The liquid form can stain the teeth. Parenteral iron has been associated with an anaphylactoid reaction. (See *Parenteral iron.*)

The Three-Step Approach

Nursing management for patients needing iron therapy includes these three steps.

Preadministration

(Recognize and analyze cues)
- Assess the patient's iron deficiency before starting therapy.
- Monitor the iron's effectiveness by evaluating the patient's hemoglobin level, hematocrit, and reticulocyte count.
- Monitor the patient's health status.
- Assess for adverse reactions and drug interactions.
- Observe the patient for delayed reactions from therapy.
- Assess the patient's and family's knowledge of drug therapy.

(Prioritize hypothesis—priority patient problems)
- Iron deficiency
- Injury risk
- Knowledge deficiency

(Generate solutions)
- The patient's iron deficiency will improve to an acceptable level.
- The patient will not encounter harm.
- The patient and family will demonstrate an understanding of drug therapy.

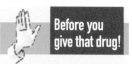
Before you give that drug!

Parenteral iron

Before administering parenteral iron, be aware that it has been associated with an anaphylactoid reaction. Administer initial test doses before a full-dose infusion to evaluate for potential reactions. Continue to monitor the patient closely because delayed reactions can occur 1 to 2 days later.

Signs and symptoms of an anaphylactoid reaction to parenteral iron include:
- arthralgia
- backache
- chest pain
- chills
- dizziness
- headache
- malaise
- fever
- myalgia
- nausea
- vomiting
- hypotension
- respiratory distress.

Medication administration
(Take action)
- Minimize skin staining with IM injections of iron by using a separate needle to withdraw the drug from its container.
- If IM or IV injections of iron are recommended, a test dose may be required in the facility.
- If administering iron IM, use a 19G or 20G needle that's 2″ to 3″ long. Inject into the upper outer quadrant of the buttock. Use the Z-track method to avoid leakage into subcutaneous tissue and staining of the skin.
- IV iron is the preferred method of parenteral administration because it results in fewer anaphylactoid reactions as well as other adverse effects. It is also used if the patient has insufficient muscle mass for deep IM injection. Examples include impaired absorption from muscle because of stasis or edema, the potential for uncontrolled IM bleeding from trauma (as in patients with hemophilia), or the need for massive and prolonged parenteral therapy (as in patients with chronic substantial blood loss).
- Assess for immediate adverse reactions and drug interactions.
- Remember to refrain from giving iron dextran with oral iron preparations.
- Promote a varied diet that is adequate in protein, calories, minerals, and electrolytes.
- Encourage foods high in iron as applicable to help delay the onset of iron deficiency anemia.
- Administer IV fluids and electrolytes as necessary to provide nutrients. Oral food intake or tube feedings are preferable to IV therapy.
- Correct underlying disorders that contribute to mineral and electrolyte deficiency or excess.
- Promote measures to relieve anorexia, nausea, vomiting, diarrhea, pain, and other signs and symptoms.
- Arrange for a nutritional consult as needed.

Postadministration
(Evaluate outcomes)
- Observe the patient for delayed reactions from therapy.
- Monitor the iron's effectiveness by evaluating the patient's hemoglobin level, hematocrit, and reticulocyte count.
- Monitor the patient's health status.
- Evaluate the patient's and family's knowledge of drug therapy. (See *Teaching about hematinic drugs*, page 431.)

> To give iron IM, use a 19G or 20G needle that's 2″ to 3″ long.

Teaching about hematinic drugs

If hematinic drugs are prescribed, review these points with the patient and caregivers:

• The best source of minerals and electrolytes is a well-balanced diet that includes a variety of foods.

• Do not take over-the-counter preparations, other drugs, or herbal remedies without first talking to the prescriber or a pharmacist. Adverse interactions can occur with hematinic drugs. For example, herbal preparations of chamomile, feverfew, and St. John's wort may inhibit iron absorption.

• Keep all mineral and electrolyte substances out of the reach of children; accidental overdose can occur.

• Keep follow-up appointments for periodic blood tests and procedures to make sure treatment is appropriate.

• Take the drug as prescribed. Iron supplements should be taken with or after meals with 8 oz (237 mL) of fluid.

• Do not crush or chew slow-release tablets or capsules. Liquid preparations can be diluted with water and sipped through a straw.

• Vitamin C increases the absorption of iron, while milk or antacids will decrease the absorption of iron (Silvestri & Silvestri, 2020).

• Rinse the mouth after taking liquid preparations to prevent staining of the teeth.

• Iron preparations may cause dark green or black stools.

• Get plenty of rest and rise slowly to avoid dizziness. Take rest periods during the day to conserve energy.

Vitamin B$_{12}$

Vitamin B$_{12}$ preparations are used to treat pernicious anemia. Common vitamin B$_{12}$ preparations include cyanocobalamin and hydroxocobalamin.

Pharmacokinetics

Vitamin B$_{12}$ is available in parenteral, oral, and intranasal forms.

A pernicious problem

A substance called *intrinsic factor*, secreted by the gastric mucosa, is needed for vitamin B$_{12}$ absorption. People who have a deficiency of intrinsic factor, such as those diagnosed with chronic autoimmune gastritis (Gwarthmey & Grogan, 2020), develop a special type of anemia known as *vitamin B$_{12}$ deficiency pernicious anemia*. It has been the common thought that those with pernicious anemia cannot take vitamin B$_{12}$ orally because they cannot absorb it; however, that is not the case. What is true is that those with vitamin B$_{12}$ deficiency pernicious anemia have severely impaired vitamin B$_{12}$ absorption; they can be treated with oral doses of vitamin B$_{12}$ but at *much* higher doses.

B$_{12}$ deficiency from poor nutritional intake is rare but has been found in people who consume a strict vegan diet for a long period of time. B$_{12}$ deficiency can also occur when intrinsic factor production is

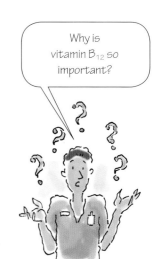

Why is vitamin B$_{12}$ so important?

limited, for example, in patients who have undergone bariatric surgery or have atrophic gastritis (Gwarthmey & Grogan, 2020).

Final destination: Liver
When cyanocobalamin is injected by the IM or subcutaneous route, it is absorbed and binds to transcobalamin II for transport to the tissues. It is then transported in the bloodstream to the liver, where 90% of the body's vitamin B_{12} supply is stored. Although hydroxocobalamin is absorbed more slowly from the injection site, its uptake in the liver may be greater than that of cyanocobalamin.

Slow release
With either drug, the liver slowly releases vitamin B_{12} as needed. It is secreted in breast milk during lactation. About 3 to 8 mcg of vitamin B_{12} are excreted in bile each day and then reabsorbed in the ileum. Within 48 hours after a vitamin B_{12} injection, 50% to 95% of the dose is excreted unchanged in urine.

Pharmacodynamics
When vitamin B_{12} is administered, it replaces vitamin B_{12} that the body normally would absorb from the diet.

A must for myelin maintenance
This vitamin is essential for cell growth and replication and for the maintenance of myelin (nerve coverings) throughout the nervous system. Vitamin B_{12} also may be involved in lipid and carbohydrate metabolism.

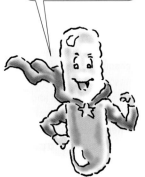

Because I'm essential for cell growth and replication and for maintaining myelin throughout the nervous system.

Pharmacotherapeutics
Cyanocobalamin and hydroxocobalamin are used to treat pernicious anemia, a megaloblastic anemia characterized by decreased gastric production of hydrochloric acid and the deficiency of intrinsic factor, a substance normally secreted by the parietal cells of the gastric mucosa that is essential for vitamin B_{12} absorption.

Common ground
Intrinsic factor deficiencies are common in patients who have undergone total or partial gastrectomies or total ileal resection. Oral vitamin B_{12} preparations are used to supplement nutritional deficiencies of the vitamin.

Drug interactions
Alcohol, aspirin (Ecotrin), aminosalicylic acid, neomycin, chloramphenicol, and colchicine (Colcrys) may decrease the absorption of oral cyanocobalamin.

Dietary sources of vitamin B_{12}
- Fortified cereals
- Meats
- Poultry
- Seafood
- Eggs
- Dairy products

Side effects/Adverse reactions

No dose-related adverse reactions occur with vitamin B_{12} therapy. However, some rare reactions may occur when vitamin B_{12} is administered parenterally.

Don't be so (hyper)sensitive

Adverse reactions to parenteral administration can include hypersensitivity reactions that could result in mild diarrhea, itching, transient rash, hives, hypokalemia, polycythemia vera, peripheral vascular thrombosis, heart failure, pulmonary edema, anaphylaxis, or even death.

The Three-Step Approach

These steps are appropriate for patients undergoing treatment with vitamin B_{12}.

Preadministration

(Recognize and analyze cues)

- Assess the patient's vitamin B_{12} deficiency before therapy.
- Monitor the patient's health status.
- Assess the patient's and family's knowledge of drug therapy.

(Prioritize hypothesis—priority patient problems)

- Altered health maintenance
- Injury risk
- Knowledge deficiency

(Generate solutions)

- The patient's vitamin B_{12} deficiency will improve as evidenced by laboratory studies.
- The risk of injury to the patient will be minimized.
- The patient and family will demonstrate an understanding of drug therapy.

Medication administration

- Promote a varied diet that is adequate in protein, calories, minerals, and electrolytes.
- Encourage foods high in iron as applicable to help delay the onset of iron deficiency anemia.
- Administer IV fluids and electrolytes as necessary to provide nutrients. Oral food intake or tube feedings are preferable to IV therapy.
- Correct underlying disorders that contribute to mineral and electrolyte deficiency or excess.
- Promote measures to relieve anorexia, nausea, vomiting, diarrhea, pain, and other signs and symptoms.
- Assess for adverse reactions and drug interactions.

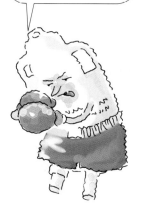

Adverse reactions to parenteral vitamin B_{12} can be a real knockout.

Postadministration

(Evaluate outcomes)

- Monitor the drug's effectiveness by evaluating the patient's hemoglobin level, hematocrit, and reticulocyte count.
- Arrange for nutritional consult as needed.
- Observe the patient for delayed reactions to therapy.
    Monitor the patient's underlying condition and neurologic signs and symptoms for signs of improvement.
- Evaluate the patient's and family's understanding of drug therapy.

> **Dietary sources of folic acid**
>
> - Enriched grain products (cereal, bean, rice)
> - Peas
> - Beans
> - Vegetables (green leafy)
> - Orange juice
> - Asparagus
> - Avocado

Folic acid

Folic acid is given to treat megaloblastic anemia caused by folic acid deficiency. This type of anemia usually occurs in infants, adolescents, pregnant and lactating women, elderly persons, alcoholics, and those with intestinal or malignant diseases. Folic acid is also used as a nutritional supplement.

Pharmacokinetics

Folic acid is absorbed rapidly in the first third of the small intestine and distributed into all body tissues. Synthetic folic acid is readily absorbed even in patients with malabsorption syndromes.

Folic acid is metabolized in the liver. Excess folate is excreted unchanged in urine, and small amounts of folic acid are excreted in feces. Folic acid is also secreted in breast milk.

Pharmacodynamics

Folic acid is an essential component for normal RBC production and growth. A deficiency in folic acid results in megaloblastic anemia and low serum and RBC folate levels.

> Three cheers for synthetic folic acid! Synthetic folic acid is readily absorbed even in patients with malabsorption syndromes.

Pharmacotherapeutics

Folic acid is used to treat folic acid deficiency. Patients who are pregnant or undergoing treatment for liver disease, hemolytic anemia, alcohol misuse, skin disorders, or renal disorders typically need folic acid supplementation. Folic acid supplementation also reduces the risk of neural tube defects during pregnancy and colon cancer (CDC, 2018). Serum folic acid levels less than 5 mg indicate folic acid deficiency.

Drug interactions

These drug interactions may occur with folic acid:

- Methotrexate (Otrexup), sulfasalazine (Azulfidine), hormonal contraceptives, aspirin (Ecotrin), triamterene (Dyrenium), pentamidine (Pentam), and trimethoprim (Primsol) reduce the effectiveness of folic acid.

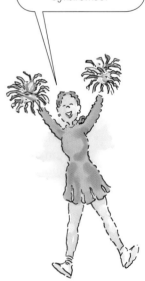

The antianticonvulsant

- In large doses, folic acid may counteract the effects of anticonvulsants, such as phenytoin (Dilantin), potentially leading to seizures.

Side effects/Adverse reactions

Side effects/adverse reactions to folic acid include:

- erythema
- itching
- rash
- anorexia
- nausea
- altered sleep patterns
- difficulty concentrating
- irritability
- overactivity.

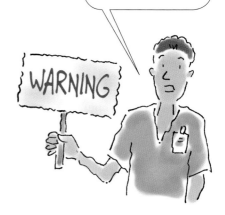

Seize this warning! Large doses of folic acid may counteract the effects of anticonvulsants.

The Three-Step Approach

These steps are appropriate for patients undergoing treatment with folic acid.

Preadministration

(Recognize and analyze cues)
- Assess the patient's folic acid deficiency before therapy.
- Assess the patient's and family's knowledge of drug therapy.

(Prioritize hypothesis—priority patient problems)
- Altered health maintenance
- Injury risk
- Knowledge deficiency

(Generate solutions)
- The patient's folic acid deficiency will improve as evidenced by laboratory studies.
- The risk of injury to the patient will be minimized.
- The patient and family will demonstrate an understanding of drug therapy.

Medication administration

(Take action)
- Promote a varied diet that is adequate in protein, calories, minerals, and electrolytes.
- Administer IV fluids and electrolytes as necessary to provide nutrients. Oral food intake or tube feedings are preferable to IV therapy.

- Correct underlying disorders that contribute to mineral and electrolyte deficiency or excess.
- Promote measures to relieve anorexia, nausea, vomiting, diarrhea, pain, and other signs and symptoms.
- If using the IM route, do not mix folic acid and other drugs in the same syringe.
- Assess for adverse reactions and drug interactions.
- Observe the patient for delayed reactions to therapy.

Postadministration
(Evaluate outcomes)
- Monitor the therapy's effectiveness by evaluating the patient's hemoglobin level, hematocrit, and reticulocyte count.
- Arrange for nutritional consult as needed.
- Monitor the patient's underlying condition for signs of improvement.
- Evaluate the patient's and family's knowledge of drug therapy.

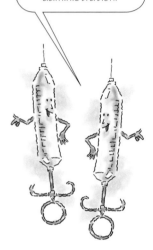

If you're using the IM route, don't mix folic acid and other drugs in the same syringe. You'll need both of us for proper administration.

Epoetin alfa and darbepoetin alfa

Erythropoietin is a substance that forms in the kidneys in response to hypoxia (reduced oxygen) and anemia. It stimulates RBC production (erythropoiesis) in the bone marrow. For the patient experiencing decreased erythropoietin production, epoetin alfa (Procrit) and darbepoetin alfa (Aranesp) are glycoproteins that are used to stimulate RBC production.

Pharmacokinetics

Epoetin alfa and darbepoetin alfa may be given subcutaneously or IV.

Reaching the peak
After subcutaneous administration, peak serum levels of epoetin alfa (Procrit) occur in 5 to 24 hours. The peak level of darbepoetin alfa (Aranesp) occurs within 24 to 72 hours. The circulating half-life is 4 to 13 hours for epoetin alfa and 49 hours for darbepoetin alfa. The therapeutic effect of these drugs lasts for several days after administration. They are eliminated through the kidneys.

Pharmacodynamics

Patients with conditions that decrease erythropoietin production (such as chronic renal failure) typically develop normocytic anemia.

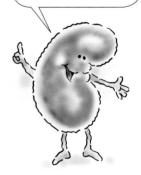

I don't know about you, but I find this discussion on erythropoietin to be incredibly stimulating.

Epoetin alfa (Procrit) and darbepoetin alfa (Aranesp) are structurally similar to erythropoietin. Therapy with these drugs corrects normocytic anemia within 5 to 6 weeks.

Pharmacotherapeutics

Epoetin alfa is used to:
- treat patients with anemia associated with chronic renal failure
- treat anemia associated with zidovudine (Retrovir) therapy in patients with human immunodeficiency virus infection
- reduce the need for allogenic blood transfusions in patients undergoing surgery.

Darbepoetin alfa is indicated for anemia associated with chronic renal failure.

Drug interactions

No known drug interactions exist.

Side effects/Adverse reactions

Hypertension is the most common adverse reaction to epoetin alfa and darbepoetin alfa. Other common adverse reactions may include:
- headache
- joint pain
- nausea and vomiting
- edema
- fatigue
- diarrhea
- seizures
- chest pain
- skin reactions at the injection site
- stroke
- dizziness
- deep vein thrombosis (DVT)
- transient ischemic attack.

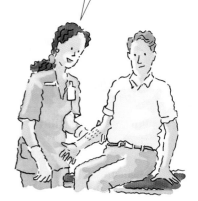

Epoetin alfa and darbepoetin alfa may cause skin reactions at the injection site.

Stop the press!

Both epoetin alfa and darbepoetin alfa increase the risk of pure red cell aplasia, myocardial infarction (MI), heart failure, stroke, cardiac arrest, and other cardiovascular events. In addition, both drugs can accelerate tumor growth and shorten life span in some oncology patients.

The Three–Step Approach

These steps are appropriate for patients undergoing treatment with epoetin alfa or darbepoetin alfa.

Preadministration

(Recognize and analyze cues)

- Assess the patient's health status.
- Assess vital signs, especially blood pressure.
- Assess the patient's and family's knowledge of drug therapy.

(Prioritize hypothesis—priority patient problems)

- Altered health maintenance
- Injury risk
- Knowledge deficiency

(Generate solutions)

- The patient's anemia will improve as evidenced by laboratory studies.
- The risk of injury to the patient will be minimized.
- The patient and family will demonstrate an understanding of drug therapy.

Medication administration

(Take action)

- Give the IV form of the drug by direct injection.
- Additional heparin may be needed to prevent blood clotting if the patient is on dialysis.
- Promote a varied diet that is adequate in protein, calories, minerals, and electrolytes.
- Encourage foods high in iron as applicable to help delay the onset of iron deficiency anemia.
- Administer IV fluids and electrolytes as necessary to provide nutrients. Oral food intake or tube feedings are preferable to IV therapy.
- Correct underlying disorders that contribute to mineral and electrolyte deficiency or excess.
- Promote measures to relieve anorexia, nausea, vomiting, diarrhea, pain, and other signs and symptoms.

Postadministration

(Evaluate outcomes)

- Monitor the drug's effectiveness by evaluating the patient's hemoglobin level, hematocrit, and reticulocyte count.
- Assess for adverse reactions and drug interactions.
- Observe the patient for delayed reactions to therapy.
- Monitor the patient's underlying condition for signs of improvement.
- Evaluate the patient's and family's knowledge of drug therapy.

Anticoagulant drugs

Anticoagulant drugs are used to reduce the ability of the blood to clot. Major categories of anticoagulant drugs include:

- heparin
- oral anticoagulants
- antiplatelet drugs
- direct thrombin inhibitors
- factor Xa inhibitors.

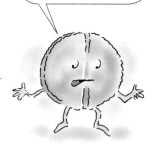

Blood trying to clot? I think not! Anticoagulant drugs reduce the blood's ability to clot.

Heparin and heparin derivatives

Heparin, prepared commercially from animal tissue, is an antithrombolytic agent used to prevent clot formation. Because it does not affect the synthesis of clotting factors, heparin cannot dissolve already formed clots.

The lightweights

Low molecular weight heparins, such as dalteparin sodium (Fragmin) and enoxaparin sodium (Lovenox), are derived by decomposing unfractionated heparin into simpler compounds. They were developed to prevent DVT, a blood clot in the deep veins (usually of the legs), in surgical patients. Their use is preferred because they can be given subcutaneously and do not require as much monitoring as unfractionated heparin.

Pharmacokinetics

Because heparin and its derivatives are not absorbed well from the GI tract, they must be administered parenterally. Unfractionated heparin is administered by continuous IV infusion or via deep subcutaneous injection. Low molecular weight heparins have the advantage of a prolonged circulating half-life. They can be administered subcutaneously once or twice daily. Distribution is immediate after IV administration, but it is not as predictable with subcutaneous injection.

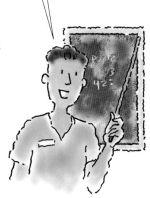

Low molecular weight heparins can be given subcutaneously and don't require as much monitoring as unfractionated heparin. So bring on those fractions!

IM is out

Heparin and its derivatives are not given IM because of the risk of local bleeding. These drugs metabolize in the liver. Their metabolites are excreted in urine. (See *Anticoagulant drugs: Heparin and heparin derivatives*, page 440.)

Pharmacodynamics

Heparin and heparin derivatives prevent the formation of new thrombi. Here's how heparin works:

- Heparin inhibits the formation of thrombin and fibrin by activating antithrombin III.

Anticoagulant drugs: Heparin and heparin derivatives

Actions
- Accelerates formation of an antithrombin III-thrombin complex
- Inactivates thrombin and prevents the conversion of fibrinogen to fibrin

Indications
- DVT
- Pulmonary embolism
- Open heart surgery
- Disseminated intravascular coagulation
- Unstable angina
- Post-MI
- Cerebral thrombosis in evolving stroke
- Left ventricular thrombi
- Heart failure
- History of embolism and atrial fibrillation

Nursing considerations
- Monitor the patient for adverse effects, such as hemorrhage, prolonged clotting time, thrombocytopenia, and hypersensitivity reactions.
- Regularly inspect the patient for bleeding gums, bruises, petechiae, epistaxis, tarry stools, hematuria, and hematemesis.
- Effects can be neutralized by protamine sulfate.
- Monitor partial thromboplastin time (PTT) regularly.

- Antithrombin III then inactivates factors IXa, Xa, XIa, and XIIa in the intrinsic and common pathways. The result is the prevention of a stable fibrin clot.
- In low doses, heparin increases the activity of antithrombin III against factor Xa and thrombin and inhibits clot formation.
- Much larger doses are necessary to inhibit fibrin formation after a clot has been formed. This relationship between dose and effect is the rationale for using low-dose heparin to prevent clotting.
- Whole blood clotting time, thrombin time, and PTT are prolonged during heparin therapy. However, these times may be only slightly prolonged with low or ultra-low preventive dosages.

Pharmacotherapeutics

Heparin may be used in many clinical situations to prevent the formation of new clots or the extension of existing clots. These situations include:
- preventing or treating venous thromboemboli, characterized by inappropriate or excessive intravascular activation of blood clotting as well as extending embolisms
- treating disseminated intravascular coagulation, a complication of other diseases that results in accelerated clotting

Monitoring heparin therapy

Therapy with unfractionated heparin requires close monitoring. Dosage adjustments may be needed to ensure therapeutic effectiveness without increasing the risk of bleeding. Monitor PTT to measure the effectiveness of unfractionated heparin therapy. Also monitor platelet count to watch for heparin-induced thrombocytopenia (HIT).

When to switch
Heparin therapy is associated with thrombocytopenia. If HIT develops, use thrombin inhibitors, such as argatroban or bivalirudin (Angiomax), instead of heparin.

- treating arterial clotting and preventing embolus formation in patients with atrial fibrillation, an arrhythmia in which ineffective atrial contractions cause blood to pool in the atria, increasing the risk of clot formation
- preventing thrombus formation and promoting cardiac circulation in an acute MI by preventing further clot formation at the site of the already formed clot.

An out-of-body experience

Heparin can be used to prevent clotting whenever the patient's blood must circulate outside the body through a machine, such as the cardiopulmonary bypass machine and hemodialysis machine, as well as during extracorporeal circulation and blood transfusions.

No bones about it

Heparin is also useful for preventing clotting during intra-abdominal or orthopedic surgery. (These types of surgery, in many cases, activate the coagulation mechanisms excessively.) In fact, heparin is the drug of choice for orthopedic surgery. (See *Monitoring heparin therapy*, page 440.)

Pulling the plug on DVT

Low molecular weight heparins are used to prevent DVT.

Drug interactions

Watch for these drug interactions in patients taking heparin or heparin derivatives:

- Because heparin and heparin derivatives act synergistically with all the oral anticoagulants, the risk of bleeding increases when the patient takes both drugs together. The prothrombin time (PT) and international normalized ratio (INR), used to monitor the effects of oral anticoagulants, may also be prolonged.
- The risk of bleeding increases when the patient takes nonsteroidal anti-inflammatory drugs (NSAIDs), iron dextran (INFeD), clopidogrel (Plavix), cilostazol, or an antiplatelet drug, such as aspirin (Ecotrin), ticlopidine, or dipyridamole (Persantine), while also receiving heparin or its derivatives.
- Drugs that antagonize or inactivate heparin and heparin derivatives include antihistamines, digoxin (Lanoxin), penicillins, cephalosporins, nitroglycerin (Nitrostat), nicotine, phenothiazines, tetracycline hydrochloride, quinidine, neomycin sulfate, and IV penicillin.
- Nicotine may inactivate heparin and heparin derivatives.
- Nitroglycerin may inhibit the effects of heparin and heparin derivatives.
- Protamine sulfate and administration of fresh frozen plasma counteract the effects of heparin and heparin derivatives.

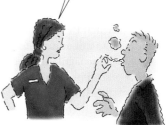

Put out that cigarette right now! Not only is smoking bad for your health but also the nicotine may inactivate heparin!

Side effects/Adverse reactions

One advantage of heparin and its derivatives is that they produce relatively few adverse reactions. These reactions can usually be prevented if the patient's PTT is maintained within the therapeutic range (1½ to 2 times the control).

Reversal of fortune

Bleeding, the most common adverse effect, can be reversed easily by administering protamine sulfate, which binds to heparin and forms a stable salt with it. Other adverse effects include bruising, hematoma formation, necrosis of the skin or other tissue, and thrombocytopenia.

The Three-Step Approach

These steps are appropriate for patients undergoing treatment with heparin or heparin derivatives.

Preadministration

(Recognize and analyze cues)
- Assess the patient for bleeding and other adverse reactions.
- Assess the patient's underlying condition before therapy.
- Monitor the patient's vital signs, hemoglobin level, hematocrit, platelet count, PT, INR, and PTT.
- Assess the patient's urine, stool, and emesis for blood.

(Prioritize hypothesis—priority patient problems)
- Bleeding risk
- Hypovolemia
- Knowledge deficiency

(Generate solutions)
- The patient will have clotting times appropriate for drug therapy.
- The patient will maintain adequate fluid volume as evidenced by vital signs and laboratory studies.
- The patient and family will demonstrate an understanding of drug therapy.

Medication administration

(Take action)
- Carefully and regularly monitor PTT. Anticoagulation is present when PTT values are 1½ to 2 times the control values.
- Do not administer heparin IM; avoid IM injections of any anticoagulant, if possible.
- Keep protamine sulfate available to treat severe bleeding caused by the drug.
- Notify the prescriber about serious or persistent adverse reactions.

- Maintain bleeding precautions throughout therapy.
- Administer IV solutions using an infusion pump, as appropriate.
- Avoid excessive IM injection of other drugs to minimize the risk of hematoma.

Postadministration
(Evaluate outcomes)
- Assess and monitor PTT. Ensure that the patient has no evidence of bleeding or hemorrhaging.
- Monitor the patient's underlying condition for signs of improvement.
- Evaluate the patient's and family's knowledge of drug therapy.

Oral anticoagulants

The major oral anticoagulant used in the United States is the coumarin compound warfarin sodium (Coumadin).

Pharmacokinetics

Warfarin is absorbed rapidly and almost completely when taken orally.

Why the delay?

Despite its rapid absorption, warfarin's effects are not seen for about 36 to 48 hours and it may take 3 to 4 days for the full effect to occur. This is because warfarin antagonizes the production of vitamin K–dependent clotting factors. Before warfarin can exhibit its full effect, the circulating vitamin K clotting factors must be exhausted.

Warfarin is bound extensively to plasma albumin, metabolized in the liver, and excreted in urine. Because warfarin is highly protein bound and metabolized in the liver, using other drugs at the same time may alter the amount of warfarin in the body. This may increase the risk of bleeding and clotting, depending on which drugs are used.

Pharmacodynamics

Oral anticoagulants alter the ability of the liver to synthesize vitamin K–dependent clotting factors, including factors II (prothrombin), VII, IX, and X. However, clotting factors already in the bloodstream

I'm extensively bound to plasma albumin. Stick with me, buddy, and you'll go places!

continue to coagulate blood until they become depleted, so anticoagulation does not begin immediately.

Pharmacotherapeutics

Oral anticoagulants are prescribed to treat thromboembolism and, in this situation, are started while the patient is still receiving heparin. Warfarin, however, may be started without heparin in outpatients at high risk for thromboembolism. (See *Anticoagulant drugs: Warfarin*.)

The chosen one

Oral anticoagulants also are the drugs of choice to prevent DVT and treat patients with prosthetic heart valves or diseased mitral valves. They sometimes are combined with an antiplatelet drug, such as aspirin (Ecotrin), clopidogrel (Plavix), or dipyridamole (Persantine), to decrease the risk of arterial clotting.

Drug interactions

Many patients who take oral anticoagulants also receive other drugs, placing them at risk for serious drug interactions:

- Many drugs, such as highly protein-bound medications, increase the effects of warfarin, resulting in an increased risk of bleeding. Examples include acetaminophen (Tylenol), allopurinol (Zyloprim), amiodarone (Pacerone), cephalosporins, cimetidine (Tagamet), ciprofloxacin (Cipro), danazol, diazoxide (Proglycem), disulfiram (Antabuse), erythromycin (Erythrocin), fluoroquinolones, glucagon, heparin, ibuprofen (Motrin), isoniazid, ketoprofen, metronidazole (Flagyl), miconazole (Monistat), neomycin, propafenone (Rythmol), propylthiouracil, quinidine, sulfonamides, tamoxifen (Soltamox), tetracyclines, thiazides, thyroid drugs, tricyclic antidepressants, and vitamin E.
- Drugs metabolized by the liver may increase or decrease the effectiveness of warfarin. Examples include barbiturates, carbamazepine (Tegretol), corticosteroids, corticotropin, mercaptopurine (Purixan), nafcillin, hormonal contraceptives containing estrogen, rifampin (Rifadin), spironolactone (Aldactone), sucralfate (Carafate), and trazodone (Oleptro).
- A diet high in vitamin K (Mephyton) reduces the effectiveness of oral anticoagulants.
- The risk of phenytoin toxicity increases when phenytoin (Dilantin) is taken with warfarin. Phenytoin may increase or decrease the effects of warfarin.

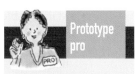

Anticoagulant drugs: Warfarin

Actions
- Inhibits vitamin K–dependent activation of clotting factors II (prothrombin), VII, IX, and X formed in the liver

Indications
- Prevention of pulmonary embolism caused by DVT, MI, rheumatic fever, prosthetic heart valves, or chronic atrial fibrillation

Nursing considerations
- Monitor the patient for adverse reactions, such as hemorrhage, prolonged clotting time, rash, fever, diarrhea, and hepatitis.
- Regularly inspect the patient for bleeding gums, bruises, petechiae, epistaxis, tarry stools, hematuria, and hematemesis.
- The drug's effects can be neutralized by vitamin K (Mephyton); however, if the liver is not capable of producing clotting factors, the vitamin K will not be effective (Dager et al., 2018).
- Monitor PT/INR regularly.

- Chronic alcohol abuse increases the risk of clotting in patients taking warfarin. Patients with acute alcohol intoxication have an increased risk of bleeding.
- Vitamin K and fresh frozen plasma reduce the effects of warfarin.

Side effects/Adverse reactions

The primary adverse reaction to oral anticoagulant therapy is minor bleeding. Severe bleeding can occur, however, with the most common site being the GI tract. Bleeding into the brain may be fatal. Bruises and hematomas may form at arterial puncture sites (for example, after a blood gas sample is drawn). Neurosis or gangrene of the skin and other tissue can occur. Warfarin is contraindicated during pregnancy.

In reverse

The effects of warfarin can be reversed with phytonadione (vitamin K_1).

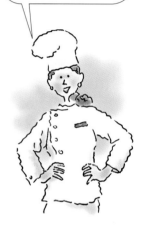

Keep an eye on your patient's diet if taking oral anticoagulants. A diet high in vitamin K reduces the effectiveness of these drugs.

The Three-Step Approach

These steps are appropriate for patients undergoing treatment with oral anticoagulants.

Preadministration

(Recognize and analyze cues)
- Assess the patient's underlying condition before starting therapy.
- Assess the patient's vital signs, hemoglobin level, hematocrit, platelet count, PT, INR, and PTT.
- Assess the patient's urine, stool, and emesis for blood prior to administration.

(Prioritize hypothesis—priority patient problems)
- Bleeding risk
- Hypovolemia
- Knowledge deficiency

(Generate solutions)
- The patient's clotting times will respond appropriately to drug therapy.
- The patient will maintain adequate fluid volume as evidenced by vital signs and laboratory studies.
- The patient and family will demonstrate an understanding of drug therapy.

Medication administration

(Take action)
- Carefully and regularly monitor PT and INR values.
- Keep vitamin K available to treat frank bleeding caused by warfarin.
- Notify the prescriber about serious or persistent adverse reactions.

Teaching about anticoagulant drugs

If anticoagulant drugs are prescribed, review these points with the patient and caregivers:

• Take the drug exactly as prescribed. If taking warfarin, take it at night.

• If taking warfarin (Coumadin), have blood drawn for PT or INR tests in the morning to ensure accurate results.

• Consult the prescriber before taking other drugs, including over-the-counter medications and herbal remedies.

• Institute ways to prevent bleeding during daily activities. For example, remove safety hazards from the home to reduce the risk of injury.

• Do not increase intake of green, leafy vegetables or other foods, or multivitamins that contain vitamin K because vitamin K may antagonize the anticoagulant effects of the drug.

• Report bleeding or other adverse reactions promptly.

• Keep appointments for blood tests and follow-up examinations.

• Report planned or known pregnancy.

• Maintain bleeding precautions throughout therapy.
• Administer the drug at the same time each day.
• Monitor the patient closely for bleeding and other adverse reactions.

Postadministration

(Evaluate outcomes)
• Observe the patient to ensure no evidence of bleeding or hemorrhaging.
• Ensure vital signs and laboratory studies indicate adequate fluid volume status.
• Evaluate the patient's and family's understanding of drug therapy. (See *Teaching about anticoagulant drugs*.)

Antiplatelet drugs

Antiplatelet drugs are used to prevent arterial thromboembolism, particularly in patients at risk for MI, stroke, and arteriosclerosis (hardening of the arteries). Antiplatelet drugs include:
• aspirin (Ecotrin)
• clopidogrel (Plavix)
• dipyridamole (Persantine)
• ticlopidine (Ticlid).

IV instances

IV antiplatelet drugs are used in the treatment of acute coronary syndromes and include the medications abciximab (ReoPro), eptifibatide (Integrilin), and tirofiban (Aggrastat).

Pharmacokinetics

Oral antiplatelet drugs are absorbed very quickly and reach peak concentration between 1 and 2 hours after administration. Aspirin maintains its antiplatelet effect for approximately 10 days, or the life of the platelet. The effects of clopidogrel last about 5 days.

Within minutes

Antiplatelet drugs administered IV are quickly distributed throughout the body. They are minimally metabolized and excreted unchanged in urine. The effects of the drugs are seen within 15 to 20 minutes of administration and last about 6 to 8 hours. Older adults and patients with renal failure may have decreased clearance of these drugs, prolonging their antiplatelet effect.

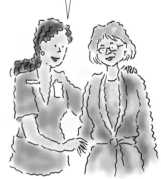

Elderly patients and patients with renal failure may have decreased clearance of antiplatelet drugs, which can prolong their antiplatelet effects.

Pharmacodynamics

Antiplatelet drugs interfere with platelet activity in different drug-specific and dosage-related ways.

Block that clot

Low dosages of aspirin appear to inhibit clot formation by blocking the synthesis of prostaglandin, which in turn prevents formation of the platelet-aggregating substance thromboxane A_2. Clopidogrel (Plavix) inhibits platelet aggregation by inhibiting platelet-fibrinogen binding.

Prevent that platelet

IV antiplatelet drugs block platelet function by inhibiting the glycoprotein IIa-IIIb receptor, which is the major receptor involved in platelet aggregation.

Dipyridamole (Persantine) may inhibit platelet aggregation through its ability to increase adenosine (Adenocard), which is a coronary vasodilator and platelet aggregation inhibitor.

In the early stages

Ticlopidine (Ticlid) inhibits the binding of fibrinogen to platelets during the first stage of the clotting cascade.

Pharmacotherapeutics

Antiplatelet drugs have many different uses.

A familiar face
Aspirin (Ecotrin) is used in patients with a previous MI or unstable angina to reduce the risk of death, and in men to reduce the risk of transient ischemic attacks (TIAs; temporary reduction in circulation to the brain).

Risky business
Clopidogrel (Plavix) is used to reduce the risk of an ischemic stroke or vascular death in patients with a history of a recent MI, stroke, or established peripheral artery disease. This drug is also used to treat acute coronary syndromes, especially in patients who undergo percutaneous transluminal coronary angioplasty (PTCA) or coronary artery bypass grafting.

Dynamic duos
Dipyridamole (Persantine) is used with a coumarin compound to prevent thrombus formation after cardiac valve replacement. Dipyridamole with aspirin has been used to prevent thromboembolic disorders in patients with aortocoronary bypass grafts (bypass surgery) or prosthetic (artificial) heart valves.

Ticlopidine (Ticlid) is used to reduce the risk of thrombotic stroke in high-risk patients (including those with a history of frequent TIAs) and in patients who have already had a thrombotic stroke. Because of the severe adverse effects, ticlopidine should only be used in patients who have not responded to or cannot use aspirin.

The list goes on
Eptifibatide (Integrilin) is indicated in the treatment of acute coronary syndrome and in those patients undergoing percutaneous coronary intervention (PCI). Tirofiban (Aggrastat) is indicated in the treatment of acute coronary syndrome. Abciximab (ReoPro) is indicated as an adjunct to PCI.

Drug interactions
Several drug interactions can occur in patients taking antiplatelet drugs:
- Antiplatelet drugs taken in combination with NSAIDs, heparin, or oral anticoagulants increase the risk of bleeding.
- Aspirin increases the risk of toxicity of methotrexate (Otrexup) and valproic acid.
- Antacids may reduce the plasma levels of ticlopidine (Ticlid).
- Cimetidine (Tagamet) increases the risk of ticlopidine toxicity and bleeding.

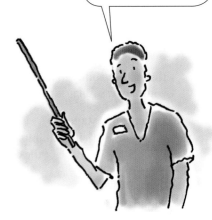

Drugs that interact with antiplatelet drugs include NSAIDs, heparin, oral anticoagulants, methotrexate, valproic acid, antacids, cimetidine, and salicylates in over-the-counter cold medicine compounds.

Don't mix and match

Because guidelines have not been established for administering ticlopidine with heparin, oral anticoagulants, aspirin, or fibrinolytic drugs, discontinue these drugs before starting ticlopidine therapy.

Side effects/Adverse reactions

Hypersensitivity reactions, particularly anaphylaxis, can occur. Bleeding is the most common adverse effect of IV antiplatelet drugs.
Side effects/adverse reactions to aspirin include:

- stomach pain
- heartburn
- nausea
- constipation
- blood in the stool
- slight gastric blood loss.

Clopidogrel may cause these adverse reactions:
- headache
- skin ulceration
- joint pain
- flulike symptoms
- upper respiratory tract infection
- thrombotic thrombocytopenic purpura is rare but potentially fatal.
  These adverse reactions may occur with ticlopidine:
- diarrhea
- nausea
- dyspepsia
- rash
- elevated liver function test results
- neutropenia.
  Dipyridamole may cause:
- headache
- dizziness
- nausea
- flushing
- weakness and fainting
- mild GI distress.

The Three-Step Approach

These steps are appropriate for patients undergoing treatment with antiplatelet drugs.

Preadministration

(Recognize and analyze cues)
- Assess the patient's underlying condition before starting therapy.
- Monitor the patient closely for bleeding and other adverse reactions.

- During long-term therapy with aspirin, monitor the patient's serum salicylate level and perform hearing assessments.
- Monitor the patient's vital signs, hemoglobin level, hematocrit, and platelet count.
- Assess the patient's urine, stool, and emesis for blood.

(Prioritize hypothesis—priority patient problems)
- Bleeding risk
- Hypovolemia
- Knowledge deficiency

(Generate solutions)
- The patient's clotting times will respond appropriately to drug therapy.
- The patient will maintain adequate fluid volume as evidenced by vital signs and laboratory studies.
- The patient and family will demonstrate an understanding of drug therapy.

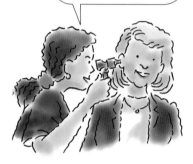

Patients receiving long-term aspirin therapy need to have their serum salicylate level monitored and their hearing checked.

Medication administration
(Take action)
- Notify the prescriber about serious or persistent adverse reactions.
- Maintain bleeding precautions throughout therapy.
- Avoid excessive IV, IM, or subcutaneous injection of other drugs to minimize the risk of hematoma.
- Give aspirin with food, milk, an antacid, or a large glass of water to reduce adverse GI reactions.
- Do not crush enteric coated products.
- Withhold the dose and notify the prescriber if bleeding, salicylism (tinnitus, hearing loss), or adverse GI reactions develop.
- Stop antiplatelet drugs 5 to 7 days before elective surgery as appropriate.

Postadministration
(Evaluate outcomes)
- Monitor the patient's clotting times to determine appropriate drug response.
- Assess regularly to ensure no evidence of bleeding or hemorrhaging.
- Evaluate the patient's and family's understanding of drug therapy.

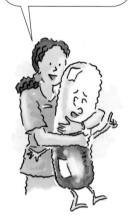

Don't crush enteric coated drugs!

Direct thrombin inhibitors

Direct thrombin inhibitors are anticoagulant drugs used to prevent the formation of harmful blood clots in the body. Dabigatran

(Pradaxa), argatroban, and bivalirudin (Angiomax) are examples of direct thrombin inhibitors.

Pharmacokinetics

Direct thrombin inhibitors are usually administered IV, typically by continuous infusion. They are metabolized by the liver. Reduced dosages may be necessary in individuals with hepatic impairment. Effects on PTT become apparent within 4 to 5 hours of administration. Platelet count recovery becomes apparent within 3 days.

When you'll reach the peak

Direct thrombin inhibitors have a rapid onset after IV bolus administration. Dabigatran (Pradaxa) plasma levels peak in 1 to 3 hours and has a half-life of 13 hours. Bivalirudin (Angiomax) reaches its peak response in 15 minutes and has a short half-life of 25 minutes. Argatroban reaches peak levels in 1 to 3 hours and a short half-life of 45 minutes, and argatroban is excreted primarily in feces through biliary secretion. Bivalirudin and dabigatran are excreted through the kidneys.

Pharmacodynamics

Direct thrombin inhibitors interfere with the blood clotting mechanism by blocking the direct activity of soluble and clot-bound thrombin. When these drugs bind to thrombin, they inhibit:
- platelet activation, granule release, and aggregation
- fibrinogen cleavage
- fibrin formation and further activation of the clotting cascade.

Creating a complex

Dabigatran (Pradaxa) binds with both free, circulating thrombin as well as the thrombin that is bound to clots. This prevents the activation of factor XIII and fibrin formation.

No chance to react

Argatroban reversibly binds to the thrombin-active site and inhibits thrombin-induced reactions, including fibrin formation; coagulation factors V, VIII, and XIII activation; protein C activation; and platelet aggregation.

Hipper than heparin

Compared with heparin, direct thrombin inhibitors have three advantages:
- They have activity against clot-bound thrombin.
- They have more predictable anticoagulant effects.
- They aren't inhibited by the platelet release reaction.

Pharmacotherapeutics

Dabigatran (Pradaxa) is used only for the prevention of stroke and embolism in patients with nonvalvular atrial fibrillation in the United States. Argatroban is used to treat HIT (heparin-induced thrombocytopenia). Argatroban is administered in combination with aspirin to patients with HIT undergoing coronary interventions, such as PTCA (percutaneous transluminal coronary angioplasty), coronary stent placement, and atherectomy. However, the safety and effectiveness of argatroban for cardiac indications have not been established for patients without HIT.

Bivalirudin bio

Bivalirudin (Angiomax) has been approved for use in patients with unstable angina who are undergoing PTCA. It should be used in conjunction with aspirin therapy.

Keep track of contraindications

Bivalirudin (Angiomax) is contraindicated in patients with cerebral aneurysm, intracranial hemorrhage, or general uncontrolled hemorrhage. In addition, the dosage may need to be reduced in those with impaired renal function because 20% of the drug is excreted unchanged in urine. Bivalirudin also increases the risk of hemorrhage in those with GI ulceration or hepatic disease. Hypertension may increase the risk of cerebral hemorrhage. Use bivalirudin with caution after recent surgery or trauma and during lactation.

Drug interactions

In addition, keep these points in mind:
- Parenteral anticoagulants should be discontinued before administering argatroban.
- Using argatroban and warfarin together has a combined effect on INR.
- If the patient previously received heparin, allow sufficient time for heparin's effect on the PTT to decrease before starting argatroban therapy.
- The safety and effectiveness of using argatroban and thrombolytic drugs together haven't been well established, but there appears to be an increased risk of allergic reaction including dyspnea, cough, and rash.

Side effects/Adverse reactions

Do not give direct thrombin inhibitors with drugs that may enhance the risk of bleeding. Patients at greatest risk for hemorrhage include those with severe hypertension; those undergoing lumbar puncture or spinal anesthesia; those undergoing major surgery, especially involving the brain, spinal cord, or eye; those with hematologic conditions associated with increased bleeding tendencies; and those with GI lesions. Use direct thrombin inhibitors cautiously in these patients.

The major adverse effect of direct thrombin inhibitors is bleeding with the possibility of major hemorrhage, although this rarely occurs.

Other adverse reactions include:
- intracranial hemorrhage
- retroperitoneal hemorrhage
- nausea, vomiting, abdominal cramps, and diarrhea
- headache
- hematoma at the IV infusion site.

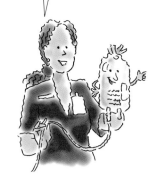

Don't give direct thrombin inhibitors with drugs that may enhance the risk of bleeding. Hemorrhage may occur.

The Three-Step Approach

These steps are appropriate for patients undergoing treatment with direct thrombin inhibitors.

Preadministration

(Recognize and analyze cues)
- Assess the patient's underlying condition before starting therapy.
- Monitor the patient closely for bleeding and other adverse reactions.
- Check PT, INR, and PTT.
- Monitor the patient's vital signs, hemoglobin level, hematocrit, and platelet count.
- Assess the patient's urine, stool, and emesis for blood.

(Prioritize hypothesis—priority patient problems)
- Bleeding risk
- Hypovolemia
- Knowledge deficiency

(Generate solutions)
- The patient's clotting times will respond appropriately to drug therapy.
- The patient will maintain adequate fluid volume as evidenced by vital signs and laboratory studies.
- The patient and family will demonstrate an understanding of drug therapy.

Medication administration

(Take action)
- Notify the prescriber about serious or persistent adverse reactions.
- Maintain bleeding precautions throughout therapy.
- Administer IV solutions using an infusion pump as appropriate: dilute solutions according to the manufacturer's recommendations.

- Avoid excessive IM, IV, or subcutaneous administration of other drugs to minimize the risk of hematoma.
- Dabigatran should only be stored in the manufacturer's supplied bottle—away from excessive moisture, heat, or cold.

Put it in reverse!

Praxbind (idarucizumab) is an FDA-approved antibody fragment that binds to free and thrombin-bound dabigatran (Pradaxa) and is given as the reversal agent in serious or life-threatening bleeding (Dager et al., 2018).

Postadministration

(Evaluate outcomes)
- Monitor the patient's clotting times to determine appropriate drug response.
- Assess regularly to ensure no evidence of bleeding or hemorrhaging.
- Ensure vital signs and laboratory studies indicate adequate fluid volume status.
- Evaluate the patient's and family's understanding of drug therapy.

Factor Xa inhibitor drugs

Factor Xa inhibitor drugs inhibit a single procoagulant target factor Xa. These drugs are administered in a fixed dose and do not require monitoring for most patients. Examples of factor Xa inhibitors are apixaban (Eliquis), edoxaban (Savaysa), fondaparinux (Arixtra), and rivaroxaban (Xarelto) (Dager et al., 2018).

Pharmacokinetics

Fondaparinux (Arixtra) is administered subcutaneously and absorbed rapidly and completely. It's excreted primarily unchanged in urine. Apixaban (Eliquis), edoxaban (Savaysa), and rivaroxaban (Xarelto) are oral factor Xa inhibitors These medications are also mostly excreted through the urine, feces, or bile. Careful monitoring of the patient's renal function (creatinine clearance) is important as dosing will need to be decreased in patients with renal insufficiency. Additional considerations include body weight and age (Dager et al., 2018).

Pharmacodynamics

Factor Xa inhibitors selectively block the active site of factor Xa, interrupting the coagulation cascade.

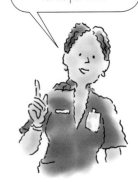

There's only one factor Xa inhibitor drug available in the United States: fondaparinux.

Pharmacotherapeutics

Currently, fondaparinux (Arixtra) is indicated for preventing DVT in patients undergoing total hip and knee replacement surgery and fractured hip surgery and for the prevention or treatment of pulmonary embolism. Apixaban (Eliquis), edoxaban (Savaysa), and rivaroxaban (Xarelto) have been approved for VTE treatment and prevention of recurrence. These medications are also approved for use of stroke and systemic embolism prevention in nonvalvular atrial fibrillation. Rivaroxaban (Xarelto) and apixaban (Eliquis) are also indicated for use of postoperative VTE prevention in knee or hip replacement surgery (Dager et al., 2018).

Drug interactions

Avoid giving factor Xa inhibitors with drugs that may enhance the risk of bleeding.

Side effects/Adverse effects

Side effects/adverse effects that can occur with factor Xa inhibitor therapy include:

- bleeding
- nausea
- anemia
- fever
- rash
- constipation
- edema.

The Three-Step Approach

These steps are appropriate for patients undergoing treatment with factor Xa inhibitor drugs.

Preadministration

(Recognize and analyze cues)
- Assess the patient's underlying condition before starting therapy.
- Monitor the patient closely for bleeding and other adverse reactions.
- Check PT, INR, and PTT.
- Monitor the patient's vital signs, hemoglobin level, hematocrit, and platelet count.
- Assess the patient's urine, stool, and emesis for blood.

(Prioritize hypothesis—priority patient problems)
- Bleeding risk
- Hypovolemia
- Knowledge deficiency

(Generate solutions)
- The patient's clotting times will respond appropriately to drug therapy.

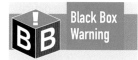

Black Box Warning

Oral Anticoagulants

All direct oral anticoagulants (such as the direct thrombin inhibitors and direct FXa inhibitors) carry a black box warning for use in patients with mechanical heart valves (Dager et al., 2018).

- The patient will maintain adequate fluid volume as evidenced by vital signs and laboratory studies.
- The patient and family will demonstrate an understanding of drug therapy.

Medication administration

(Take action)

- Administer fondaparinux (Arixtra) by subcutaneous injection into fatty tissue only, rotate injection sites.
- Do not mix the drug with other injections or infusions.
- Notify the prescriber about serious or persistent adverse reactions.
- Maintain bleeding precautions throughout therapy.
- Avoid excessive IV, IM, or subcutaneous administration of other drugs to minimize the risk of hematoma.

Put it in reverse!

Andexxa (coagulation factor Xa [recombinant], inactivated) is an FDA-approved factor Xa decoy protein that binds to factor Xa inhibitors and neutralizes the effects. This medication is currently approved for reversal of rivaroxaban (Xarelto) and apixaban (Eliquis) (Dager et al., 2018).

Postadministration

(Evaluate outcomes)

- Monitor the patient's clotting times to determine appropriate drug response.
- Assess regularly to ensure no evidence of bleeding or hemorrhaging.
- Ensure vital signs and laboratory studies indicate adequate fluid volume status.
- Evaluate the patient's and family's understanding of drug therapy.

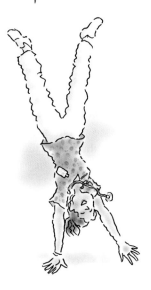

I don't think this is quite what they mean when they say to "rotate" injection sites for subcutaneous administration of fondaparinux!

Thrombolytic drugs

Thrombolytic drugs are used to dissolve an existing clot or a thrombus, commonly in an acute or emergency situation. Some of the thrombolytic drugs currently used include alteplase (Activase), reteplase (Retavase), and Tenecteplase (TNKase).

Pharmacokinetics

After IV or intracoronary administration, thrombolytic drugs are distributed immediately throughout the circulation, quickly activating plasminogen (a precursor to plasmin, which dissolves fibrin clots).

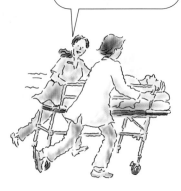

Thrombolytic drugs are commonly used in acute or emergency situations.

How alteplase helps restore circulation

When a thrombus forms in an artery, it obstructs the blood supply, causing ischemia and necrosis. Alteplase (Activase) can dissolve a thrombus in either the coronary or the pulmonary artery, restoring blood supply to the area beyond the blockage.

Obstructed artery
A thrombus blocks blood flow through the artery, causing distal ischemia.

Inside the thrombus
Alteplase enters the thrombus, which consists of plasminogen bound to fibrin. Alteplase binds to the fibrin-plasminogen complex, converting the inactive plasminogen into active plasmin. This active plasmin digests the fibrin, dissolving the thrombus. As the thrombus dissolves, blood flow resumes.

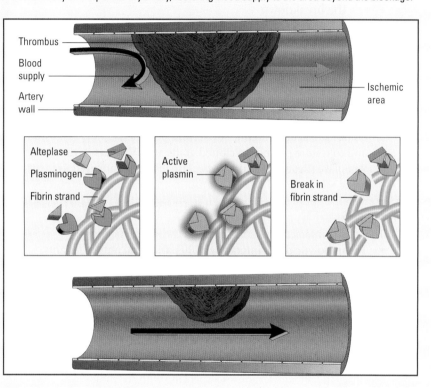

In the blink of an eye

Alteplase (Activase), tenecteplase (TNKase), and reteplase (Retavase) are cleared rapidly from circulating plasma, primarily by the liver. These drugs do not appear to cross the placental barrier.

Pharmacodynamics

Thrombolytic drugs convert plasminogen to plasmin, which lyses (dissolves) thrombi, fibrinogen, and other plasma proteins. (See *How alteplase helps restore circulation*.)

Pharmacotherapeutics

Thrombolytic drugs have several uses. They are used to treat certain thromboembolic disorders (such as acute MI, acute ischemic stroke, and peripheral artery occlusion) and have also been used to dissolve thrombi in arteriovenous cannulas (used in dialysis) and IV catheters to reestablish blood flow. (See *Thrombolytic drugs: Alteplase*.)

Here's the breakdown

Thrombolytic drugs are the drugs of choice to break down newly formed thrombi. They seem most effective when administered within 6 hours after the onset of symptoms.

To be more specific...

In addition, each drug has specific uses:
- Alteplase (Activase) is used to treat acute MI, pulmonary embolism, acute ischemic stroke, and peripheral artery occlusion and to restore patency to clotted grafts and IV access devices.
- Reteplase (Retavase) and tenecteplase (TNKase) are used to treat acute MI.

Drug interactions

These drug interactions can occur with thrombolytic drugs:
- Thrombolytic drugs interact with heparin, oral anticoagulants, antiplatelet drugs, and NSAIDs to increase the patient's risk of bleeding.
- Aminocaproic acid inhibits streptokinase and can be used to reverse its fibrinolytic effects.

Side effects/Adverse reactions

The major reactions associated with the thrombolytic drugs are bleeding and allergic responses, especially with streptokinase.

The Three-Step Approach

These steps are appropriate for patients undergoing treatment with thrombolytic drugs.

Preadministration

(Recognize and analyze cues)
- Assess the patient's underlying condition before starting therapy.
- Monitor the patient closely for bleeding and other adverse reactions.
- Check PT, INR, and PTT.

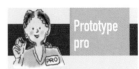

Thrombolytic drugs: Alteplase

Actions
- Dissolves clots by converting plasminogen to plasmin

Indications
- Pulmonary embolism
- Acute MI

Nursing considerations
- Monitor the patient for adverse effects, such as arrhythmias, bleeding, pulmonary edema, and hypersensitivity reactions.
- Monitor the patient's vital signs frequently.
- Monitor the patient frequently for bleeding.

- Monitor the patient's vital signs, hemoglobin level, hematocrit, and platelet count.
- Assess the patient's urine, stool, and emesis for blood.
- Assess the patient's cardiopulmonary status, including the electrocardiogram and vital signs, before and during therapy.

(Prioritize hypothesis—priority patient problems)
- Altered perfusion
- Hypovolemia
- Knowledge deficiency
- Bleeding risk

(Generate solutions)
- The patient's cardiopulmonary assessment findings will improve.
- The patient will maintain adequate fluid volume as evidenced by vital signs and laboratory studies.
- The patient and family will demonstrate an understanding of drug therapy.

Medication administration

(Take action)
- Notify the prescriber about serious or persistent adverse reactions.
- Maintain bleeding precautions throughout therapy.
- Monitor the patient for internal bleeding and check puncture sites frequently.
- Administer IV solutions using an infusion pump as appropriate; reconstitute solutions according to facility protocol.
- Avoid excessive IM, IV, or subcutaneous administration of other drugs to minimize the risk of hematoma.
- Administer heparin with thrombolytics according to facility protocol.
- Have antiarrhythmics available; monitor cardiac status closely.
- Avoid invasive procedures during thrombolytic therapy.

Postadministration

(Evaluate outcomes)
- Monitor cardiopulmonary assessment findings for improved perfusion.
- Assess regularly to ensure no evidence of bleeding or hemorrhaging.
- Ensure vital signs and laboratory studies indicate adequate fluid volume status.
- Evaluate the patient's and family's understanding of drug therapy.

Quick quiz

1. Which administration method for parenteral iron helps avoid leakage into subcutaneous tissue?
   A. Z-track method
   B. IM injection into the deltoid
   C. Subcutaneous injection
   D. Intradermal injection

Answer: A. The Z-track method helps to avoid leakage into subcutaneous tissue and staining of the skin.

2. Which laboratory value would the nurse assess for a patient receiving heparin therapy?
   A. Complete blood count
   B. PTT
   C. Arterial blood gas levels
   D. Hemoglobin level

Answer: B. PTT should be monitored to measure the effectiveness of heparin therapy.

3. Which adverse reaction is experienced most often with IV antiplatelet drugs?
   A. Nausea
   B. Joint pain
   C. Headache
   D. Bleeding

Answer: D. Bleeding is the most common adverse effect of IV antiplatelet drugs.

4. The nurse is caring for a patient who is experiencing life-threatening bleeding from trauma. This patient is also on warfarin. Which medication will the nurse anticipate administering?
   A. Vitamin K
   B. Folic acid
   C. Plasma
   D. Oral charcoal

Answer: A. Vitamin K is the reversal agent of Coumadin.

5. What is the only FDA-approved reversal agent for reversal of serious and life-threatening bleeding for a patient taking apixaban?
   A. Vitamin K
   B. Andexxa
   C. Idarucizumab
   D. Fresh frozen plasma

Answer: B. Andexxa is the only FDA-approved reversal agent for rivaroxaban and apixaban. Andexxa works by neutralizing the effects of the medication.

Scoring

 If you answered all five questions correctly, magnificent! You're on top when it comes to managing clots.

 If you answered four questions correctly, way to go! You're in the know about drugs and blood flow.

If you answered fewer than two questions correctly, stay calm. Another look at this chapter with efficiency should reverse any deficiencies.

Suggested References

Andres, E., & Serraj, K. (2012). Optimal management of pernicious anemia. *Journal of Blood Medicine*, 3, 97–103. http://www.ncbi.nlm.nih.gov/pmc/articles/PMC3441227/

Burchum, J. R., & Rosenthal, L. D. (2019). *Lehne's pharmacology for nursing care* (10th ed.). St. Louis, MO: Elsevier.

Centers for Disease Control and Prevention. (2018, April 18). *Folic acid*. Retrieved from www.cdc.gov/ncbddd/folicacid

Centers for Disease Control and Prevention. (2020, December 11). *Iron*. Retrieved from https://www.cdc.gov/nutrition/infantandtoddlernutrition/vitamins-minerals/iron.html

Dager, W. E., Gulseth, M. P., & Nutescu, E. A. (2018). *Anticoagulation therapy: A clinical practice guide* (2nd ed.). ASHP Publications.

Garzon, S., Cacciato, P. M., Certelli, C., Salvaggio, C., Magliarditi, M., & Rizzo, G. (2020). Iron deficiency anemia in pregnancy: Novel approaches for an old problem. *Oman Medical Journal*, 35(5), e166. https://doi.org/10.5001/omj.2020.108.

Gwarthmey, K. G., & Grogan, J. (2020). Nutritional neuropathies. *Muscle & Nerve*, 62, 13–29. https://doi.org 10.1002/mus.26783

Silvestri, L. A., & Silvestri, A. E. (2020). *Saunders comprehensive review for the NCLEX-RN examination* (8th ed.). Elsevier.

Witt, D. M., Nieuwlaat, R., Clark, N. P., Ansell, J., Holbrook, A., Skov, J., Shehab, N., … Guyatt, G. (2018). American Society of Hematology 2018 guidelines for management of venous thromboembolism: Optimal management of anticoagulation therapy. *Blood Advances*, 22(2), 3257–3291. https://doi.org/10.1182/bloodadvances.2018024893

Chapter 13

Endocrine drugs

Just the facts

In this chapter, you'll learn:

◆ classes of drugs that affect the endocrine system

◆ uses and varying actions of these drugs

◆ absorption, distribution, metabolization, and excretion of these drugs

◆ drug interactions and adverse reactions to these drugs.

Drugs and the endocrine system

The endocrine system consists of organs and glands that are located throughout the body. This system secretes substances called "hormones." Hormones are natural chemicals that travel through the circulatory system to their target tissues. Hormones help balance and maintain the physiologic stability of the body. The body secretes hormones based on body response and feedback systems (Ignatavicius et al., 2021).

A delicate balance

Together with the central nervous system, the endocrine system regulates and integrates the body's metabolic activities and maintains homeostasis (the body's internal chemical equilibrium). The drug types that treat endocrine system disorders include:

- natural hormones and their synthetic analogues, such as insulin and glucagon
- hormonelike substances
- drugs that stimulate or suppress hormone secretion.

The endocrine system helps maintain the body's internal equilibrium.

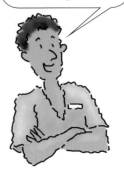

Antidiabetic drugs and glucagon

Insulin, a pancreatic hormone, and oral antidiabetic drugs are classified as *hypoglycemic drugs* because they lower blood glucose levels. Glucagon, another pancreatic hormone, is classified as a *hyperglycemic drug* because it raises blood glucose levels.

Low insulin = high glucose

Diabetes mellitus is a chronic disease of insulin deficiency or resistance. It is characterized by disturbances in carbohydrate, protein, and fat metabolism. This leads to elevated glucose levels in the body. The disease comes in two primary forms that are recognized by the American Diabetes Association (ADA) type 1 and type 2 diabetes (ADA, 2020a). (See *Common types of diabetes mellitus.*)

Insulin

Insulin is secreted by the beta cells of the pancreas as a response to an increase in blood glucose (McCuistion et al., 2020). Patients with type 1 diabetes require an external source of insulin to control blood glucose levels. Insulin may also be given to patients with type 2 diabetes in certain situations.

Pick a rate, any rate

Types of insulin include:
- rapid-acting: lispro (Humalog), aspart (Novolog), and glulisine (Apidra)
- short-acting: regular insulin (Humulin R) or (Novolin R)
- intermediate-acting: NPH insulin (Humulin N) or (Novolin N)
- long-acting: glargine (Lantus), detemir (Levemir), and degludec (Tresiba).

Pharmacokinetics

Insulin is not effective when taken orally because the GI tract breaks down the protein molecule before it reaches the bloodstream.

Common types of diabetes mellitus

Type 1 diabetes mellitus
- Characterized by destruction of pancreatic beta cells.
- Insulin is not secreted by the pancreas.
- Can be autoimmune or idiopathic.
- Treated with insulin.

Type 2 diabetes mellitus
- Heterogeneous group of conditions characterized by cellular insulin resistance. Can include progressive loss of beta cell insulin secretion.
- Multifactorial risk factors including age, family history, obesity, inactivity, race, and gestational diabetes.
- Treated with lifestyle changes (diet and exercise) and oral or injectable antidiabetic drugs.

Skin deep

However, all insulins can be given by subcutaneous injection. Absorption of subcutaneous insulin varies according to the injection site, the blood supply, and the degree of tissue hypertrophy at the injection site.

In the IV league

Regular insulin is typically given subcutaneously but may be given other routes such as an IV bolus, an IV infusion, or an IM injection.

Far and wide

After absorption, insulin is distributed throughout the body. Insulin-responsive tissues are located in the liver, fat, and muscle. Insulin is metabolized primarily in the liver and, to a lesser extent, in the kidneys and muscle. It is excreted in feces and urine (Katzung, 2018).

Pharmacodynamics

Insulin is an anabolic or building hormone that promotes:

- storage of glucose as glycogen (see *How insulin aids glucose uptake,* page 465.)
- an increase in protein and fat synthesis
- a deceleration of the breakdown of glycogen, protein, and fat
- a balance of fluids and electrolytes.

Extracurricular activity

Although it has no antidiuretic effect, insulin can correct the polyuria (excessive urination) and polydipsia (excessive thirst) associated with the osmotic diuresis that can occur with hyperglycemia by decreasing the blood glucose level. Insulin also facilitates the movement of potassium from the extracellular fluid into the cell.

Pharmacotherapeutics

Insulin is indicated for:

- type 1 diabetes
- type 2 diabetes when other methods of controlling blood glucose levels have failed or are contraindicated
- type 2 diabetes when blood glucose levels are elevated during periods of emotional or physical stress (such as during infection, surgery, or medication therapy)
- type 2 diabetes when oral antidiabetic drugs are contraindicated because of pregnancy or hypersensitivity.

Calming complications

Insulin is also used to treat two complications of diabetes: diabetic ketoacidosis (DKA) and hyperglycemic-hyperosmolar state (HHS). (DKA) is characterized by inadequate insulin and generation of ketoacids in the liver. DKA is more

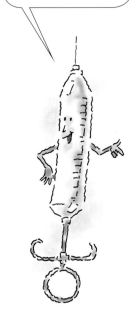

The amount of insulin absorbed depends on the injection site, the patient's blood supply, and the degree of tissue hypertrophy at the injection site.

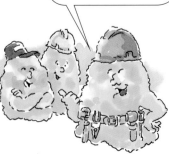

As building hormones, insulin can store glucose as glycogen, increase protein and fat synthesis, and balance fluid and electrolytes!

Pharm function

How insulin aids glucose uptake

These illustrations show how insulin allows a cell to use glucose for energy.

1. Glucose cannot enter the cell without the aid of insulin.

2. Normally produced by the beta cells of the pancreas, insulin binds to the receptors on the surface of the target cell. Insulin and its receptor first move to the inside of the cell, which activates glucose transporter channels to move to the surface of the cell.

3. These channels allow glucose to enter the cell. The cell can then use the glucose for metabolism.

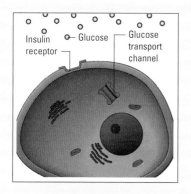

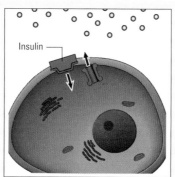

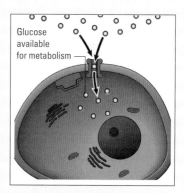

common with type 1 diabetes. HHS is more common with type 2 diabetes and is characterized by decreased insulin and severe dehydration (Ignatavicius et al., 2021).

Nondiabetic duty

Insulin is also used to treat severe hyperkalemia (elevated serum potassium levels) in patients without diabetes. Potassium moves with glucose from the bloodstream into the cell, lowering serum potassium levels. (See *Hypoglycemic drugs: Insulin,* page 466.)

Drug interactions

Some drugs interact with insulin, altering its ability to decrease the blood glucose level; other drugs directly affect glucose levels:

- Anabolic steroids, salicylates, alcohol, sulfa drugs, angiotensin-converting enzyme inhibitors, propranolol (Inderal), and

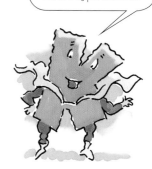

Insulin can be used in patients without diabetes to treat severe hyperkalemia.

Hypoglycemic drugs: Insulin

Actions
• Increases glucose transport across muscle and fat cell membranes to reduce blood glucose levels
• Promotes conversion of glucose to glycogen (its storage form)
• Triggers amino acid uptake and conversion to protein in muscle cells and inhibits protein degradation
• Stimulates triglyceride formation and inhibits the release of free fatty acids from adipose tissue
• Stimulates lipoprotein lipase activity, which converts circulating lipoproteins to fatty acids

Indications
• Type 1 diabetes

• Adjunct treatment in type 2 diabetes
• DKA
• HHS

Nursing considerations
• Assess the patient's blood sugar and hemoglobin A1C before initiating therapy and as needed during therapy.
• Monitor the patient for adverse effects, such as hypoglycemia and hypersensitivity reactions.
• Evaluate the patient for learning readiness and self-care ability. These are vital for the patient to administer their own insulin.

monoamine oxidase (MAO) inhibitors may increase the hypoglycemic effect of insulin.
• Corticosteroids, oral contraceptives, sympathomimetic drugs, isoniazid, thyroid hormones, niacin, furosemide, and thiazide diuretics may reduce the effects of insulin, resulting in hyperglycemia.
• Beta-adrenergic blockers may prolong the hypoglycemic effect of insulin and may mask signs and symptoms of hypoglycemia.

Side effects/adverse reactions

Adverse reactions to insulin include:
• hypoglycemia (below-normal blood glucose levels)
• Somogyi effect (hypoglycemia followed by rebound hyperglycemia)
• hypersensitivity reactions
• lipodystrophy (disturbance in fat deposition)
• insulin resistance.

The Three-Step Approach

Nursing management for the patient receiving treatment with insulin therapy includes these three steps.

Preadministration

(Recognize and analyze cues)

- Assess the patient's glucose level before therapy and regularly thereafter.
- Assess the patient's hemoglobin A1C level before therapy and regularly thereafter.
- Monitor the patient's urine ketone level when the glucose level is elevated.

(Priority hypothesis—priority patient problems)

- Altered health maintenance
- Injury risk
- Malnutrition risk
- Knowledge deficiency

(Generate solutions)

- The patient's glucose levels will be maintained within prescribed limits.
- The patient will not be injured or harmed.
- The patient will adhere to the ADA nutrition guidelines.
- The patient and family will demonstrate an understanding of drug therapy.

Medication administration

(Take action)

- Extensive and ongoing patient and family teaching is necessary for patient with diabetes.
- Blood sugar monitoring and insulin administration teaching are imperative to achieve patient goals and health.
- Use regular insulin in patients with circulatory collapse, DKA, or hyperkalemia.
- Insulin resistance may develop; large insulin doses are needed to control signs and symptoms of diabetes in these cases. For severe insulin resistance (when a patient's daily dose is greater than 200 units), U-500 insulin is available as regular insulin (concentrated). Be cautious in the storage of U-500 insulin because of the danger of severe overdose if given accidentally to other patients.
- Do not use insulin that has changed color or become clumped or granular.
- Check the expiration date on the vial before using.
- If administering IV, use only regular insulin. Inject directly at the ordered rate into the vein, through an intermittent infusion device, or into a port close to the IV access site. If giving continuous infusion, infuse the drug diluted in normal saline solution at the prescribed rate.
- If administering subcutaneously, pinch a fold of skin with the fingers starting at least 30 (7.6 cm) apart and insert the needle at a

45- to 90-degree angle. Press but don't rub the site after injection. Rotate and chart injection sites to avoid overuse of one area. A patient with diabetes may achieve better control if injection sites are rotated within the same anatomic region.

- Lispro insulin has a rapid onset of action and should be given within 15 minutes of meals

Mix it up

The key players: Insulins that can be mixed

- Rapid-acting
  - Lispro (Humalog), aspart (Novolog), and glulisine (Apidra)
- Short-acting
  - Regular insulin (Humulin R or Novolin R)
- Intermediate-acting
  - NPH insulin (Humulin N or Novolin N) (ADA, 2020b)

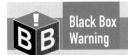

Preparing for practice: Humulin R U-500

Humulin R U-500 is a high alert drug. It is 5 times more potent than U-100 insulin. Humulin R U-500 should only be administered using a KwikPen or a green capped U-500 insulin syringe.

Mixing tips

- Long-acting insulins cannot be diluted or mixed with any other insulin or solution or given IV.
- Regular insulin may be mixed with NPH insulin in any proportion. When mixing regular insulin with NPH insulin, always draw up regular insulin into the syringe first.
- Whenever NPH is mixed with regular insulin in the same syringe, give the mixture immediately to avoid a loss of potency.
- Switching from separate injections to a prepared mixture may alter the patient's response.

Highs and lows

- A patient with type 1 diabetes prone to DKA, severely ill, and newly diagnosed with very high glucose levels may require hospitalization and IV treatment with regular fast-acting insulin.
- Notify the prescriber of sudden changes in glucose levels, dangerously high or low levels, or ketosis.
- Be prepared to provide supportive measures if the patient develops DKA or HHS.

Sustaining snacks

- Treat hypoglycemic reactions with an oral form of rapid-acting glucose (if the patient can swallow) or with glucagon or IV glucose (if the patient cannot be roused). Follow administration with a complex carbohydrate snack when the patient is awake, and then, determine the cause of the reaction.

Teaching about insulin

See Education edge: Teaching template in Chapter 3 page 38 for general teaching for all medications. Specific points to review with patients and family for insulin therapy:

- Insulin relieves signs and symptoms but does not cure the disease; therapy is lifelong.
- Understanding proper techniques and equipment for glucose monitoring is essential for determining insulin dosage and success of therapy.
- Follow the prescribed therapeutic regimen; adhere to specific diet, weight reduction if appropriate, and exercise.
- Adhere to recommended personal hygiene programs—including daily foot inspection—and consult with the prescriber about ways to avoid infection.
- Review the timing of injections and eating with the health care team; do not skip meals.

- Accuracy of drug measurement is very important, especially with concentrated regular insulin. Aids, such as a magnifying sleeve or dose magnifier, may improve accuracy.
- Don't alter the order in which insulin types are mixed or change the model or brand of the syringe or needle used.
- Learn to recognize signs and symptoms of hyperglycemia and hypoglycemia and what to do if they occur.
- Wear or carry medical identification at all times.
- Have carbohydrates (glucose tablets or candy) on hand for emergencies.

- Make sure that the patient is following an appropriate diet and exercise program. Expect to adjust the insulin dosage when other aspects of the regimen are altered.
- Discuss with the health care team how to handle nonadherence.
- Teach the patient and family members how to monitor glucose levels and administer insulin. (See *Teaching about insulin.*)

Postadministration

(Evaluate outcomes)
- Monitor the immediate effectiveness of the patient's treatment regimen by evaluating glucose level.
- Monitor long-term effectiveness of the patient's treatment regimen by evaluating the patient's hemoglobin A1C.
- Monitor the patient for signs and symptoms of hypoglycemia.
- Monitor the patient's glucose level more frequently if the patient is under stress, medically unstable, recently diagnosed with diabetes, undergoing dietary changes, under physician orders to have nothing by mouth, experiencing nausea and vomiting, or taking drugs that can interact with insulin.
- Monitor the patient's overall health status.
- Promote use of the ADA dietary guidelines to maintain the patient's nutritional needs.
- Evaluate the patient's and family's knowledge of insulin therapy and diabetes care. (See *Teaching about insulin.*)

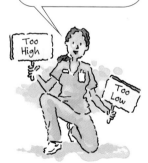

Notify the prescriber if your patient develops glucose levels that are dangerously high or low.

Oral antidiabetic drugs and beyond

Available oral antidiabetic drugs include:
- biguanide drugs (metformin [Glucophage])
- second-generation sulfonylureas drugs (glipizide [Glucotrol], glyburide [DiaBeta], and glimepiride [Amaryl]) (first-generation drugs are no longer used on patients)
- thiazolidinedione drugs (pioglitazone [Actos] and rosiglitazone [Avandia])
- alpha-glucosidase inhibitors (acarbose [Precose] and miglitol [Glyset])
- meglitinides (repaglinide [Prandin] and nateglinide [Starlix])
- dipeptidyl peptidase 4 (DPP-4) inhibitors (sitagliptin [Januvia], saxagliptin [Onglyza], linagliptin [Tradjenta], and alogliptin [Nesina])
- sodium-glucose cotransport inhibitors (canagliflozin [Invokana], dapagliflozin [Farxiga], empagliflozin [Jardiance], and ertugliflozin [Steglatro]).

Pharmacokinetics

Most oral antidiabetic drugs are absorbed well from the GI tract, are distributed via the bloodstream throughout the body, primarily metabolized by the liver, and excreted mostly in the urine with some excreted in feces.

Prototype pro

Oral antidiabetic drugs: Glyburide

Actions
- Stimulates insulin release from the pancreatic beta cells and reduces glucose output by the liver.
- Extrapancreatic effect increases peripheral sensitivity to insulin and causes mild diuretic effect.

Indications
- Type 2 diabetes

Nursing considerations
- Monitor the patient for adverse effects, such as hypoglycemia, hypersensitivity reactions, and hematologic disorders.
- Educate the patient about timing dosing before meals.
- During times of stress, the patient may need insulin; monitor for hypoglycemia.
- Avoid use of alcohol, which produces a disulfiramlike reaction.
- Advise against starting new supplements or medication without consulting their health care provider.

Pharmacodynamics

It is believed that oral antidiabetic drugs produce actions within and outside the pancreas (extrapancreatic) to regulate blood glucose.

To the pancreas…

Oral antidiabetic drugs stimulate pancreatic beta cells to release insulin in a patient with a minimally functioning pancreas. Within a few weeks to a few months of starting sulfonylureas, pancreatic insulin secretion drops to pretreatment levels, but blood glucose levels remain normal or near normal. Most likely, the actions of the oral antidiabetic drugs outside of the pancreas are responsible for maintaining this glucose control.

… and beyond!

Oral antidiabetic drugs provide several extrapancreatic actions to decrease and control blood glucose. They can go to work in the liver and decrease glucose production (gluconeogenesis) there. Also, by increasing the number of insulin receptors in the peripheral tissues, they provide more opportunities for the cells to bind sufficiently with insulin, initiating the process of glucose metabolism.

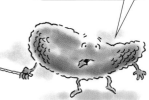

If the pancreas isn't functioning properly, it's believed that oral antidiabetic drugs can temporarily stimulate it to release insulin.

Let's get specific

These oral antidiabetic drugs produce specific actions:

- Metformin (Glucophage) decreases liver production of glucose and intestinal absorption of glucose and improves insulin sensitivity.
- Glipizide (Glucotrol), glyburide (DiaBeta), and glimepiride (Amaryl) decrease glucose production in the liver and increase the tissue response to insulin.
- Pioglitazone (Actos) and rosiglitazone (Avandia) improve insulin sensitivity.
- Acarbose (Precose) and miglitol (Glyset) inhibit enzymes, delaying glucose absorption.
- Repaglinide (Prandin) and nateglinide (Starlix) stimulate the beta cells of the pancreas to release insulin.
- Sitagliptin (Januvia), saxagliptin (Onglyza), linagliptin (Tradjenta), and alogliptin (Nesina) slow the breakdown of intestinal hormones that allow insulin levels to increase after a meal.
- Canagliflozin (Invokana), dapagliflozin (Farxiga), empagliflozin (Jardiance), and ertugliflozin (Steglatro) lower blood sugar by causing the kidneys to excrete sugar from the body in the urine.

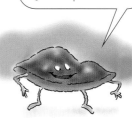

Oral antidiabetic drugs also work in the liver to decrease glucose production.

Pharmacotherapeutics

Oral antidiabetic drugs are indicated for patients with type 2 diabetes if diet and exercise cannot control blood glucose levels. These drugs are not effective in patients with type 1 diabetes because the pancreatic beta cells are not functioning at a minimal level.

Calling all combos

Combinations of an oral antidiabetic drug and insulin therapy may be indicated for some patients who do not respond to either drug alone.

Drug interactions

Hypoglycemia and hyperglycemia are the main risks when oral antidiabetic drugs interact with other drugs.

Low blow

Hypoglycemia may occur when sulfonylureas are combined with alcohol, anabolic steroids, gemfibrozil (Lopid), MAO inhibitors, salicylates, sulfonamides, fluconazole (Diflucan), cimetidine (Tagamet), warfarin, and ranitidine (Zantac). It may also occur when metformin (Glucophage) is combined with cimetidine (Tagamet), nifedipine (Procardia), and vancomycin (Vancocin). Hypoglycemia is less likely to occur when metformin (Glucophage) is used as a single agent.

High fly

Hyperglycemia may occur when sulfonylureas are taken with corticosteroids, rifampin, sympathomimetics, and thiazide diuretics. Metformin (Glucophage) administration with iodinated contrast dyes can result in acute renal failure. Doses should be withheld in patients undergoing procedures that require IV contrast dyes.

Side effects/adverse reactions

Hypoglycemia is a major adverse reaction to oral antidiabetic drugs, especially when combination therapy is used.

Side effects/adverse reactions specific to sulfonylureas include:
- nausea
- epigastric fullness
- blood abnormalities
- fluid retention
- rash
- hyponatremia
- photosensitivity.

Side effects/adverse reactions to metformin include:
- metallic taste
- nausea and vomiting
- abdominal discomfort.
  Alpha-glucosidase inhibitors may cause these reactions:
- elevated liver enzymes
- abdominal pain
- diarrhea

- gas.
  Thiazolidinediones may cause:
- elevated liver enzymes
- weight gain
- swelling.
  Meglitinides may cause these reactions:
- headache
- diarrhea.
  DPP-4 inhibitors may cause these reactions:
- headache
- nasopharyngitis.
  Sodium-glucose cotransport inhibitors may cause these
reactions:
- candidiasis
- cystitis/vaginitis
- nasopharyngitis.

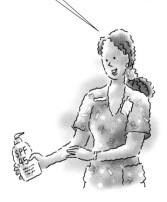

Encourage sun protection for patients taking sulfonylureas. They can cause photosensitivity.

The Three-Step Approach

Nursing management for patients undergoing treatment with oral antidiabetic medications includes these three steps.

Preadministration

(Recognize and analyze cues)
- Assess the patient's baseline blood glucose and hemoglobin A1C before beginning therapy and regularly. Keep in mind that the patient may require glucose monitoring several times daily.

(Prioritize hypothesis—priority patient problems)
- Altered health maintenance
- Hyperglycemic risk
- Hypoglycemia risk
- Knowledge deficiency

(Generate solutions)
- The patient's blood glucose level will be maintained within normal limits.
- The patient's hemoglobin A1C will reach and stay at goal set by the patient and provider.
- The patient and family members will demonstrate an understanding of glucose monitoring and drug therapy.

Medication administration

(Take action)
- Most oral antidiabetic drugs require specific administration timing.

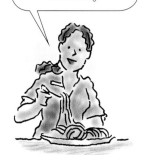

The first bite is just right. Alpha-glucosidase inhibitors should be taken with the first bite of each main meal three times daily.

Timing is everything

- Give sulfonylureas 30 minutes before the morning meal (once-daily dosing) or 30 minutes before morning and evening meals (twice-daily dosing).
- Give metformin with morning and evening meals.
- Alpha-glucosidase inhibitors should be taken with the first bite of each main meal three times daily.
- Meglitinides and sodium-glucose cotransport inhibitors should be taken before meals as ordered.
- A patient who is taking thiazolidinediones and alpha-glucosidase inhibitors should have liver enzyme levels measured at the start of therapy, every 2 months for the first year of therapy and periodically thereafter.
- A patient transferring from one oral antidiabetic drug to another (except chlorpropamide) usually does not need a transition period.
- If the patient switches insulin therapy to oral antidiabetics, they will need monitoring at least three times daily before meals.
- Treat hypoglycemic reactions with an oral form of rapid-acting carbohydrates (if the patient can swallow) or with glucagon or IV glucose (if the patient can't swallow or is comatose). Follow up treatment with a complex carbohydrate snack when the patient is awake, and determine the cause of the reaction.
- Anticipate that the patient may need insulin therapy during periods of increased stress, such as with infection, fever, surgery, or trauma. Increase monitoring, especially for hyperglycemia, during these situations.
- Make sure that adjunct therapies, such as diet and exercise, are being used appropriately.
- Ensure that the patient is adequately hydrated.
- Teach the patient how and when to monitor glucose levels and to recognize signs and symptoms of hyperglycemia and hypoglycemia. (See *Teaching about antidiabetic drugs*, page 475.)

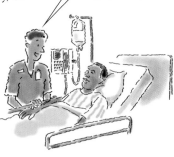

Patients using oral antidiabetics may need insulin therapy during times of stress, such as when they have surgery.

Postadministration
(Evaluate outcomes)

- Observe for any adverse reactions and drug interactions.
- Evaluate the patient's glucose control by analyzing blood glucose readings and hemoglobin A1C over time.
- Evaluate the patient's and family's knowledge of oral antidiabetic therapy. (See *Teaching about antidiabetic drugs*, page 475.)

Other antidiabetic drugs

Incretin mimetics (glucagon-like peptide-1 agonists) are injectable drugs that are utilized for patients with type 2 diabetes. These drugs work in several ways including enhancing beta cell insulin secretion, suppression of glucagon secretion, and increased feelings of fullness

Teaching about antidiabetic drugs

See Education edge: Teaching template in Chapter 3 page 38 for general teaching for all medications. Specific points to review with patients and family for antidiabetic drugs:

- Therapy relieves signs and symptoms but does not cure the disease.
- Follow the prescribed therapeutic regimen; adhere to specific diet, weight reduction, exercise, and personal hygiene programs, and consult with the prescriber about ways to avoid infection.
- Know how and when to monitor glucose levels.
- Learn to recognize signs and symptoms of hyperglycemia and hypoglycemia and what to do if these occur.
- Do not change the dosage without the prescriber's consent.
- Report adverse reactions.
- Do not take other drugs, including over-the-counter drugs and herbal remedies, without first checking with the prescriber.
- Avoid consuming alcohol during drug therapy.
- Wear or carry medical identification at all times.

and satiety when eating. These medications should not be used in place of insulin (McCuistion et al., 2020).

- Incretin mimetics (glucagon-like peptide-1 agonists) (dulaglutide [Trulicity], exenatide [Byetta], liraglutide [Victoza], lixisenatide [Adlyxin], and semaglutide [Ozempic])

Amylin is an amino acid that is secreted from the pancreas with insulin. It works to slow stomach emptying, regulate glucagon, and reduce food intake. This helps to regulate postmeal blood glucose and decrease appetite (Dungan, 2020). The amylin analog pramlintide is approved for use in both type 1 and type 2 diabetes.

- Amylin analog (pramlintide [Symlin])

Glucagon

Glucagon, a hyperglycemic drug that raises blood glucose levels, is a hormone normally produced by the alpha cells of the islets of Langerhans in the pancreas. When adequate stores of glycogen are present, glucagon can raise glucose levels in patients with severe hypoglycemia.

Pharmacokinetics

After subcutaneous, IM, or IV injection, glucagon is absorbed rapidly. It is distributed throughout the body, although its effect occurs primarily in the liver.

Here, there, and (almost) everywhere

Glucagon is degraded extensively by the liver, kidneys, and plasma and at its tissue receptor sites in plasma membranes. It is removed from the body by the liver and kidneys.

Pharmacodynamics

Glucagon regulates the rate of glucose production through:

- glycogenolysis, the conversion of glycogen back into glucose by the liver
- gluconeogenesis, the formation of glucose from free fatty acids and proteins
- lipolysis, the release of fatty acids from adipose tissue for conversion to glucose.

Pharmacotherapeutics

Glucagon is used for emergency treatment of severe hypoglycemia. It is also used during radiologic examination of the GI tract to reduce GI motility.

Drug interactions

Glucagon interacts adversely with oral anticoagulants, increasing the tendency to bleed.

Side effects/adverse reactions

Adverse reactions to glucagon are rare.

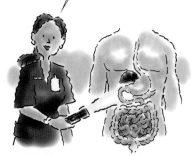

Glucagon is used during radiologic examination of the GI tract to reduce GI motility. How illuminating!

The Three-Step Approach

Nursing management for patients requiring treatment with glucagon includes these three steps.

Preadministration

(Recognize and analyze cues)

- Assess the patient's baseline blood glucose and hemoglobin A1C before beginning therapy.
- Assess the patient's baseline health status.

(Prioritize hypothesis—priority patient problems)

- Altered health maintenance
- Hyperglycemia risk
- Knowledge deficiency

(Generate solutions)

- The patient will recover and maintain blood glucose within normal limits.

- The patient and family will express understanding of signs and symptoms and treatment of hypo/hyperglycemia.
- The patient and family members will demonstrate an understanding of drug therapy.

Medication administration
(Take action)

- Assess the patient's blood glucose level regularly. Increase monitoring during periods of increased stress (infection, fever, surgery, or trauma).
- For IM and subcutaneous use, reconstitute the drug in a 1-unit vial with 1 mL of diluent; reconstitute the drug in a 10-unit vial with 10 mL of diluent.
- For IV administration, a drip infusion, such as dextrose solution, which is compatible with glucagon, may be used. The drug forms precipitate in chloride solutions. Inject drug into the vein at a rate of 1 mg/minute (Skidmore-Roth, 2020).
- Arouse the lethargic patient as quickly as possible. Give additional carbohydrates orally to prevent a secondary hypoglycemic episode, and then, determine the cause of the reaction.
- Notify the prescriber that the patient's hypoglycemic episode required glucagon use.
- Be prepared to provide emergency intervention if the patient doesn't respond to glucagon administration. An unstable, hypoglycemic patient with diabetes may not respond to glucagon; give IV dextrose 50% instead.
- Notify the prescriber if the patient cannot retain some form of sugar for 1 hour because of nausea or vomiting.

Postadministration
(Evaluate outcomes)

- Observe the patient closely for effects of medication.
- Monitor the patient's glucose level after medication administration.
- Evaluate the patient's and family's knowledge of glucagon.
- Evaluate the patient's and family's knowledge of hypo/hyperglycemia signs and symptoms and treatment.

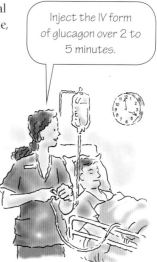

Inject the IV form of glucagon over 2 to 5 minutes.

Thyroid and antithyroid drugs

Thyroid and antithyroid drugs function to correct thyroid hormone deficiency (hypothyroidism) and thyroid hormone excess (hyperthyroidism).

Thyroid drugs

Thyroid drugs, used for hormone replacement, are typically synthetic and may contain triiodothyronine (T_3), thyroxine (T_4), or both.

Synthesized from sodium

Synthetic thyroid drugs actually are the sodium salts of the L-isomers of the hormones. These synthetic hormones include:
- levothyroxine sodium (Synthroid), which contains T_4
- liothyronine sodium (Triostat), which contains T_3.

Pharmacokinetics

Thyroid hormones are absorbed variably from the GI tract, distributed in plasma, and bound to serum proteins. They are metabolized through deiodination, primarily in the liver, and excreted unchanged in feces.

Pharmacodynamics

The principal pharmacologic effect is an increased metabolic rate in body tissues. Thyroid hormones affect protein and carbohydrate metabolism and stimulate protein synthesis. They promote gluconeogenesis and increase the use of glycogen stores (Katzung, 2018).

Taken to heart

Thyroid hormones increase heart rate and cardiac output (the amount of blood pumped by the heart each minute). They may even increase the heart's sensitivity to catecholamines and increase the number of beta-adrenergic receptors in the heart (stimulation of beta receptors in the heart increases heart rate and contractility).

More flow

Thyroid hormones may increase blood flow to the kidneys and increase the glomerular filtration rate (the amount of plasma filtered through the kidneys each minute) in patients with hypothyroidism, producing diuresis. (See *Thyroid hormones: Levothyroxine*, page 479.)

Pharmacotherapeutics

Thyroid drugs act as replacement or substitute hormones in these situations:
- to treat the many forms of hypothyroidism
- with antithyroid drugs to prevent goiter formation (an enlarged thyroid gland) and hypothyroidism
- to differentiate between primary and secondary hypothyroidism during diagnostic testing
- to treat papillary or follicular thyroid carcinoma.

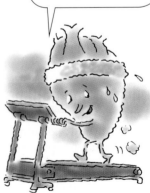

Talk about increasing productivity! Thyroid hormones increase my rate and output in addition to increasing the metabolic rate of body tissues.

Prototype pro

Thyroid hormones: Levothyroxine

Actions
- Levothyroxine works in cells to stimulate metabolism in all body tissues by increasing gluconeogenesis and protein synthesis, and by mobilizing glycogen stores. Thyroid hormone receptors are found in the pituitary, liver, kidney, heart, skeletal muscles, lungs, and intestines (Eghtedari & Correa, 2020).

Indications
- Thyroid hormone replacement

- Myxedema coma
- Cretinism

Nursing considerations
- Monitor the patient for side effects/adverse effects, such as nervousness, insomnia, tremor, tachycardia, palpitations, angina, dysrhythmias, thyroid storm, and cardiac arrest.
- Levothyroxine is prescribed in micrograms (mcg): medication errors can occur if written in another unit. Verify dose and order to avoid error.

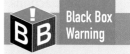

Black Box Warning

Preparing for practice: Levothyroxine

Use with extreme caution in elderly patients and in patients with cardiovascular disorders.

A winning choice

Levothyroxine (Synthroid) is the drug of choice for thyroid hormone replacement and thyroid-stimulating hormone (TSH) suppression therapy.

Drug interactions

Thyroid drugs interact with several common drugs:
- They increase the effects of oral anticoagulants, increasing the risk for bleeding.
- Bile acid sequestrants including cholestyramine (Questran) and colestipol (Colestid) reduce the absorption of thyroid hormones.
- Phenytoin (Dilantin) may accelerate metabolism of levothyroxine.
- Taking thyroid drugs with digoxin (Lanoxin) may reduce serum digoxin levels, increasing the risk of dysrhythmias or heart failure.
- Carbamazepine (Tegretol), phenytoin (Dilantin), phenobarbital, and rifampin increase thyroid hormone metabolism, reducing effectiveness.
- Serum theophylline levels may increase when theophylline is administered with thyroid drugs.

Side effects/adverse reactions

Most adverse reactions to thyroid drugs result from toxicity.

Gut reactions

Side effects/adverse reactions in the GI system include diarrhea, abdominal cramps, weight loss, and increased appetite.

Cardiac concerns

Side effects/adverse reactions in the cardiovascular system include palpitations, sweating, rapid heart rate, increased blood pressure, angina, and dysrhythmias.

Effects all around

Signs and symptoms of toxic doses include:
- headache
- tremor
- insomnia
- nervousness
- fever
- heat intolerance
- menstrual irregularities.

The Three-Step Approach

Nursing management for the patient being treated with thyroid medications includes these three steps.

Preadministration

(Recognize and analyze cues)
- Assess the patient's condition before therapy and regularly thereafter. Normal levels of T_4 should occur within 24 hours, followed by a threefold increase in the T_3 level in 3 days.
- Assess the patient's and family's knowledge of drug therapy.

(Prioritize hypothesis—priority patient problems)
- Altered health maintenance
- Injury risk
- Knowledge deficiency

(Generate solutions)
- The patient's thyroid levels will reach and remain within normal limits.
- The patient remains free from signs and symptoms of toxicity.
- The patient and family members will demonstrate an understanding of drug therapy.

Medication administration

(Take action)
- Assess for adverse reactions and drug interactions.
- Monitor the patient's pulse rate and blood pressure.

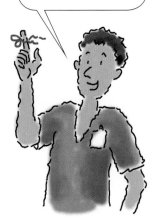

Remember, there is a narrow therapeutic range for thyroid drugs. Educate patients that thyroid level checks are important to maintain optimum therapeutic results.

- In a patient with coronary artery disease receiving thyroid hormone, watch for possible coronary insufficiency.
- Thyroid hormone dosages vary widely. Begin treatment at the lowest level, adjusting to higher doses according to the patient's symptoms and laboratory data, until a euthyroid state is reached.
- When changing from levothyroxine to liothyronine, stop levothyroxine and then start liothyronine. The dosage is increased in small increments after residual effects of levothyroxine disappear. When changing from liothyronine to levothyroxine, start levothyroxine several days before withdrawing liothyronine to avoid relapse.
- Give thyroid hormones at the same time each day, preferably in the morning, to prevent insomnia. This medication should be taken on an empty stomach.
- Thyroid drugs may be supplied either in micrograms (mcg) or in milligrams (mg). Do not confuse these dose measurements.
- Thyroid hormones alter thyroid function test results. A patient taking levothyroxine who needs radioactive iodine uptake studies must discontinue the drug 4 weeks before the test.
- A patient taking a prescribed anticoagulant with thyroid hormones usually needs a reduced anticoagulant dosage.
- If the patient has diabetes, they may need an increased antidiabetic dosage when starting the thyroid hormone replacement.
- Instruct the patient never to stop the drug abruptly. Therapy is usually lifelong.

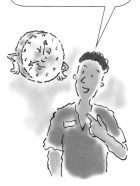

Give thyroid hormones at the same time each day, preferably in the morning, to prevent insomnia.

Postadministration
(Evaluate outcomes)
- Observe and monitor for adverse reactions and drug interactions.
- Evaluate the patient's thyroid hormone levels.
- The patient sustains no injury from adverse reactions.
- Monitor the patient for signs of thyrotoxicosis or inadequate dosage, including diarrhea, fever, irritability, listlessness, rapid heartbeat, vomiting, and weakness.
- Monitor prothrombin time (PT) and international normalized ratio. Patients taking anticoagulants usually need lower doses.
- Evaluate the patient's and family's knowledge of drug therapy.

Antithyroid drugs

A number of drugs act as antithyroid drugs, or *thyroid antagonists*. Used for patients with hyperthyroidism (thyrotoxicosis), these drugs include:
- thioamides, which include propylthiouracil (PTU) and methimazole (Tapazole)

- iodides, which include stable iodine and radioactive iodine (prophylaxis for patient radiation exposure).

Pharmacokinetics

Thioamides and iodides are absorbed through the GI tract, concentrated in the thyroid, and metabolized by conjugation. They are excreted in urine.

Pharmacodynamics

Drugs used to treat hyperthyroidism work in different ways.

Stopping synthesis

Thioamides block iodine's ability to combine with tyrosine, thereby preventing thyroid hormone synthesis (Katzung, 2018).

Inhibited by iodine

Stable iodine inhibits hormone synthesis through the Wolff-Chaikoff effect, in which excess iodine decreases the formation and release of thyroid hormone (Ross, 2020).

Reduced by radiation

Radioactive iodine reduces hormone secretion by destroying thyroid tissue through induction of acute radiation thyroiditis (inflammation of the thyroid gland) and chronic gradual thyroid atrophy. Acute radiation thyroiditis usually occurs 3 to 10 days after administering radioactive iodine (Katzung, 2018). Chronic thyroid atrophy may take several years to appear.

Pharmacotherapeutics

Antithyroid drugs commonly are used to treat hyperthyroidism, especially Graves' disease (hyperthyroidism caused by autoimmunity), which accounts for 60% to 80% of all cases (Pokhrel & Bhusal, 2020).

Thioamides

Propylthiouracil (PTU), which lowers serum T_3 levels faster than methimazole (Tapazole), is usually used for rapid improvement of severe hyperthyroidism.

Good for gravidas

Propylthiouracil (PTU) is preferred in the first trimester of pregnancy. Methimazole (Tapazole) is used in the second and third trimesters. There have been some reported side effects with methimazole. Both of these drugs are used cautiously in patients who are pregnant or lactating.

Propylthiouracil (PTU) and methimazole (Tapazole) are distributed in breast milk. Patients receiving these drugs should make a plan with their health care provider before starting therapy.

Once a day

Because methimazole (Tapazole) blocks thyroid hormone formation for a longer time, it is better suited for administration once per day to a patient with mild to moderate hyperthyroidism. Therapy may continue for 12 to 24 months before remission occurs.

Iodides

To treat hyperthyroidism, the thyroid gland may be removed by surgery or destroyed by radiation. Before surgery, stable iodine is used to prepare the gland for surgical removal by firming it and decreasing its vascularity. Stable iodine is also used after radioactive iodine therapy to control signs and symptoms of hyperthyroidism while the radiation takes effect.

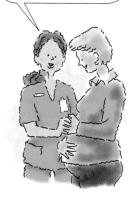

Propylthiouracil use is preferred in pregnant women because its rapid action reduces transfer of the drug across the placenta…

Drug interactions

Iodide preparations may react synergistically with lithium (Lithobid), causing hypothyroidism. Other interactions with antithyroid drugs are not clinically significant.

Side effects/adverse reactions

The most serious adverse reaction to thioamide therapy is agranulocytosis (McCuistion et al., 2020). Hypersensitivity reactions may also occur.

(Not) a spoonful of sugar

The iodides can cause an unpleasant brassy taste and burning sensation in the mouth, increased salivation, and painful swelling of the parotid glands.

The Three-Step Approach

Nursing management for patients undergoing treatment with antithyroid medications includes these three steps.

 Black Box Warning

Preparing for practice: Iodine

Rare, but be aware…
Rarely, IV iodine administration can cause an acute hypersensitivity reaction. Radioactive iodine also can cause a rare but acute reaction 3 to 14 days after administration.

Preadministration

(Recognize and analyze cues)
- Assess the patient's condition and thyroid function tests before therapy begins.

(Prioritize hypothesis—priority patient problems)
- Altered health maintenance
- Activity intolerance
- Injury risk
- Knowledge deficiency

(Generate solutions)
- The patient's thyroid levels will stabilize and settle within normal limits.
- The patient will reach desired activity level.
- The patient will encounter no harm.
- The patient and family will demonstrate an understanding of drug therapy.

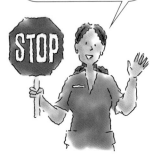

Stop the drug and notify the prescriber if a severe rash or enlarged cervical lymph nodes develop.

Medication administration

(Take action)
- Give propylthiouracil (PTU) several times a day due to its short half-life. Methimazole (Tapazole) is usually given once a day.
- Monitor for sore throat or fever with propylthiouracil (PTU).
- Give fruit juice to dilute the strong taste of iodine solution.
- Observe the patient for immediate and delayed reactions from the drug therapy.
- If adverse GI reactions occur, monitor the patient's hydration status.
- Monitor the patient for fatigue and activity intolerance.

A rash decision
- Discontinue the drug and notify the prescriber if the patient develops a severe rash or enlarged cervical lymph nodes.

Postadministration

(Evaluate outcomes)
- Monitor the patient's activity tolerance during therapy and report changes.
- Watch for signs of hypothyroidism (depression, cold intolerance, nonpitting edema) and adjust the dosage as directed.
- Monitor complete blood count (CBC) as directed to detect impending leukopenia, thrombocytopenia, and agranulocytosis.
- Evaluate the patient's and family's knowledge of thyroid and antithyroid therapy. (See *Teaching about thyroid and antithyroid drugs*, page 485.)

Teaching about thyroid and antithyroid drugs

See Education edge: Teaching template in Chapter 3 page 38 for general teaching for all medications. Specific points to review with patients and family for thyroid or antithyroid drugs:

- Take the drug exactly as prescribed, at the same time each day, preferably in the morning before breakfast, to maintain constant hormone levels. Taking the drug in the morning prevents insomnia.
- Report signs and symptoms of thyroid hormone overdose (chest pain, palpitations, sweating, nervousness) or aggravated cardiovascular disease (chest pain, dyspnea, tachycardia).
- If taking antithyroid drugs, report skin eruptions (signs of hypersensitivity), fever, sore throat, or mouth sores (early signs of agranulocytosis).
- Ask the prescriber about using iodized salt and eating shellfish, especially if taking antithyroid medications, to avoid possible toxic levels of iodine.

- If a stable response has been achieved, don't change drug brands.
- Children may lose hair during the first months of therapy; this is a temporary reaction.
- Report unusual bleeding or bruising.
- Keep follow-up appointments and have thyroid levels tested regularly.
- Do not use other drugs, over-the-counter products, or herbal remedies without first consulting with the prescriber or a pharmacist.

Pituitary drugs

Pituitary drugs are natural or synthetic hormones that mimic the hormones produced by the pituitary gland. The pituitary drugs consist of two groups:

1. **Anterior pituitary drugs**: may be used diagnostically or therapeutically to control the function of other endocrine glands, such as the thyroid gland, adrenals, ovaries, and testes.
2. **Posterior pituitary drugs**: may be used to regulate fluid volume and stimulate smooth muscle contraction in selected clinical situations.

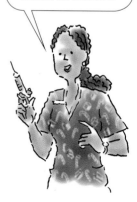

Anterior pituitary drugs control the function of endocrine glands. Posterior pituitary drugs regulate fluid volume and stimulate smooth muscle contraction.

Anterior pituitary drugs

The protein hormones produced in the anterior pituitary gland regulate growth, development, and sexual characteristics by stimulating the actions of other endocrine glands. Anterior pituitary drugs include:

- adrenocorticotropics, which include corticotropin, corticotropin repository (H.P. Acthar), and cosyntropin (Cortrosyn)

- somatropin (Genotropin) growth hormone
- gonadotropics, which include chorionic gonadotropin and menotropins (Menopur)
- thyrotropics, which include TSH and thyrotropin alfa (Thyrogen).

Pharmacokinetics

Anterior pituitary drugs are not given orally because they are destroyed in the GI tract. Some of these hormones can be administered topically, but most require injection.

Sometimes slower than mother nature

Usually, natural hormones are absorbed, distributed, and metabolized rapidly. Some analogues, however, are absorbed and metabolized more slowly. Anterior pituitary hormone drugs are metabolized at the receptor site and in the liver and kidneys. The hormones are excreted primarily in urine.

Pharmacodynamics

Anterior pituitary drugs exert a profound effect on the body's growth and development. The hypothalamus controls secretions of the pituitary gland. In turn, the pituitary gland secretes hormones that regulate secretions or functions of other glands.

Production managers

The concentration of hormones in the blood helps determine the hormone production rate. Increased hormone levels inhibit hormone production while decreased levels raise production and secretion. Anterior pituitary drugs, therefore, control hormone production by increasing or decreasing the body's hormone levels.

Pharmacotherapeutics

The clinical indications for anterior pituitary hormone drugs are diagnostic and therapeutic:

- Corticotropin and cosyntropin (Cortrosyn) are used diagnostically to differentiate between primary and secondary failure of the adrenal cortex.
- Corticotropin is used as an anti-inflammatory drug in allergic responses and can decrease symptoms of multiple sclerosis exacerbations.
- Somatropin (Genotropin) is used to treat pediatric patients with growth failure due to an inadequate secretion of endogenous growth hormone.
- In males, chorionic gonadotropin is used to evaluate testosterone production, treat hypogonadism, and treat cryptorchidism (undescended testes).

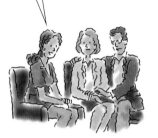

Chorionic gonadotropin and menotropins are used to induce ovulation for women during fertility treatment.

- In women, chorionic gonadotropin and menotropins (Menopur) are used to help induce ovulation during infertility treatments.
- Thyrotropin alfa (Thyrogen) is a synthetic TSH used to treat and evaluate treatment for thyroid cancer.

Drug interactions

Anterior pituitary drugs interact with several different types of drugs:
- Administering immunizations to a person receiving corticotropin increases the risk of neurologic complications and may reduce the antibody response.
- Enhanced potassium loss may occur when diuretics are taken with corticotropins.
- Barbiturates, phenytoin (Dilantin), and rifampin increase the metabolism of corticotropin, reducing its effects.
- Estrogen increases the effect of corticotropin.
- Taking estrogens, amphetamines, and lithium (Lithobid) with cosyntropin can alter results of adrenal function tests.
- Amphetamines and androgens (concurrently) administered with somatropin (Genotropin) may promote epiphyseal (cartilaginous bone growth plate) closure.
- Concurrent use of somatropin (Genotropin) and corticosteroids inhibits the growth-promoting action of somatropin (Genotropin).
- Increased insulin and oral antidiabetic doses may be needed with corticotropin.

Side effects/adverse reactions

The major adverse reactions to pituitary drugs are hypersensitivity reactions. Long-term corticotropin use can cause Cushing's syndrome.

The Three-Step Approach

Nursing management for patient undergoing treatment with anterior pituitary drugs includes these three steps.

Preadministration

(Recognize and analyze cues)
- Assess the patient's underlying condition before therapy and regularly during therapy.

(Prioritize hypothesis—priority patient problems)
- Altered health maintenance
- Altered body image perception
- Knowledge deficiency

(Generate solutions)
- The patient's underlying condition will improve.
- The patient will discuss and express feelings about their body image.

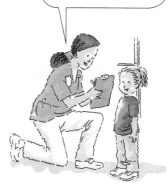

Children taking anterior pituitary drugs should have their growth assessed regularly.

- The patient and family members will demonstrate an understanding of the diagnostic test or drug therapy ordered.

Medication administration

(Take action)

- Administer the drug as prescribed and monitor for effects.
- If administering corticotropin IV, dilute it in 500 mL of dextrose 5% in water and infuse over 8 hours.
- If administering corticotropin gel, warm it to room temperature and draw it into a large needle. Replace the needle with a 21G or 22G needle. Give slowly as a deep IM injection. Warn the patient that the injection is painful.
- Refrigerate reconstituted solution and use it within 24 hours.
- Assess for hypersensitivity and allergic reactions and have adrenal responsiveness verified before starting corticotropin treatment.

Postadministration

(Evaluate outcomes)

- Assess for adverse reactions and drug interactions.
- Note and record weight changes, fluid exchange, and resting blood pressures until the minimal effective dosage is achieved.
- Assess neonates of corticotropin-treated mothers for signs of hypoadrenalism.
- With somatropin (Genotropin), observe the patient for signs of glucose intolerance, hyperglycemia, and hypothyroidism. Periodic thyroid function tests may be required.
- Counteract edema with a low-sodium, high-potassium diet; nitrogen loss, with a high-protein diet; and psychotic changes, with a reduction in corticotropin dosage or use of sedatives.
- Monitor the patient for stress. Unusual stress may require additional use of rapidly acting corticosteroids. When possible, gradually reduce the corticotropin dosage to the smallest effective dosage to minimize induced adrenocortical insufficiency. Therapy can be restarted if a stressful situation, such as trauma, surgery, or severe illness, occurs shortly after stopping the drug.
- For children, monitor height and blood with regular checkups. Radiologic studies may also be needed.
- Monitor the patient for changes in body image.
- Evaluate the patient's and family's knowledge of drug therapy.

Posterior pituitary drugs

Posterior pituitary hormones are synthesized in the hypothalamus and stored in the posterior pituitary, which, in turn, secretes the hormones into the blood. Posterior pituitary drugs include:

- all forms of antidiuretic hormone (ADH), such as desmopressin acetate (DDAVP) and vasopressin (Vasostrict)
- the oxytocic drug oxytocin (Pitocin).

Pharmacokinetics

Because enzymes in the GI tract can destroy all protein hormones, these drugs cannot be given orally. Posterior pituitary drugs may be given by injection or intranasal spray (Katzung, 2018).

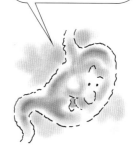

> Posterior pituitary drugs can't be given orally because enzymes in the GI tract destroy protein hormones.

ADH on the move

ADH is distributed throughout extracellular fluid and does not appear to bind with protein. Most of the drug is metabolized rapidly in the liver and kidneys. It is excreted in urine.

Slower (or maybe faster) by a nose

Like other natural hormones, oxytocin (Pitocin) is absorbed, distributed, and metabolized rapidly. However, when oxytocin (Pitocin) is administered intranasally, absorption is erratic.

Pharmacodynamics

Under neural control, posterior pituitary hormones affect:
- smooth muscle contraction in the uterus, bladder, and GI tract
- fluid balance through kidney reabsorption of water
- blood pressure through stimulation of the arterial wall muscles.

On the rise

ADH increases cAMP, which increases the permeability of the tubular epithelium in the kidneys, promoting reabsorption of water. High dosages of ADH stimulate contraction of blood vessels, increasing blood pressure (Katzung, 2018).

Less…and more

Desmopressin (DDAVP) reduces diuresis and promotes clotting by increasing the plasma level of factor VIII (antihemophilic factor).

Mother's little helper

In a pregnant woman, oxytocin may stimulate uterine contractions by increasing the permeability of uterine cell membranes to sodium ions. It can also stimulate lactation through its effect on mammary glands.

Pharmacotherapeutics

Desmopressin (DDAVP) is the drug of choice for patients with neurogenic diabetes insipidus (an excessive loss of urine caused by a brain lesion or injury that interferes with ADH synthesis or release) (Katzung, 2018). However, it does not effectively treat nephrogenic diabetes insipidus (caused by renal tubular resistance to ADH).

The long and short of ADH therapy

Short-term desmopressin (DDAVP) is indicated for patients with transient diabetes insipidus after head injury or surgery. Therapy may be lifelong for patients with idiopathic hormone deficiency.

The dirt on desmopressin

Desmopressin (DDAVP) is the drug of choice for chronic ADH deficiency. It is also indicated for primary nocturnal enuresis. Desmopressin (DDAVP) is administered intranasally, has a long duration of action, and a relative lack of adverse effects.

A lesson on vasopressin

Used for short-term therapy, vasopressin (Vasostrict) elevates blood pressure in patients with hypotension caused by lack of vascular tone. High-dose vasopressin (Vasostrict) can be given during a pulseless cardiac arrest in place of epinephrine (Katzung, 2018). Additionally, vasopressin (Vasostrict) may be used for transient polyuria resulting from ADH deficiency related to neurosurgery or head injury.

Partum me, is this the OB?

Oxytocin (Pitocin) is used to:
* induce labor
* complete incomplete abortions
* treat preeclampsia, eclampsia, and premature rupture of the membranes
* control bleeding and uterine relaxation after delivery
* hasten uterine shrinking after delivery
* stimulate lactation.

It is a chore

Oxytocin (Pitocin) is used to induce or support the labor process only when:
* vaginal delivery is indicated
* the fetus is mature
* the fetal position is favorable
* critical care facilities and an experienced clinician are immediately available.

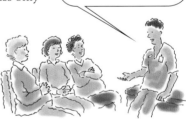

Oxytocin may be used under certain conditions to induce or support the labor process.

Drug interactions

Various drugs may interact with posterior pituitary drugs:
* Alcohol, demeclocycline, and lithium (Lithobid) may decrease ADH activity of desmopressin (DDAVP) and vasopressin (Vasostrict).
* Carbamazepine (Tegretol) and cyclophosphamide (Cytoxan) increase ADH activity.

- Synergistic effects may occur when barbiturates are used concurrently with ADH, leading to coronary insufficiency or dysrhythmias.
- Cyclophosphamide (Cytoxan) may increase the effect of oxytocin (Pitocin).
- Concurrent use of vasopressors (anesthetics, ephedrine, methoxamine) and oxytocin (Pitocin) increases the risk of hypertensive crisis and postpartum rupture of cerebral blood vessels.

Side effects/adverse reactions

Hypersensitivity reactions are the most common adverse reactions to posterior pituitary drugs. Desmopressin (DDAVP) and vasopressin (Vasostrict) can cause:

- seizures
- anaphylaxis
- anxiety
- hyponatremia (low serum sodium levels)
- water intoxication
- headache
- transient edema.
  Adverse reactions to synthetic ADH are rare.

"Expecting" some problems

Synthetic oxytocin (Pitocin) can cause adverse reactions for pregnant women, including:

- seizures
- cardiac dysrhythmias
- bleeding after delivery
- GI disturbances
- sweating
- headache
- dizziness
- ringing in the ears
- severe water intoxication.

The Three-Step Approach

Nursing management for patients undergoing treatment with posterior pituitary hormones includes these three steps.

Preadministration

(Recognize and analyze cues)

- Obtain a history of the patient's underlying condition before starting therapy.
- Assess the patient for baseline measurements and labs as appropriate before starting therapy.

(Prioritize hypothesis—priority patient problems)
- Electrolyte imbalance risk
- Altered health maintenance
- Knowledge deficiency

(Generate solutions)
- The patient's fluid and electrolyte levels will remain within normal limits throughout treatment.
- The patient will show increased engagement in their care process and treatment course.
- The patient and family will demonstrate an understanding of drug therapy.

Medication administration

(Take action)
- Administer the drug according to the prescriber's instructions and monitor for effect.
- Monitor the patient carefully for hypertension and water intoxication when giving ADH drugs. Seizures, coma, and death can occur from water intoxication. Watch for excessively elevated blood pressure or lack of response to the drug, which may be indicated by hypotension. Weigh the patient daily.
- Desmopressin (DDAVP) injection should not be used to treat severe cases of von Willebrand's disease or hemophilia A with factor VIII levels of 0% to 5%.
- When desmopressin (DDAVP) is used to treat diabetes insipidus, the dosage or frequency of administration may be adjusted according to the patient's fluid output. Morning and evening doses are adjusted separately for adequate diurnal rhythm of water turnover.
- Teach the patient and the caregivers how to properly measure and inhale the intranasal form of ADH. (See *Teaching about ADH.*)
- The patient and family will demonstrate an understanding of drug therapy.

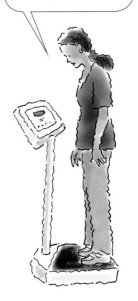

Patients taking posterior pituitary drugs should be weighed daily.

Ban the bolus
- Oxytocin is administered only by IV infusion, not by IV bolus.
- When administering oxytocin, monitor and record uterine contractions, heart rate, blood pressure, intrauterine pressure, fetal heart rate, and blood loss every 15 minutes. Also monitor the patient's fluid intake and output. Antidiuretic effect may lead to fluid overload, seizures, and coma.
- Have magnesium sulfate (20% solution) available for relaxation of the myometrium when administering oxytocin.
- If contractions are less than 2 minutes apart, if they are above 50 mm Hg, or if they last 90 seconds or longer, stop oxytocin infusion, turn the patient on her left side, and notify the prescriber.

Teaching about ADH drugs

See Education edge: Teaching template in Chapter 3 page 38 for general teaching for all medications. Specific points to review with patients and family if an ADH drug is prescribed:

• Clear the nasal passages before using the drug intranasally.

• Report such conditions as nasal congestion, allergic rhinitis, or upper respiratory tract infection; a dosage adjustment may be needed.

• If using subcutaneous desmopressin (DDAVP), rotate injection sites to avoid tissue damage.

• Drink only enough water to satisfy thirst.

• Monitor fluid intake and output.

• Wear or carry medical identification indicating that you are using ADH.

Postadministration

(Evaluate outcomes)

• Observe the patient for any medication reactions.

• Assess the effectiveness of ADH medications by checking the patient's fluid intake and output, serum and urine osmolality, and urine specific gravity.

• Evaluate the patient's and family's knowledge of drug therapy and reeducate as appropriate. (*See Teaching about ADH drugs.*)

• Monitor electrolyte levels based on drug given.

• Ensure that the patient has the resources necessary to make lifestyle changes related to health maintenance.

• Evaluate the patient's and family's knowledge of ADH drug therapy.

Estrogens

Estrogens mimic the physiologic effects of naturally occurring female sex hormones. They are used to correct estrogen-deficient states and, along with hormonal contraceptives, to prevent pregnancy.

Natural and synthetic estrogens

Estrogens that treat endocrine system disorders include:

• natural conjugated estrogenic substances (estradiol [Estrace] and estropipate)

• synthetic estrogens (esterified estrogens, estradiol cypionate, estradiol valerate, and ethinyl estradiol).

Pharmacokinetics

Estrogens are absorbed well and distributed throughout the body. Metabolism occurs in the liver, and the metabolites are excreted primarily by the kidneys.

Pharmacodynamics

The exact mechanism of action of estrogen is not clearly understood. It is believed to increase synthesis of deoxyribonucleic acid, ribonucleic acid, and protein in estrogen-responsive tissues in the female breast, urinary tract, and genital organs (Katzung, 2018). (See *Estrogens: Conjugated estrogenic substances.*)

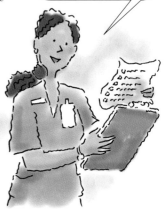

Vasomotor menopausal symptoms also known as "HOT FLASHES" can be treated with hormone replacement therapy.

Pharmacotherapeutics

Estrogens are prescribed:
- primarily for hormone replacement therapy in postmenopausal women to relieve symptoms caused by loss of ovarian function
- less commonly for hormone replacement therapy in women with primary ovarian failure or female hypogonadism (reduced hormonal secretion by the ovaries) and in patients who have undergone removal of ovaries

Prototype pro

Estrogens: Conjugated estrogenic substances

Actions
- Increases synthesis of deoxyribonucleic acid, ribonucleic acid, and protein in responsive tissues
- Reduces release of follicle-stimulating hormone and luteinizing hormone from the pituitary gland

Indications
- Abnormal uterine bleeding
- Palliative treatment of breast cancer at least 5 years after menopause
- removal of ovaries
- Primary ovarian failure
- Osteoporosis
- Hypogonadism
- Vasomotor menopausal symptoms
- Atrophic vaginitis, kraurosis vulvae

- Palliative treatment of inoperable prostate cancer
- Vulvar and vaginal atrophy

Nursing considerations
- Monitor the patient for adverse reactions, including seizures, thromboembolism and increased risk of stroke, pancreatitis, pulmonary embolism, myocardial infarction.
- Educate the patient about increased risk for endometrial cancer, hepatic adenoma, and breast cancer.
- Because of the risk of thromboembolism, therapy should be discontinued at least 1 month before procedures that may cause prolonged immobilization or thromboembolism, such as knee or hip surgery.
- Give oral forms at mealtime or at bedtime (if only once-daily dose is required) to minimize nausea.

- palliatively to treat advanced, inoperable breast cancer in postmenopausal women and prostate cancer in men.

Drug interactions

Relatively few drugs interact with estrogens:
- Estrogens may decrease the effects of anticoagulants, increasing the risk of blood clots.
- Carbamazepine (Tegretol), phenytoin (Dilantin), barbiturates, antibiotics, primidone (Mysoline), and rifampin reduce estrogen's effectiveness.
- Estrogens interfere with the absorption of dietary folic acid, which may result in a folic acid deficiency.

Side effects/adverse reactions

Adverse reactions to estrogens include:
- hypertension
- thromboembolism (blood vessel blockage caused by a blood clot)
- thrombophlebitis (vein inflammation associated with clot formation)
- stroke
- depression
- myocardial infarction
- vaginal bleeding.

The Three-Step Approach

Nursing management for patients undergoing treatment with estrogens includes these three steps.

Preadministration

(Recognize and analyze cues)
- Assess and obtain a history of the patient's underlying condition before therapy and reassess regularly thereafter.
- Ensure that the patient has a thorough physical examination before starting estrogen therapy.

(Prioritize hypothesis—priority patient problems)
- Nausea/GI upset risk
- Venous thromboembolism risk
- Knowledge deficiency

(Generate solutions)
- The patient will remain free of GI upset while taking estrogen preparation.
- The patient will remain free of thrombus and related issues (stroke, heart attack, etc.).
- The patient and family will demonstrate an understanding of drug therapy.

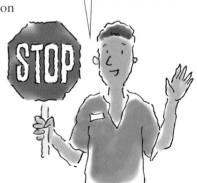

Stop estrogen therapy if a thromboembolic event is suspected.

Medication administration

(Take action)

- Notify the pathologist about the patient's estrogen therapy when sending specimens for evaluation.
- Keep in mind that estrogens often are given cyclically (once daily for 3 weeks, followed by 1 week without drugs).
- Administer the drug as prescribed and monitor for effects.
- Stop drug and notify the prescriber if a thromboembolic event is suspected. Be prepared to provide supportive care as indicated.
- Teach the patient how to apply estrogen ointments or transdermal estrogen or how to insert an intravaginal estrogen suppository. Also, inform the patient of the signs and symptoms that accompany a systemic reaction to ointments. (See *Teaching about estrogens.*)

Postadministration

- Observe the patient for immediate and delayed reactions from therapy.

Education edge

Teaching about estrogens

See Education edge: Teaching template in Chapter 3 page 38 for general teaching for all medications. Specific points to review with patients and family if estrogens are prescribed:

- When taken orally, take with meals or at bedtime to relieve nausea. Nausea usually disappears with sustained therapy.
- Review how to apply estrogen ointments or transdermal estrogen.
- Be aware of signs and symptoms that accompany a systemic reaction to ointments.
- Use sanitary pads instead of tampons when using the suppository.
- Stop taking the drug immediately if pregnancy occurs (estrogens can harm the fetus).
- Do not breast-feed during estrogen therapy.
- If receiving cyclic therapy for postmenopausal symptoms, withdrawal bleeding may occur during the week off. However, fertility is not restored, and ovulation does not occur.
- Medical supervision is essential during prolonged therapy.

- Males on long-term therapy may experience temporary gynecomastia and impotence, which will disappear when therapy ends.
- Report abdominal pain; pain, numbness, or stiffness in the legs or buttocks; pressure or pain in the chest; shortness of breath; severe headaches; vision disturbances (such as blind spots, flashing lights, or blurriness); vaginal bleeding or discharge; breast lumps; swelling of hands or feet; yellow skin and sclera; dark urine; or light-colored stools to the prescriber immediately.
- If diabetic, report symptoms of hyperglycemia or glycosuria.
- Keep follow-up appointments for gynecologic examinations, clinical breast examinations, and mammography. Perform breast self-examinations as instructed.

- Ensure that the patient understands the risk factors, signs, and symptoms related to thromboembolism.
- Promote measures to relieve nausea, vomiting, and other adverse reactions.
- Monitor the patient regularly to detect improvement or worsening of symptoms.
- Assess for adverse reactions and drug interactions.
- Evaluate the patient's and family's knowledge of drug therapy
- Ensure that estrogens are used for the shortest time necessary for postmenopausal symptoms.

Year in, year out
- A patient receiving long-term therapy should have yearly breast, pelvic, and physical examinations. Periodically monitor lipid levels, blood pressure, body weight, and liver function.
- If the patient has diabetes mellitus, watch closely for loss of glucose control.
- If the patient is also receiving a warfarin-type anticoagulant, monitor PT. If ordered, adjust the anticoagulant dosage.

Quick quiz

1. The nurse is caring for a patient with hyperkalemia. Which type of insulin will the nurse anticipate administering?
   A. NPH insulin
   B. Lispro insulin
   C. Regular insulin
   D. Glargine insulin

Answer: C. Use regular insulin in a patient with circulatory collapse, DKA, or hyperkalemia. NPH, lispro and glargine insulins are not used in treating hyperkalemia.

2. A patient is prescribed glyburide (DiaBeta). When will the nurse instruct the patient to take the medication?
   A. At bedtime
   B. Right after dinner
   C. 2 hours after eating
   D. Just prior to breakfast

Answer: D. Glyburide (DiaBeta) should be administered before the morning meal to prevent nighttime hypoglycemic reactions.

3. After a head injury, a patient has developed diabetes insipidus. Which medication will the nurse anticipate being prescribed?
   A. Oxytocin (Pitocin)
   B. Vasopressin (Vasostrict)
   C. Desmopressin (DDAVP)
   D. Carbamazepine (Tegretol)

Answer: C. Desmopressin (DDAVP) mimics the actions of endogenous ADH and therefore helps to treat the symptoms of diabetes insipidus caused by head trauma. Oxytocin is used to induce labor and support the labor process. Vasopressin may be used for transient polyuria resulting from ADH deficiency related to neurosurgery or head injury. Carbamazepine is an anticonvulsant agent.

4. A nurse is managing an oxytocin infusion for a patient in labor. When would the nurse stop the infusion?
   A. When contractions stop.
   B. When contractions begin.
   C. Contractions are less than 2 minutes apart.
   D. Contractions last between 10 and 20 seconds.

Answer: C. When contractions are less than 2 minutes apart, oxytocin should be stopped, the patient placed on the left side, and the provider notified.

5. A nurse is teaching a patient about estrogen therapy. Which would the nurse include in the teaching?
   A. Continue use during pregnancy.
   B. Use tampons instead of sanitary pads.
   C. Avoid breast-feeding when taking estrogens.
   D. Take the estrogen medication on an empty stomach.

Answer: C. Patients on estrogen therapy should be taught to avoid breast-feeding during estrogen, use sanitary pads instead of tampons, take estrogen with food or meals, and not to use during pregnancy.

Scoring

☆☆☆   If you answered all five questions correctly, perfect! There's no end to your endocrine drug knowledge!

☆☆   If you answered three or four questions correctly, marvelous! You've done your homework on homeostasis and hormones.

☆   If you answered fewer than three questions correctly, don't sink too low. You can always give the chapter another go.

Suggested References

American Diabetes Association (ADA). (2020a). *Diabetes: The path to understanding starts here.* Retrieved from https://diabetes.org/diabetes

American Diabetes Association (ADA). (2020b). *Insulin basics.* Retrieved from https://www.diabetes.org/healthy-living/medication-treatments/insulin-other-injectables/insulin-basics

Dungan, K. (2020). Amylin analogs for the treatment of diabetes mellitus. In I. B. Hirsch & J. E. Mulder (Eds.), *UpToDate.* Retrieved from https://www.uptodate.com/contents/amylin-analogs-for-the-treatment-of-diabetes-mellitus

Eghtedari, B., & Correa, R. (2020). Levothyroxine. In *StatPearls.* Treasure Island, FL: StatPearls Publishing. Retrieved from https://www.ncbi.nlm.nih.gov/books/NBK539808/

Ignatavicius, D. D., Workman, M. L., Rebar, C. R., & Heimgartner, N. M. (2021). *Medical-surgical nursing: Concepts for interprofessional collaborative care* (10th ed.). St. Louis, MO: Elsevier.

Katzung, B. G. (2018). *Basic and clinical pharmacology* (14th ed.). New York, NY: McGraw-Hill Education.

Martin, K. A., & Barbieri, R. L. (2020). Treatment of menopausal symptoms with hormone therapy. In J. E. Mulder & W. F. Crowley (Eds.), *UpToDate.* Retrieved from https://www.uptodate.com/contents/treatment-of-menopausal-symptoms-with-hormone-therapy

McCuistion, L. E., Vuljoin-DiMaggio, K., Winton, M. B., & Yeager, J. J. (2020). *Pharmacology: A patient-centered nursing process approach* (10th ed.). St. Louis, MO: Elsevier.

Pokhrel, B., & Bhusal, K. (2020). Graves' disease. In *StatPearls.* Treasure Island, FL: StatPearls Publishing. Retrieved from https://www.ncbi.nlm.nih.gov/books/NBK448195/

Ross, D. S. (2020). Iodine in the treatment of hyperthyroidism. In J. E. Mulder & D. S. Cooper (Eds.), *UpToDate.* Retrieved from https://www.uptodate.com/contents/iodine-in-the-treatment-of-hyperthyroidism

Skidmore-Roth, L. (2020). *Nursing drug reference* (33rd ed.). St. Louis, MO: Elsevier.

Chapter 14

Sensory drugs

Just the facts

In this chapter, you'll learn:

◆ classes of drugs used to treat ophthalmic and otic disorders

◆ uses and actions of these drugs

◆ absorption, distribution, metabolization, and excretion of these drugs

◆ drug interactions, side effects, and adverse reactions to these drugs.

Ophthalmic drugs

Drugs used for eye conditions can be classified into several types. These types include:
- antiallergic
- anesthetics
- anti-infectives
- anti-inflammatories
- lubricants
- mydriatics and cycloplegics
- drugs to lower intraocular pressure (IOP).

Most of these drugs are administered topically unless otherwise noted in the discussion. The three-step approach for safe administration of all ophthalmic drugs is presented in page 511.

Antiallergic

Oh my itchy eyes!

Itchy eyes can often be caused by allergens. Antiallergic ophthalmic drugs consist of anti-histamines and mast cell stabilizers. Antiallergic medications work to decrease eye irritation and itching. They are typically used to treat allergic conjunctivitis and keratitis. Common medications include:
- alcaftadine (Lastacaft)
- azelastine

- bepotastine (Bepreve)
- cetirizine (Zerviate)
- cromolyn
- epinastine
- ketotifen
- lodoxamide (Alomide)
- Nedocromil (Alocril)
- olopatadine.

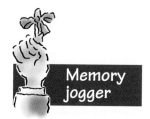

Pharmacokinetics

These agents typically have minimal systemic absorption. Azelastine, ketotifen, and olopatadine, however, are metabolized by the liver. They are primarily excreted in urine, feces, and occasionally bile.

Pharmacodynamics

Antihistamines selectively block histamine receptors, which prevents histamine release from mast cells. Mast cell stabilizers also inhibit histamine release by preventing mast cell degranulation.

Are you crying???

While there are no significant drug interactions in this drug class, the most common side effect is ocular burning and tearing. Occasionally, headache, fatigue, and pharyngitis may occur.

Another thing....

- Cromolyn can cause pancytopenia, so monitor those blood counts!
- Educate your patient that lodoxamide can cause corneal ulcer and ocular edema.

Anesthetics

Anesthetics are used to anesthetize the cornea to allow for application of instruments to measuring intraocular pressure (IOP), to remove foreign bodies or sutures, for conjunctival or corneal scraping, and for tear duct manipulation.

Anesthetic eyedrops, or numbing medications, include:
- proparacaine (Alcaine)
- tetracaine.

Pharmacokinetics

These medications are metabolized in plasma and excreted in urine.

Pharmacodynamics

Anesthetic eyedrops prevent irritation and transmission of nerve impulses by inhibiting sodium ion channels and stabilizing the membranes of nerve cells.

Side effects/Adverse reactions

Side effects include corneal opacities, delayed corneal healing, eye pain, redness, and contact dermatitis. Rarely, drugs in this class can cause seizures and central nervous system (CNS) depression, so be sure to educate your patient on this. There are no significant drug interactions with this class.

Anti-infectives

Anti-infective ophthalmic drugs are used to treat conditions such as corneal ulcers or conjunctivitis caused by bacterial, fungal, or viral organisms. Common anti-infective or antibiotic drugs include:

- azithromycin (AzaSite)
- bacitracin
- ciprofloxacin (Ciloxan)
- erythromycin
- gentamicin
- levofloxacin
- natamycin (Natacyn)
- ofloxacin (Ocuflox)
- sulfacetamide (Bleph-10)
- tobramycin (Tobrex)
- trifluridine (Viroptic)
- trimethoprim-polymyxin B (Polytrim).

Pharmacokinetics

Ciprofloxacin, ofloxacin, and polymyxin B/trimethoprim are metabolized in the liver minimally and so are not absorbed much systemically. Depending on the agent, they are primarily unchanged in urine (40% to 50%), feces (20% to 35%), or bile (4% to 8%).

Erythromycin, azithromycin, and sulfacetamide are mostly metabolized by the liver with minimal system absorption. Bacitracin, gentamicin, natamycin, tobramycin, and trifluridine are not absorbed systemically. Tobramycin is excreted in urine unchanged.

Pharmacodynamics

Most of these drugs work to either kill (bactericidal) or inhibit the growth of bacteria or viruses (bacteriostatic). Erythromycin, azithromycin, and bacitracin can be both bactericidal and bacteriostatic. Natamycin is an antifungal, binding to cell membrane sterols and increasing permeability. Trifluridine works as an antiviral by inhibiting DNA synthesis.

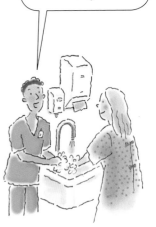

Remember, with anti-infective eyedrops, they are used to treat an infection. Be very careful to wash your hands and do not allow the tip of the eyedrops to contact the eye.

Side effects/Adverse reactions

Common reactions to anti-infective ophthalmic drugs include itching, application site burning, ocular irritation, and conjunctivitis.
- Azithromycin, ciprofloxacin, levofloxacin, and polymyxin B/ trimethoprim can rarely cause superinfections.
- Watch for Stevens-Johnson syndrome with sulfacetamide and tobramycin administration.

Anti-inflammatories

Anti-inflammatory ophthalmic drugs are used to treat inflammatory disorders and hypersensitivity-related conditions of the cornea, iris, conjunctiva, sclera, and anterior uvea. These drugs can be classified into steroidal and nonsteroidal anti-inflammatories.

Steroidal

Steroidal drugs decrease the immune response at sites of inflammation, causing reduced oozing of fluids and reduced edema, redness, and scarring. Steroidal drugs include:
- dexamethasone
- fluorometholone (FML)
- loteprednol (Lotemax)
- prednisolone (Pred Mild).

Pharmacokinetics

Dexamethasone is metabolized locally in the liver with minimal systemic absorption. Dexamethasone and prednisolone are excreted primarily in urine. Loteprednol and prednisolone are locally metabolized locally. All of these agents have minimal systemic absorption.

Drug interactions

Use caution when ophthalmic steroids are given with voclosporin as the combination could raise blood pressure and increase the risk of serious infection. Monitor your patient closely if they are on multiple forms of steroids (inhaled, oral, etc.), as the additive effects could lead to Cushing's syndrome.

Side effects/Adverse reactions

Stinging and burning are common reactions. With prolonged use, there is increased susceptibility to secondary ocular infection, glaucoma, and delayed corneal healing.

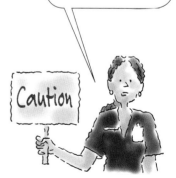

Beware of prolonged use of steroidal eyedrops. While they do not have a high systemic absorption, they can make it easier to develop an eye infection and delay overall healing in the eye.

Nonsteroidal

Nonsteroidal medications are used to decrease inflammation and itching. They help treat ocular inflammation after cataract or corneal refractive surgery.

Nonsteroidal drugs include:
- diclofenac (Voltaren)
- ketorolac (Acular).

Pharmacokinetics

These drugs are metabolized in the liver and are primarily excreted in urine and to a lesser extent in bile.

Pharmacodynamics

How these medications work are not fully understood, but they are thought to inhibit cyclooxygenase, reducing prostaglandin and thromboxane synthesis.

Drug interactions

These medications should not be combined with enoxaparin or fondaparinux when possible due to increased risk for postoperative ocular bleeding. This can also happen to a lesser extent with medications such as sertraline, penicillin G, garlic, and aspirin.

Side effects/Adverse reactions

Common side effects include ocular irritation, corneal opacification, keratitis, and blurred vision. More serious reactions can include corneal ulcers, vitreous detachment, and delayed ocular wound healing.

Lubricants

Ophthalmic lubricants are used to moisten the eye surface. Most lubricant formulations can be found over-the-counter. Some common examples include:
- carboxymethylcellulose (Refresh)
- hydroxypropyl cellulose (Lacrisert)
- polyvinyl alcohol (Tears Again).

Pharmacokinetics

These drugs are not metabolized or systemically absorbed.

Pharmacotherapeutics

These drugs act as artificial tears to lubricate the cornea. They can also work to protect the cornea during diagnostic procedures and can moisten contact lenses.

Do your eyes feel like the sand? Dry and itchy?

Side effects/Adverse reactions

Most side effects are limited to ocular irritation, photophobia, and transient blurred vision.

Mydriatics and cycloplegics

Mydriatics and cycloplegics are utilized to perform diagnostic eye examinations, can be used for procedures on the eye, and are also used to treat conditions involving the iris. Mydriatics dilate the eye, and cycloplegics temporarily paralyze eye muscles. Examples in this class include:

- atropine sulfate (Isopto Atropine)
- cyclopentolate hydrochloride (Cyclogyl)
- phenylephrine
- tropicamide (Mydriacyl).

Some of these drugs also come in combination forms such as hydroxyamphetamine/tropicamide (Paremyd) or phenylephrine/ketorolac (Omidria).

Pharmacokinetics

Atropine is metabolized in the liver. It is excreted primarily in urine.

It is not understood how cyclopentolate and tropicamide are metabolized or excreted. Phenylephrine is metabolized in the liver, but its excretion is unknown.

Pharmacodynamics

Atropine, cyclopentolate, and tropicamide antagonize acetylcholine receptors, inhibiting the response of iris sphincter and ciliary body muscles, causing paralysis and preventing accommodation for near vision.

Phenylephrine stimulates alpha-adrenergic receptors, resulting in dilation and vasoconstriction.

Drug interactions

Atropine, cyclopentolate, and tropicamide should not be combined with clozapine due to risk of paralytic ileus or with inhaled revefenacin due to additive anticholinergic effects. Atropine and phenylephrine can also decrease the effectiveness of some medications used for hypertension such as valsartan and amlodipine and can increase the risk of hypertension when used in combination with ibuprofen, caffeine, and modafinil.

Cyclopentolate and tropicamide combined with clomipramine can increase anticholinergic adverse effects.

Phenylephrine should be avoided in cocaine users due to the risk for severe vasoconstriction and heart arrhythmias. This medication should also not be used in combination with MAO inhibitors such as selegiline and phenelzine.

Side effects/Adverse reactions

Common reactions include blurred vision, ocular irritation, conjunctivitis, increased intraocular pressure, and photophobia. Be on the lookout for seizures, tachycardia, and respiratory depression with atropine, cyclopentolate, and tropicamide. Phenylephrine can also cause reflex bradycardia and, rarely, subarachnoid hemorrhage and myocardial infarction.

My pressure is rising!!

Increased intraocular pressure is associated with several eye conditions such as glaucoma. Medications that lower intraocular pressure (IOP) include:

- beta-adrenergic blockers
- carbonic anhydrase inhibitors
- prostaglandin analogues
- alpha-adrenergic agonists
- cholinergic agents
- rho kinase inhibitors
- osmotic agents.

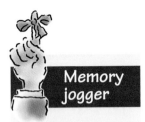

Memory jogger

Glaucoma refers to a group of eye conditions that can lead to blindness. Glaucoma is most often associated with high pressure in the eye. Open-angle glaucoma is the most common and often has no symptoms other than slow visual deterioration. Many eye medications can be used to lower intraocular pressure, which can prevent vision loss.

Beta-adrenergic blockers

Beta-adrenergic blockers prevent and control elevated IOP and are used for acute angle-closure and open-angle glaucoma. These drugs include:

- betaxolol (Betoptic S)
- carteolol
- levobunolol (Betagan)
- timolol maleate (Betimol).

Pharmacokinetics

These drugs are metabolized in the liver. They are excreted primarily in urine.

Betaxolol has minimal systemic absorption, but this information is unknown with carteolol. Levobunolol and timolol are possibly absorbed systemically, as well.

Pharmacodynamics

Beta-blockers may decrease aqueous humor formation by blocking the nerve endings that produce this fluid. Betaxolol selectively antagonizes beta-1 adrenergic receptors. Carteolol, levobunolol, and timolol all antagonize beta-1 and beta-2 adrenergic receptors nonselectively.

Drug interactions

This class of drugs should not be used with clonidine, quinidine, or verapamil due to risk of AV block and bradycardia. Their use should be monitored closely when combined with medications such as canagliflozin, tadalafil, or ropinirole, as they can all cause hypotension.

Side effects/Adverse reactions

Betaxolol can cause ocular discomfort, keratitis, and blurred vision. Be on the lookout for symptoms of heart failure, heart block, and bronchospasm. Carteolol shares many of these side effects and can also cause corneal staining, ptosis, and thyrotoxicosis. Serious adverse effects of levobunolol and timolol include cardiac arrest, cerebral ischemia, and Raynaud's phenomenon.

Carbonic anhydrase inhibitors

Carbonic anhydrase inhibitors are used to treat open-angle glaucoma or ocular hypertension. This class of drugs includes:
- brinzolamide (Azopt)
- dorzolamide (Trusopt).

Pharmacokinetics

Both medications are absorbed systemically, but its metabolic process is unknown. They are excreted primarily in urine.

Pharmacodynamics

As their name implies, these drugs inhibit the action of carbonic anhydrase in the ciliary processes, thus decreasing aqueous humor production.

Drug interactions

These medications should not be combined with other carbonic anhydrase inhibitors such as acetazolamide or topiramate, as taking these drugs together can increase the risk of adverse reactions.

Side effects/Adverse reactions

Brinzolamide and dorzolamide can cause dermatitis, blepharitis, and ocular discomfort commonly. More severe adverse effects can include Stevens-Johnson syndrome and toxic epidermal necrolysis.

Prostaglandin analogues

Prostaglandin analogues are considered first line of treatment for open-angle glaucoma due to their once-daily dosing and low risk of systemic side effects.

Drugs in this class include:
- bimatoprost (Lumigan)
- latanoprost (Xalatan)
- tafluprost (Zioptan)
- travoprost (Travatan Z).

Pharmacokinetics

Bimatoprost metabolizes through oxidation, *N*-demethylation, and glucuronidation. It is primarily excreted in urine. Latanoprost is metabolized locally and in the liver. It is excreted primarily in urine. Tafluprost is metabolized through oxidation and conjugation. Its excretion is unknown. Travoprost is metabolized through beta-oxidation.

There is minimal systemic absorption with this class of medications.

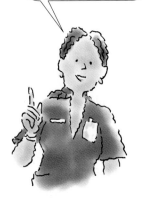

It's the first line of treatment! You only have to use these drops once a day- easy, peasy!

Pharmacodynamics

Prostaglandin analogues decrease IOP by increasing aqueous outflow through trabecular meshwork and/or the uveoscleral tract.

Drug interactions

There are no significant drug-drug interactions in this group.

Side effects/Adverse reactions

Bimatoprost, travoprost, and tafluprost can cause photophobia, dry eyes, cataracts, and macular edema.

Latanoprost has adverse effects including ocular burning, blepharitis, angina, and can reactivate herpes simplex keratitis.

Alpha-adrenergic agonists

Adrenergic blockers may reduce aqueous humor formation and increase outflow to prevent and control elevated IOP and open-angle glaucoma.
- Apraclonidine (Iopidine)
- Brimonidine (Alphagan P)

Pharmacokinetics

The metabolism and excretion of apraclonidine is unknown. Brimonidine is metabolized by the liver primarily and renally excreted. Both medications have some level of systemic absorption.

Pharmacodynamics

Adrenergic blockers may reduce aqueous humor formation and increase outflow by stimulating alpha-adrenergic receptors.

Drug interactions

Apraclonidine is contraindicated with MAO inhibitors and with linezolid as these combinations can lead to hypertensive crisis. It should also be avoided with iobenguane I 131 as it can decrease levels of the drug in targeted tissues. Exercise caution when used in conjunction with beta-blockers, as bradycardia and hypotension can occur.

Brimonidine interacts with several medications that can cause central nervous system (CNS) and respiratory depression including midazolam, promethazine, thalidomide, and hydrocodone.

Side effects/Adverse reactions

Apraclonidine can cause dizziness, bradycardia, dry eyes, asthma, and corneal erosion. Brimonidine can cause hypertension, dizziness, and conjunctivitis.

Cholinergic agonists

Cholinergic agonists are used to treat acute angle-closure glaucoma and to prevent elevated IOP postoperatively.

Drugs in this class include:
- carbachol (Miostat)
- pilocarpine (Isopto Carpine).

Pharmacokinetics

Pilocarpine uses neuronal synapses and plasma for metabolism. It is excreted renally. The pharmacokinetics of carbachol is unknown.

Pharmacodynamics

These drugs stimulate and contract the sphincter muscle of the iris through cholinergic receptor sites, constricting the pupil and improving aqueous flow.

Drug interactions

Carbachol should not be used in combination with eyedrops such as bromfenac, diclofenac, or ketorolac due to a decrease in intraocular cholinergic effects.

Pilocarpine is contraindicated with dicyclomine, as the combination may decrease efficacy of the drug and increase IOP. Other medications such as pyridostigmine, doxepin, and hydroxyzine should be used with caution as they can decrease pilocarpine's effectiveness.

Side effects/Adverse reactions

Carbachol can cause flushing, epigastric discomfort, retinal detachment, and corneal opacification. Adverse effects of pilocarpine include blurred vision, impaired dark adaptation, tearing, and retinal detachment.

Rho kinase inhibitors

Rho kinase inhibitors are used to treat open-angle glaucoma or ocular hypertension. *Currently*, there is only one medication in this class: netarsudil (Rhopressa).

Pharmacokinetics

Netarsudil is metabolized through ocular esterases. There is minimal systemic absorption. Its mechanism of excretion is unknown.

Pharmacodynamics

It is thought to work by improving aqueous outflow through the trabecular meshwork, but the exact mechanism is unknown.

Drug interactions

There are no known drug interactions.

Side effects/Adverse reactions

Netarsudil can cause ocular redness, corneal staining, and keratitis.

Osmotic agents

Osmotic agents are used to prepare for intraocular surgery and treat refractory acute glaucoma. This drug class is only available through intravenous administration, and mannitol (Osmitrol) is the most commonly used of these drugs.

Pharmacokinetics

Mannitol is metabolized by the liver minimally. It is excreted mostly in urine unchanged.

Pharmacodynamics

Osmotic agents reduce the volume of vitreous humor and decrease IOP by elevating the glomerular filtrate osmolarity.

Drug interactions

Mannitol has many drug interactions that can result in nephrotoxicity and neurotoxicity, including acyclovir, amphotericin, liraglutide, methotrexate, and cyclosporine.

Side effects/Adverse reactions

Serious side effects can occur with mannitol use including heart failure, seizures, CNS depression, and pulmonary edema. More commonly, it may be associated with hypotension, dehydration, and polyuria.

The Three-Step Approach

Nursing management for patients prescribed ophthalmic medications includes these three steps.

Preadministration

(Recognize and analyze cues)
- Assess the patient's vision, understanding of the disease (that is, glaucoma, conjunctivitis) or upcoming procedure (that is, dilation), and understanding of the medication before starting therapy.

(Prioritize hypothesis—priority patient problems)
- Visual impairment
- Infection risk
- Knowledge deficiency

(Generate solutions)
- The patient's vision will remain stable or improve with therapy.
- The patient will not develop or experience worsening infection.
- The patient and family will demonstrate an understanding of drug therapy.

Medication administration

(Take action)
- Wash your hands prior to administration of eye medication.
- Check to ensure that contacts are not being worn during medication administration.
- If indicated, agitate the bottle gently. If the bottle has been refrigerated, warm it between your hands.
- Ensure that the tip of the dropper does not touch any part of the eye.
- Ensure that the tip of the dropper stays clean.
- If more than one drop is prescribed in a particular eye, wait 5 minutes before instilling the next drop to allow proper dosing and absorption.
- Have the patient tilt their head backward while sitting or lying down with the head supported. Place the index finger just below the lower lid and gently pull down to form a pocket.

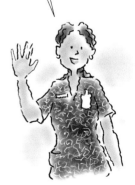

Be patient between those drops! Wait 5 minutes between to allow for absorption!

- Have the patient look up and squeeze one drop into the pocket of the lower lid. Instruct the patient not to blink or wipe their eye. It is okay to blot around the eye to remove any excess medication.
- If an ointment is prescribed, place ¼ to ½ inch line into the pocket of the lower lid.
- The patient should keep their eye closed for 1 to 3 minutes. Punctal occlusion may also be performed. (See *Teaching about punctal occlusion*.)
- Assess for immediate adverse reactions and drug interactions.

Postadministration
(Evaluate outcomes)
- Observe the patient for delayed reactions from therapy.
- Monitor glaucoma medication effectiveness by occasionally evaluating the patient's intraocular pressure (IOP).
- Monitor the patient for improvement in symptoms.
- Evaluate the patient's and family's knowledge of drug therapy and proper medication administration if the patient is being discharged.

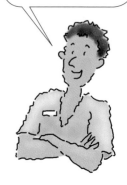

> Keep your eyes closed for 1 to 3 minutes after using eyedrops.

Teaching about punctal occlusion

If eyedrops are prescribed, review these points with the patient and caregivers:
- Punctal occlusion involves closing the eyes after instilling an eyedrop and placing a finger gently on the inner side of the eye (bridge of the nose) for 1 to 2 minutes.
- This is a simple maneuver that can be used to make sure that the medication is effectively absorbed in the eye by preventing drainage into the nasolacrimal duct and then the nose.
- This technique also helps prevent systemic absorption of the eye medication.

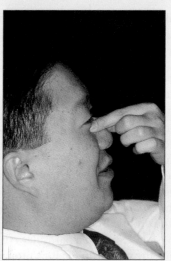

Reprinted image with permission from Rhee, D. (2018). *Glaucoma*. Philadelphia, PA: Wolters Kluwer Health.

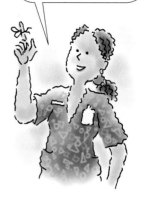

> Remember to go to the eye doctor for regular check-ups! You cannot feel the pressure in your eyes; it has to be measured, just like your blood pressure. Routine follow-up care can save your vision!

The ears are next...can you hear me?

Otic drugs

Topical medications used for common ear conditions can be classified into several groups including:
- cerumenolytics
- antiseptics
- antiseptic and glucocorticoid combinations
- anti-infective and glucocorticoid combinations
- glucocorticoids.

Cerumenolytics

Cerumenolytics are used to aid in cerumen (ear wax) removal. One of the most common drugs in this class is carbamide peroxide (Debrox), which is available over-the-counter.

Pharmacokinetics

This drug is not metabolized or excreted by the body and has minimal systemic absorption.

Pharmacodynamics

Carbamide peroxide releases oxygen to soften ear wax. It also may have mild antibacterial effects.

Side effects/Adverse reactions

There are no known drug interactions. Side effects of carbamide peroxide include local irritation and, with prolonged use, superinfection.

Antiseptics

Antiseptics are used to treat and prevent bacterial and fungal otitis externa. Acetic acid 2% is a common antiseptic.

Pharmacokinetics

Acetic acid uses intracellular metabolism and has limited systemic absorption. It is excreted via urine.

Pharmacodynamics

This agent is bactericidal, fungicidal, and acts as an astringent to acidify the ear canal.

Side effects/Adverse reactions

There are no known drug interactions. Common side effects include burning, stinging, and irritation of the ear canal.

Antiseptic and glucocorticoid combinations

Combination drugs such as antiseptic and glucocorticoid combinations are used to treat otitis externa with intact eardrum. One agent in this class is acetic acid 2% and hydrocortisone 1% otic solution (Vosol HC).

Pharmacokinetics

Acetic acid is metabolized intracellularly and excreted through urine. Hydrocortisone is metabolized by the liver and excreted in urine.

Pharmacodynamics

Acetic acid is bactericidal and fungicidal and acidifies the ear canal. Hydrocortisone works as an anti-inflammatory, but the exact mechanism is unknown.

Side effects/Adverse reactions

There are no known drug interactions. Side effects of this drug class include burning, stinging, and irritation at the site of application.

Anti-infectives

Anti-infectives are used to treat infections in and of the ear. Only two antibiotic otic preparations are currently available. They are:
- ciprofloxacin 0.2% otic solution (Cetraxal otic)
- ofloxacin 0.3% otic solution.

Pharmacokinetics

The metabolism of ciprofloxacin is unknown, although there is little to no systemic absorption. Ofloxacin is metabolized by the liver minimally, and there is little systemic absorption.

Pharmacodynamics

These medications, both fluoroquinolones, are bactericidal through inhibiting DNA gyrase and topoisomerase IV.

Pharmacotherapeutics

Ciprofloxacin is used to treat acute bacterial otitis externa, especially for those infections due to *P. aeruginosa* or *S. aureus*. Ofloxacin is used for otitis externa and for treatment of chronic suppurative otitis media. It can be used if the tympanic membrane is not intact.

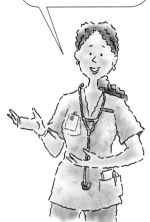

Ear infections can be painful! To decrease the discomfort of cold drops in the ear, roll the bottle between your hands for a moment to warm the drops. Never heat the drops.

Side effects/Adverse reactions

There are no known drug interactions. These drugs can cause pain at the application site, itching, headache, and, rarely, superinfection. If the tympanic membrane is perforated, ofloxacin can cause changes in taste.

Anti-infective and glucocorticoid combinations

Combination drugs such as anti-infectives and glucocorticoid combinations are used to treat acute bacterial infections such as otitis externa.

Drugs in this class include:
- ciprofloxacin 0.3% and dexamethasone 0.1% otic suspension (Ciprodex)
- ciprofloxacin 0.2% and hydrocortisone 1% otic suspension (Cipro HC)
- neomycin 0.35%, polymyxin B 10,000 units/mL, and hydrocortisone 0.5% otic suspension.

Pharmacokinetics

For combination medications, the metabolism and excretion will depend on the individual drugs.

Ciprofloxacin is partially metabolized by the liver and is excreted primarily in urine. Dexamethasone has unknown metabolic and excretory processes.

Hydrocortisone and prednisolone are metabolized by the liver and are excreted by urine.

Neomycin is not metabolized by the body. It is excreted in the feces 97% unchanged; the rest is absorbed systemically. The metabolism of polymyxin B is unknown. It is excreted by urine.

Pharmacodynamics

Ciprofloxacin/dexamethasone otic and ciprofloxacin/hydrocortisone are bactericidal. Ciprofloxacin inhibits DNA gyrase and topoisomerase IV.

Dexamethasone, hydrocortisone, and prednisolone have anti-inflammatory actions that aren't entirely understood.

Neomycin is bactericidal and works by binding to the bacterial 30S ribosomal subunit, which blocks protein synthesis.

Polymyxin B is bactericidal, increasing cell wall permeability.

Pharmacotherapeutics

Ciprofloxacin/dexamethasone is used for infections caused by *P. aeruginosa* or *S. aureus*. Ciprofloxacin/hydrocortisone can be used for these bacteria and also for *P. mirabilis*.

Neomycin/polymyxin B/hydrocortisone otic treats otitis externa and other infections such as those that occur postmastoidectomy.

Drug interactions

No significant drug interactions exist for most of these agents.

Side effects/Adverse reactions

Side effects include ear pain and secondary infection. A serious side effect of ciprofloxacin/hydrocortisone is hypoacusis (hearing loss). Neomycin/polymyxin B/hydrocortisone otic may cause ototoxicity.

Glucocorticoids

Glucocorticoids (steroids) used in the ear are used to treat otitis externa from eczema. Steroids used in the ear include fluocinolone 0.01% (DermOtic Oil).

Pharmacokinetics

Fluocinolone is metabolized by the liver and is also excreted in urine.

Pharmacodynamics

The exact mechanism of action of this drug class is unknown.

Drug interactions

When combined with canagliflozin or dulaglutide, prolonged fluocinolone can decrease the efficacy of these diabetic medications.

Side effects/Adverse reactions

Fluocinolone can cause dryness, burning, and itching at the application site. Also be aware of Cushing's syndrome and elevated blood sugar with this medication.

The Three-Step Approach

Nursing management for patients prescribed otic medications includes these three steps.

Preadministration
(Recognize and analyze cues)
- Assess the patient's hearing, understanding of the condition being treated, and understanding of the medication before starting therapy.

(Prioritize hypothesis—priority patient problems)
- Hearing impairment
- Infection risk
- Knowledge deficiency

(Generate solutions)
- The patient's hearing will remain stable or improve with therapy.
- The patient will not develop or experience worsening infection.
- The patient and family will demonstrate an understanding of drug therapy.

Medication administration

(Take action)
- Wash your hands prior to administration of ear medication.
- Warm the medication between your hands to decrease discomfort that could be caused by cold drops in the ear.
- Ensure that the tip of the dropper stays clean.
- Have the patient tilt their head to the side or have them lie on their side. Gently pull the ear up and back for adults. For children, gently pull the lower ear down and back. Give the number of drops prescribed. (See *Teaching about ear drops in adults and children*.)
- Pull the earlobe up and down so all the drops navigate into the ear. Keep the head tilted for 2 to 5 minutes to help with absorption. Excess medication can be blotted away.
- Assess for immediate adverse reactions and drug interactions.

Education edge

Teaching about ear drops in adults and children

Because of anatomy changes in the ear as we grow, administration of ear medication is different in children than in adults.

- When administering ear drops to a child, pull the bottom of the ear down and back gently.

- When administering ear drops to an adult, pull the top of the ear up and back gently.

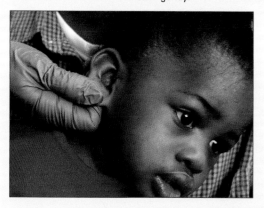

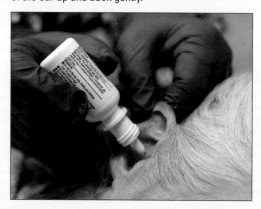

Reprinted images with permission from Taylor, C. R., Lillis, C., et al. (2008). *Fundamentals of nursing: The art and science of nursing care* (9th ed.). Philadelphia, PA: Lippincott Williams & Wilkins.

Postadministration

(Evaluate outcomes)
- Observe the patient for delayed reactions from therapy.
- Monitor medication effectiveness by having the patient return for otoscopic examination in a few days if needed.
- Monitor the patient for improvement in symptoms.
- Evaluate the patient's and family's knowledge of drug therapy and proper medication administration if the patient is being discharged.

Quick quiz

1.   In what way do mast cell stabilizers prevent histamine release?
  A.   Inhibiting mast cell degranulation
  B.   Indirectly binding to pathogens
  C.   Engulfing cellular debris
  D.   Promoting mast cell degranulation

Answer: A. Mast cell stabilizers inhibit mast cell degranulation, which prevents the release of histamine.

2.   Which medication will the nurse anticipate in the treatment of acute bacterial otitis externa due to *P. aeruginosa* or *S. aureus*?
  A.   Betaxolol
  B.   Ciprofloxacin
  C.   Natamycin
  D.   Latanoprost

Answer: B. Ciprofloxacin/dexamethasone is used for infections caused by *P. aeruginosa* or *S. aureus*.

3.   Which side effect will the nurse anticipate with long-term use of ophthalmic steroids? Select all that apply.
  A.   Secondary ocular infection
  B.   Glaucoma
  C.   Ototoxicity
  D.   Delayed corneal healing
  E.   Stinging

Answer: A, B, D, E. Ototoxicity is not an anticipated side effect of long-term use of steroid eyedrops.

4. Which teaching will the nurse provide regarding punctal occlusion?
    A. Prevents medication from draining into the nasal passages
    B. Promotes systemic absorption of medications
    C. Is a permanent occlusion of the tympanic membrane
    D. Must be performed with the patient lying down to be effective

Answer: A. This technique promotes absorption of the medication in the eye and helps minimize systemic absorption.

5. Which drug class will the nurse anticipate using first for acute open-angle glaucoma?
    A. Carbonic anhydrase inhibitors
    B. Rho kinase inhibitors
    C. Cholinergic agonists
    D. Prostaglandin analogues

Answer: D. Prostaglandin analogues.

Scoring

☆☆☆ If you answered all five questions correctly, fantastic! You're all eyes and ears!

☆☆ If you answered four questions correctly, congrats! You obviously had a good eye for learning this information!

☆ If you answered fewer than four questions correctly, don't worry. Just give yourself another look over this chapter and recheck the results.

Suggested References

Epocrates. (2021). *Drug lookup.* Retrieved from https://online.epocrates.com/drugs

Glaucoma Research Foundation. (2020). *Medication guide.* Retrieved from https://www.glaucoma.org/treatment/medication-guide.php

Healthline. (2016). *How to use ear drops.* Retrieved from https://www.healthline.com/health/general-use/how-to-use-ear-drops

Jacobs, S. (2020). Open-angle glaucoma: Treatment. *UptoDate.* Retrieved March 9, 2020 from https://www.uptodate.com/contents/open-angle-glaucoma-treatment?search=glaucoma%20treatment&source=search_result&selectedTitle=1~150&usage_type=default&display_rank=1

Joint Commission on Allied Health Personnel in Ophthalmology. (2013). *Best practices procedure for instillation of eye drops.* Retrieved from http://documents.jcahpo.org/EyeLights/0413/EyeDrop_Ointment_Checklist.pdf

Tenney, S., Patel, R., & Thorell, W. (2020). *Mannitol.* National Center for Biotechnology Information, U.S. National Library of Medicine. Retrieved from https://www.ncbi.nlm.nih.gov/books/NBK470392/#:~:text=Mannitol%20may%20be%20used%20to%20reduce%20intraocular%20pressure%20when%20given,and%20into%20t he%20intravascular%20space

Chapter 15

Psychotropic drugs

Just the facts

In this chapter, you'll learn:

◆ classes of drugs that alter thoughts, feelings and behaviors, and promote sleep

◆ uses and varying actions of these drugs

◆ absorption, distribution, metabolization, and excretion of these drugs

◆ drug interactions and adverse reactions to these drugs.

Drugs and psychiatric disorders

This chapter discusses drugs that are used to treat various sleep, psychological, and psychiatric disorders, including anxiety, anxiety disorders, mood disorders including depression, attention deficit hyperactivity disorder (ADHD), and psychotic disorders.

Sedative and hypnotic drugs

Sedatives are central nervous depressants that slow down brain activity resulting in slowed activity and relaxation. Some degree of drowsiness commonly accompanies sedative use.

You're getting very sleepy...

When given in large doses, sedatives are considered *hypnotic drugs*, which induce a state that facilitates sleep. The three main classes of synthetic drugs used as sedatives and hypnotics are:

1. benzodiazepines
2. barbiturates
3. nonbenzodiazepine-nonbarbiturate drugs.

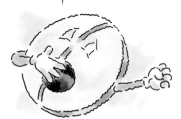

When given in large doses, sedatives facilitate sleep.

Benzodiazepines

In addition to treating anxiety and insomnia, benzodiazepines can be used to treat agitation, seizures, muscle spasms, and alcohol withdrawal. They can also be used as premedication for medical or dental procedures.

"Chill" pills

Benzodiazepines used primarily for their primary or secondary sedative or hypnotic effects include the following:

Drugs primarily used for both the sedative and/or hypnotic effects include:

- alprazolam (Xanax)
- clonazepam (Klonopin)
- diazepam (Valium)
- lorazepam (Ativan).
  Drugs primarily used for the hypnotic effect include:
- estazolam (no trade name at the time of publication)
- flurazepam (no trade name at the time of publication)
- temazepam (Restoril)
- zaleplon (Sonata).

Pharmacokinetics

Benzodiazepines (BZDs) are absorbed rapidly and completely from the GI tract and distributed widely in the body. Penetration into the brain is rapid. The rate of absorption determines how quickly the drug will work. Specific benzodiazepines have different rates of onset and duration of action which help guide which one may be more effective in certain clinical situations. Benzodiazepines are usually categorized as short, intermediate, or long acting.

The ins and outs

Benzodiazepines are usually given orally but may be given parenterally in certain situations, such as when a patient needs immediate sedation. All benzodiazepines are metabolized in the liver and excreted primarily in urine. Some benzodiazepines have active metabolites, which may give them a longer action.

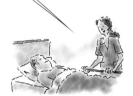

Benzodiazepines increase total sleep time and decrease the number of awakenings.

Pharmacodynamics

Researchers believe that benzodiazepines produce a calming effect by enhancing the binding of gamma-aminobutyric acid (GABA) in the ascending reticular activating system (RAS) of the brain. This RAS is associated with wakefulness and attention and includes the cerebral cortex and limbic, thalamic, and hypothalamic levels of the central nervous system (CNS). (See *How benzodiazepines work*, page 522.)

How benzodiazepines work

These illustrations show how benzodiazepines work at the cellular level.

Speed and passage

The speed of impulses from a presynaptic neuron across a synapse is influenced by the amount of chloride in the postsynaptic neuron. The passage of chloride ions into the postsynaptic neuron depends on the inhibitory neurotransmitter called *gamma-aminobutyric acid* or *GABA*.

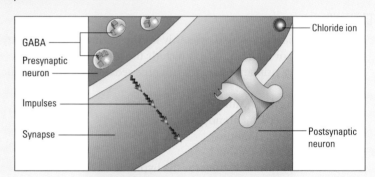

It binds

When GABA is released from the presynaptic neuron, it travels across the synapse and binds to GABA receptors on the postsynaptic neuron. This binding opens the chloride channels, allowing chloride ions to flow into the postsynaptic neuron and causing the nerve impulses to slow down.

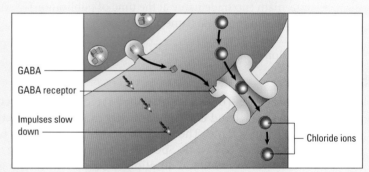

It slows brain activity

Benzodiazepines bind to receptors on or near the GABA receptor, enhancing the effect of GABA and allowing more chloride ions to flow into the postsynaptic neuron. This depresses the nerve impulses, causing them to slow down or stop.

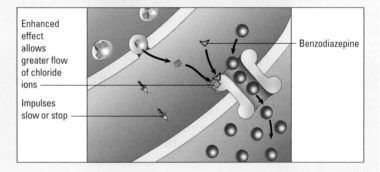

Snooze inducer

Benzodiazepines change how the brain manages sleep cycles. They also potentially induce tolerance. Therefore, long-term use of these drugs to treat insomnia is not recommended. Treatment for insomnia should always include nonpharmacological sleep hygiene strategies in addition to any medication.

Prototype pro

Benzodiazepines: Alprazolam (exemplar drug)

Actions
- Acts at the limbic, thalamic, and hypothalamic levels of the CNS
- Enhances or facilitates the action of GABA, an inhibitory neurotransmitter in the CNS
- Produces anxiolytic, sedative, hypnotic, skeletal muscle relaxant, and anticonvulsant effects
- Produces CNS depression

Indications
- Anxiety (acute)
- Anxiety disorders, including panic disorders

Nursing considerations
- Teach the patient that benzodiazepines have a potential for addiction, tolerance, and physical dependence; therefore, they must be used only as directed and for the shortest amount of time possible.
- Monitor the patient for adverse reactions, such as drowsiness, dizziness, weakness, and slowed breathing. Other adverse reactions can include:
  - decreased cognitive functioning
  - anterograde amnesia (forgetting events that occur after dosing)
- paradoxical reaction (excitation, increased anxiety/agitation, aggression, and behavioral disinhibition).
- Closely monitor older adults and those with a history of a substance use disorder or a severe respiratory condition if they are prescribed this drug.
- Use cautiously in pregnancy; these drugs are not usually recommended during breast-feeding.
- Recognize that this drug is classified under schedule IV of the Controlled Substance Act.
  - There is an FDA **black box warning** about the risk of abuse, misuse, addiction, physical dependence, and withdrawal reactions to improve the safe use of benzodiazepine drug class (Pfizer, 2021).
- When discontinuing benzodiazepines taken regularly for a long time, follow the health care provider's order to taper the dose slowly over several weeks to prevent seizures and other withdrawal symptoms.

Pharmacotherapeutics

Clinical indications for benzodiazepines include:
- treating acute anxiety states and anxiety disorders, like panic disorder
- treating insomnia (short-term only)
- treating alcohol withdrawal symptoms
- treating status epilepticus
- producing skeletal muscle relaxation
- promoting relaxation prior to surgery.

Drug interactions

- CNS depressants (such as alcohol, barbiturates, and anticonvulsants) may cause additive CNS depression.
- Concurrent use of opioids can lead to a significantly increased risk for respiratory depression and death when used with benzodiazepines.
- Some benzodiazepines may increase the serum digoxin level, resulting in potential digoxin toxicity.

A lethal combination

When benzodiazepines are taken with other CNS depressants, especially alcohol, the result is enhanced sedative and CNS depressant effects. These can include a reduced level of consciousness (LOC), impaired mental state, reduced muscle coordination, ataxia, slurred speech, respiratory depression, and death. The drug flumazenil can be used as an antidote to reverse the CNS depression from a benzodiazepine overdose.

Hormonal contraceptives may reduce the metabolism of some benzodiazepines inducing toxicity and increase the metabolism of others resulting in decreased effectiveness.

Adverse reactions

Benzodiazepines may cause the following:
- CNS depression
  - sedation
  - decreased cognitive function
  - dizziness
  - ataxia (impaired ability to coordinate movement).
- Paradoxical response and amnesia (mentioned previously)

Feeling a little out of it?

Unintentional daytime sedation, residual drowsiness, impaired reaction time on awakening, and rebound insomnia may also occur.

Older adult alert!

Benzodiazepines should be used with caution in older adults. Decreased protein-drug binding and decreased renal and hepatic clearance makes them much more sensitive to these drugs. These drugs increase the risk of falls and mental confusion in this population. If they must be used, the health care provider will start the patient at a lower dosage and gradually increase it.

The Three-Step Approach

Nursing management for patients receiving benzodiazepine therapy includes these three steps. Be certain to pay particular attention to the type of benzodiazepine being given, and personalize care accordingly.

Preadministration

(Recognize and analyze cues)

- Conduct a baseline physical assessment before therapy begins and watch for significant changes.
- Assess level of anxiety prior to administration so that comparison can be done afterward to determine efficacy.
- Observe baseline liver, renal, and hematopoietic function test results.

(Prioritize hypothesis—priority patient problems)

- Anxiety
- Potential for respiratory depression

(Generate solutions)

- Anxiety will be decreased.
- Respiratory depression will not occur.

Medication administration

(Take action)

- Determine whether the patient is taking other medication that could depress the respiratory system; collaborate with the health care provider if necessary to confirm the need for benzodiazepine treatment.
- Offer additional nonpharmacological methods to decrease anxiety or to facilitate sleep.
- If hospitalized, make sure that the patient has a call light in hand. Remind not to get out of bed without calling for a nurse.
- Ensure that the room is free from clutter that may increase the risk for falls.

Postadministration

(Evaluate outcomes)

- Conduct a follow-up assessment to determine if anxiety has decreased (or if sleep has been achieved).

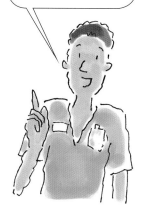

Be careful! Taking benzodiazepines with other CNS depressants such as alcohol increases sedative and CNS depressant effects.

- Monitor closely for changes in breathing and any signs of respiratory depression.
- If given over time, monitor liver, renal, and hematopoietic function test results.

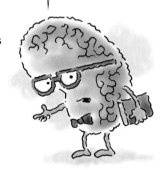

Are you paying attention? Barbiturates reduce overall CNS alertness.

Barbiturates

The major pharmacologic action of barbiturates is to reduce overall CNS alertness. Barbiturates used as sedatives and hypnotics include:

- phenobarbital (no trade name at the time of publication); its main use is to treat or prevent seizures
- secobarbital (Seconal; this drug is not available at the time of publication due to being on back order without a release date) (American Society of Hospital Pharmacists, 2021).

The highs and lows

Low doses of barbiturates depress the sensory and motor cortex in the brain, causing drowsiness. High doses may cause respiratory depression and death because of their ability to depress all levels of the CNS.

Pharmacokinetics

Barbiturates are absorbed well from the GI tract. They're distributed rapidly, metabolized by the liver, and excreted in urine.

Pharmacodynamics

Like sedatives and hypnotics, barbiturates depress the sensory cortex of the brain; decrease motor activity; alter cerebral function; and produce drowsiness, sedation, and sleep. These drugs appear to act throughout the CNS; however, the reticular activating system of the brain, which is responsible for wakefulness, is a particularly sensitive site. (See *Barbiturates: Phenobarbital,* page 527.)

Pharmacotherapeutics

Barbiturates were used somewhat commonly in the past to treat anxiety or insomnia. With many more drugs on the market today that are safer to treat these conditions, barbiturates are not frequently used for this purpose unless other methods of treatment have failed. Because of their sedative and hypnotic properties, these drugs are more commonly used for:

- seizures unresponsive to other anticonvulsant agents
- preoperative sedation and anesthesia induction.

Prototype pro

Barbiturates: Phenobarbital

Actions
- Induces an imbalance in central inhibitory and facilitatory mechanisms, which influence cerebral cortex and reticular formation
- Decreases presynaptic and postsynaptic membrane excitability
- Produces all levels of CNS depression (mild sedation to coma to death)
- Facilitates the action of GABA, an inhibitory neurotransmitter in the CNS
- Exerts a central effect, which depresses respiration and GI motility
- Reduces nerve transmission and decreases excitability of the nerve cell as its principal anticonvulsant mechanism of action
- Raises the seizure threshold

Indications
- Epilepsy
- Febrile seizures
- Need for sedation

Nursing considerations
- This drug is contraindicated in pregnancy and should be used cautiously in mothers who are breast-feeding.
- Monitor for adverse reactions, such as drowsiness, lethargy, hangover, respiratory depression, apnea, Stevens-Johnson syndrome, and angioedema.
- Don not withdraw the drug abruptly; if the patient is prone to seizures, they may worsen.
- Watch for signs of toxicity including labored breathing and/or wheezing, clammy skin, and cyanosis. These can quickly progress to a comatose state.

A little too good
Tolerance to barbiturates occurs even more rapidly than tolerance to benzodiazepines. Physical dependence may occur even with a small daily dosage.

Drug interactions

Barbiturates may negatively interact with many other drugs by increasing or decreasing the blood level of the other drug, leading to increased toxicity or decreased effectiveness. Always consult the health care provider before initiating a new drug. Common adverse drug-drug interactions can occur with:
- CNS depressants, including sedatives, hypnotics, benzodiazepines, antihistamines, and opioids (these may cause excessive CNS depression which can be fatal)
- anticonvulsant medications such as phenytoin
- birth control pills (which can become less effective)
- oral anticoagulants
- antiretrovirals
- corticosteroids.

Yikes! It says here that using methoxyflurane and barbiturates together may stimulate production of metabolites that are toxic to the kidneys.

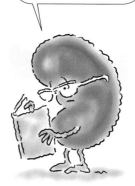

Adverse reactions

Barbiturates may have widespread adverse effects.

Draining the brain

CNS reactions include:

- drowsiness
- lethargy
- headache
- depression and thoughts of suicide
- mental status changes, anxiety, agitation, and hallucinations (rare).

"Heart-y" responses

Cardiovascular effects include:

- mild bradycardia
- hypotension.

"Air" ways

Respiratory effects include:

- hypoventilation
- spasm of the larynx (voice box) and bronchi
- reduced rate of breathing
- severe respiratory depression.

And everything else

Other reactions include:

- vertigo
- nausea and vomiting
- diarrhea
- epigastric pain
- allergic reactions, such as hives, itching, tightness of chest, and/or swelling
- peeling and blistering of skin
- tolerance and withdrawal symptoms with prolonged use.

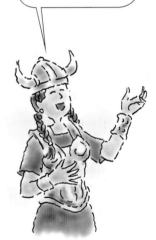

Barbiturates can cause spasm of the voice box—but I need to keep my voice box spasm-free. LAAA!

The Three–Step Approach

Nursing management for patients receiving barbiturate therapy follows the same principles as the three-step approach for patients receiving benzodiazepine therapy. A key concept to remember when administering a barbiturate drug in parenteral form is to avoid extravasation, which may cause local tissue damage and tissue necrosis; inject IV or deep IM only. Don't exceed 5 mL for any IM injection site to avoid tissue damage. Also, be prepared to resuscitate. Too-rapid IV administration may cause respiratory depression, apnea, laryngospasm, or hypotension.

Teaching about barbiturates

If barbiturates are prescribed, review these points with the patient and caregiver:
• Barbiturates can cause tolerance and physical or psychological dependence.
• Take the drug exactly as prescribed. Do not take other drugs, including over-the-counter drugs or herbal remedies, without the prescriber's approval.
• Do not drink alcohol while taking this drug.
• Morning drowsiness is common after therapeutic use of barbiturates.
• Avoid hazardous tasks, driving a motor vehicle, operating machinery, and making important decisions while taking the drug. Review other safety measures with your health care provider to prevent injury.
• Do not stop taking the drug abruptly; contact your health care provider to determine how to wean off the medication.

• Notify your health care provider if you plan to become pregnant. These drugs are contraindicated in pregnancy.
• Barbiturates can lessen the effectiveness of hormonal contraceptives. Consider using other birth control methods while taking a barbiturate.
• Seek emergency care for skin eruptions or other significant adverse effects such as shallow breathing, numbness (especially in the extremities), or mental status changes.
• Contact your health care provider if weight loss or muscle weakness, numbness in hands or feet, or mental status changes occur (other than expected drowsiness).

Nonbenzodiazepine drugs ("Z drugs")

Nonbenzodiazepines, also called "Z drugs," act as hypnotics for short-term treatment of simple insomnia. These drugs do not have antianxiety, muscle relaxant, or antiepileptic properties.
These drugs include:
• eszopiclone
• zaleplon
• zolpidem.

Shoring up sleep for the short term

Nonbenzodiazepines are usually intended for short-term use. Zolpidem, however, has been shown by evidence to be safe to use for long-term management if needed (Sanofi, 2018). Teach the patient to work with their health care provider to find the best sleep solutions.

Pharmacokinetics

Nonbenzodiazepines are absorbed rapidly from the GI tract. They're metabolized in the liver and excreted in urine.

Pharmacodynamics

The mechanism of action for nonbenzodiazepines isn't fully known. They appear to enhance the action of GABA in the CNS.

Pharmacotherapeutics

Nonbenzodiazepines are typically used for:
- treatment of simple insomnia.

Drug interactions

Drug interactions involving nonbenzodiazepines primarily occur when they are used with other CNS depressants (including alcohol). The additive CNS depression can result in drowsiness, respiratory depression, stupor, coma, and death.

Adverse reactions

Some common adverse reactions involving nonbenzodiazepines include:
- nausea and vomiting
- gastric irritation
- daytime drowsiness and increased fall risk
- mental status changes including unusual behavior, like eating or driving a vehicle while in a sleeping state.

The Three-Step Approach

Nursing management for patients receiving nonbenzodiazepines, also called "Z drugs," follows the same principles as the three-step approach for patients receiving benzodiazepine or barbiturate therapy. A key concept to remember when administering a nonbenzodiazepine drug is to diligently educate the patient about safety measures such as not taking the medication until being in bed for the night. The patient must also be taught to refrain from operating machinery, driving, and making important decisions until they have secured at least 8 hours of sleep following administration of a nonbenzodiazepine drug. Also teach the patient to have roommates or family members monitor for abnormal behavior such as sleep walking, sleep eating, and driving without recollection; these are potential side effects of Z drugs that must be reported to the health care provider immediately.

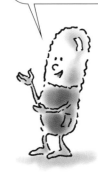

Nonbenzodiazepines-nonbarbiturates are used for short-term treatment of insomnia and for sedation before surgery or EEG studies.

Antianxiety drugs

Antianxiety drugs, also called *anxiolytics*, include some of the most prescribed drugs in the United States. They can be used to treat acute anxiety and anxiety disorders. The three main types of antianxiety drugs are:
- benzodiazepines
- barbiturates (less commonly used as anxiolytics)
- buspirone.

Experiencing drug déjà vu?

Benzodiazepines and barbiturates were discussed earlier in this chapter regarding their sedative and hypnotic use, but they can also be used to treat anxiety. Due to the high potential for addiction, they are not commonly used in this way; however, recognize that there are patients who have been prescribed these drugs for many years that still may be taking them. Most health care providers continue to work diligently to wean patients from these drugs when they are used to treat anxiety and to move the patient to medication with a much lower side effect profile that still provides relief.

The "am" list

As noted in the earlier section, recall that common benzodiazepines (ending in "am") include:

- alprazolam (Xanax)
- clonazepam (Klonopin)
- diazepam (Valium)
- lorazepam (Ativan).

Taking the edge off

Benzodiazepines decrease anxiety by acting on the limbic system and other areas of the brain that help regulate emotion, as well as depress the CNS. (See important information about patient teaching in the *Teaching about antianxiety drugs*.)

Education edge

Teaching about antianxiety drugs

If antianxiety drugs are prescribed, review these points with the patient and caregiver:

- These drugs help relieve symptoms temporarily; they do not cure or solve the underlying issue that induces anxiety. Counseling or psychotherapy can be helpful to address root cause issues.
- Teach other methods to promote relaxation, such as physical exercise and stress management techniques.
- Identify factors that contribute to symptoms. Avoiding caffeine, cold medications, appetite suppressants, and other stimulating medications can help reduce symptoms of anxiety.
- Notify all health care providers about drugs and over-the-counter products you're taking to avoid being prescribed medications with similar effects.
- Avoid hazardous activities that require alertness and psychomotor coordination until the CNS effects of the drug are known.

- Avoid alcohol consumption (which increases CNS depression) and smoking (which decreases effectiveness) while taking the drug.
- Don't take other drugs, over-the-counter products, or herbal remedies without first consulting the health care provider to avoid adverse drug-drug interactions.
- Take the drug exactly as prescribed; don't stop taking it without working directly with your health care provider.
- Dependence on the drug may occur if the drug is taken longer than directed or in excess of the prescribed amount. Dependence is also possible if taken exactly as directed, so work with your health care provider if long-term management of anxiety is needed.
- Take the drug later in the day or at night as indicated to help decrease daytime drowsiness.

Buspirone

Buspirone is in a class of drugs known as *azaspirodecanedione derivatives*. This drug's structure and mechanism of action differ from those of other antianxiety drugs.

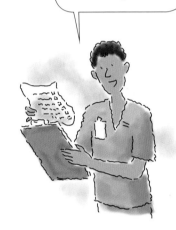

Buspirone has less potential for dependence or abuse than other anxiolytic drugs.

Advantages

Buspirone has several advantages, including:
- less sedating than benzodiazepines and barbiturates
- less of a synergistic CNS depressant effect when taken with alcohol or sedative-hypnotics (although use with alcohol or sedative-hypnotic drugs should still be discouraged)
- less potential for dependence or abuse.

Pharmacokinetics

Buspirone is absorbed rapidly, undergoes extensive first-pass effect, and is metabolized in the liver to at least one active metabolite. The drug is eliminated in urine and feces.

Pharmacodynamics

Although the exact mechanism of action of buspirone remains unknown, buspirone's anxiolytic effect is associated with enhanced serotonergic activity in the brain's anxiety and fear circuitry. Buspirone also seems to impact the availability of dopamine.

Pharmacotherapeutics

Buspirone is used to treat generalized anxiety disorder. Patients who haven't received benzodiazepines in the past seem to respond better to buspirone. The drug is also effective for panic disorder, generalized phobias, and obsessive-compulsive disorders.

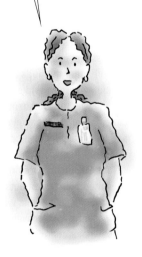

Buspirone's onset of action is slow but effective.

Slow as a tortoise

Because of its slow onset of action, which may take up to several weeks, buspirone is ineffective when quick relief from anxiety is needed.

Drug interactions

Unlike other antianxiety drugs, buspirone doesn't have a toxic additive effect with alcohol or other CNS depressants. Nevertheless, concurrent use of alcohol and buspirone is discouraged. When buspirone is given with MAO inhibitors, malignant hypertensive reactions may occur. Carefully review the patient's regular medications, and notify the health care provider if an MAO inhibitor is prescribed.

Adverse reactions

The most common reactions to buspirone include:
- dizziness
- light-headedness
- insomnia
- rapid heart rate
- palpitations
- headache
- nausea.

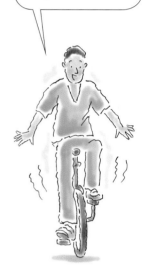

Tell the patient to avoid activities that require alertness and psychomotor coordination until the CNS effects of buspirone are known.

The Three-Step Approach

Nursing management for patients receiving a benzodiazepine, a barbiturate, or buspirone for anxiety follows the same principles as the three-step approach for patients receiving benzodiazepine or barbiturate therapy for insomnia (see Chapter 7). Again, remind the patient of safety considerations, to refrain from performing activities that require alertness, and to report unusual side effects to the health care provider.

Antidepressant and mood stabilizer drugs

Antidepressant drugs and mood stabilizer drugs are used to treat mood disturbances.

Fasts facts on antidepressants
- **All antidepressants** have a delayed onset. It takes 1 to 4 weeks or longer for antidepressants to relieve mood symptoms, although side effects may occur immediately.
- **Certain antidepressants** can precipitate a manic episode (experiencing feelings of heightened energy, creativity, and euphoria) in susceptible individuals.
- **Some antidepressants** are also frequently used as first-line treatment for anxiety disorders.
- **All antidepressants** have the potential side effect of increased the risk for developing suicidal thinking, especially in teenagers and young adults.

One pole versus two poles
Unipolar (one pole) disorders are characterized by periods of clinical depression and are treated with:
- selective serotonin reuptake inhibitors (SSRIs)
- serotonin-norepinephrine reuptake inhibitors (SNRIs)
- tricyclic antidepressants (less commonly)
- MAO inhibitors (much less commonly).

Bipolar depression (two poles) is characterized by periods of mania (elevated mood and heightened energy and creativity) and periods of depression (extreme sadness, guilt, and hopelessness). It is treated with:

- lithium (Lithobid)
- valproate (Depakote)
- quetiapine (Seroquel)
- lamotrigine (Lamictal).

SSRIs

Selective serotonin reuptake inhibitors (SSRIs) are a group of antidepressants that have fewer adverse effects, as compared to other subclasses of antidepressants. They are first-line therapy for treatment of clinical depression and anxiety disorders. Some of the SSRIs currently available are:

- citalopram (Celexa)
- escitalopram (Lexapro)
- fluoxetine (Prozac)
- fluvoxamine (Luvox)
- paroxetine (Paxil)
- sertraline (Zoloft).

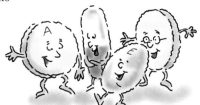

Good news! SSRIs are very effective in the treatment of depression!

Pharmacokinetics

SSRIs are absorbed almost completely after oral administration and are highly protein bound. They're primarily metabolized in the liver and excreted in urine.

Pharmacodynamics

SSRIs inhibit the neuronal reuptake of the neurotransmitter serotonin. (See *Selective serotonin reuptake inhibitors: Sertraline*, page 535.)

Pharmacotherapeutics

SSRIs are used to treat major depressive disorder, obsessive-compulsive disorder, and certain anxiety disorders.

Here's the (SSRI) scoop

SSRIs have been shown to be effective is treatment of select eating disorders, personality disorders, and impulse control disorders. These drugs can also be used as an adjunct treatment for persistent pain.

Drug interactions

Drug interactions with SSRIs are associated with their ability to competitively inhibit a liver enzyme that is responsible for oxidation of numerous drugs, including tricyclic antidepressants; antipsychotics,

Prototype pro

Selective serotonin reuptake inhibitors: Sertraline

Actions
Selectively inhibits the reuptake of serotonin (5HT) at the presynaptic membrane

Indications
• Major depressive disorder
• Obsessive-compulsive disorder
• Panic disorder
• Posttraumatic stress disorder
• Premenstrual dysphoric disorder
• Social anxiety disorder

Nursing considerations
• All antidepressants increase the risk of developing suicidal thinking, especially in patients who are teens or young adults. Teach the patient and caregiver to report any mood changes or suicidal thoughts.
• Teach about common side effects including anxiety, agitation, insomnia, nausea, diarrhea, headache, and sexual dysfunction.
• Teach about symptoms associated with internal bleeding and hyponatremia; these are rare adverse reactions that require notification to the health care provider.
• Encourage the patient to take the drug in the morning to prevent insomnia and with food to minimize gastrointestinal side effects.
• Caution the patient to avoid hazardous activities that require alertness and psychomotor coordination until the CNS effects of the drug are known.

carbamazepine, warfarin, lithium, benzodiazepines, and some antiarrhythmics. St. John's wort, an herbal supplement, also causes this same interaction and should be avoided while taking an SSRI.

Watch out for the SHIVERS

A toxic adverse effect of SSRIs is the development of **serotonin syndrome**. This syndrome develops when too much serotonin accumulates in the body, which is often the result of a drug interaction between two serotonergic drugs (Boyer, 2021). It can also occur during regular therapeutic dosing of an SSRI (although rare) or as the result of intentional overdose. **This is a life-threatening condition that requires immediate intervention**. Use the word SHIVERS to help remember the symptoms:

• Shivering
• Hyperreflexia (and muscle rigidity)
• Increased temperature
• Vital signs instability
• Encephalopathy (agitation, delirium, confusion)
• Restlessness (and impaired coordination)
• Sweating (diaphoresis)

Remember to assess for SHIVERS if you suspect serotonin syndrome.

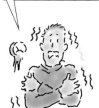

Danger ahead!

As noted above, although serotonin syndrome can occur when treatment when an SSRI is initiated or increased in dosage, it is seen most often when one serotonergic drug is taken with other one. Taking the following substances with an SSRI increase the risk of developing this syndrome:

- MAO inhibitors (strong risk)
- Other antidepressants, especially SNRIs and bupropion
- Antimigraine medication
- Pain medication, especially opioids
- Antinausea medications
- Herbal supplements, especially St. John's wort
- Over-the-counter cold and cough medication
- Illegal drugs (amphetamines, cocaine, etc.)

If you suspect a patient has serotonin syndrome, hold the next dose of medication, and contact the health care provider immediately.

Adverse reactions

Common side effects associated with SSRI use include anxiety, gastrointestinal upset, dry mouth, insomnia, somnolence, and sexual dysfunction. Remember the seven S's when assessing for side effects or adverse reactions:

- Stomach upset (nausea, vomiting, and diarrhea)
- Sexual dysfunction (anorgasmia, especially in women, and delayed ejaculation)
- Serotonin syndrome
- Sleep difficulties (insomnia)
- Suicidal thoughts
- Stress (anxiety, agitation)
- Size increase (weight gain)

Caution patients who are pregnant or considering pregnancy to talk with their health care provider about use of SSRIs. Venlafaxine specifically has been associated with certain birth defects, especially heart defects, when used during pregnancy (Anderson et al., 2020).

Teach patients about the possible adverse reaction of hyponatremia. Symptoms include nausea and vomiting, confusion, fatigue, muscle spasms or cramping, and restlessness. This condition develops more often in older adults who have high cardiac comorbidities (Lien, 2018).

Finally, teach that abrupt discontinuation of SSRIs can cause unpleasant symptoms for patients. (See important information about *SSRI discontinuation syndrome*, page 537.) Patients must work with their health care provider to determine the best course of action for weaning and discontinuation.

SSRI discontinuation syndrome

Abrupt discontinuation of SSRIs may result in a condition called *SSRI discontinuation syndrome*. This syndrome occurs in approximately 20% of patients who engage in an abrupt stoppage of medication or a marked decrease in dose (Gabriel & Sharma, 2017). Of all SSRIs, discontinuation syndrome occurs most frequently with paroxetine (Paxil) and least frequently with fluoxetine (Prozac) (Gabriel & Sharma).

The mnemonic FINISH summarizes symptoms:
- **F**lulike symptoms: lethargy, fatigue, headache, achiness
- **I**nsomnia (with vivid dreams)
- **N**ausea
- **I**mbalance (dizziness, vertigo)
- **S**ensory disturbances (burning, tingling feelings)
- **H**yperarousal (anxiety, irritability, tremors, aggression, and crying spells)

How to deal

This syndrome is self-limited. With treatment, it usually resolves within 2 to 3 weeks. Tapering the drug dosage slowly over several weeks can help prevent it.

Black Box Warning

Antidepressants

SSRIs and all antidepressants have a "black box warning" of an increased risk of developing suicide ideation and aggression, especially in children and adolescents with a diagnosis of major depressive disorder. Teach patients (and caregivers, as appropriate) symptoms to monitor for and to report these symptoms immediately to the health care provider. Clearly, if a patient is expressing suicidal intentions or actions, emergent care is needed.

The Three-Step Approach

Nursing management for patients receiving SSRI therapy includes these three steps. Be certain to pay particular attention to the type of SSRI being given, and personalize care accordingly.

Preadministration

(Recognize and analyze cues)
- Conduct a baseline physical assessment before therapy begins and watch for significant changes.
- Assess level of depression prior to administration so that comparison can be done afterward to determine efficacy.
- Recognize that older adults may be started on a lower dose of an antidepressant.
- Assess for the presence of suicidal ideation (especially in adolescents and younger adults).

(Prioritize hypothesis—priority patient problems)
- Mood alteration
- Potential for suicidal ideation (especially if the patient is a child, adolescent, or young adult)

(Generate solutions)
- Depressive mood will be alleviated.
- Suicidal ideation will not occur.

Medication administration

(Take action)
- Determine whether the patient is taking other medication that could increase the risk for serotonin syndrome.
- Offer additional nonpharmacological methods to address depression (for example, increase physical activity, observe proper nutrition, find activities to do that may alleviate the focus on depressed mood).
- If hospitalized, make sure that the patient has a call light in hand. Remind not to get out of bed without calling for a nurse until the effects of the drug are known.
- Ensure that the room is free from clutter that may increase the risk for falls.

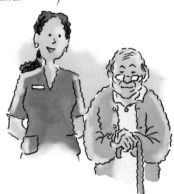

Older adults may need a lower starting dose of an SSRI.

Postadministration

(Evaluate outcomes)
- Conduct a follow-up assessment to determine if depressive symptoms have decreased.
- Monitor closely for any sign of suicidal ideation.
- Ensure that the patient and caregivers understand drug therapy. (See *Teaching about SSRIs*, page 539.)

Teaching about SSRIs

If SSRIs are prescribed, review these points with the patient and caregivers:
• Take the drug as directed; do not stop taking the drug even when symptoms resolve. SSRIs are usually given for at least several months to a year, and sometimes longer.
• Follow up with your health care provider regularly to monitor efficacy of treatment and to discuss whether the drug should be discontinued by tapering after sufficient relief is experienced.
• Relief from symptoms may not occur until 1 to 4 weeks after the drug is started; don't stop taking the drug prematurely.

• Don't take other drugs, over-the-counter products, or herbal remedies without first consulting with the prescriber. Serious drug interactions may occur.
• Tell other health care providers that you're taking an SSRI to avoid toxic drug interactions.
• Take the drug in the morning to help avoid insomnia or nervousness, unless otherwise directed.
• Report excessive drowsiness, dizziness, or other adverse reactions (especially symptoms associated with serotonin syndrome and hyponatremia) to the health care provider.
• Counseling or psychotherapy, support groups, stress management techniques, and relaxation techniques are recommended in addition to drug therapy.

Monoamine oxidase (MAO) inhibitors

Monoamine oxidase (MAO) inhibitors were the first antidepressant drugs to be used. Although they are no longer first-line therapy, they are often used for treatment-resistant depression and other disorders (for example, depression with atypical features) (Hirsch & Birnbaum, 2021). There are two isomers of monoamine oxidase, MAO-A and MAO-B. MAO-A metabolizes serotonin, epinephrine, and norepinephrine, while MAO-B metabolizes dopamine (Hirsch & Birnbaum, 2021).

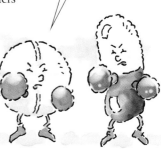

There are two isomers: MAO-A and MAO-B.

Pharmacokinetics

MAO inhibitors are absorbed rapidly and completely from the GI tract and are metabolized in the liver to inactive metabolites. These metabolites are excreted mainly by the GI tract and, to a lesser degree, by the kidneys.

Pharmacodynamics

MAO inhibitors appear to work by inhibiting monoamine oxidase, a widely distributed enzyme that normally metabolizes many neurotransmitters, including norepinephrine and serotonin. This action makes more norepinephrine, dopamine, and serotonin available to the receptors, thereby relieving the symptoms of depression.

Pharmacotherapeutics

Indications for MAO inhibitors include treatment-resistant depression, depression with atypical features, panic disorder, social anxiety disorder, and unresponsive dysthymia (Hirsch & Birnbaum, 2021). These drugs are prescribed much less frequently than other antidepressants because of the necessary dietary precautions that must be taken and the high risk of toxic drug-drug interactions.

Atypical depression

MAO inhibitors are also thought to be effective in treatment of atypical depression. Symptoms associated with this condition include mood reactivity and two or more secondary symptoms, which may be hyperphagia, hypersomnia, weight gain or increased appetite, leaden paralysis, or interpersonal sensitivity to rejection (Cuijpers et al., 2017).

Battling the blues

MAO inhibitors are often prescribed for treatment-resistant depression (symptoms of clinical depression that do not respond to other antidepressants or therapies). Certain drugs like selegiline (Zelapar) can be used in the treatment of Parkinson's disease. These medications inhibit the breakdown of dopamine, thereby prolonging its action in the brain, which provides some relief of Parkinson's symptoms (University of California San Francisco, 2021).

Drug interactions

MAO inhibitors interact with many drugs. Be sure to take a thorough history, asking the patient what other medications are taken and if any supplements or herbal preparations are used. Report these to the health care provider.

- Taking MAO inhibitors with CNS stimulants, such as amphetamines, methylphenidate, levodopa, or sympathomimetics, or nonamphetamine appetite suppressants may increase catecholamine release, causing hypertensive crisis.
- Clinical symptoms of a hypertensive crisis include increased blood pressure and heart rate, an acute occipital headache, nausea, and diaphoresis.
- Using MAO inhibitors with other subclasses of antidepressants, such as SSRIs, SNRIs, TCAs, or atypical antidepressants may result in an elevated body temperature, excitation, seizures, and serotonin syndrome. (See *Pharm fact alert: Stopping MAO inhibitors*, page 541.)
- MAO inhibitors may enhance the hypoglycemic effects of antidiabetic drugs.
- Administering MAO inhibitors with prescription pain medication, such as methadone and meperidine, may result in excitation, hypertension or hypotension, extremely elevated body temperature, and coma.

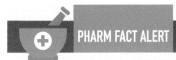

PHARM FACT ALERT

Stopping MAO inhibitors

If a patient is switching from another antidepressant (other than fluoxetine) to an MAO inhibitor, a waiting period of 2 weeks is recommended before starting the MAO inhibitor. If the patient is switching from fluoxetine to an MAO inhibitor, a waiting period of 5 to 6 weeks is recommended before starting the MAO inhibitor (Soreide et al., 2017).

Eat, drink, and…be careful

Certain foods can interact with MAO inhibitors and produce severe reactions. The most serious reactions involve tyramine-rich foods such as chocolate, red wine, aged cheese, smoked or processed meats, fermented foods, fava beans, and soybean and soybean-based foods. Caffeine can increase the stimulation side effects of MAO inhibitors. Selegiline (Zelapar), when delivered via transdermal patch, has less severe food-drug interactions; however, caution should still be exercised, and patients must be made aware of symptoms of hypertensive crisis (Selegiline: Drug Information, 2021).

Adverse reactions

Some of the following adverse reactions associated with MAO inhibitors include:

- hypertensive crisis (when taken with tyramine-rich foods or which may result from certain drug-drug interactions)
- serotonin syndrome (arising from drug-drug interactions, especially other antidepressants)
- orthostatic hypotension
- restlessness, drowsiness, dizziness, and insomnia
- headache
- constipation, anorexia, and nausea and vomiting
- weakness and joint pain
- dry mouth
- blurred vision
- peripheral edema
- urine retention and transient impotence
- rash
- skin and mucous membrane hemorrhage
- mental status changes including suicidal thoughts.

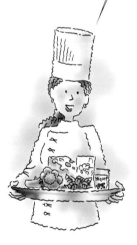

Patients taking MAO inhibitors need to watch what they eat. Tyramine-rich foods—such as aged cheese—can interact with these drugs and produce hypertensive crisis.

The Three-Step Approach

Nursing management for patients receiving MAOI therapy is the same as the three steps to administering SSRIs, with a few additional key points:

- Remind the patient to work with the prescriber if the medication regimen is changed or discontinued at any time.
- If the patient is to have surgery, teach to collaborate with the health care provider and anesthesia provider about how to manage MAOI therapy. There are conditions in which MAOI drugs are continued prior to surgery, and other conditions in which discontinuation 2 weeks prior to surgery is recommended (Muluk et al., 2021).
- Teach that severe hypertension can occur with use of an MAOI, so to monitor blood pressure regularly. If a patient is treated in an agency, be aware that phentolamine or nitroprusside may be used to address severe hypertension (Garcia & Santos, 2021).
- Teach to avoid tyramine-rich foods. (See *Teaching about MAO inhibitors.*) These precautions should be observed 10 to 14 days after stopping the drug (at the health care provider's discretion).

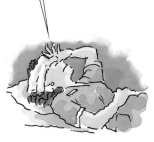

Signs of MAO inhibitor overdose include a severe headache, nausea and vomiting, sweating, tachycardia, vision changes, shortness of breath, and confusion.

Education edge

Teaching about MAO inhibitors

If MAO inhibitors are prescribed, review these points with the patient and caregivers:

- Teach the patient to avoid foods high in tyramine (such as chocolate, red wine, aged cheese, smoked or processed meats, fermented foods, fava beans, and soybean and soybean-based foods) as well as large amounts of caffeine.
- Sit up for 1 minute before getting out of bed, or from sitting to standing, to avoid dizziness when changing position.
- Avoid overexertion because MAO inhibitors may suppress the pain from angina.

- Always consult your health care provider before taking other prescription or over-the-counter drugs. Severe adverse effects can occur if MAO inhibitors are taken with cold or allergy medications or diet aids.
- Consider using a medication alert bracelet or necklace to communicate that you are taking an MAO inhibitor.
- Continue to take the medication even when symptoms of depression resolve. Don't stop taking the drug suddenly.

Tricyclic antidepressants (TCAs)

TCAs are used to treat depression. They include:

- amitriptyline (Elavil)
- amoxapine (no trade name at the time of publication)
- desipramine (Norpramin)
- doxepin (Silenor)
- imipramine hydrochloride (Tofranil)
- nortriptyline (Pamelor)
- protriptyline (no trade name at the time of publication)
- trimipramine (no trade name at the time of publication).

Pharmacokinetics

All of the TCAs are active pharmacologically, and some of their metabolites are also active. They're absorbed completely when taken orally but undergo first-pass effect.

Passing it on

With first-pass effect, a drug passes from the GI tract to the liver, where it's partially metabolized before entering the circulation. TCAs are metabolized extensively in the liver and eventually excreted in urine as inactive compounds. Only small amounts of active drug are excreted in urine.

Half-life concerns

The extreme fat solubility of these drugs accounts for their wide distribution throughout the body, slow excretion, and long half-lives. This long half-life increases the risk for lethality if they are taken in overdose.

Pharmacodynamics

Researchers believe that TCAs increase the amount of norepinephrine, serotonin, or both in the CNS by preventing their reuptake (reentry) into the storage granules in the presynaptic nerves. Preventing reuptake results in increased levels of these neurotransmitters in the synapses, relieving depression. TCAs also block acetylcholine and histamine receptors.

Now, just relax. I'm here to prevent your reuptake of norepinephrine and serotonin, which should help you feel less depressed.

Pharmacotherapeutics

TCAs are used primarily to treat episodes of major depressive disorder (MDD). They're especially effective in treating depression of insidious onset accompanied by weight loss, anorexia, or insomnia. Symptom relief usually begins 1 to 4 weeks after starting the medication.

Working together

TCAs may be helpful when used with a mood stabilizer in treating acute episodes of clinical depression in patients with type 1 bipolar disorder. TCAs should never be used alone for patients with bipolar disorder, as the risk for exacerbation of mania symptoms increases.

Additional assistance

TCAs are also used to prevent migraine headaches (usually doxepin or amitriptyline) and to treat conditions such as (Moraczewski & Aedma, 2020):

- panic disorder with agoraphobia
- neuropathic pain (for example, diabetic neuropathy, postherpetic neuralgia)
- obsessive-compulsive disorder
- enuresis
- nocturia
- mixed urinary incontinence
- fibromyalgia (after other treatments have been ineffective).

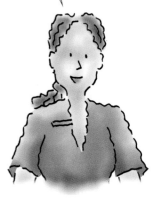

TCAs don't mix well with a number of other drugs.

Prototype pro

Tricyclic antidepressants: Amitriptyline

Actions
- Inhibits the reuptake of norepinephrine and serotonin in CNS nerve terminals (presynaptic neurons), thus enhancing the concentration and activity of neurotransmitters in the synaptic cleft.

Indication
- Major depressive disorder

Nursing considerations
- Monitor for side effects such as dizziness or drowsiness, constipation, xerostomia, blurred vision, orthostatic hypotension, and urinary retention. Teach that an increased anticholinergic effect (in the form of more serious blurred vision, tachycardia, and urine retention) can occur if TCAs are taken anticholinergic drugs.

- Teach about adverse reactions, such as an increased risk for bleeding if taken with anticoagulants, EKG changes (QRS prolongation)—especially dose-related changes, hyponatremia, serotonin syndrome if taken with other serotonergic drugs, and possible increase in risk of suicidal thinking and behaviors.
- Because tricyclic antidepressants are lethal in overdose due to their long half-life, monitor inpatients closely for suicidal ideation.
- Teach to work with the health care provider to gradually reduce the dosage over several weeks when discontinuing this drug.
- Warn to avoid hazardous activities that require alertness and psychomotor coordination until the CNS effects of the drug are known.

Drug interactions

TCAs interact with several commonly used drugs:

- TCAs increase the catecholamine effects of amphetamines and sympathomimetics, leading to hypertension.
- Barbiturates increase the metabolism of TCAs and decrease their blood levels.
- Cimetidine (Tagamet) impairs the metabolism of TCAs by the liver, increasing the risk of toxicity.
- Alcohol blocks the antidepressant action of TCAs while increasing sedation.
- Use of epinephrine (Adrenalin, Auvi-Q, EpiPen) or clonidine (Catapres, Catapres-TTS-1, Catapres TTS-2, Catapres TTS-3, Kapvay) and TCAs can cause dangerously high blood pressure.
- Use of acetylcholine-blocking drugs can lead to paralytic ileus.

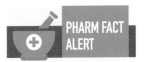

PHARM FACT ALERT

Temperature's rising

Using TCAs concurrently with MAO inhibitors and/ or St. John's wort can cause serotonin syndrome.

Dangerous blood pressure elevations can occur when TCAs are combined with clonidine.

Adverse reactions

Remember the adverse effects of TCAs by remembering the mnemonic TCASS:

- Thrombocytopenia (rare)
- Cardiac
  - ○ Arrhythmias
  - ○ Orthostatic hypotension
  - ○ Myocardial infarction
- Anticholinergic and antihistamine
  - ○ Tachycardia
  - ○ Dry mouth
  - ○ Blurry vision
  - ○ Urinary retention and constipation
  - ○ Sexual dysfunction
- Seizure
- Sedation

The Three-Step Approach

Nursing management for patients receiving TCA therapy is the same as the three steps to administering SSRIs, with a few additional key points:

- Prior to administration, patients should be assessed for underlying cardiovascular disease, as TCAs can induce adverse cardiac reactions.
- Monitor blood pressure (BP) carefully if the patient is hospitalized, and teach outpatients to monitor their own BP and report abnormal values to the health care provider.

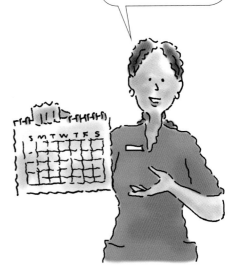

The prescriber will work with the patient to wean TCAs gradually over several weeks to avoid a rebound effect or other adverse reactions.

Teaching about TCAs

If TCAs are prescribed, review these points with the patient and caregivers:
• Recognize that the full therapeutic effect of taking a TCA may not occur for several weeks.
• Take the drug exactly as prescribed. Don't increase the dosage, stop the drug, or take another drug (including over-the-counter drugs and herbal remedies) without discussing this with your health care provider.
• To avoid dizziness, sit upright for a minute before getting out of bed.
• Because an overdose with TCAs can be fatal, store this drug safely away from children.
• Avoid alcohol while taking TCAs.

• Avoid hazardous tasks that require mental alertness until the drug's full effects are known.
• Sedation is a usual side effect, so take the drug at night.
• Excessive time spent in sunlight, under heat lamps, or in tanning beds may cause rashes and abnormal hyperpigmentation; use sunscreen appropriately and avoid these sources of exposure when possible.
• If you have diabetes, monitor your glucose level carefully because the drug may alter it.
• Chew sugarless gum, suck on hard candy or ice chips, or use artificial saliva to relieve dry mouth.

Other drugs that relieve depression

There are a variety of other subclasses of antidepressants in use today. Some include:
• bupropion (Wellbutrin, Zyban), an aminoketone drug
• venlafaxine (Effexor) and duloxetine (Cymbalta), serotonin-norepinephrine reuptake inhibitors (SNRIs)
• trazodone (no trade name at the time of publication), a triazolopyridine derivative drug.

Pharmacokinetics

The paths these antidepressants take through the body may vary:
• Bupropion (Wellbutrin, Zyban) is well absorbed from the GI tract and metabolized by the liver. Its metabolites are excreted by the kidneys. It appears to be highly bound to plasma proteins.
• Venlafaxine (Effexor) and duloxetine (Cymbalta) are rapidly absorbed after oral administration, metabolized in the liver, and excreted in urine.
• Trazodone (no trade name at the time of publication) is well absorbed from the GI tract, distributed widely in the body, and

metabolized by the liver. It is excreted mainly in urine. The rest is excreted in feces.

Pharmacodynamics

Much about how these drugs work has yet to be fully understood.

Rethinking reuptake

- Bupropion (Wellbutrin, Zyban) inhibits the reuptake of the neurotransmitter dopamine and norepinephrine; it is thought to affect monoamine uptake (Huecker et al., 2021).
- Venlafaxine (Effexor) and duloxetine (Cymbalta) are thought to potentiate neurotransmitter activity in the CNS by inhibiting the neural reuptake of serotonin and norepinephrine.
- Trazodone (no trade name at the time of publication) is thought to exert antidepressant effects by inhibiting the reuptake of norepinephrine and serotonin in the presynaptic neurons.

Pharmacotherapeutics

These miscellaneous drugs are all used to treat depression.
- Bupropion (Wellbutrin, Zyban) is also used to aid in smoking cessation and seasonal affective disorder.
- Venlafaxine (Effexor) is also used to treat generalized anxiety, social anxiety, and panic disorder.
- Duloxetine (Cymbalta) is also used to treat peripheral neuropathy, fibromyalgia, and chronic musculoskeletal pain.
- Trazodone (no trade name at the time of publication) may also be effective in treating aggressive behavior and panic disorder. In low doses, trazodone is a useful treatment for insomnia because of its sedative effects.

Drug interactions and contraindications

All of these antidepressants may have serious, potentially fatal reactions when combined with MAO inhibitors. Each of these drugs also carries individual, specific risks when used with other drugs:
- Bupropion (Wellbutrin, Zyban) is contraindicated for patients with an increased risk of seizures, such as those with anorexia nervosa or traumatic brain injury (TBI).
- Bupropion (Wellbutrin, Zyban), when combined with levodopa, phenothiazines, or TCAs, increases the risk of adverse reactions, including seizures.
- Bupropion (Wellbutrin, Zyban) should not be given with venlafaxine (Effexor), as the risk for seizure development increases.
- Venlafaxine (Effexor) should not be given with amphetamine/dextroamphetamine (Adderall), as venlafaxine increases the amphetamine effects resulting in racing thoughts, anxiety, and restlessness.

- Trazodone (no trade name at the time of publication) may increase serum levels of digoxin and phenytoin. Its use with antihypertensive drugs may cause significantly increased hypotensive effects. CNS depression may be enhanced if trazodone is administered with other CNS depressants.
- Trazodone (no trade name at the time of publication) and venlafaxine (Effexor) should not be given together, as there is an increased risk of serotonin syndrome.

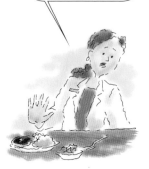

Several of the antidepressants can cause nausea. No, thank you!

Adverse reactions

Adverse reaction	Bupropion blues	Venlafaxine variances and duloxetine downfalls	Trazodone trouble
Cardiovascular	Tachycardia	Vasodilation/flushing	Cardiac arrhythmias Orthostatic hypotension
Central nervous system	Headache Insomnia Seizures	Headache Dizziness	Dizziness Drowsiness Headache
Gastrointestinal	Anorexia Constipation Nausea and vomiting	Anorexia Nausea Weight loss	Nausea and vomiting
Psychiatric	Agitation Restlessness	Abnormal dreams Agitation Anxiety	Anxiety
Other	Diaphoresis	Diaphoresis Hyponatremia Sexual dysfunction	Priapism (rare)

Bupropion should be taken in the morning. Otherwise, insomnia may result, and I'm tired of counting sheep.

The Three-Step Approach

Nursing management for patients receiving therapy with antidepressants such as bupropion, venlafaxine, duloxetine, and trazodone is the same as the three steps to administering SSRIs, recognizing that care must be personalized based on the type of drug prescribed.

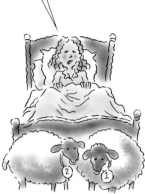

Lithium (Lithobid)

Lithium (Lithobid) is a mood stabilizer used to prevent or treat mania associated with bipolar disorder. The discovery of lithium was a milestone in treating this condition.

Pharmacokinetics

When taken orally, lithium (Lithobid) is absorbed rapidly and completely and is distributed to body tissues. Lithium (Lithobid) isn't metabolized and is excreted from the body unchanged primarily through the kidneys.

Pharmacodynamics

Lithium's exact mechanism of action is unknown.

Curbing catecholamines

One pharmacodynamic theory regarding lithium (Lithobid) states that symptoms associated with bipolar disorder occur due to catecholamine variances. In bipolar disorder, the patient is affected by swings between the excessive catecholamine stimulation of mania and the diminished catecholamine stimulation of depression. A few of the ways it may regulate catecholamine release in the CNS include:

- increasing norepinephrine and serotonin uptake
- reducing the release of norepinephrine from the synaptic vesicles (where neurotransmitters are stored) in the presynaptic neuron
- inhibiting norepinephrine's action in the postsynaptic neuron.

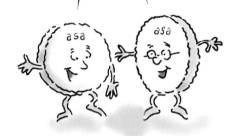

Excessive catecholamine stimulation results in mania; Diminished catecholamine stimulation causes depression.

Lithium tablets may regulate catecholamine release to treat mania and bipolar disorders.

Pharmacotherapeutics

Lithium (Lithobid) is used to treat manic and mixed episodes associated with bipolar disorder and as maintenance treatment for this condition.

Drug interactions

Lithium (Lithobid) has a narrow therapeutic margin of safety. A blood level that is even slightly higher than the therapeutic level can be dangerous. Serious interactions with other drugs can occur because of this narrow therapeutic range:

- The risk of lithium toxicity increases when lithium is taken with thiazide and loop diuretics and nonsteroidal anti-inflammatory drugs (NSAIDs).
- Administration of lithium with haloperidol, phenothiazines, and carbamazepine may produce an increased risk of neurotoxicity.
- Lithium may increase the hypothyroid effects of potassium iodide.
- Sodium bicarbonate may increase lithium excretion, reducing its effects.
- Lithium's effects are reduced when taken with theophylline.

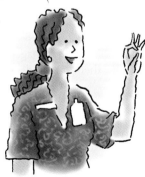

Lithium has a narrow therapeutic margin. A blood level even a little higher than the therapeutic level can be dangerous.

Salt at fault?

A patient on a severe salt-restricted diet, or who is dehydrated or experiencing a significant loss of sodium through something like excessive sweating or diarrhea, is susceptible to lithium toxicity. On the other hand, an increased intake of sodium may reduce the therapeutic effects of lithium.

Adverse reactions

Common adverse reactions to short-term use of lithium include:
- drowsiness
- diarrhea
- dizziness
- headache
- increase in thirst
- muscle weakness
- nausea and vomiting
- tremors
- weight gain.

Adverse effects seen after long-term use include hypothyroidism and, rarely, renal toxicity.

Toxic times

If there is a suspicion of toxicity, hold a dose of the medication and assure that blood levels of lithium are drawn, contacting the health care provider if an order needs to be placed. Symptoms of lithium toxicity include severe nausea, vomiting, and diarrhea, and neurological findings such as (Perrone & Chattergee, 2020):
- ataxia
- confusion
- encephalopathy
- myoclonic jerks
- nonconvulsive status epilepticus
- progressive muscle weakness
- seizures
- tremors that continue or worsen.

The Three-Step Approach

Nursing management for patients receiving lithium (Lithobid) therapy includes these three steps.

Preadministration

(Recognize and analyze cues)
- Determine if the patient is pregnant before initiative or administering lithium (Lithobid). This drug is teratogenic.
- Assure that a baseline ECG, thyroid and kidney studies, and electrolyte levels have been ordered and obtained. Thyroid and kidney function must be regularly monitored.

- Assess level of depression prior to administration so that comparison can be done afterward to determine efficacy.
- Monitor lithium blood levels 8 to 12 hours after the first or most recent dose, usually before the morning dose. Lithium blood levels must also be regularly monitored during maintenance therapy.

(Prioritize hypothesis—priority patient problems)
- Mood alteration
- Potential for drug toxicity

(Generate solutions)
- Depressed mood will be alleviated.
- Drug toxicity will not occur.

Medication administration

(Take action)
- Determine whether the patient is taking other medication that could affect lithium (Lithobid) therapy.
- Assess if the patient will comply with long-term lab work requirements, as monitoring ongoing lithium blood levels is crucial to safe use of the drug. Lithium (Lithobid) should not be given to a patient who can't have blood levels checked regularly.
- Give the drug with plenty of water and meals to minimize GI side effects and metallic taste.
- Teach about side effects that can occur with regular administration, as well as toxicity. (See *Teaching about lithium [Lithobid]*.)

Education edge

Teaching about lithium (Lithobid)

If lithium is prescribed, review these points with the patient and caregivers:
- Take the drug with plenty of water and meals to minimize GI upset.
- Lithium has a narrow therapeutic margin of safety. A blood level that is even slightly high can be dangerous.
- Watch for signs and symptoms of toxicity, such as nausea, diarrhea, vomiting, tremor, drowsiness, muscle weakness, and ataxia. Withhold one dose of the drug and contact your health care provider.
- Do not stop the drug abruptly. Work closely with your health care provider to determine how to proceed to discontinue the drug if needed.
- Expect transient nausea, polyuria, and thirst during the first few days of therapy.

- Make all health care providers aware that you are taking this drug, as it should not be given with diuretics and NSAIDs that may be prescribed. Talk with your health care provider before taking over-the-counter medications, as well.
- Avoid activities that require alertness and good psychomotor coordination until the drug's CNS effects are known.
- Do not abruptly change your sodium intake.
- Notify your health care provider if you plan to become pregnant.
- Wear or carry medical identification that states you are taking this drug.

Postadministration

(Evaluate outcomes)

- Conduct a follow-up assessment to determine if mood alterations have decreased.
- Monitor glucose level closely, as lithium (Lithobid) may alter glucose tolerance in a patient with diabetes.
- Monitor (and teach to monitor) lithium blood levels for therapeutic index, which is usually 0.6 to 1.2 mmol/L.

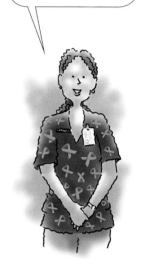

Antipsychotic drugs can treat psychotic symptoms that occur with various disorders.

Antipsychotic drugs

Antipsychotic drugs can control psychotic symptoms (delusions, hallucinations, paranoia, and thought disorders) that can occur with schizophrenia spectrum disorders, mania, and other psychoses.

The name game

Drugs used to treat psychoses may be called:

- *antipsychotic*, because they can lessen and sometimes eliminate signs and symptoms of psychoses
- *neuroleptic*, because they depress nerve functions in the brain.

One…or the other

Regardless of what they're called, all antipsychotic drugs belong to one of two major groups:

- first-generation antipsychotics (also called typical)
- second-generation antipsychotics (also called atypical).

Typical antipsychotics

Typical antipsychotics, which include phenothiazines and nonphenothiazines, can be broken down into smaller classifications.

Typical antipsychotics have been around for a long time.

Sort and separate

Many clinicians believe that the phenothiazines should be treated as three distinct drug classes because of the differences in the adverse reactions they cause:

- *Aliphatics* primarily cause sedation and anticholinergic effects and are low-potency drugs. They include drugs such as chlorpromazine (Thorazine).
- *Piperazines* primarily cause extrapyramidal reactions and include fluphenazine decanoate, fluphenazine hydrochloride, perphenazine, and trifluoperazine hydrochloride. None of these drugs have trade names at the time of publication.

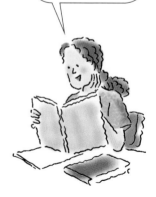

- *Piperidines* primarily cause sedation and anticholinergic and cardiac effects and include thioridazine (no trade name at the time of publication).

Pharmacokinetics

Although typical antipsychotics are absorbed erratically, they are very lipid-soluble and highly protein-bound. Therefore, they are distributed to many tissues and are highly concentrated in the brain. All typical antipsychotics are metabolized in the liver and excreted in urine and bile.

Effects keep going and going

Because fatty tissues slowly release accumulated phenothiazine metabolites into the plasma, phenothiazines may produce effects up to 3 months after they're discontinued.

Pharmacodynamics

Although the mechanism of action of typical antipsychotics isn't understood fully, researchers believe that these drugs work by blocking postsynaptic dopaminergic receptors in the brain.

Blocking...

The antipsychotic effect of phenothiazines and nonphenothiazines arises from receptor blockade in the limbic system. Their antiemetic effects result from receptor blockade in the chemoreceptor trigger zone located in the brain's medulla.

... and stimulating

Phenothiazines also stimulate the extrapyramidal system (motor pathways that connect the cerebral cortex with the spinal nerve pathways). Antiparkinsonian drugs, such as benztropine, beta-blockers, anticholinergics, and/or antihistamines can be used to manage extrapyramidal (EP) adverse effects. (See *Phenothiazines: Chlorpromazine*, page 554.)

Pharmacotherapeutics

Phenothiazines are used primarily to:
- treat schizophrenia spectrum disorders
- calm patients who are severely anxious, agitated, or aggressive.

Haloperidol (Haldol) and pimozide (no trade name at the time of publication) are approved to treat Tourette's syndrome.

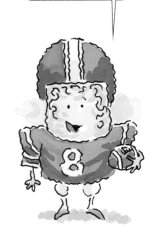

Typical antipsychotic drugs block postsynaptic dopaminergic receptors in the brain. See if you can tackle that concept!

Phenothiazines: Chlorpromazine

Actions
- Functions as a dopamine antagonist by blocking postsynaptic dopamine receptors in various parts of the CNS
- Produces antiemetic effects by blocking the chemoreceptor trigger zone
- Produces varying degrees of anticholinergic and alpha-adrenergic receptor blocking actions

Indications
- Psychotic symptoms (for example, severe aggression or agitation, hallucinations, delusions)
- Manic episodes associated with bipolar disorder
- Schizophrenia
- Severe nausea and vomiting
- Severe behavioral concerns in children (combativeness, explosive hyperexcitability)
- Intractable hiccups

Nursing considerations
- Monitor for adverse reactions and extrapyramidal symptoms (ranging from akathisia to tardive dyskinesia).
- Monitor for symptoms of neuroleptic malignant syndrome (NMS), a life-threatening emergent condition that requires immediate recognition and care (Wijdicks, 2019). Symptoms can be recognized by the acronym FEVER:
  - **F**ever (high elevated temperature)
  - **E**ncephalopathy with sudden mental status changes
  - **V**ital sign instability
  - **E**nzyme elevation (CPK)
  - **R**igidity (of muscles)
- Elevated liver enzyme levels that progress to obstructive jaundice usually indicate an allergic reaction.
- Don't withdraw the drug abruptly; gradually reduce the dosage over several weeks based on the health care provider's orders.
- Teach to avoid hazardous activities and decisions that require alertness and psychomotor coordination until the drug's CNS effects are known.

Serious business
Phenothiazines interact with many different types of drugs and may have serious effects:
- Increased CNS depressant effects, such as stupor, may occur when they're taken with CNS depressants.
- Taking anticholinergic drugs with phenothiazines may result in increased anticholinergic effects, such as dry mouth and constipation, and potentially reduce the antipsychotic effects of phenothiazines.
- Phenothiazines may reduce the antiparkinsonian effects of levodopa.

- Concurrent use with lithium may increase the risk of neurotoxicity.
- The threshold for seizures is lowered when phenothiazines are used.
- Phenothiazines may increase the serum levels of TCAs and beta-adrenergic blockers.
- Drugs that inhibit the cytochrome P-450 2D6 isoenzyme and drugs known to prolong the QTc interval should be avoided when taking phenothiazines.

Voted less likely to interact

Nonphenothiazines interact with fewer drugs than phenothiazines. Their dopamine-blocking activity can inhibit the effect of levodopa. Haloperidol (Haldol) may boost the effects of lithium, producing encephalopathy (brain dysfunction).

Adverse reactions

Phenothiazines have side effects including weight gain, glucose abnormalities, dystonia, akathisia, tardive dyskinesia, and extrapyramidal symptoms (EPS). EPS may appear after the first few days of therapy; tardive dyskinesia may occur after several years of treatment. Neuroleptic malignant syndrome (NMS) is a life-threatening concern. (See *Phenothiazines: Chlorpromazine*, page 554.) Use of phenothiazines may also cause pink or brown discoloration of urine.

Shared traits

Most nonphenothiazines cause the same adverse reactions as phenothiazines.

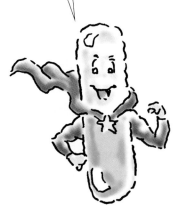

I'm not your run-of-the-mill antipsychotic. I block the activity of two receptors, dopamine and serotonin.

Second-generation antipsychotics

Second-generation (atypical) antipsychotics are drugs designed to treat numerous psychiatric conditions. They include:
- clozapine (Clozaril)
- lurasidone (Latuda)
- olanzapine (Zyprexa)
- risperidone (Risperdal)
- quetiapine (Seroquel)
- ziprasidone (Geodon)
- brexpiprazole (Rexulti)
- aripiprazole (Abilify).

Pharmacokinetics

Atypical antipsychotics are absorbed after oral administration. They are metabolized by the liver. Metabolites of many second-generation antipsychotics are inactive, whereas risperidone (Risperdal) has an active metabolite. They are highly plasma protein–bound and eliminated in urine, with a small portion eliminated in feces.

Pharmacodynamics

Second-generation antipsychotics typically block the dopamine receptors but to a lesser extent than the first-generation antipsychotics, resulting in far fewer extrapyramidal adverse effects. Additionally, they also block serotonin receptor activity. These combined actions help to treat positive and negative symptoms associated with schizophrenia.

Pharmacotherapeutics

Atypical antipsychotics are considered the first line of treatment for patients with schizophrenia spectrum disorders because of equal or improved effectiveness and improved tolerability. They are also used to treat acute agitation, bipolar disorder (often as adjunctive to lithium or valproate), irritability (associated with autistic disorder), and treatment-resistant depression (Jibson, 2021).

Watch the route

Second-generation antipsychotics have multiple routes of administration. The various drugs are available in different forms, such as:

- fast dissolving oral tablets; these are helpful for patients who may be resistant to taking medication that must be swallowed
- oral pill, liquid formulation, parenteral form; administration via these routes are shorter acting, so the dose must be taken regularly for full effectiveness
- long-acting intramuscular injection—this formulation lasts 2 to 4 weeks and is helpful for patients who have challenges adhering to treatment
- very long-acting IM injection—this formulation lasts up to 4 months and is again helpful for patients with challenges adhering to treatment.

Drug interactions

Drugs that alter the P-450 enzyme system will alter the metabolism of some atypical antipsychotics.

Dopamine effects

Atypical antipsychotics counteract the effects of levodopa and other dopamine agonists.

And the rest of the story…

Combining second-generation antipsychotics with other drugs has the potential to increase the blood level of the drug leading to toxicity or decrease the blood level of the drug making them less effective. There are numerous interactions, so the health care provider must be consulted before initiating a new medication. Examples of drug interactions that may occur include the following:

- Second-generation antipsychotics taken with antihypertensives may potentiate hypotensive effects.
- Second-generation antipsychotics taken with benzodiazepines or CNS depressants (including alcohol) may enhance CNS depression.
- Smoking when taking second-generation antipsychotics may increase clearance of olanzapine and other antipsychotics making them less effective due to the influence of nicotine.

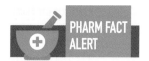

PHARM FACT ALERT

Teach that when taking an antipsychotic drug, exposure to sunlight, heat lamps, or tanning beds may cause photosensitivity reactions.

Adverse reactions

All antipsychotics have the potential to produce multiple adverse reactions because they affect many receptors. Although second-generation antipsychotic drugs have fewer side effects than first-generation antipsychotics, it is still important to monitor for these effects, and report findings to the health care provider. Examples include:

- CNS effects (sedation and/or respiratory depression when given in large doses; seizures)
- antiadrenergic effects (orthostatic hypotension, dizziness, fatigue)
- anticholinergic effects (dry mouth, blurry vision, urinary retention, constipation, tachycardia)
- extrapyramidal symptoms (EPS) (dystonia, parkinsonism, akathisia, tardive dyskinesia)
- metabolic/endocrine effects (dyslipidemia, weight gain, hyperglycemia—all of which increases the risk for cardiovascular disease)
- neuroleptic malignant syndrome (NMS)
- hematologic effects (blood dyscrasias)
- cardiovascular effects (prolonged QT interval).

The Three-Step Approach

Nursing management for patients receiving first-generation **or** second-generation antipsychotic therapy includes these three steps.

Preadministration

(Recognize and analyze cues)
- Assure that a baseline diagnostic testing has been collected per the health care provider's order. This may include a complete blood count, metabolic panel, and EKG.

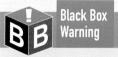

Black Box Warning

Antipsychotics

Antipsychotics can increase the risk of death (cardiovascular or infectious disease) when prescribed for a patient with dementia. These drugs are not approved for use in patients with dementia-related psychosis.

- Obtain baseline vital signs and weight, as initial values are needed when monitoring blood pressure, pulse rate, and weight following administration.
- Assess symptoms prior to administration so that comparison can be done afterward to determine efficacy.
- An annual formal assessment of drug-related abnormal muscle movements is standard practice when a patient is taking an antipsychotic drug. The Abnormal Involuntary Movement Scale (AIMS) is a short, evidence-based screening tool that can be used. This can be performed more frequently as needed, particularly if a patient is experiencing the onset of tardive dyskinesia, which requires early intervention.

(Prioritize hypothesis—priority patient problems)
- Mood alteration
- Potential for significant adverse effects of drug therapy

(Generate solutions)
- Psychotic symptoms will be alleviated.
- Adverse effects will not occur.

Medication administration

(Take action)
- Do not withdraw medication abruptly. Although physical dependence doesn't occur with antipsychotic drugs, rebound worsening of psychotic symptoms is possible and many drug effects may persist.
- Teach to avoid activities that require alertness and psychomotor coordination until the drug's CNS effects are known.
- Teach to avoid alcohol while taking antipsychotics.
- Teach to refrain from stopping the drug abruptly unless severe adverse reactions occur; consult with the health care provider for direction.
- Monitor for NMS and EPS; intervene immediately if either condition is suspected.
- Thoroughly explain potential side effects, especially NMS and EPS; emphasize the need to seek help immediately if NMS symptoms arise and to report EPS symptoms or involuntary movements to the health care provider right away.

Postadministration

(Evaluate outcomes)
- Conduct a follow-up assessment to determine if psychotic symptoms (or reason for drug therapy) have decreased.
- Recognize that acute dystonic reactions should be treated quickly with intravenous diphenhydramine.
- Recommend the use of sugarless gum or hard candy to help relieve dry mouth.

Extrapyramidal symptoms may appear after the first few days of antipsychotic therapy.

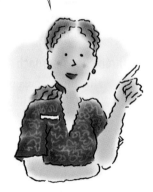

Stimulants

Stimulants are used to treat attention deficit hyperactivity disorder (ADHD), a condition characterized by inattention, impulsiveness, and hyperactivity. There are many types of stimulants. Select examples include:

- dextroamphetamine (Dexedrine)
- methylphenidate (Ritalin, Concerta, Quillivant)
- mixed amphetamine salts (Mydayis)
- combination products (for example, Adderall, which is a combination of amphetamine and dextroamphetamine).

Some prescribers recommend using stimulants only for periods needed and stopping the drug for a brief period, such as when children are on summer break from school, to reassess the need for therapy. Other health care providers recommend always continuing on the medication to maintain focus and control ADHD-related behaviors.

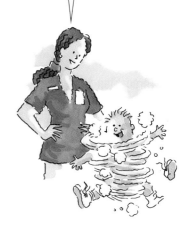

> Stimulants are the treatment of choice for ADHD, helping to decrease impulsiveness and hyperactivity.

Pharmacokinetics

Stimulants are absorbed well from the GI tract and are distributed widely in the body. Methylphenidate, however, undergoes significant first-pass effect. Stimulants are metabolized in the liver and excreted primarily in urine.

Pharmacodynamics

Stimulants are believed to work by increasing levels of dopamine and norepinephrine, by blocking the reuptake of dopamine and norepinephrine, by enhancing the presynaptic release, or by inhibiting MAO.

Pharmacotherapeutics

Stimulants are the treatment of choice for ADHD. They are helpful in improving attention span, which can lead to improved school or work performance and decreased impulsivity and hyperactivity.

Drug interactions

Stimulants should not be used within 14 days of discontinuing an MAO inhibitor. Also, methylphenidate may decrease the effect of guanethidine (Minoxidil) and increase the effects of TCAs, warfarin (Coumadin), and some anticonvulsants. Use of over-the-counter cold medications and sympathomimetics should be avoided due an increased stimulant effect.

Adverse reactions

Stimulant use increases the risk for development of a substance use disorder, so close monitoring of the patient is required. Stimulants may affect growth, so monitor children closely for height and weight changes. With short-acting stimulants, there is a risk for insomnia if the medication is given later in the day.

Dextroamphetamine drawbacks and methylphenidate misfortune

Adverse reactions include:

- CNS stimulation (restlessness, tremors, insomnia, seizure)
- cardiac effects (tachycardia, palpitations, arrhythmias)
- gastrointestinal effects (weight loss from decreased appetite, dry mouth, unpleasant taste, abdominal discomfort, diarrhea)
- rare effects (rash, thrombocytopenia, development of psychosis).

The Three-Step Approach

Nursing management for patients receiving stimulant therapy includes these three steps.

Preadministration

(Recognize and analyze cues)

- Assess symptoms prior to administration so that comparison can be done afterward to determine efficacy.
- Obtain a baseline weight (as stimulants can incite weight loss due to anorexia).
- Determine the patient's normal sleeping pattern (as stimulants given later in the day may affect sleep).

(Prioritize hypothesis—priority patient problems)

- Concentration and/or behavioral alterations
- Potential for sleep and nutrition alterations

(Generate solutions)

- Concentration will improve, while behavioral alterations will be alleviated.
- Sleep and nutrition status will not be adversely affected.

Medication administration

(Take action)

- Administer as prescribed; if late-day dosing affects sleep, collaborate with the health care provider to potentially select a different stimulant.
- Teach to take only as prescribed, as misuse may cause psychological dependence or habituation, especially in a patient with a history of a substance use disorder.
- Teach to avoid drinks containing caffeine, which increases the effects of amphetamines and related amines.

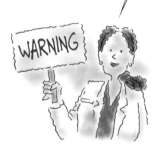

Stimulant misuse increases the risk for addiction, so monitor the patient closely for adherence to the prescribed dose.

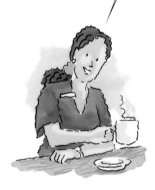

Hold the lattes for patients taking stimulants! Caffeine increases the effects of these drugs.

Postadministration

(Evaluate outcomes)

- Conduct a follow-up assessment to determine if concentration has improved and/or behavioral concerns have decreased.
- Encourage attention to appropriate nutrition due to side effect of anorexia.

Quick quiz

1. A patient taking haloperidol calls the telehealth nurse reporting a fever and muscle rigidity. Which information will the nurse communicate?

    A. Stop the drug and go to the closest emergency department.
    B. Take your temperature every 4 hours for the next 24 hours.
    C. Push fluids and symptoms should resolve within 2 to 3 days.
    D. Skip the next dose of medication and call back tomorrow.

Answer: A. Fever and muscle rigidity are symptoms associated with neuroleptic malignant syndrome (NMS), a medical emergency requiring immediate treatment. Taking the temperature, pushing fluids, and skipping the next dose of medication are all instructions that delay treatment of NMS, which can be fatal if care is not sought.

2. A patient taking tranylcypromine (Parnate) has received dietary teaching from the nurse. When return demonstrating food selections, which patient choice requires the nurse to intervene?

    A. Fresh fish, carrots, vanilla pudding
    B. Apple juice, fries, fresh pineapple
    C. Hamburger, salad, milkshake
    D. Yogurt, salami, sliced avocado

Answer: D. Salami, yogurt, and avocados are tyramine-rich foods. Patients taking an MAO inhibitor such as tranylcypromine (Parnate) must avoid foods high in tyramine to prevent a hypertensive crisis. Fish, carrots, vanilla pudding, apple juice, fries, pineapple, hamburgers, salad, and milkshakes are not rich in tyramine, so these choices do not require the nurse to intervene.

3. Which adverse effect of fluoxetine (Prozac) will the nurse emphasize when teaching a patient who will begin taking this drug?

    A. Tremors
    B. Bradykinesia
    C. Sexual dysfunction
    D. Tardive dyskinesia

Answer: C. Fluoxetine (Prozac) is an SSRI drug. This category of drugs is often associated with sexual dysfunction. Tremors, bradykinesia, and tardive dyskinesia are extrapyramidal symptoms usually associated with antipsychotic medications.

4. A nurse is caring for a patient who has been taking sertraline (Zoloft) for several months. Which **priority** assessment finding will the nurse report to the health care provider?
  A. Diarrhea
  B. Fever
  C. Dizziness
  D. Insomnia

Answer: B. Symptoms of serotonin syndrome align with the SHIVERS acronym: Shivering, Hyperreflexia, *Increased temperature*, Vital signs instability, Encephalopathy, Restlessness, Sweating. Therefore, the fever must be reported as the priority to the health care provider. Diarrhea, dizziness, and insomnia are expected side effects associated with sertraline (Zoloft).

5. The health care provider is planning to place a 61-year-old patient on amitriptyline (no trade name at the time of publication) for depression. Which diagnostic test does the nurse anticipate will be ordered before drug therapy begins?
  A. Electrocardiogram
  B. Complete blood count
  C. Basic metabolic panel
  D. CT scan of the head

Answer: A. Amitriptyline (no trade name at the time of publication) can cause dose-dependent cardiac changes including QRS prolongation and arrhythmias; the nurse will anticipate that an electrocardiogram will be performed as a baseline before drug therapy begins. In the absence of other health concerns, a complete blood count, basic metabolic panel, and CT of the head would not be necessary prior to beginning amitriptyline.

Scoring

✰✰✰ If you answered all five questions correctly, great job! You're solid with this drug class.

✰✰ If you answered four questions correctly, you did just fine! There's no reason for you to feel badly.

✰ If you answered one to three questions correctly, stay calm. A quick review of the chapter will be helpful.

Suggested References

American Society of Hospital Pharmacists. (2021). *Secobarbital capsules*. Retrieved from https://www.ashp.org/Drug-Shortages/Current-Shortages/Drug-Shortage-Detail.aspx?id=517&loginreturnUrl=SSOCheckOnly

Amitriptyline: Drug information. (2021). In *UpToDate*. Waltham, MA: UpToDate.

Anderson, K., Lind, J., & Simeone, R. (2020). Maternal use of specific antidepressants during early pregnancy and the risk of selected birth defects. *JAMA Psychiatry, 77*(12), 1246–1255.

Boyer, E. (2021). Serotonin syndrome (serotonin toxicity). In S. Traub (Ed.), *UpToDate*. Waltham, MA: UpToDate.

Chokhawala, K., & Stevens, L. (2021). Antipsychotic medications. In *StatPearls* [Internet]. Treasure Island, FL: StatPearls Publishing. Retrieved from https://www.ncbi.nlm.nih.gov/books/NBK519503/

Cuijpers, P., Weitz, E., Lamers, F., Penninx, B. W., Twisk, J., DeRubeis, R. J., … & Hollon, S. D. (2017). Melancholic and atypical depression as predictor and moderator of outcome in cognitive behavior therapy and pharmacotherapy for adult depression. *Depression and Anxiety, 34*(3), 246–256.

Epocrates Online. (2021). *Desipramine*. Retrieved from https://online.epocrates.com/drugs/1611/desipramine/Black-Box-Warnings

Farzam, K., Faizy, R., & Saadabadi, A. (2021). Stimulants [Updated 2021 March 10]. In *StatPearls* [Internet]. Treasure Island, FL: StatPearls Publishing. Retrieved from https://www.ncbi.nlm.nih.gov/books/NBK539896/#_NBK539896_pubdet

Gabriel, M., & Sharma, V. (2017). Antidepressant discontinuation syndrome. *Canadian Medical Association Journal, 189*(21), E747.

Garcia, E., & Santos, C. (2021). Monoamine oxidase inhibitor toxicity. In *StatPearls* [Internet]. Treasure Island, FL: StatPearls Publishing. Retrieved from https://www.ncbi.nlm.nih.gov/books/NBK459386/

Hirsch, M., & Birnbaum, R. (2021). Monoamine oxidase inhibitors (MAOIs): Pharmacology administration, safety, and side effects. In P. Roy-Byrne (Ed.), *UpToDate*. Waltham, MA: UpToDate.

Huecker, M., Smiley, A., & Saadabadi, A. (2021). Bupropion [Updated 2021 April 19]. In *StatPearls* [Internet]. Treasure Island, FL: StatPearls Publishing. Retrieved from https://www.ncbi.nlm.nih.gov/books/NBK470212/

Jibson, M. (2021). Second-generation antipsychotic medications: Pharmacology, side effects, and administration. In S. Marder (Ed.), *UpToDate*. Waltham, MA: UpToDate.

Lien, Y. (2018). Antidepressants and hyponatremia. *The American Journal of Medicine, 131*(1), 7–8.

Moraczewski, J., & Aedma, K. (2020). Tricyclic antidepressants [Updated 2020 Dec 07]. In *StatPearls* [Internet]. Treasure Island, FL: StatPearls Publishing. Retrieved from https://www.ncbi.nlm.nih.gov/books/NBK557791/

Muluk, V., Cohn, S., & Whinney, C. (2021). Perioperative medication management. In A. Auerbach & N. Holt (Eds.), *UpToDate*. Waltham, MA: UpToDate.

Perrone, J., & Chattergee, P. (2020). Lithium poisoning. In S. Traub (Ed.), *UpToDate*. Waltham, MA: UpToDate.

Pfizer. (2021). Xanax (alprazolam), CIV boxed warning. Retrieved from https://www. pfizermedicalinformation.com/en-us/xanax/boxed-warning

Sanofi. (2018). *New data support long-term use of AMBIEN CR™ (zolpidem tartrate extended-release) tablets CIV for up to 24 weeks.* Retrieved from http://www. news.sanofi.us/press-releases?item=118389

Selegiline: Drug Information. (2021). In UpToDate, Lexicomp® database. Waltham, MA.

Soreide, K., Ward, K., & Bostwick, J. (2017). Strategies and solutions for switching antidepressants. *Psychiatry Times, 34*(12).

University of California San Francisco. (2021). *Monoamine oxidase B (MAO-B) inhibitors.* Retrieved from https://pdcenter.ucsf.edu/monoamine-oxidase-b-mao-b-inhibitors

Wijdicks, E. (2019). Neuroleptic malignant syndrome. In M. Aminoff (Ed.), *UpToDate*. Waltham, MA: UpToDate.

Chapter 16

Anti-infective drugs

Just the facts

In this chapter, you'll learn:

◆ classes of drugs that act as anti-infectives

◆ uses and varying actions of these drugs

◆ absorption, distribution, metabolization, and excretion of these drugs

◆ drug interactions and adverse reactions to these drugs.

Drugs and infection

When infection attacks the body, anti-infective drugs can help address the concern. Four main types of anti-infective drugs exist: antibacterial, antiviral, antitubercular, and antifungal. Other classes include antiprotozoals and antiparasitics. Due to the abundance of trade names for these types of drugs, *only select drugs in this chapter may have a trade name listed.* These lists are not exhaustive, so consult a current electronic drug database for the most up-to-date trade names associated with drugs.

Selecting an anti-infective drug

Selection of an appropriate anti-infective drug to treat a specific infection involves several important factors that the health care provider considers:

- First, the microorganism must be isolated and identified—generally through growing a culture.
- Its susceptibility to various drugs must be determined. Because culture and sensitivity results take 48 hours, broad treatment typically starts at assessment and is then reevaluated when test results are obtained.
- The location of the infection must be considered. For therapy to be effective, an adequate concentration of the anti-infective drug must be delivered to the infection site.

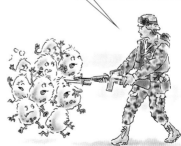

When infection attacks, anti-infective drugs can help you win the battle. Get back!

The rise of the resistance movement

Indiscriminate use of anti-infective drugs has serious consequences. Unnecessary exposure of organisms to these drugs encourages the emergence of resistant strains. These resistant strains are likely to do far more damage than their predecessors.

Anti-infective drugs should be reserved for patients with infections caused by susceptible organisms and should be used in high enough doses and for an appropriate period. New anti-infective drugs should be reserved for severely ill patients with serious infections that don't respond to conventional drugs.

- Finally, the cost of the drug as well as its potential adverse effects and the possibility of patient allergies must be considered.

Preventing pathogen resistance

The usefulness of anti-infective drugs is limited by the pathogens that may develop resistance to a drug's action.

The mutants strike back

Resistance is the ability of a microorganism to live and grow in the presence of an anti-infective drug. Resistance usually results from genetic mutation of the microorganism. (See *The rise of the resistance movement*.)

Antibacterial drugs

Antibacterial drugs, also known as *antibiotics*, are drugs that either kill bacteria or inhibit the growth of bacteria. They're mainly used to treat systemic (involving the whole body rather than a localized area) bacterial infections. Antibacterial drugs include:
- aminoglycosides
- penicillins
- cephalosporins
- tetracyclines
- clindamycin (Cleocin)
- macrolides
- vancomycin (Vancocin)
- carbapenems
- monobactams
- fluoroquinolones

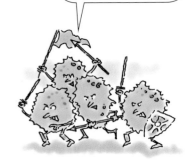

When anti-infective drugs are used indiscriminately, our resistance grows.

- sulfonamides
- nitrofurantoin
- linezolid (Zyvox).

Aminoglycosides

Aminoglycosides are bactericidal (they destroy bacteria). They're effective against:
- gram-negative bacilli
- some aerobic gram-positive bacteria
- mycobacteria
- some protozoa.

Naming names

Aminoglycosides currently in use include:
- amikacin sulphate
- gentamicin sulphate
- neomycin sulfate
- paromomycin sulfate
- plazomicin
- streptomycin sulfate
- tobramycin sulfate.

Pharmacokinetics

Because aminoglycosides are absorbed poorly from the GI tract, they're usually given parenterally except neomycin, which is given orally for preoperative bowel cleansing. After IV or IM administration, aminoglycoside absorption is rapid and complete.

Flowing with extracellular fluid

Aminoglycosides are distributed widely in extracellular fluid. They readily cross the placental barrier but don't cross the blood-brain barrier.

You're kidney-ing me!

Aminoglycosides aren't metabolized. They're excreted primarily by the kidneys, so the half-life will increase as kidney function decreases.

Pharmacodynamics

Aminoglycosides act as bactericidal drugs against susceptible organisms by binding to the bacteria's 30S subunit, a specific ribosome in the microorganism, thereby interrupting protein synthesis and causing the bacteria to die.

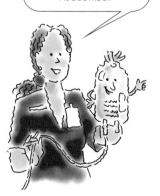

Aminoglycosides kill bacteria by binding to their 30S subunit ribosomes.

Reasons behind resistance

Bacterial resistance to aminoglycosides may be related to:

- failure of the drug to cross the cell membrane
- altered binding to ribosomes
- destruction of the drug by bacterial enzymes.

Penetration power provided by penicillin

Some gram-positive enterococci resist aminoglycoside transport across the cell membrane. When penicillin is used with aminoglycoside therapy, the cell wall is altered, allowing the aminoglycoside to penetrate the bacterial cell. In combination therapy, penicillin should be given first. (See *Aminoglycosides: Gentamicin.*)

Pharmacotherapeutics

Aminoglycosides are most useful in treating:

- infections caused by gram-negative bacilli
- serious nosocomial (hospital-acquired) infections, such as gram-negative bacteremia (abnormal presence of microorganisms in the bloodstream), peritonitis (inflammation of the peritoneum, the membrane that lines the abdominal cavity), and pneumonia in critically ill patients
- urinary tract infections (UTIs) caused by enteric bacilli that are resistant to less toxic antibacterial drugs, such as penicillins and cephalosporins
- infections of the central nervous system (CNS) and the eye (treated with local instillation).

Prototype pro

Aminoglycosides: Gentamicin

Actions

- Inhibits protein synthesis by binding directly to the 30S ribosomal subunit; usually bactericidal

Indications

- Serious infections caused by susceptible organisms
- Prevention of endocarditis during GI and genitourinary procedures or surgery

Nursing considerations

- Monitor the patient for adverse effects, such as ototoxicity, nephrotoxicity, anaphylaxis, thrombocytopenia, and agranulocytosis.
- Peak gentamicin levels occur 1 hour after IM injection and 30 minutes after IV infusion; check trough levels before the next dose.

Combo care

Aminoglycosides are often used in combination with other antibiotics to treat complicated infections such as septicemia, urinary tract infections, endocarditis, and intra-abdominal infections.

Taming strains

Individual aminoglycosides may be used for a specific reason. Examples include:

- Streptomycin is active against many strains of mycobacteria, including *Mycobacterium tuberculosis*, although is now considered second-line for the treatment of this disease.
- Amikacin, gentamicin, and tobramycin are active to varying degrees against *Acinetobacter*, *Enterobacter*, *Haemophilus influenzae*, *Pseudomonas aeruginosa*, and *Serratia*.
- Neomycin is given orally to suppress intestinal bacteria before surgery and is active against *Escherichia coli* infectious diarrhea.

When the drug's a dud

Aminoglycosides are inactive against anaerobic bacteria.

Drug interactions

There are many medications that can interact with the aminoglycosides. Reference a current electronic database to confirm interactions.

Amplified effects

Aminoglycosides administered with neuromuscular blockers such as succinylcholine increase neuromuscular blockade, resulting in increased muscle relaxation and respiratory distress.

Toxic mix

Toxicity to the kidneys may result in renal failure, which is usually reversible. The risk of renal toxicity increases with drugs such as cyclosporine, amphotericin B, acyclovir, additional aminoglycosides, naproxen, and some chemotherapeutic agents. Caution should also be used with warfarin, as this combination can increase the risk of bleeding.

Oh dear, those poor ears

The symptoms of ototoxicity caused by aminoglycosides may be masked by antiemetic drugs and preexisting hearing loss. Loop diuretics taken with aminoglycosides increase the risk of ototoxicity. Hearing loss may occur in varying degrees and may be irreversible.

Side effects/Adverse reactions

Serious adverse reactions limit the use of aminoglycosides and include:

- neuromuscular reactions, ranging from peripheral nerve toxicity to neuromuscular blockade
- ototoxicity
- renal toxicity.

Oral report

More common adverse reactions to oral aminoglycosides include:

- nausea
- vomiting
- fatigue.

The Three-Step Approach

Nursing management for patients prescribed aminoglycosides includes these three steps.

Preadministration

(Recognize and analyze cues)

- Obtain the patient's allergy history.
- Obtain culture and sensitivity tests before giving the first dose; therapy may begin pending test results. Check these tests periodically to assess the drug's efficacy.
- Obtain baseline vital signs, electrolyte levels, weight, hearing ability, and renal function before and during therapy.
- Assess for drug interactions and adverse reactions.

(Prioritize hypothesis—priority patient problems)

- Compromise in immunity due to infection
- Potential for injury

(Generate solutions)

- The infection will resolve without injury to the patient.

Medication administration

(Take action)

- Double check the route of delivery.
- If prescribed IM, administer drug into a large muscle mass (ventral gluteal); rotate injection sites to minimize tissue injury. Apply ice to the injection site to relieve pain.
- Follow the manufacturer's instructions for reconstitution, dilution, and storage of medications; check expiration dates.
- Don't add or mix other drugs if prescribed as an IV infusion. If other drugs must be given IV, temporarily stop infusion of the primary drug.

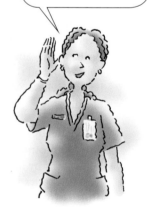

Because of the potential for ototoxicity, make sure you assess the patient's hearing ability before and during therapy with aminoglycosides.

- Because too-rapid IV administration may cause neuromuscular blockade, carefully read the recommendations for infusing time.
- For patients prescribed gentamicin, draw blood to check for the peak level 1 hour after IM injection (30 minutes to 1 hour after IV infusion); for the trough level, draw a sample just before the next dose. Peak gentamicin levels above 12 mcg/mL and trough levels above 2 mcg/mL may increase the risk of toxicity. Time and date all blood samples. Don't use a heparinized tube to collect blood samples because it interferes with results.
- Assess for immediate adverse reactions and drug interactions.

Postadministration
(Evaluate outcomes)
- Keep the patient well hydrated to minimize chemical irritation of the renal tubules.
- Notify the health care provider of signs and symptoms of decreasing renal function or changes in hearing.
- Be aware that 8 hours of hemodialysis removes up to 50% of gentamicin from blood. Scheduled dosages may need to be adjusted accordingly.
- Be aware that therapy usually continues for 7 to 10 days. If no response occurs in 3 to 5 days, therapy may be stopped and new specimens may be obtained for culture and sensitivity testing. It is also common for aminoglycosides to be stopped in favor of less toxic antibiotics once sensitivities are available.

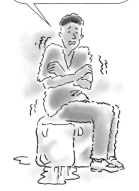

Brrr! Applying ice can help relieve pain at an IM injection site.

Penicillins

Penicillins remain one of the most important and useful antibacterial drugs, despite the availability of numerous others. The penicillins can be divided into three groups:
- natural penicillins: penicillin G (Pfizerpen) and penicillin V potassium
- antistaphylococcal penicillins: nafcillin, oxacillin, and dicloxacillin
- broad-spectrum penicillins: second-generation ampicillin, amoxicillin, and fourth-generation piperacillin (Zosyn).

Pharmacokinetics

After oral administration, penicillins are absorbed mainly in the duodenum and the upper jejunum of the small intestine.

Affecting absorption
Absorption of oral penicillin varies and depends on such factors as:
- particular penicillin used
- pH of the patient's stomach and intestine
- presence of food in the GI tract.

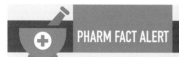

PHARM FACT ALERT

Most penicillins should be given on an empty stomach (1 hour before or 2 hours after a meal) to enhance absorption. Penicillins that can be given without regard to meals include amoxicillin, penicillin V, and amoxicillin-clavulanate (Augmentin).

Well traveled

Penicillins are distributed widely to most areas of the body, including the lungs, liver, kidneys, muscle, bone, and placenta. High concentrations also appear in urine, making penicillins useful in treating urinary tract infections.

Exit route

Penicillins are metabolized to a limited extent in the liver to inactive metabolites. Most penicillins are excreted 60% unchanged by the kidneys. Nafcillin and oxacillin, however, are excreted in bile.

Pharmacodynamics

Penicillins are usually bactericidal in action. They bind reversibly to several enzymes outside the bacterial cytoplasmic membrane. These enzymes, known as *penicillin-binding proteins* (PBPs), are involved in cell wall synthesis and cell division. Interference with these processes inhibits cell wall synthesis, causing rapid destruction of the cell.

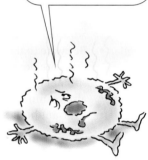

Can't build walls! Can't divide! Too many PBPs attacked by penicillins!

Pharmacotherapeutics

No other class of antibacterial drugs provides as wide a spectrum of antimicrobial activity as the penicillins. As a class, they cover gram-positive, gram-negative, and anaerobic organisms, although specific penicillins are more effective against specific organisms.

IM: A solution for the insoluble

Penicillin is given by IM injection when oral administration is inconvenient or a patient's compliance is questionable. Because long-acting preparations of penicillin G (penicillin G benzathine or Bicillin L-A and penicillin G procaine) are relatively insoluble, they must be administered by the IM route. (See *Natural penicillins: Penicillin G sodium,* page 573.)

Drug interactions

Penicillins may interact with various drugs:
- Probenecid increases the plasma concentration of penicillins.
- Penicillins reduce tubular secretion of methotrexate in the kidneys, increasing the risk of methotrexate toxicity.

Prototype pro

Natural penicillins: Penicillin G sodium

Actions
- Inhibits cell wall synthesis during microorganism multiplication
- Resists penicillinase enzymes produced by bacteria that convert penicillins to inactive penicilloic acid

Indications
- Bacterial infection caused by non–penicillinase-producing strains of gram-positive and gram-negative aerobic cocci, spirochetes, or certain gram-positive aerobic and anaerobic bacilli

Nursing considerations
- Monitor the patient for adverse effects, such as seizures, anaphylaxis, leukopenia, and thrombocytopenia.
- Monitor for signs of superinfection, including yeast infections and *Clostridium difficile* colitis.
- Obtain a specimen for culture and sensitivity tests before giving the first dose. Therapy may begin pending results.

- Tetracyclines reduce the bactericidal action of penicillins.
- The effectiveness of hormonal contraceptives is reduced when they're taken with penicillins. If applicable, advise the patient to use a reliable alternative method of contraception in addition to hormonal contraceptives during antibiotic therapy.
- Penicillins can also increase the bleeding risks of anticoagulants as they prolong bleeding time by decreasing vitamin K.
- Penicillins may precipitate or worsen hyperkalemia and hypernatremia.
- Aminoglycosides and clavulanic acid increase the anti-infective actions of penicillins.

Adverse reactions

Hypersensitivity reactions are the major adverse reactions to penicillins, including:
- anaphylactic reactions
- serum sickness (a hypersensitivity reaction occurring 1 to 2 weeks after injection of a foreign serum)
- drug fever
- various skin rashes.

GI didn't know this could happen

Adverse GI reactions associated with oral penicillins include:
- oral candidiasis
- nausea and vomiting
- diarrhea.

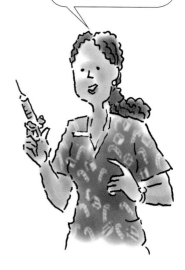

Penicillin can be given IM when oral administration isn't appropriate, or a patient's adherence to therapy is a concern.

I'm all nerves

CNS reactions may include:

- lethargy
- hallucinations
- anxiety or depression
- confusion
- seizures.

The Three-Step Approach

Nursing management for patients prescribed penicillin therapy includes these three steps.

Preadministration

(Recognize and analyze cues)

- Obtain a history of the course of infection before therapy; reassess for improvement regularly thereafter.
- Assess the patient's allergy history. Ask clarifying questions to confirm whether previous reactions were true hypersensitivity reactions or adverse reactions (such as GI distress) that the patient interpreted as an allergy.
- Obtain culture and sensitivity tests before giving the first dose; therapy may begin pending test results. Repeat these tests periodically to assess the drug's effectiveness.
- Obtain baseline vital signs, electrolytes, and renal function studies.
- Assess the patient's baseline consciousness and neurologic status when giving high doses; CNS toxicity can occur.
- Because of coagulation abnormalities, monitor prothrombin time (PT), international normalized ratio (INR), and platelet counts, and assess the patient for signs of occult or frank bleeding.
- Clarify route of delivery. Recognize that certain penicillins (e.g., penicillin G benzathene injection) must never be injected into a vein, as this can be lethal.

(Prioritize hypothesis—priority patient problems)

- Compromise in immunity due to infection
- Potential for dehydration

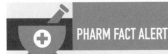

PHARM FACT ALERT

Penicillins such as amoxicillin and ampicillin can produce pseudomembranous colitis (diarrhea caused by a change in the flora of the colon or an overgrowth of a toxin-producing strain of *C. difficile*).

(Generate solutions)
- The infection will resolve and the patient will not become dehydrated.

Medication administration

(Take action)
- Give penicillins at least 1 hour before bacteriostatic antibacterial drugs (such as tetracyclines), as these drugs inhibit bacterial cell growth and decrease the rate of penicillin uptake by bacterial cell walls.
- Follow the manufacturers' directions for reconstituting, diluting, and storing drugs; check expiration dates.
- Give oral penicillins at least 1 hour before or 2 hours after meals to enhance GI absorption. Some penicillins can be given without regard to food.
- Refrigerate oral suspensions; shake well before administering to ensure the correct dosage.
- Give an IM dose deep into a large muscle mass (gluteal or midlateral thigh), rotate injection sites to minimize tissue injury, and apply ice to the injection site to relieve pain.
- With IV infusions, don't add or mix another drug, especially an aminoglycoside, which becomes inactive if mixed with a penicillin. If other drugs must be given IV, temporarily stop infusion of the primary drug.
- Infuse an IV drug continuously or intermittently (over 30 minutes). Rotate the infusion site every 48 hours. Carefully read labels for dilution instructions for an intermittent IV infusion.

Teach your patient when to take oral penicillin, as some must be taken <u>without</u> food and some should be taken <u>with</u> food.

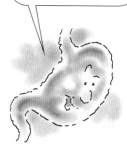

Postadministration

(Evaluate outcomes)
- Monitor continuously for possible allergic reactions. A patient who has never had a penicillin hypersensitivity reaction may still have future allergic reactions.
- Monitor patients receiving long-term therapy for possible superinfection (especially older adults, individuals who are debilitated, and those receiving immunosuppressants or radiation).
- Monitor hydration status if adverse GI reactions occur.
- Provide patient education. (See *Teaching about anti-infective therapy*, page 576.)

Just because a patient hasn't had an allergic reaction to penicillin before doesn't mean he won't have one in the future. Make sure you monitor for possible allergic reactions during penicillin therapy.

 Lifespan Lightbulb

Older adults are more susceptible to the development of a superinfection when taking penicillin than younger individuals. Monitor them closely!

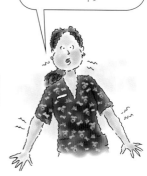

Teaching about anti-infective therapy

If anti-infective therapy is prescribed, review these points with the patient and caregivers:

- Take this drug exactly as prescribed. Some drugs should be taken on an empty stomach 1 hour before or 2 hours after meals. Food may decrease drug absorption.
- Complete the entire prescribed regimen even if you begin to feel better. Comply with instructions for around-the-clock scheduling, and keep follow-up appointments.

- Report unusual reactions, such as a rash, fever, or chills. These may be signs and symptoms of hypersensitivity to the drug.
- If using hormonal contraceptives, use an additional form of contraception during drug therapy, as anti-infective drugs can decrease the efficacy of these drugs.
- Store the drug appropriately; some drugs may need refrigeration.

First-generation cephalosporins: Cefazolin

Actions
- Inhibits cell wall synthesis, promoting osmotic instability
- Usually are bactericidal

Indications
- Infection caused by susceptible organisms including mostly select gram-positive and gram-negative aerobes

Nursing considerations
- Obtain a specimen for culture and sensitivity tests before giving the first dose. Therapy may begin pending results.
- Monitor for adverse effects, such as diarrhea, hematologic disorders, rash, and hypersensitivity reactions.
- With large doses or prolonged treatment, monitor for superinfections.

Cephalosporins

Cephalosporins are grouped into generations according to their effectiveness against different organisms, their characteristics, and their development:

- First-generation cephalosporins include cefadroxil, cefazolin sodium, and cephalexin hydrochloride monohydrate (Keflex). (See *First-generation cephalosporins: Cefazolin.*)
- Second-generation cephalosporins include cefaclor, cefotetan (Cefotan), cefoxitin, cefprozil, cefuroxime axetil, and cefuroxime sodium.
- Third-generation cephalosporins include cefdinir, cefixime (Suprax), cefotaxime sodium, cefpodoxime proxetil, ceftazidime (Fortaz), and ceftriaxone sodium.
- Fourth-generation cephalosporins include cefepime hydrochloride (Maxipime).
- Fifth-generation cephalosporins include cefiderocol (Fetroja) and ceftaroline fosamil (Teflaro).

Similar components = similar reactions

Because penicillins and cephalosporins are chemically similar (they both have what's called a *beta-lactam* molecular structure), cross-sensitivity can occur. This means that someone who has had a true reaction to penicillin is also at risk for having a reaction to cephalosporins.

Pharmacokinetics

Many cephalosporins are administered parenterally because they aren't absorbed from the GI tract. Some cephalosporins are absorbed from the GI tract and can be administered orally, but food usually decreases their absorption rate more than the amount absorbed. Some cephalosporins (for example, oral cefuroxime and cefpodoxime) actually have increased absorption when given with food.

No service to the CNS

After absorption, cephalosporins are distributed widely, although first- and second-generation drugs aren't distributed well in the CNS.

Crossing the line

Cefuroxime (second-generation) and the third-generation drugs cefotaxime, ceftizoxime, ceftriaxone, and ceftazidime cross the blood-brain barrier. Cefepime (fourth-generation) also crosses the blood-brain barrier. Ceftaroline (fifth-generation) appears to penetrate into cerebrospinal fluid (CSF); this phenomenon is still being studied (Cies et al., 2020).

Much ado about metabolism

Many cephalosporins aren't metabolized at all. Cefotaxime is metabolized to the nonacetyl form, which provides less antibacterial activity than the parent compound. To a small extent, ceftriaxone is metabolized in the intestines to inactive metabolites, which are excreted via the biliary system.

Making an exit

All cephalosporins are excreted primarily unchanged by the kidneys with the exception of ceftriaxone, which is excreted in feces via bile.

There's always an exception to the rule! Although the absorption of oral cephalosporins usually decreases when given with food, the absorption of oral cefuroxime and cefpodoxime increases with food.

Pharmacodynamics

Like penicillins, cephalosporins inhibit cell wall synthesis by binding to the bacterial PBP enzymes located on the cell membrane. After the drug damages the cell wall by binding with the PBPs, the body's natural defense mechanisms destroy the bacteria. (See *How cephalosporins attack bacteria*, page 578.)

Pharmacotherapeutics

The five generations of cephalosporins have particular therapeutic uses:
- First-generation cephalosporins, which act primarily against gram-positive organisms, may be used as alternative therapy in a patient who's allergic to penicillin, depending on how sensitive

Pharm function

How cephalosporins attack bacteria

The antibacterial action of cephalosporins depends on their ability to penetrate the bacterial wall and bind with proteins on the cytoplasmic membrane, as shown below.

> Cephalosporins penetrate and bind. That's how they wipe me out!

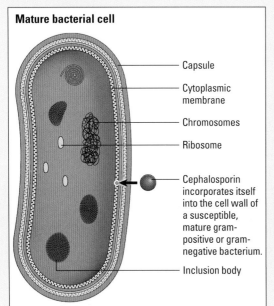

Mature bacterial cell

- Capsule
- Cytoplasmic membrane
- Chromosomes
- Ribosome
- Cephalosporin incorporates itself into the cell wall of a susceptible, mature gram-positive or gram-negative bacterium.
- Inclusion body

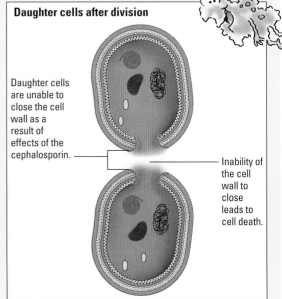

Daughter cells after division

Daughter cells are unable to close the cell wall as a result of effects of the cephalosporin.

Inability of the cell wall to close leads to cell death.

to penicillin the person is. They're also used to treat staphylococcal and streptococcal infections, including pneumonia, cellulitis (skin infection), and osteomyelitis (bone infection).

- Second-generation cephalosporins act against gram-negative bacteria. Cefoxitin and cefotetan are the only cephalosporins effective against anaerobes (organisms that live without oxygen) as seen in pressure injuries or intra-abdominal sepsis. The oral medications may help in treating otitis, sinusitis, and respiratory infections.
- Third-generation cephalosporins act on infections caused by *H. influenzae*, streptococci, and *Moraxella catarrhalis*. They are also more active than the other generations against gram-negative bacteria such as *E. coli*, *Proteus mirabilis*, and *Klebsiella*.
- Fourth-generation cephalosporins are active against a wide range of gram-positive and gram-negative bacteria.

- Fifth-generation cephalosporins are aimed at treating resistant strains of gram-positive and gram-negative bacteria present in acute bacterial skin infections (including methicillin-resistant *Staphylococcus aureus*—MRSA) and many strains of community-acquired bacterial pneumonia. They are not, however, active against *Pseudomonas*.

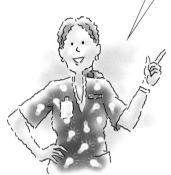

Cephalosporins and alcohol don't mix. Acute alcohol intolerance can occur, even 3 days after stopping the drug.

Drug interactions

Patients receiving cefotetan who drink alcoholic beverages with or up to 72 hours after taking a dose may experience acute alcohol intolerance. Signs and symptoms include headache, flushing, dizziness, nausea, vomiting, or abdominal cramps within 30 minutes of alcohol ingestion. This reaction can occur up to 3 days after discontinuing the antibiotic.

Other interactions

Uricosurics (drugs to relieve gout), such as probenecid, can reduce kidney excretion of some cephalosporins. Proton pump inhibitors and other drugs for acid reflux such as famotidine (Pepcid AC and Pepcid Complete, which are over-the-counter drugs) and cimetidine (Tagamet HB, which is also available over-the-counter) may decrease the efficacy of some cephalosporins, as well.

Adverse reactions

Adverse reactions to cephalosporins include:
- confusion
- seizures
- nausea
- vomiting
- diarrhea.

Bleeding concerns

Some cephalosporins such as cefotetan and ceftriaxone may be associated with a prolonged prothrombin time and partial thromboplastin time, leading to an increased risk of bleeding. Populations at risk include elderly, debilitated, malnourished, and immunocompromised patients and those with renal impairment, hepatic disease, or impaired vitamin K synthesis or storage. Warfarin dosing may also need to be adjusted while on cephalosporin therapy.

Systemically speaking

Hypersensitivity reactions are the most common systemic adverse reactions to cephalosporins and include hives, itching, rash, and (in rare cases) anaphylaxis.

The Three-Step Approach

Nursing management for patients undergoing treatment with a cephalosporin drug is similar to that of management of patients receiving other anti-infective therapies. Remember to administer cephalosporins at least 1 hour before bacteriostatic antibacterial drugs (tetracyclines, erythromycins, and chloramphenicol); by decreasing cephalosporin uptake by bacterial cell walls, the antibacterial drugs inhibit bacterial cell growth. Monitor renal function laboratory values, and PT and platelet counts while on this type of medication regimen. As with any drug administration, be certain to pay particular attention to the type of drug being given, and personalize care. (See *Teaching about cephalosporins.*)

> Review the patient's allergy history to help determine if previous reactions to cephalosporins were true hypersensitivity reactions.

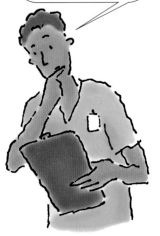

Tetracyclines

Tetracyclines are broad-spectrum antibacterial drugs. Doxycycline (Vibramycin) and minocycline (Minocin) are the most commonly used drugs in this class. Tetracycline hydrochloride is also widely used. In recent years, development of tetracycline analogues has led to development of a group of medications called glycylcyclines. These include tigecycline (Tygacil), eravacycline (Xerava), sarecycline (Seysara), and omadacycline (Nuzyra).

Pharmacokinetics

Tetracyclines are absorbed from the duodenum and stomach when taken orally. They're distributed widely into body tissues and fluids and concentrated in bile. Additionally, these medications cross the placenta. Tetracycline is excreted primarily by the kidneys. Doxycycline and tigecycline are mostly excreted in feces. Minocycline undergoes enterohepatic recirculation.

Education edge

Teaching about cephalosporins

Teaching about cephalosporins is similar to teaching about other anti-infective therapies. Additional key items to teach include:

- Don't consume alcohol in any form within 72 hours of treatment with certain cephalosporins.
- Eat yogurt or consider probiotics to prevent intestinal superinfection resulting from the drug's suppression of normal intestinal flora.

Pharmacodynamics

All tetracyclines are primarily bacteriostatic, meaning they inhibit the growth or multiplication of bacteria. They penetrate the bacterial cell by an energy-dependent process or through passive diffusion. Within the cell, they bind primarily to a subunit of the ribosome, inhibiting the protein synthesis required for maintaining the bacterial cell. The long-acting compounds doxycycline and minocycline provide more action against various organisms than other tetracyclines. (See *Tetracyclines: Tetracycline hydrochloride.*)

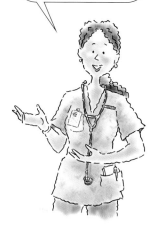

Tetracyclines inhibit bacteria growth or multiplication.

Pharmacotherapeutics

Tetracyclines cover a wide range of organisms, including:
- gram-positive and gram-negative aerobic and anaerobic bacteria
- spirochetes
- mycoplasmas
- rickettsiae
- chlamydiae
- some protozoa.
  Tetracyclines are used to treat:
- Rocky Mountain spotted fever
- Q fever
- Lyme disease
- nongonococcal urethritis caused by *Chlamydia.*
  Additionally, tigecycline has activity against vancomycin-resistant enterococci (VRE), *Listeria, Pasteurella multocida,* and *Acinetobacter baumannii.*

Prototype pro

Tetracyclines: Tetracycline hydrochloride

Actions
- Bacteriostatic, although may be bactericidal against certain organisms
- Binds reversibly to 30S ribosomal subunit, inhibiting bacterial protein synthesis

Indications
- Infection caused by susceptible organisms located in the respiratory, GI, and urinary tracts.
- *Syphilis* and *Chlamydia*

Nursing considerations
- Obtain a specimen for culture and sensitivity tests before giving the first dose. Therapy may begin pending results.
- Monitor the patient for adverse effects, such as nausea, diarrhea, hematologic disorders, Stevens-Johnson syndrome, rash, photosensitivity, and hypersensitivity reactions.
- With large doses or prolonged treatment, monitor the patient for superinfections.

Two-timing

Combination therapy with a tetracycline and rifampin is the most effective treatment for brucellosis.

Facial effects

Tetracyclines in low dosages effectively treat acne because they decrease the fatty acid content of sebum.

Drug interactions

Tetracyclines can reduce the effectiveness of hormonal contraceptives, which may result in breakthrough bleeding or ineffective contraception. Patients taking hormonal contraceptives should use a reliable, secondary method of contraception before and throughout treatment. Tetracyclines may also decrease the bactericidal action of penicillin.

Affecting other pharmacodynamics

Other interactions commonly affect the ability of tetracyclines to move through the body:

- Aluminum, calcium, and magnesium antacids reduce the absorption of oral tetracyclines.
- Iron salts, bismuth subsalicylate, and zinc sulfate reduce the absorption of doxycycline and tetracycline. Reduced absorption can be prevented by separating doses of tetracyclines and these agents by 2 to 3 hours.
- Barbiturates, carbamazepine, and phenytoin increase the metabolism and reduce the antibiotic effect of doxycycline.

Lifestyle considerations

- Sun exposure should be avoided with tetracyclines as photosensitivity is common.
- Alcohol reduces the effectiveness of doxycycline and should be avoided.

Adverse reactions

Tetracyclines produce many of the same adverse reactions as other antibacterials, including:

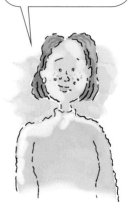

Low dosages of tetracyclines are used to treat acne.

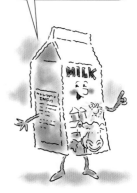

Tetracyclines can also interact with milk!

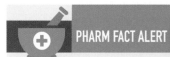

PHARM FACT ALERT

Tetracyclines, with the exception of doxycycline and minocycline, may also interact with milk and milk products, which bind with the drugs and prevent their absorption. To prevent decreased absorption, administer the tetracycline 1 hour before or 2 hours after meals.

- superinfection
- nausea and vomiting
- abdominal distress and distention
- diarrhea.
  Other adverse reactions include:
- photosensitivity reactions (red rash on areas exposed to sunlight)
- hepatic and/or renal toxicity
- discoloration of permanent teeth and tooth enamel hypoplasia in fetuses and children (doxycycline may be the only exception if used for short-term treatment of a disorder)
- possible impaired fetal skeletal development if taken during pregnancy.

The Three-Step Approach

Nursing management for patients undergoing treatment with a tetracycline is similar to that of management of patients receiving other anti-infective therapies. Remind patients to refrain from use of antacids, iron compounds, and dairy products, which can impair absorption. Giving a tetracycline drug with water helps to facilitate passage to the stomach. Do not give a tetracycline within 1 hour of bedtime to prevent esophageal reflux. As with any drug administration, be certain to pay particular attention to the drug being given, and personalize administration and teaching. (See *Teaching about tetracyclines*.)

Clindamycin (Cleocin)

Clindamycin is a derivative of another drug, lincomycin. Because of its high potential for causing serious adverse effects, clindamycin is prescribed only when there's no therapeutic alternative or if the patient is allergic to penicillins. It's used for various gram-positive and anaerobic organisms.

Pharmacokinetics

When taken orally, clindamycin is absorbed well and distributed widely in the body. It's metabolized by the liver and excreted by the kidneys and biliary pathways.

Pharmacodynamics

Clindamycin inhibits bacterial protein synthesis and may also inhibit the binding of bacterial ribosomes. At therapeutic concentrations, clindamycin is primarily bacteriostatic against most organisms.

Pharmacotherapeutics

Because of its potential for causing serious toxicity and pseudomembranous colitis (characterized by severe diarrhea,

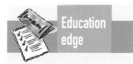

Education edge

Teaching about tetracyclines

Teaching about tetracyclines is similar to teaching about other anti-infective therapies. Additional key items to teach include:
- Don't take the drug with food, milk or other dairy products, sodium bicarbonate, or iron compounds because they may interfere with absorption.
- Wait 3 hours after taking a tetracycline before taking an antacid.
- Avoid direct exposure to sunlight and use a sunscreen to help prevent photosensitivity reactions.
- Monitor teeth; report any discoloration, even subtle changes, immediately.

abdominal pain, fever, and mucus and blood in feces), clindamycin is prescribed only in a few clinical situations in which safer alternative antibacterials aren't available:

- It's potent against most aerobic gram-positive organisms, including staphylococci and streptococci (except *Enterococcus faecalis*).
- It may be used as an alternative to penicillin in treating staphylococcal infections in patients who are allergic to penicillin.

Drug interactions

Clindamycin has neuromuscular blocking properties and may enhance the blocking action of neuromuscular blockers. This can lead to profound respiratory depression. Macrolides and chloramphenicol bind to the same site as clindamycin and should not be given together. Additionally, drugs that are strong inducers of CYP3A4 metabolism such as rifampin can decrease serum concentrations of clindamycin if given together.

Adverse reactions

Pseudomembranous colitis may occur with clindamycin use. This syndrome can be fatal and requires prompt discontinuation of the drug as well as aggressive fluid and electrolyte management. Although this is the most serious reaction to clindamycin and limits its use, other reactions may also occur, such as:

- diarrhea
- stomatitis (mouth inflammation)
- nausea
- vomiting
- hypersensitivity reactions.

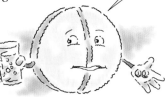

Because of its high potential for causing serious adverse effects, clindamycin is a last resort.

The Three-Step Approach

Nursing management for patients undergoing treatment with clindamycin is similar to that of management of patients receiving other anti-infective therapies. Key additional actions include:

- Monitor renal, hepatic, and hematopoietic functions during prolonged therapy.
- Give the capsule form with a full glass of water to prevent dysphagia.
- Recognize that IM injections may raise creatine kinase levels in response to muscle irritation.

As with any drug administration, be certain to pay particular attention to the drug being given and personalize care.

Macrolides

Macrolides are used to treat many common infections. They include erythromycin and its derivatives, such as:

- erythromycin ethylsuccinate (EryPed)
- erythromycin lactobionate (Erythrocin).

Other macrolides include:
- azithromycin (Zithromax)
- clarithromycin
- fidaxomicin (Dificid).

Pharmacokinetics

Because erythromycin is acid sensitive, it must be buffered or have an enteric coating to prevent destruction by gastric acid. Erythromycin is absorbed in the duodenum. It's distributed to most tissues and body fluids except, in most cases, cerebrospinal fluid (CSF).

Following many paths

Erythromycin is metabolized by the liver and excreted in bile in high concentrations; small amounts are excreted in urine. It also crosses the placental barrier and is secreted in breast milk.

Something in common

Azithromycin is rapidly absorbed by the GI tract and is distributed throughout the body. It readily penetrates cells but doesn't readily enter the CNS. Like erythromycin, azithromycin is excreted mostly in bile; small amounts are excreted in urine.

Wide ranging

Clarithromycin is rapidly absorbed and widely distributed and is excreted in urine.

With or without

Fidaxomicin may be taken without regard to food intake. This drug stays local in the GI tract where it is metabolized through hydrolysis and excreted in feces.

Pharmacodynamics

Macrolides inhibit ribonucleic acid (RNA)-dependent protein synthesis by acting on a small portion of the ribosome, much like clindamycin.

Pharmacotherapeutics

Macrolides have a range of therapeutic uses:
- They provide a broad spectrum of antimicrobial activity against gram-positive and gram-negative bacteria, including *Campylobacter, Treponema, Mycoplasma,* and *Chlamydia*.
- They are effective against group A streptococci. Traditionally, macrolides have also been used for pneumococcal infections; however, due to increased resistance, they are now used to cover potential atypical infections of the lower respiratory tract in combination with other antibiotics.
- *Staphylococcus aureus* is sensitive to erythromycin; however, resistant strains have appeared.

First in class

- Macrolides are drugs of choice for *Mycoplasma pneumoniae*, *Legionella*, and *Bordetella pertussis*.
- Fidaxomicin is specifically indicated only for infection caused by *C. difficile*.

More tolerable

In patients who are allergic to penicillin, azithromycin is effective for infections produced by group A beta-hemolytic streptococci or *Streptococcus pneumoniae*. It may also be used to treat gonorrhea in patients who can't tolerate penicillin G or a tetracycline. Topical erythromycin may also be used to treat minor staphylococcal infections of the skin.

Broad-spectrum benefits

These broad-spectrum antibacterial drugs (drugs that cover a wide range of organisms) have multiple therapeutic actions:

- Azithromycin and clarithromycin have a broader range of activity than erythromycin.
- Clarithromycin and azithromycin both provide activity against *Haemophilus influenzae* and *Mycobacterium avium* complex. Additionally, they are usually active against groups A, B, C, and G *Streptococcus*.
- Azithromycin is commonly used to treat sexually transmitted diseases such as those caused by *N. gonorrhoeae* (combination therapy), *Chlamydia trachomatis*, and *Haemophilus ducreyi* (chancroid).
- Clarithromycin has been used in combination with penicillin and proton pump inhibitors to treat *Helicobacter pylori*–induced duodenal ulcer disease, although some resistance has been shown.

Drug interactions

Macrolides may cause these drug interactions:

- Erythromycin, azithromycin, and clarithromycin can increase theophylline levels in patients receiving high dosages of theophylline, increasing the risk of toxicity.
- Clarithromycin may increase the concentration of carbamazepine when the drugs are used together.
- Macrolides when coadministered with colchicine in those with renal or hepatic impairments may cause colchicine toxicity.
- This drug class should not be given with cisapride or pimozide due to a combined potential for an increased QT interval.

Adverse reactions

Although macrolides have few adverse effects, they may produce:

- epigastric distress
- nausea and vomiting

- diarrhea (especially with large doses)
- rashes
- fever
- eosinophilia (an increase in the number of eosinophils, a type of WBC)
- anaphylaxis.

The Three-Step Approach

Nursing management for patients undergoing treatment with a macrolide is similar to that of management of patients receiving other anti-infective therapies. Key additional actions include:
- Give the oral form with a full glass of water 1 hour before or 2 hours after meals to enhance absorption.
- Remember that coated tablets may be taken with meals.
- Tell the patient not to drink fruit juice when taking a macrolide drug.
- Teach that chewable erythromycin tablets shouldn't be swallowed whole.
- Monitor hepatic function (increased levels of alkaline phosphatase, alanine aminotransferase, aspartate aminotransferase, and bilirubin may occur). Erythromycin derivatives can cause varying degrees of hepatotoxicity.

As with any drug administration, be certain to pay particular attention to the specific drug being given and personalize care.

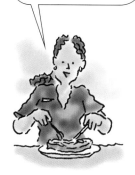

It's okay to take coated tablets with meals.

Vancomycin (Vancocin)

Vancomycin hydrochloride is used increasingly to treat methicillin-resistant *S. aureus*, which has become a major concern worldwide. Because of the emergence of vancomycin-resistant enterococci, this drug must be used judiciously. As a rule of thumb, it should be used only when culture and sensitivity test results confirm the need for it.

Pharmacokinetics

Because vancomycin is absorbed poorly from the GI tract, it must be given IV to treat systemic infections. An oral form of vancomycin is used to treat pseudomembranous colitis or *C. difficile* colitis. Remember, however, that IV vancomycin can't be used in place of oral vancomycin and vice versa. The two forms aren't interchangeable.

Flowing with fluids

Vancomycin diffuses well into pleural (around the lungs), pericardial (around the heart), synovial (joint), and ascitic (in the peritoneal cavity) fluids.

And then what happens?

The metabolism of vancomycin is unknown. Approximately 85% of the dose is excreted unchanged in urine within 24 hours; the rate is directly related to creatinine clearance. A small amount may be eliminated through the liver and biliary tract.

Pharmacodynamics

Vancomycin inhibits bacterial cell wall synthesis, damaging the bacterial plasma membrane. When the bacterial cell wall is damaged, the body's natural defenses can attack the organism.

Pharmacotherapeutics

Vancomycin has several therapeutic uses:
- It's active against aerobic gram-positive organisms, such as *Staphylococcus aureus*, *Staphylococcus epidermidis*, *Streptococcus pyogenes*, *Enterococcus*, and *Streptococcus pneumoniae*.

Staving off staph
- The IV form is the therapy of choice for patients with serious resistant staphylococcal infections who are hypersensitive to penicillins.

Coping with colitis
- The oral form is used for patients with antibiotic-associated *C. difficile* colitis as the first-line of therapy.

Penicillin alternative
- When used with an aminoglycoside, vancomycin can also serve as treatment for *E. faecalis* endocarditis in patients who are allergic to penicillin; however, this combination is used infrequently due to risk of nephrotoxicity.

Drug interactions

Vancomycin may increase the risk of toxicity when administered with other drugs toxic to the kidneys and organs of hearing, such as aminoglycosides, amphotericin B, cisplatin, bacitracin, and polymyxin B.

Adverse reactions

Adverse reactions to vancomycin, although rare, include:
- hypersensitivity and anaphylactic reactions
- drug fever
- eosinophilia
- neutropenia (reduced number of neutrophils, a type of WBC)
- hearing loss (transient or permanent), especially in excessive doses, such as when it's given with other ototoxic drugs

- nephrotoxicity
- vancomycin flushing syndrome.

Slow it down!

Severe hypotension may occur with rapid IV administration of vancomycin and may be accompanied by a red rash with flat and raised lesions on the face, neck, chest, and arms (vancomycin flushing syndrome Martel, Jamil, & King (2021)). Carefully read instructions for rate of administration.

The Three-Step Approach

Nursing management for patients undergoing treatment with vancomycin is similar to that of management of patients receiving other anti-infective therapies. Key additional actions include:
- Obtain hearing evaluation and kidney function studies before therapy and repeat during therapy.
- Monitor serum levels regularly, especially in older adults, premature neonates, and those with decreased renal function.
- For IV infusion, carefully read instructions for dilution and infusion.
- Do not give this drug intramuscularly!
- If vancomycin flushing syndrome occurs because the drug is infused too rapidly, stop the infusion and report this finding to the health care provider.
- Refrigerate an IV solution after reconstitution and use it within 96 hours.
    As with any drug administration, be certain to pay particular attention to the drug being given and personalize care.

Carbapenems

Carbapenems are a class of beta-lactam antibacterials that include:
- imipenem-cilastatin sodium (a combination drug) (Primaxin)
- meropenem (Merrem)
- ertapenem (Invanz).

Super-sized spectrum of activity

The antibacterial spectrum of activity for this class of drug is broader than that of other antibacterial drugs studied to date. Because of this broad spectrum of activity, it's used for serious or life-threatening infection, especially gram-positive and gram-negative nosocomial infections.

Pharmacokinetics

The pharmacokinetic properties of carbapenems vary slightly.

Lifespan Lightbulb

When giving vancomycin to an older adult or neonate, continually assess serum levels, as they are more sensitive to this drug than younger adults!

Enabling imipenem's effects

Imipenem is given with cilastatin because imipenem alone is rapidly metabolized in the tubules of the kidneys, rendering it ineffective. After parenteral administration, imipenem-cilastatin sodium is distributed widely. It's metabolized by several mechanisms and excreted primarily in urine.

Follow the ertapenem road

Ertapenem is completely absorbed after IV administration and is more highly protein bound than the other two carbapenems. It's metabolized by hydrolysis and excreted mainly in urine.

Sights on the CNS and elsewhere

After parenteral administration, meropenem is distributed widely, including to the CNS. Metabolism is insignificant; most of the drug is excreted unchanged in urine.

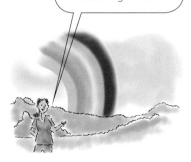

Because of its broad spectrum of activity, imipenem-cilastatin is used for serious or life-threatening infection.

Pharmacodynamics

Imipenem-cilastatin sodium, ertapenem, and meropenem are usually bactericidal. They exert antibacterial activity by inhibiting bacterial cell wall synthesis.

Pharmacotherapeutics

Imipenem-cilastatin sodium has the broadest spectrum of activity of currently available beta-lactam antibacterial drugs:

- It's effective against aerobic gram-positive species, such as *Streptococcus*, *Staphylococcus aureus*, and *Staphylococcus epidermidis*.
- It inhibits most *Enterobacter* species.
- It inhibits *P. aeruginosa* (although resistance is rising) and most anaerobic species, including *Bacteroides fragilis*.
- It may be used to treat serious health care–associated infections and infections in immunocompromised patients caused by mixed aerobic and anaerobic organisms.

Meropenem marvels

Meropenem is indicated for treatment of intra-abdominal infections as well as for management of bacterial meningitis caused by susceptible organisms.

Enter ertapenem

Ertapenem's spectrum of activity includes intra-abdominal, skin, urinary tract, and gynecologic infections as well as community-acquired pneumonias caused by various gram-positive, gram-negative, and anaerobic organisms. Due to its long half-life, this medication can be dosed once daily, which may be a desirable benefit.

Drug interactions

These drug interactions may occur with carbapenems:

- Taking probenecid with imipenem-cilastatin sodium increases the serum concentration of cilastatin and slightly increases the serum concentration of imipenem.
- Probenecid may cause meropenem and ertapenem to accumulate to toxic levels.
- Imipenem-cilastatin can increase bleeding risk in those also on warfarin therapy.
- This drug class can also decrease valproic acid levels and so should be avoided in patient on this anticonvulsant medication.

Adverse reactions

Common adverse reactions to imipenem-cilastatin sodium, ertapenem, and meropenem include:

- nausea and vomiting
- diarrhea
- hypersensitivity reactions such as rashes (particularly in patients with known hypersensitivity to penicillins)
- seizures.

Ertapenem extras

Ertapenem may also cause:

- hypotension
- altered mental status
- respiratory distress
- death.

The Three-Step Approach

Nursing management for patients undergoing treatment with a carbapenem is similar to that of management of patients receiving other anti-infective therapies. Key additional actions include:

- Don't give the drug by direct IV bolus injection; reconstitute it as directed and infuse per the instructions. If nausea occurs, slow the infusion.
- When reconstituting the powder form, shake it until the solution is clear. Solutions may range from colorless to yellow; variations of color within this range don't affect the drug's potency. After reconstitution, the solution is stable for 10 hours at room temperature and for 48 hours when refrigerated.
- Reconstitute the drug for an IM injection per the package directions (for example, for ertapenem with 1% lidocaine hydrochloride [without epinephrine] as directed).
- Some patients may develop seizures when taking a carbapenem drug; the health care provider will often prescribe anticonvulsants

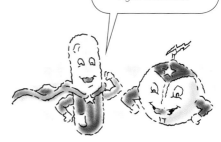

What a pair! Imipenem-cilastatin sodium is used with an aminoglycoside to fight *E. faecalis*.

in this case. Institute seizure precautions. If seizures persist despite using anticonvulsants, notify the health care provider, who may discontinue the drug.

As with any drug administration, be certain to pay particular attention to the drug being given and personalize care.

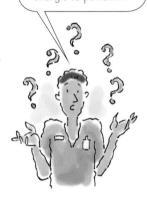

What do you do when a patient is allergic to penicillin?

Monobactams

Monobactams are used when a patient is allergic to penicillins and cephalosporins. They bind and inhibit enzymes like other antibacterial drugs, but their composition is slightly different. Aztreonam (Azactam) is the first member in this class of antibacterial drugs and the only one currently available. It's a synthetic monobactam with a narrow spectrum of activity that includes many gram-negative aerobic bacteria.

Pharmacokinetics

After parenteral administration, aztreonam is rapidly and completely absorbed and widely distributed. It's metabolized partially and excreted primarily in urine as unchanged drug.

Pharmacodynamics

Aztreonam's bactericidal activity results from inhibition of bacterial cell wall synthesis. It binds to the PBP-3 of susceptible gram-negative bacteria, inhibiting cell wall division and resulting in lysis.

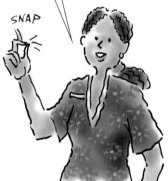

Use a monobactam instead!

SNAP

Pharmacotherapeutics

Aztreonam is indicated in a range of therapeutic situations:
- It's effective against a variety of gram-negative aerobic organisms, including *P. aeruginosa* (although some resistant strains emerge with therapy).
- It's effective against most strains of *E. coli*, *Enterobacter*, *Klebsiella pneumoniae*, *Klebsiella oxytoca*, *P. mirabilis*, *Serratia marcescens*, *H. influenzae*, and *Citrobacter*.
- It's used to treat complicated and uncomplicated UTIs, septicemia, and lower respiratory tract; skin and skin structure; intra-abdominal; and gynecologic infections caused by susceptible gram-negative aerobic bacteria.
- It's usually active against gram-negative aerobic organisms that are resistant to antibiotics hydrolyzed by beta-lactamases. (Beta-lactamase is an enzyme that makes an antibacterial drug ineffective.)

When experience doesn't count

Aztreonam shouldn't be used alone as empirical therapy (treatment based on clinical experience rather than on medical data) in seriously ill patients who may have a gram-positive bacterial infection or a mixed aerobic-anaerobic bacterial infection.

Drug interactions

Aztreonam may interact with several other drugs:

- Probenecid increases serum levels of aztreonam by prolonging the tubular secretion rate of aztreonam in the kidneys.
- Synergistic or additive effects occur when aztreonam is used with aminoglycosides or other antibiotics, such as cefoperazone, cefotaxime, clindamycin, and piperacillin.
- Potent inducers of beta-lactamase production (such as cefoxitin and imipenem) may inactivate aztreonam. Concomitant use isn't recommended.
- Taking aztreonam with clavulanic acid–containing antibiotics may produce synergistic or antagonistic effects, depending on the organism involved.

Adverse reactions

Adverse reactions to aztreonam include:

- diarrhea
- hypersensitivity and skin reactions
- hypotension
- nausea and vomiting
- transient electrocardiogram (ECG) changes (including ventricular arrhythmias)
- transient increases in serum liver enzymes.

The Three-Step Approach

Nursing management for patients undergoing treatment with a monobactam drug is similar to that of management of patients receiving other anti-infective therapies. Key additional actions include:

- Although patients who are allergic to penicillins or cephalosporins may not be allergic to aztreonam, closely monitor patients who have had an immediate hypersensitivity reaction to these antibacterial drugs.
- To give an IV bolus dose, inject the drug slowly per the package directions.
- Recognize that doses larger than 1 g should be administered via IV.

- Give infusions over 20 minutes to 1 hour.
- Give IM injections deep into a large muscle mass, such as the upper outer quadrant of the gluteus maximus or the lateral aspect of the thigh.
- Teach the patient receiving the drug IM that pain and swelling may develop at the injection site.

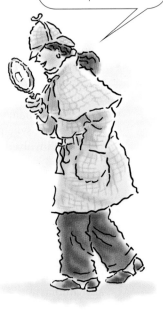

> Evidence of whether an infection is progressing or resolving can be found in the patient's culture report and WBC, as well as by monitoring their temperature.

Fluoroquinolones

Fluoroquinolones are structurally similar synthetic antibacterial drugs. They are broad-spectrum antibiotics and are effective against many organisms; however, their use has more recently been limited due to potential adverse effects. This class of drugs includes:

- ciprofloxacin (Cipro)
- delafloxacin (Baxdela)
- gemifloxacin (Factive)
- levofloxacin
- moxifloxacin hydrochloride (Avelox)
- ofloxacin (Floxin).
  A couple of fluoroquinolones are formulated only for ophthalmic use:
- besifloxacin (Besivance)
- gatifloxacin (Zymar).

Pharmacokinetics

After oral administration, fluoroquinolones are absorbed well. They aren't highly protein bound, are minimally metabolized in the liver, and are excreted primarily in urine.

Pharmacodynamics

Fluoroquinolones interrupt deoxyribonucleic acid (DNA) synthesis during bacterial replication by inhibiting DNA gyrase, an essential enzyme of replicating DNA. As a result, the bacteria can't reproduce.

Pharmacotherapeutics

Fluoroquinolones can be used to treat a wide variety of infections such as anthrax, typhoid, and mycobacteria including tuberculosis. Each drug in this class also has specific indications:

- Ciprofloxacin has the best activity against aerobic gram-negative bacilli such as *E. coli*, *Klebsiella*, and *Proteus*. It also is active against *Pseudomonas*. It can be used to treat UTIS, pneumonia, intra-abdominal infections, bone/joint infections, and prostatitis.
- Levofloxacin and moxifloxacin have better activity against gram-positive organisms such as *Staphylococcus aureus*, some streptococci

strains, and some coagulase-negative staphylococci. Despite this, fluoroquinolones are usually not used to treat infections caused by these organisms.

- Levofloxacin and moxifloxacin are also active against respiratory organisms such as *Streptococcus pneumoniae, H. influenzae*, and *M. catarrhalis*. Additionally, it works well against *Legionella, Mycoplasma*, and *Chlamydia*.
- Moxifloxacin has good activity against some anaerobes, as well.
- Ofloxacin is used to treat selected sexually transmitted diseases (not typically first line), lower respiratory tract infections, UTIs, and prostatitis.
- Otic ofloxacin is used to treat infections of the middle ear and swimmer's ear.
- Ophthalmic ofloxacin, besifloxacin, and gatifloxacin solution (drops) are used to treat conjunctivitis.
- Gemifloxacin is used in the treatment of bacterial exacerbations of chronic bronchitis and mild to moderate community-acquired pneumonia. It can also be used in combination with azithromycin to treat gonococcal infections.
- Delafloxacin can be used for skin/skin structure bacterial infections and for community-acquired pneumonia.

Drug interactions

Several drug interactions may occur with the fluoroquinolones:
- Administration with antacids that contain magnesium or aluminum hydroxide results in decreased absorption of the fluoroquinolone.
- Some fluoroquinolones, such as ciprofloxacin and ofloxacin, interact with xanthine derivatives, such as aminophylline and theophylline, increasing the plasma theophylline concentration and the risk of theophylline toxicity.
- Giving ciprofloxacin or gemifloxacin with probenecid results in decreased kidney elimination of these fluoroquinolones, increasing their serum concentrations and half-lives. It also can cause QT prolongation.
- Drugs that prolong the QT interval such as antiarrhythmics should be avoided during fluoroquinolone therapy if possible.
- NSAIDs may lower seizure threshold when given in combination with fluoroquinolones.

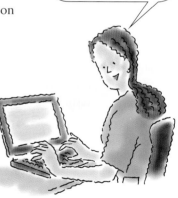

Fluoroquinolones are at the head of the class when it comes to treating UTIs!

Adverse reactions

Fluoroquinolones are well tolerated by most patients, but some adverse effects may occur, including:
- infection with *C. difficile*
- nausea and vomiting

- peripheral neuropathy
- ruptured tendons and tendinitis
- hepatotoxicity
- blurred vision
- tinnitus.

Special populations

Use of this drug class should be avoided in patients with myasthenia gravis as their neuromuscular-blocking activity may exacerbate muscle weakness. Fluoroquinolones should also be avoided in those with risk factors for or known aortic aneurysm. Caution should be used in patients with diabetes due to risk of hypoglycemia.

Blister in the sun

Moderate to severe phototoxic reactions have occurred with direct and indirect sunlight and with artificial ultraviolet lights, both with and without sunscreen. These types of light should be avoided while the patient is on fluoroquinolone therapy and for several days after cessation of therapy.

The Three-Step Approach

Nursing management for patients undergoing treatment with fluoroquinolones is similar to that of management of patients receiving other anti-infective therapies. Key additional actions include:

- Oral forms may be given 2 hours after meals, 2 hours before meals, or 6 hours after taking antacids, sucralfate, or products that contain iron (such as vitamins with mineral supplements).
- Dilute the drug for IV use as directed and monitor for adverse effects. Infuse slowly over 1 hour into a large vein.

Education edge

Teaching about fluoroquinolones

Teaching about fluoroquinolones is similar to teaching about other anti-infective therapies. Additional key items to teach include:

- Take the oral form 2 hours before or after meals.
- Take prescribed antacids at least 2 hours after taking the drug.
- Drink plenty of fluids to reduce the risk of crystalluria.
- Avoid hazardous tasks that require alertness, such as driving, until the drug's CNS effects are known.

- Hypersensitivity reactions may occur even after the first dose. If a rash or other allergic reactions develop, stop the drug immediately and notify the health care provider.
- Stop breast-feeding during treatment or consult with the health care provider about taking a different drug.

- Provide teaching *per Teaching about fluoroquinolones*, page 596. As with any drug administration, be certain to pay particular attention to the type of drug being given and personalize care.

Sulfonamides

Sulfonamides were the first effective systemic antibacterial drugs. They include:
- mafenide (Sulfamylon)
- sulfacetamide (Bleph-10)
- trimethoprim and sulfamethoxazole (Bactrim)
- sulfadiazine (Silvadene)
- sulfasalazine (Azulfidine).

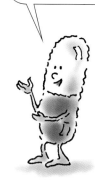

Monitor patients with diabetes who are taking sulfonamindes, as these drugs can increase the hypoglycemic effect of antidiabetic drugs.

Pharmacokinetics

Most sulfonamides are well absorbed and widely distributed in the body. They're metabolized in the liver to inactive metabolites and excreted by the kidneys.

A fluid situation

Because crystalluria and subsequent stone formation may occur during the metabolic excretory phase, adequate fluid intake is highly recommended during oral sulfonamide therapy.

Pharmacodynamics

Sulfonamides are bacteriostatic drugs that prevent the growth of microorganisms by inhibiting folic acid production. The decreased folic acid synthesis decreases the number of bacterial nucleotides and inhibits bacterial growth.

Pharmacotherapeutics

Sulfonamides are commonly used to treat acute UTIs. With recurrent or chronic UTIs, the infecting organism may not be susceptible to sulfonamides. Therefore, the choice of therapy should be based on bacteria susceptibility tests.

Other targets

Sulfonamides also are used to treat infections caused by *Nocardia asteroides* and *Toxoplasma gondii*. In addition, sulfonamides exhibit a wide spectrum of activity against gram-positive and gram-negative bacteria.

Winning combination

Trimethoprim and sulfamethoxazole (a combination of a sulfa drug and a folate antagonist) are used for various other infections, such as *Pneumocystis jirovecii* pneumonia, acute otitis media (due to *H. influenzae* and *S. pneumoniae*), and acute exacerbations of chronic bronchitis (due to *H. influenzae* and *S. pneumoniae*). (See *Sulfonamides: Trimethoprim and sulfamethoxazole*.)

Drug interactions

Sulfonamides have few significant interactions:
- They increase the hypoglycemic effects of the sulfonylureas (oral antidiabetic drugs), which may decrease blood glucose levels.
- When taken with methenamine, they may lead to the development of crystals in the urine.
- Trimethoprim and sulfamethoxazole may increase the anticoagulant effect of coumarin anticoagulants.
- Trimethoprim and sulfamethoxazole plus cyclosporine increase the risk of kidney toxicity.

Adverse reactions

These adverse reactions may occur with sulfonamides:
- Excessively high doses of less water-soluble sulfonamides can produce crystals in the urine and deposits of sulfonamide crystals in the renal tubules; however, this complication isn't a problem with the newer water-soluble sulfonamides.

Prototype pro

Sulfonamides: Trimethoprim and sulfamethoxazole

Actions
- Is bacteriostatic (mechanism of action correlates directly with the structural similarities it shares with para-aminobenzoic acid)
- Inhibits biosynthesis of folic acid, thus inhibiting susceptible bacteria that synthesize folic acid

Indications
- Infections of the urinary tract, respiratory tract, and ear caused by susceptible organisms
- Chronic bacterial prostatitis
- Prevention of recurrent UTI in natal sex women and of "traveler's diarrhea"

Nursing considerations
- Obtain a specimen for culture and sensitivity tests before giving the first dose. Therapy may begin pending results.
- Monitor the patient for adverse effects, such as seizures, nausea, vomiting, diarrhea, hematologic disorders, Stevens-Johnson syndrome, toxic nephrosis, and hypersensitivity reactions.
- Reduced dosages are needed in patients with renal and hepatic impairment.
- With large dosages or prolonged treatment, monitor the patient for superinfections.

- Hypersensitivity reactions may occur and appear to increase as the dosage increases.
- A reaction that resembles serum sickness may occur, producing fever, joint pain, hives, bronchospasm, and leukopenia (reduced WBC count).
- Photosensitivity may occur.

The Three-Step Approach

Nursing management for patients undergoing treatment with a sulfonamide is similar to that of management of patients receiving other anti-infective therapies. Key additional actions include:

- Assess the patient's history of allergies, especially to sulfonamides or to drugs containing sulfur (such as thiazides, furosemide, and oral sulfonylureas).
- Assess for adverse reactions and drug interactions; patients with acquired immunodeficiency syndrome (AIDS) have a much higher risk of adverse reactions.
- Give an oral dose with 8 oz (237 mL) of water. Give 3 to 4 L of fluids daily, depending on the drug. Urine output should be at least 1,500 mL daily to ensure proper hydration. Inadequate urine output can lead to crystalluria or tubular deposits of the drug.
- Provide teaching included in *Teaching about sulfonamides.*

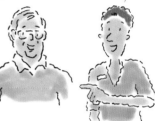

Patients with diabetes need to watch their glucose levels when taking sulfonamides. Sulfonamides increase the hypoglycemic effects of oral antidiabetic drugs.

Education edge

Teaching about sulfonamides

Teaching about sulfonamides is similar to teaching about other anti-infective therapies. Additional key items to teach include:

- Take the oral form with a full glass of water and drink plenty of fluids. The tablet may be crushed and swallowed with water to ensure maximal absorption.
- Report signs and symptoms of hypersensitivity and other adverse reactions, such as bloody urine, difficulty breathing, rash, fever, chills, or severe fatigue.
- Avoid direct sun exposure and use a sunscreen to help prevent photosensitivity reactions.
- Sulfonamides may increase the effects of oral antidiabetic drugs.
- Sulfasalazine may cause an orange-yellow discoloration of urine or the skin and may permanently stain soft contact lenses yellow.

Nitrofurantoin (Macrodantin)

Nitrofurantoin is a drug that has higher antibacterial activity in acidic urine. It's commonly used to treat acute and chronic UTIs.

Pharmacokinetics

After oral administration, nitrofurantoin is absorbed rapidly and well from the GI tract. Taking the drug with food enhances its bioavailability.

Form facts

Nitrofurantoin is available in a monohydrate and a macrocrystalline form. The monohydrate form is absorbed more slowly because of slower dissolution and thus causes less GI distress.

Oh where oh where does nitrofurantoin go?

Nitrofurantoin is 20% to 60% protein bound. It crosses the placental barrier and is secreted in breast milk. It's also distributed in bile. Nitrofurantoin is partially metabolized by the liver, and 30% to 50% is excreted unchanged in urine.

Pharmacodynamics

Usually bacteriostatic, nitrofurantoin may become bactericidal, depending on its urinary concentration and the susceptibility of the infecting organisms.

Zapping bacterial energy

Although its exact mechanism of action is unknown, nitrofurantoin appears to inhibit the formation of acetyl coenzyme A from pyruvic acid, thereby inhibiting the energy production of the infecting organism. Nitrofurantoin also may disrupt bacterial cell wall formation.

Pharmacotherapeutics

Because the absorbed drug concentrates in urine, nitrofurantoin is used to treat UTIs. Nitrofurantoin isn't effective against systemic bacterial infections.

Can't handle the kidneys

Nitrofurantoin isn't useful in treating pyelonephritis or perinephric (around the kidney) diseases.

Drug interactions

Nitrofurantoin has few significant interactions:
- When combined with lidocaine or dapsone, can increase the risk of methemoglobinemia.

- Bremelanotide, exenatide, and magnesium citrate can reduce nitrofurantoin absorption.
- Nitrofurantoin may decrease the efficacy of hormonal contraceptives.

Adverse reactions

Adverse reactions to nitrofurantoin include:
- GI irritation
- anorexia
- nausea and vomiting
- diarrhea
- dark yellow or brown urine
- abdominal pain
- chills
- fever
- joint pain
- anaphylaxis
- hypersensitivity reactions involving the skin, lungs, blood, and liver.

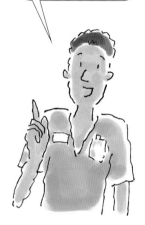

Fortunately, nitrofurantoin has few significant drug interactions.

The Three-Step Approach

Nursing management for patients undergoing treatment with nitrofurantoin is similar to that of management of patients receiving other anti-infective therapies. Key additional actions include:
- Assess the patient's allergy history, especially allergies to sulfonamides or to drugs containing sulfur (such as thiazides, furosemide, and oral sulfonylureas).
- Give the drug with food or milk to minimize GI distress.
- Monitor urine cultures; treatment continues for 3 days after urine specimens become sterile.
- Monitor CBC and pulmonary status regularly.
- Monitor intake and output. This drug may turn urine brown or dark yellow.
  As with any drug administration, be certain to pay particular attention to the type of drug being given and personalize care.

Oxazolidinones

Linezolid (Zyvox) and tedizolid (Sivextro) are synthetic antibacterials. They are used primarily in treatments involving aerobic gram-positive bacteria but also used for treatment of certain gram-negative and anaerobic organisms.

Pharmacokinetics

Linezolid may be administered via IV or by mouth without regard to food and easily distributed into tissues. Its metabolic pathways are not

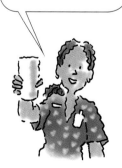

Give nitrofurantoin with food or milk to minimize GI distress.

fully understood. They undergo minimal oxidation, and excretion is completed primarily through nonrenal pathways.

Pharmacodynamics

The oxazolidinones bind to bacterial RNA, preventing the formation of materials necessary for bacterial reproduction (bacteriostatic).

Pharmacotherapeutics

- This class of drugs is potent against most select aerobic gram-positive organisms, including *Enterococcus faecium* (vancomycin-resistant isolates only), *Staphylococcus aureus* (including methicillin-resistant isolates), *Streptococcus agalactiae*, *Streptococcus pneumoniae*, and *Streptococcus pyogenes*.
- Linezolid is used primarily to treat nosocomial pneumonia, community-acquired pneumonia, and complicated and uncomplicated skin and skin structure infections. Linezolid is also used in the treatment of vancomycin-resistant *E. faecium* infections.
- Tedizolid is currently used for treatment of skin and skin structure infections. Since this drug is newer, research is ongoing regarding its use in the treatment of ventilator-associated pneumonia and other gram-positive infections.

Drug interactions

Linezolid is a reversible, nonselective inhibitor of monoamine oxidase (MAO). Do not give linezolid concurrently or within 2 weeks of taking any MAO inhibitors. Tedizolid can increase atorvastatin levels, increasing risk of myopathy and rhabdomyolysis. Atorvastatin should be held during tedizolid administration if possible unless CK can be monitored.

Adverse reactions

Myelosuppression has been noted with administration of oxazolidinones. This may include anemia, leukopenia, pancytopenia, and thrombocytopenia. Peripheral and optic neuropathy was noted in some patients on extended therapy.

Because of the potential for serotonin syndrome, linezolid should only be considered for those taking serotonin-based antidepressants when no other drugs are available. In this case, the serotonin-based drug should be stopped and the patient should be closely monitored for signs and symptoms related to the syndrome. Other reactions may also occur, such as:

- diarrhea
- headache
- nausea
- vomiting
- anemia
- hypersensitivity reactions.

The Three-Step Approach

Nursing management for patients undergoing treatment with linezolid is similar to that of management of patients receiving other anti-infective therapies. Key additional actions include:

- Don't refrigerate a reconstituted oral solution because it will thicken. The drug is stable for 3 weeks at room temperature.
- Inspect IV bags visually for particulate matter prior to infusion. It is ok if the solution is slightly yellowed.

As with any drug administration, be certain to pay particular attention to the type of drug being given and personalize care.

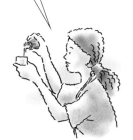

Don't refrigerate reconstituted oral clindamycin because it will thicken.

Antiviral drugs

Antiviral drugs are used to prevent or treat viral infections ranging from influenza to human immunodeficiency virus (HIV). The major antiviral drug classes used to treat systemic infections include:

- nucleoside analogues
- pyrophosphate analogues
- influenza A and syncytial virus drugs
- nucleoside analogue reverse transcriptase inhibitors (NRTIs)
- nonnucleoside reverse transcriptase inhibitors (NNRTIs)
- nucleotide reverse transcriptase inhibitors
- protease inhibitors
- hepatitis B virus (HBV) and hepatitis C virus (HCV) drugs.

Nucleoside analogues

Nucleoside analogues are a group of drugs used to treat various viral syndromes that can occur in immunocompromised patients, including herpes simplex virus (HSV) and cytomegalovirus (CMV). Drugs in this class include:

- acyclovir (Zovirax)
- cidofovir
- famciclovir
- ganciclovir (Cytovene)
- valacyclovir hydrochloride (Valtrex)
- valganciclovir hydrochloride (Valcyte)
- ribavirin (Rebetol).

Ribavirin is a nucleoside analogue developed for the treatment of chronic hepatitis C (CHC) and a main treatment for respiratory syncytial virus (RSV). Information regarding ribavirin is found in the "Influenza A and syncytial virus drugs" section below.

Pharmacokinetics

Each of these synthetic nucleosides travels its own route through the body. For example:

- When given orally, acyclovir absorption is slow and only 15% to 30% complete. Acyclovir is distributed throughout the body and metabolized primarily inside the infected cells; most of the drug is excreted in urine.
- Cidofovir is administered only by IV and must be accompanied by probenecid to facilitate metabolism and decrease risk of nephrotoxicity. Even with probenecid, most of cidofovir is excreted unchanged in urine within 24 hours of administration.
- Famciclovir is less than 20% bound to plasma proteins. It's extensively metabolized in the liver and excreted in urine.
- Ganciclovir is administered IV because it's absorbed poorly from the GI tract. Most of ganciclovir isn't metabolized and is excreted unchanged by the kidneys.

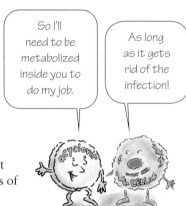

A true convert

- Valacyclovir is converted to acyclovir during its metabolism and has pharmacokinetic properties similar to those of acyclovir.
- Valganciclovir is metabolized in the intestinal wall and liver to ganciclovir; however, interchanging the two drugs isn't effective.

Pharmacodynamics

The action of these drugs also varies:

- Acyclovir enters virus-infected cells, where it's changed through a series of steps to acyclovir triphosphate. Acyclovir triphosphate inhibits virus-specific DNA polymerase, an enzyme necessary for viral growth, thus disrupting viral replication.
- Cidofovir becomes cidofovir diphosphate as an intercellular metabolite. It inhibits viral DNA synthesis at concentrations much lower than those needed to inhibit human DNA growth.
- On entry into virus-infected cells, ganciclovir is converted to ganciclovir triphosphate, which is thought to produce its antiviral activity by inhibiting viral DNA synthesis.
- Famciclovir enters viral cells (HSV types 1 and 2, varicella-zoster), where it inhibits DNA polymerase, viral DNA synthesis, and, thus, viral replication.
- Valacyclovir rapidly converts to acyclovir, and acyclovir then becomes incorporated into viral DNA and inhibits viral DNA polymerase, thus inhibiting viral multiplication.
- Valganciclovir is converted to ganciclovir, which inhibits replication of viral DNA synthesis of CMV.

Pharmacotherapeutics

Acyclovir is an effective antiviral drug that causes minimal toxicity to cells. Oral acyclovir is used primarily to treat initial and recurrent HSV type 2 infections. (See *Antivirals: Acyclovir.*)

IV instances

IV acyclovir is used to treat:

- severe initial HSV type 2 infections in patients with normal immune systems
- initial and recurrent skin and mucous membrane HSV type 1 and 2 infections in immunocompromised patients
- herpes zoster infections (shingles) caused by the varicella-zoster virus in immunocompromised patients
- disseminated varicella-zoster virus in immunocompromised patients
- varicella infections (chickenpox) caused by the varicella-zoster virus in immunocompromised patients.

Rounding out the group

Other nucleoside analogues have their own therapeutic uses:

- Ganciclovir is used to treat CMV retinitis in immunocompromised patients, including those with AIDS, other CMV infections (such as encephalitis), and HSV.
- Famciclovir is used to treat acute herpes zoster, genital herpes, and recurrent herpes simplex in HIV-infected patients.
- Valacyclovir is effective against herpes zoster, genital herpes, and herpes labialis.
- Cidofovir and valganciclovir are used to treat CMV retinitis in patients who have HIV.
- Valganciclovir is also used as CMV prophylaxis in heart, kidney, and pancreas transplants.

Drug interactions

Combination with many medications such as cisplatin, lithium, or methotrexate could lead to myelosuppression and nephrotoxicity.

Tearing into tissue cells

- Taking ganciclovir with drugs that are damaging to tissue cells, such as pentamidine isethionate, flucytosine, vincristine, vinblastine, doxorubicin, and amphotericin B, inhibits replication of rapidly dividing cells in the bone marrow, GI tract, skin, and sperm-producing cells.

Prototype pro

Antivirals: Acyclovir

Actions
- Interferes with DNA synthesis and inhibits viral multiplication

Indications
- HSV types 1 and 2
- Varicella
- Herpes zoster (shingles)

Nursing considerations
- Monitor the patient for adverse effects, such as malaise, headache, encephalopathy, renal failure, thrombocytopenia, and pain at the injection site.

- Cidofovir should not be administered with potentially nephrotoxic agents, such as aminoglycosides, amphotericin B, foscarnet, IV pentamidine, vancomycin, and nonsteroidal anti-inflammatory drugs (NSAIDs).
- Imipenem-cilastatin sodium increases the risk of seizures when taken with ganciclovir or valganciclovir.
- Zidovudine increases the risk of granulocytopenia (reduced number of granulocytes, a type of WBC) when taken with ganciclovir. Zidovudine should be held or reduced by 50% when administered with cidofovir. Discuss this with the health care provider to assure that the patient is dosed appropriately.

Adverse reactions

Treatment with nucleoside analogues may cause these adverse reactions:
- Reversible kidney impairment may occur with rapid IV injection or infusion of acyclovir.
- Headache, nausea, vomiting, and diarrhea are common reactions to oral acyclovir.
- Hypersensitivity reactions may occur with acyclovir.
- Nephrotoxicity is the most frequent adverse reaction with cidofovir, occurring in more than half the patients.
- Granulocytopenia and thrombocytopenia are the most common adverse reactions to ganciclovir.
- Famciclovir and valacyclovir may cause headache and nausea.
- Valganciclovir may cause seizures, retinal detachment, neutropenia, and bone marrow suppression.

The Three-Step Approach

Nursing management for patients undergoing treatment with a nucleoside analogue is similar to that of management of patients receiving other anti-infective therapies. Key additional actions include:

Preadministration

- Monitor renal and hepatic function, CBC, and platelet count regularly.
- Monitor the patient's mental status when giving the drug via IV. Encephalopathic changes are more likely to occur in patients with neurologic disorders or in those who have had neurologic reactions to cytotoxic drugs.
- Provide appropriate patient teaching. (See *Teaching about antiviral drug therapy*, page 607.)

As with any drug administration, be certain to pay particular attention to the type of drug being given and personalize care.

Teaching about antiviral drug therapy

If antiviral drug therapy is prescribed, review these points with the patient and caregivers:
• The drug therapy that has been prescribed effectively manages viral infection but may not eliminate it or cure it.
• Maintain immunizations against viral infections as indicated.
• This drug therapy won't prevent the infection from spreading to others. Use proper techniques to prevent the spread of infection. For example, avoid sexual intercourse when visible lesions are present,

always wash hands after touching lesions, practice safer sex by using a condom, and avoid sharing IV needles.

If the patient is taking antiretroviral drugs, review these additional points:
• Effective treatment of HIV requires drug therapy with several drugs that may have multiple daily doses. Missing doses decreases blood levels of the drugs, which results in increased HIV replication (this is called a "higher viral load"). This can result in drug-resistant viral strains.

• Don't take other drugs, over-the-counter products, or herbal preparations without first consulting the health care provider. They may make anti-HIV drugs less effective or more toxic.
• Adverse effects may vary depending on the specific drugs used; request information about the adverse effects and what to do if they occur.
• Have regular tests, such as viral load, CD4+ cell count, CBC, and renal and hepatic function, as indicated.

Pyrophosphate analogues

Pyrophosphate analogues target pyrophosphate-binding sites of certain viruses. Foscarnet sodium (Foscavir) is one such drug that's used to treat cytomegalovirus (CMV) retinitis in patients with AIDS. It's also used to treat acyclovir-resistant HSV infections in immunocompromised patients.

Pharmacokinetics

Foscarnet is poorly bound to plasma proteins. In patients with normal kidney function, the majority of foscarnet is excreted unchanged in urine.

Pharmacodynamics

Foscarnet prevents viral replication by selectively inhibiting DNA polymerase.

Pharmacotherapeutics

Foscarnet's primary therapeutic use is treating CMV retinitis in patients with AIDS. It's also occasionally used in combination with ganciclovir for patients who have relapsed with either drug.

Drug interactions

Foscarnet has a few drug interactions:

- Foscarnet and pentamidine together increase the risk of hypocalcemia and toxicity to the kidneys.
- Using foscarnet along with other drugs that alter serum calcium levels may result in hypocalcemia.
- The risk of kidney impairment increases when drugs toxic to the kidneys, such as amphotericin B and aminoglycosides, are taken with foscarnet. Because of the risk of kidney toxicity, patients should be aggressively hydrated during treatment.

Adverse reactions

Adverse reactions to foscarnet may include:

- fatigue
- depression
- fever
- confusion
- headache
- numbness and tingling
- dizziness
- seizures
- nausea and vomiting
- diarrhea
- abdominal pain
- granulocytopenia
- leukopenia
- involuntary muscle contractions
- neuropathy
- difficulty breathing
- rash
- altered kidney function
- hypocalcemia, hypophosphatemia, and hypokalemia.

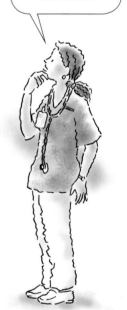

That's quite a list of adverse reactions…

The Three-Step Approach

Nursing management for patients undergoing treatment with a pyrophosphate analogue is similar to that of management of patients receiving other anti-infective therapies. Key additional actions include:

- Give the drug over at least 1 hour using an infusion pump. To minimize renal toxicity, ensure adequate hydration before and during the infusion.
- Monitor renal and hepatic function, CBC, and platelet count regularly.
- Monitor creatinine clearance two to three times weekly during induction and at least once every 1 to 2 weeks during maintenance.

Eyeing electrolyte levels
- Monitor for tetany and seizures with abnormal electrolyte levels; the drug may cause a dose-related transient decrease in ionized serum calcium, which may not be reflected in laboratory values.
- Monitor the patient's mental status. Encephalopathic changes are more likely in patients with neurologic disorders or in those who have had neurologic reactions to cytotoxic drugs.
    As with any drug administration, be certain to pay particular attention to the type of drug being given and personalize care.

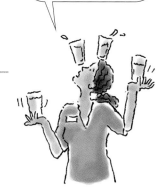

To minimize renal toxicity, ensure adequate hydration before and during foscarnet infusion.

Influenza A and syncytial virus drugs

Influenza A and syncytial virus drugs include:
- oseltamivir (Tamiflu)
- inhaled zanamivir (Relenza)
- peramivir (Rapivab)
- baloxavir (Xofluza)
- ribavirin (Rebetol)
- amantadine (Gocovri)
- rimantadine hydrochloride (an amantadine derivative) (Flumadine).

Pharmacokinetics

After oral administration, amantadine, rimantadine, and oseltamivir are well absorbed in the GI tract and widely distributed throughout the body. Amantadine is eliminated primarily in urine; rimantadine is extensively metabolized and then excreted in urine. Ninety-nine percent of oseltamivir is excreted renally. Baloxavir is excreted in bile.

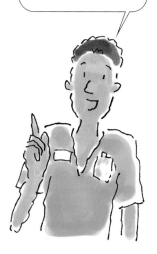

Aerosolized ribavirin is only administered by ventilator with a small particle aerosol generator.

Take a deep breath
Aerosolized ribavirin (Virazole) and inhaled zanamivir are administered by inhalation with a ventilator. Absorption of aerosolized ribavirin varies widely based between plasma and respiratory tract sections. Its highest concentrations are found in the respiratory tract and in red blood cells (RBCs). Zanamivir is inhaled, with a small portion of the drug being absorbed systemically. It is primarily excreted unchanged in the urine.

Swallow this
Ribavirin capsules are rapidly absorbed after administration and are distributed in plasma. Ribavirin is metabolized in the liver and by RBCs and then excreted primarily by the kidneys, with some excreted in feces.

Don't swallow this

Peramivir is given IV and is not significantly metabolized. Ninety percent of the drug is cleared unchanged through the kidneys.

Pharmacodynamics

Influenza A and syncytial virus drugs act in various ways:

- Although its exact mechanism of action is unknown, amantadine appears to inhibit an early stage of viral replication.
- Rimantadine inhibits viral RNA and protein synthesis.
- The mechanism of action of ribavirin isn't known completely, but the drug's metabolites inhibit viral DNA and RNA synthesis, subsequently halting viral replication.
- Peramivir, oseltamivir, and zanamivir inhibit the enzyme that allows viral particles to be released and to spread from infected cells.

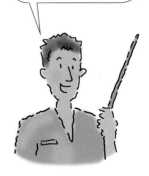

Peramivir, oseltamivir, baloxavir, and zanamivir are used for treatment of influenza in the United States.

Pharmacotherapeutics

These drugs are used to treat influenza and syncytial viruses. Note that amantadine and rimantadine were used in the very recent past to prevent and treat respiratory tract infections caused by strains of the influenza A virus; however, they are no longer recommended for this treatment due to increasing resistance.

Offering a little more protection

Peramivir, oseltamivir, baloxavir, and zanamivir are the recommended drugs for treatment of the influenza in the United States. Oseltamivir, zanamivir, and baloxavir are used for treatment and prophylaxis from influenza A and B. Peramivir is indicated for acute cases of influenza A and B in those 18 years or older.

Hep C remedy

Ribavirin can be used in combination with interferon alfa-2B to treat hepatitis C infection in adults; however, with the emergence of new medications proven to be more efficacious and also due to side effects, this combination is used much less frequently.

Drug interactions

These drug interactions may occur with amantadine:

- Taking anticholinergics with amantadine increases adverse anticholinergic effects.
- Amantadine given with the combination drug hydrochlorothiazide and triamterene results in decreased urine excretion of amantadine, resulting in increased amantadine levels.
- Amantadine and trimethoprim levels are increased when used together. The combination can also increase the risk for psychosis.

Not a troublemaker
No clinically significant drug interactions have been documented with rimantadine.

Intoxicating
Ribavirin has few interactions with other drugs:
- Ribavirin reduces the antiviral activity of zidovudine; using these drugs together may cause blood toxicity.
- Taking ribavirin and digoxin together can cause digoxin toxicity, producing such effects as GI distress, CNS abnormalities, and cardiac arrhythmias.

Adverse reactions
Rimantadine and amantadine share similar adverse reactions; however, those resulting from rimantadine tend to be less severe. Adverse reactions include:
- anorexia
- anxiety
- confusion
- depression
- fatigue
- forgetfulness
- hallucinations
- hypersensitivity reactions
- insomnia
- irritability
- nausea
- nervousness
- psychosis.

Oseltamivir and zanamivir also share adverse reactions. They include:
- headache
- nausea, vomiting, and diarrhea
- bronchitis
- dizziness.

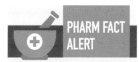

PHARM FACT ALERT

Live-attenuated influenza vaccines (LAIVs) should be avoided for 2 weeks before and at least 48 hours after administration of peramivir, oseltamivir, or zanamivir due to their antiviral properties.

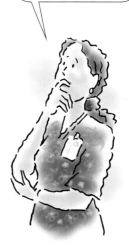

What was it? It was just on the tip of my tongue... something about amantadine and rimantadine causing forgetfulness...

Anaphylaxis and hypersensitivity
Anaphylaxis and hypersensitivity are the main adverse reactions reported with peramivir and baloxavir. Stevens-Johnson syndrome has been reported with administration of peramivir.

Ribavirin reactions
Adverse reactions to ribavirin include:
- apnea (lack of breathing)
- cardiac arrest

- hypotension
- pneumothorax (air in the pleural space, causing the lung to collapse)
- worsening of respiratory function.

The Three-Step Approach

Nursing management for patients undergoing treatment with influenza A and syncytial virus drugs is similar to that of management of patients receiving other anti-infective therapies. Key additional actions include:
- If the patient has a history of heart failure, watch closely for exacerbation or recurrence during amantadine therapy.
- Warn the patient with parkinsonism not to stop the drug abruptly; doing so could cause a parkinsonian crisis.
  As with any drug administration, be certain to pay particular attention to the type of drug being given and personalize care.

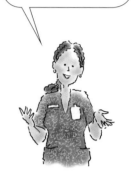

Patients with a history of heart failure should be watched for exacerbation or recurrence of the condition during amantadine therapy.

Nucleoside Reverse Transcriptase Inhibitors (NRTIs)

NRTIs are used to treat advanced HIV infections. Drugs in this class include:
- zidovudine (Retrovir)
- didanosine (Videx EC)
- abacavir sulfate (Ziagen)
- lamivudine (Epivir)
- emtricitabine (Emtriva).

Pharmacokinetics

Each of the NRTIs has its own pharmacokinetic properties.

A familiar path

Zidovudine is well absorbed from the GI tract, widely distributed throughout the body, metabolized by the liver, and excreted by the kidneys.

Buffed up

Because didanosine is degraded rapidly in gastric acid, didanosine tablets and powder contain a buffering drug to increase pH. The exact route of metabolism isn't fully understood. Approximately one half of an absorbed dose is excreted in urine.

Abracad-abacavir

Abacavir is rapidly and extensively absorbed after oral administration. It's distributed in the extravascular space, and about 50% binds with plasma proteins. Abacavir is metabolized by the cytosolic enzymes and is excreted primarily in urine with the remainder excreted in feces.

Ride the rapids

Lamivudine is rapidly absorbed after administration and is excreted by the kidneys. Emtricitabine is rapidly and extensively absorbed after oral administration. It's also excreted by the kidneys.

Pharmacodynamics

NRTIs must undergo conversion to their active metabolites to produce their action. For example:

- Zidovudine is converted by cellular enzymes to an active form, zidovudine triphosphate, which prevents viral DNA from replicating. (See *How zidovudine works,* page 614.)
- Didanosine undergoes cellular enzyme conversion to its antiviral metabolites to block HIV replication.
- Abacavir is converted to an active metabolite that inhibits the activity of HIV-1 transcriptase by competing with a natural component and incorporating into viral DNA.
- Lamivudine is converted in the cells to its active metabolite, which inhibits viral DNA replication.
- Emtricitabine inhibits the enzyme reverse transcriptase and thus inhibits viral DNA replication.

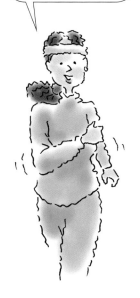

NRTIs must undergo conversion to their active metabolites to produce their action. Talk about keeping active!

Pharmacotherapeutics

NRTIs are used to treat HIV and AIDS as well as HBV.

Common combinations

NRTIs are often used in combination with other antiretrovirals to treat HIV infection, most often in pairs. For example, Combivir is a combination therapy that includes lamivudine and zidovudine. Trizivir is a combination therapy that includes abacavir, lamivudine, and zidovudine.

The vein game

Zidovudine is the only NRTI that can be given IV. The IV form of zidovudine is used as part of a multidrug regimen in hospitalized patients who can't take oral drugs. It's also used to prevent transmission of HIV from mother to fetus and to treat AIDS-related dementia.

Drug interactions

NRTIs may be responsible for a number of drug interactions:

- Potentially fatal lactic acidosis (increased lactic acid production in the blood) and severe hepatomegaly (enlargement of the liver) with steatosis (accumulation of fat) have occurred in patients taking NRTIs alone or with other antiretrovirals. This tends to happen more in women (HIV.info.NIH.gov, 2021). Obesity and prolonged NRTI exposure may be additional risk factors.

Pharm function

How zidovudine works

Zidovudine inhibits replication of HIV. The first two illustrations show how HIV invades cells and then replicates itself. The bottom illustration shows how zidovudine blocks viral transformation.

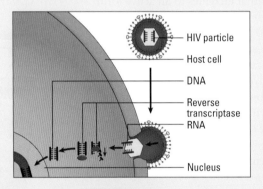

HIV particle
Host cell
DNA
Reverse transcriptase
RNA
Nucleus

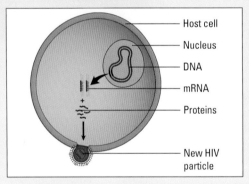

Host cell
Nucleus
DNA
mRNA
Proteins
New HIV particle

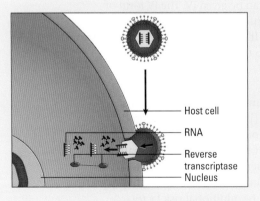

Host cell
RNA
Reverse transcriptase
Nucleus

- An increased risk of cellular and kidney toxicity occurs when zidovudine is taken with such drugs as flucytosine, vincristine, vinblastine, doxorubicin, interferon, and ganciclovir.
- Taking zidovudine with probenecid increases the risk of toxicity of either drug.
- Didanosine may reduce the absorption of tetracyclines, delavirdine, and fluoroquinolones.
- Abacavir levels increase with alcohol consumption.

Plays well with others

Emtricitabine has no clinically significant drug interactions when used in combination with indinavir, famciclovir, and tenofovir.

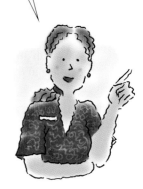

Lactic acidosis and severe hepatomegaly with steatosis can occur in patients taking NRTIs.

Adverse reactions

Adverse reactions to zidovudine and lamivudine include:
- blood-related reactions
- headache and fever
- dizziness
- muscle pain
- rash
- nausea and vomiting
- abdominal pain and diarrhea.

Details on didanosine

Didanosine may cause:
- nausea and vomiting
- abdominal pain and constipation or diarrhea
- stomatitis
- unusual taste or loss of taste
- dry mouth
- pancreatitis
- headache, peripheral neuropathy, or dizziness
- muscle weakness or pain
- rash and itchiness
- hair loss.

Didanosine

Abacavir may cause potentially fatal hypersensitivity reactions. Emtricitabine may cause severe hepatomegaly and lactic acidosis.

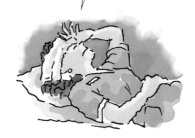

Several of the NRTIs can cause headache.

The Three-Step Approach

Nursing management for patients undergoing treatment with NRTIs is similar to that of management of patients receiving other anti-infective therapies. Key additional actions include:

- Monitor renal and hepatic function, CBC, and platelet count regularly.
- Monitor the patient's mental status when giving drugs IV. Encephalopathic changes are more likely in patients with neurologic disorders or in those who have had neurologic reactions to cytotoxic drugs.
- Take safety precautions if adverse CNS reactions occur. For example, place the bed in a low position, raise the bed rails, and supervise ambulation and other activities.
- Provide appropriate patient teaching. As an example, see *Teaching about zidovudine therapy*.
  As with any drug administration, be certain to pay particular attention to the type of drug being given and personalize care.

Nonnucleoside reverse transcriptase inhibitors (NNRTIs)

NNRTIs are used in combination with other antiretrovirals to treat HIV infection. The drugs in this class include:
- doravirine (Pifeltro)
- efavirenz (Sustiva)
- etravirine (Intelence)
- nevirapine (Viramune)
- rilpivirine (Edurant).

Pharmacokinetics

Efavirenz, etravirine, doravirine, and rilpivirine are highly protein bound after absorption and distribution. Nevirapine is widely distributed throughout the body. Efavirenz, doravirine, nevirapine, and rilpivirine are metabolized by the cytochrome P450 liver enzyme system; etravirine is metabolized by CYP3A4, CYP2C9, and CYP2C19 enzymes. All of these drugs are excreted in urine and feces.

Pharmacodynamics

Nevirapine, etravirine, and doravirine bind to the reverse transcriptase enzyme, preventing it from exerting its effect. Efavirenz and rilpivirine compete for the enzyme through noncompetitive inhibition.

Pharmacotherapeutics

NNRTIs are used in combination with other antiretrovirals in HIV treatment; nevirapine is specifically indicated for patients whose clinical condition and immune status have deteriorated.

Drug interactions

These drug interactions may occur with NNRTIs:
- Nevirapine may decrease the activity of protease inhibitors and hormonal contraceptives; don't use these drugs together.

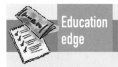

Teaching about zidovudine therapy

If zidovudine therapy is prescribed, review these points with the patient and caregivers:

- Blood transfusions may be needed during treatment because the drug commonly causes a low RBC count.
- Compliance with the twice daily dosage schedule is important for oral administration. Use reminders, such as an alarm on a smart phone, to avoid missing doses.
- Notify your health care provider if you are taking other medication. Other drugs, including other drugs used to treat AIDS, may interfere with zidovudine's effectiveness.
- For pregnant women infected with HIV, drug therapy only reduces the risk of HIV transmission to neonates. Long-term risks to infants are unknown.

- Coadministration of rifampin and doravirine is contraindicated as rifampin decreases exposure of doravirine by more than 70%.

Drug levels can drop....
- Indinavir and etravirine levels are decreased when administered with efavirenz.

No, no, no!
- Combining rilpivirine with a number of drugs can reduce effectiveness and possibly lead to resistance. Do not coadminister rilpivirine with anticonvulsants, antimycobacterials, proton pump inhibitors, dexamethasone, or St. John's wort.

Adverse reactions

Adverse reactions to NNRTIs include:
- headache
- dizziness
- asthenia
- nausea and vomiting
- diarrhea.

Rash response
In addition, nevirapine has been associated with a rash that may be life threatening. If a rash occurs, hold the next dose of the drug and immediately report this finding to the health care provider.

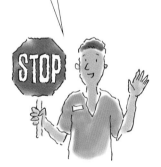

Patients taking nevirapine may develop a severe, life-threatening rash. If this happens, stop the drug.

The Three-Step Approach
Nursing management for patients undergoing treatment with NNRTIs is similar to that of management of patients receiving NRTI therapy. As with any drug administration, be certain to pay particular attention to the type of drug being given and personalize care.

A nucleoside reverse transcriptase inhibitor and a nucleotide analogue

Tenofovir (Viread), a nucleoside reverse transcriptase inhibitor, is approved for HIV treatment. Adefovir (Hepsera), a nucleotide analogue, is prescribed for the treatment of HBV. They work similarly to the NNRTIs.

Pharmacokinetics
Tenofovir is absorbed better after a high-fat meal. The absorption of adefovir is unaffected by the lack or presence of food. They are

then distributed in small amounts into plasma and serum proteins. Metabolism isn't thought to be mediated by cytochrome P450 liver enzymes, and the drugs are excreted by the kidneys.

Pharmacodynamics

Tenofovir competes with substrates and is subsequently incorporated into the DNA chain, thus halting HIV replication. Adefovir competes with HBV DNA in the same manner causing DNA chain termination.

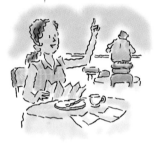

Tenofovir is absorbed better after a high-fat meal. Waiter! I'll have butter with that baked potato.

Pharmacotherapeutics

Tenofovir is used to treat HIV infection in combination with other drugs. Adefovir, used for HBV treatment, should never be given with tenofovir or any combination drug containing tenofovir.

Drug interactions

These drug interactions may occur with tenofovir:
* Drugs that are eliminated through the kidneys or that decrease renal function may increase levels of the drugs when given concurrently.
* Didanosine concentrations increase when given with tenofovir; watch for didanosine-based adverse effects.

Adverse reactions

Adverse reactions to tenofovir include:
* nausea and vomiting
* diarrhea
* anorexia
* abdominal pain.

The most common adverse reaction with adefovir is weakness.

Handle with care

Potentially fatal lactic acidosis and severe hepatomegaly with steatosis have occurred in patients taking these drugs alone or with other antiretrovirals. Most patients were natal sex women. Obesity and previous NRTI exposure may also be risk factors. Patients with preexisting liver disease should take this drug with caution. Suspend treatment if hepatotoxicity is suspected.

Patients with preexisting liver disease should take tenofovir with caution.

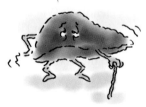

The Three–Step Approach

Nursing management for patients undergoing treatment with these two drugs is similar to that of management of patients receiving treatment with a NRTI drug. As with any drug administration, be certain to pay particular attention to the type of drug being given and personalize care.

Protease inhibitors

Protease inhibitors are drugs that act against the HIV enzyme protease, preventing it from dividing a larger viral precursor protein into the active smaller enzymes that the HIV virus needs to fully mature. The result is an immature, noninfectious cell. Two new protease inhibitors utilize the same mechanism to disrupt HCV viral replication. Drugs in this group include:

- saquinavir mesylate (Invirase)
- nelfinavir mesylate (Viracept)
- ritonavir (Norvir)
- lopinavir (Kaletra)
- fosamprenavir (Lexiva)
- atazanavir sulfate (Reyataz)
- tipranavir (Aptivus)
- darunavir (Prezista).

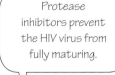

Protease inhibitors prevent the HIV virus from fully maturing.

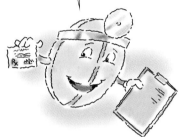

Pharmacokinetics

Protease inhibitors have different pharmacokinetic properties.

Saquinavir's story

Saquinavir mesylate is poorly absorbed from the GI tract. It's widely distributed, highly bound to plasma proteins, metabolized by the liver, and excreted mainly by the kidneys.

Nelfinavir notables

Nelfinavir's bioavailability (the degree to which it becomes available to target tissue after administration) isn't known. Food increases its absorption. It's highly protein bound, metabolized in the liver, and excreted primarily in feces.

Ritonavir review

Ritonavir is well absorbed, metabolized by the liver, and broken down into at least five metabolites. It's mainly excreted in feces, with some elimination through the kidneys.

One complements the other

Lopinavir is extensively metabolized by the liver's cytochrome P450 system. Lopinavir is only manufactured as a combination drug with ritonavir. When given together, ritonavir inhibits the metabolism of lopinavir, leading to increased plasma lopinavir levels. They are used in combination because of their positive effects on HIV RNA levels and CD4+ counts. This combination is typically not recommended due to issues with its potency and toxicity.

All about amprenavir

Fosamprenavir is metabolized in the liver to active and inactive metabolites and is minimally excreted in urine and feces.

As a group

Atazanavir and darunavir are combination drugs, used frequently with ritonavir or cobicistat (Evotaz). Nelfinavir, saquinavir, and fosamprenavir are older drugs in this class that are not used as often due to toxicity. Tipranavir is also rarely used. These drugs should be administered with food to maximize absorption with the exception of tipranavir, which is not food dependent for absorption. These drugs utilize the CY3PA pathway for metabolism. The group is primarily metabolized in the liver with biliary excretion through feces.

At last, atazanavir

Atazanavir is rapidly absorbed and is metabolized in the liver by the cytochrome P450 3A (CYP3A) pathway. The drug is excreted mainly in feces and urine.

Pharmacodynamics

All of these drugs inhibit the activity of HIV or HCV proteases and prevent the cleavage (division) of viral polyproteins.

Pharmacotherapeutics

Protease inhibitors are used in combination with other antiretroviral agents to treat HIV, and now, HCV infections. (See *Raltegravir (Isentress), dolutegravir sodium (Tivicay), enfuvirtide (Fuzeon), and maraviroc (Selzentry), "Other inhibitors,"* page 621.)

Drug interactions

Protease inhibitors may interact with many drugs. Here are some common interactions:
- Saquinavir mesylate may decrease the effectiveness of hormonal contraceptives.
- Ritonavir, atazanavir, darunavir, and tipranavir should not be given with drugs that inhibit or induce CYP3A pathways. They may significantly affect the absorption and plasma concentrations of either the protease inhibitor or the contraindicated drug. Drug-drug interaction should be checked frequently before and during therapy.
- Didanosine decreases gastric absorption of indinavir; give these drugs at least 1 hour apart.
- Rifampin markedly reduces plasma concentrations of most protease inhibitors, including atazanavir.

Raltegravir (Isentress), dolutegravir sodium (Tivicay), enfuvirtide (Fuzeon), and maraviroc (Selzentry): "Other inhibitors"

Four newer drugs have been approved for treatment of HIV: dolutegravir and raltegravir, both integrase inhibitors (INSTIs); enfuvirtide, a fusion inhibitor; and maraviroc, a CCR5 blocking entry inhibitor. All are indicated for patients who have strains of HIV that are resistant to multiple antiretroviral drugs. However, to work effectively, they must be combined with other HIV drugs.

Raltegravir's role

Raltegravir blocks the activity of integrase, an enzyme that hides HIV's DNA. When integrase is blocked, the HIV's DNA can't combine with the healthy cell's DNA.

So far, raltegravir seems to have few interactions with other drugs, although plasma levels of raltegravir are decreased when it's taken with rifampin. Adverse effects include diarrhea, nausea, headache, and an elevated creatine kinase level. Raltegravir also increases the risk of opportunistic infections; monitor the patient for indications of such an infection.

Maraviroc moves in

Maraviroc works by binding to a protein on the membrane of CD4 cells called *CCR5*, which blocks HIV from attaching to CD4 cells. When maraviroc instead of HIV is bound to CD4 cells, HIV can't infect these cells.

Maraviroc interacts with some drugs: Anticonvulsants and rifampin can decrease levels of maraviroc in the bloodstream. Conversely, clarithromycin, ketoconazole, and itraconazole can increase maraviroc levels. Maraviroc can also interact with other HIV medications, so dosages must be adjusted accordingly.

Adverse effects include cough, fever, respiratory tract infections, rash, muscle and joint pain, stomach pain, and diarrhea. Some patients have experienced systemic allergic reactions and, later, liver toxicity. Keep in mind that maraviroc should be used cautiously in patients at risk for cardiovascular events such as myocardial infarction. Patients are also at increased risk for developing opportunistic infections and malignancies.

Dolutegravir's duty

Dolutegravir blocks strand transfer in the HIV DNA replication process by binding to the integrase active site. It is administered in combination with other antiretroviral drugs. Its bioavailability is unknown and does not depend on food consumption. Primarily, it is excreted unchanged in feces.

Some other antivirals decrease the bioavailability of dolutegravir. Rifampin also reduces the drug availability. Coadministration with anticonvulsants, such as oxcarbazepine, phenytoin, phenobarbital, and carbamazepine, should be avoided. St. John's wort is contraindicated. Drugs containing cations, such as magnesium, aluminum, calcium, or iron, should be given outside a 2-hour window of dolutegravir. Metformin availability is increased with coadministration, and its dosage should be reduced during treatment.

The most common adverse reactions with dolutegravir are insomnia, fatigue, and headache. Monitor for signs of hypersensitivity, exacerbations of underlying hepatic disease, and immune reconstitution syndrome.

Enfuvirtide's function

Enfuvirtide is a drug used in the combination treatments designed to fight HIV. It interferes with entry of HIV into cells by inhibiting fusion of viral and cellular membranes. Enfuvirtide has largely bioavailable following injection. It is bound to and distributed predominantly by albumin in plasma. No elimination studies on humans have been completed.

No drug-drug interactions have been identified with enfuvirtide aside from decreased efficacy when combined with orlistat. Injection site reactions in the form of pain or discomfort, erythema, nodules or cysts, or ecchymosis have been noted. Other common reactions include diarrhea, nausea, and fatigue.

- Nelfinavir may greatly increase plasma levels of amiodarone, ergot derivatives, midazolam, rifabutin, quinidine, and triazolam.
- Carbamazepine, phenobarbital, and phenytoin may reduce the effectiveness of nelfinavir.
- Protease inhibitors may increase sildenafil concentrations and result in sildenafil-associated adverse reactions, including hypotension, vision changes, and priapism (a persistent, possibly painful erection).
- Atazanavir may prolong the PR interval. Drugs that prolong the PR interval, such as calcium channel blockers (diltiazem, for example) and beta-adrenergic blockers (atenolol, for example), should be used cautiously with atazanavir.
- Atazanavir shouldn't be administered with benzodiazepines such as midazolam and triazolam because of the potential for increased sedation or respiratory depression.
- Atazanavir shouldn't be administered with ergot derivatives, such as ergotamine and dihydroergotamine because life-threatening ergot toxicity can result, causing peripheral vasospasm and ischemia of the extremities.
- St. John's wort may reduce plasma concentrations of atazanavir.
- Ritonavir may increase plasma nelfinavir levels.

Adverse reactions

Adverse reactions depend on the type of protease inhibitor used:
- Saquinavir mesylate may cause dizziness, an increase in triglyceride and lipid levels, changes in body fat, anxiety, blurred vision, diarrhea, constipation or abdominal discomfort, night sweats, sleeplessness, or bleeding gums.
- Ritonavir's adverse reactions include muscle weakness, nausea, diarrhea, vomiting, anorexia, abdominal pain, and taste perversion.
- Nelfinavir may cause seizures, suicidal ideation, diarrhea, pancreatitis, hepatitis, hypoglycemia, or allergic reactions.
- Fosamprenavir may cause paresthesia, nausea, vomiting, loose stools, hyperglycemia, or rash.
- Reactions to combination therapy with lopinavir and ritonavir include encephalopathy, deep vein thrombosis, diarrhea, nausea, hemorrhagic colitis, and pancreatitis.
- Atazanavir may cause hepatotoxicity, arrhythmias, or lactic acidosis.

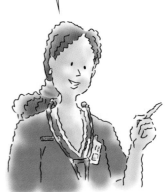

Adverse reactions to protease inhibitors vary from drug to drug. Make sure you familiarize yourself with the specific reactions of the drug your patient is taking.

Very similar

Tipranavir and darunavir both contain a sulfonamide moiety. Caution should be taken with administration of these drugs to patients with known sulfa allergies. Common adverse reactions for this group include:

- nausea, vomiting, and/or diarrhea
- headache
- rash
- fatigue
- abdominal pain.

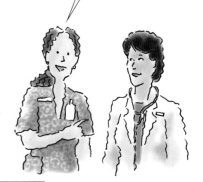

Notify the health care provider if the patient develops serious or persistent adverse reactions to a protease inhibitor.

The Three-Step Approach

Nursing management for patients undergoing treatment with protease inhibitors is similar to that of management of patients receiving other drugs that are designed to treat HIV and HBV. It is important to check the blood sugar levels of patients with diabetes taking saquinavir mesylate. As with any drug administration, be certain to pay particular attention to the type of drug being given and personalize care.

More HBV and HCV drugs

In addition to those already mentioned, there are remaining drugs of different classes indicated for the treatment of HBV and HCV. Interferon alfa-2b (Intron A) is a biological response modifier. Entecavir (Baraclude) is a guanosine nucleoside analogue. A nucleotide analogue inhibitor for the treatment of HCV is sofosbuvir (Sovaldi). Lastly, virus proliferation inhibitors include peginterferon alfa-2a (Pegasys) and peginterferon alfa-2b (PegIntron).

Black Box Warning

HBV or HCV

Carefully check labels for any drug that is indicated for treatment of HBV or HCV. Many carry black box warnings for various reasons. As an example, entecavir has a black box warning that notes these concerns (Epocrates, 2021a):

- Severe acute exacerbations of hepatitis B may occur (even months later) if a patient discontinues antihepatitis B therapy.
- This drug is not recommended for patients who have HIV in addition to hepatitis B who are not on highly active antiretroviral therapy, as resistance to HIV nucleoside reverse transcriptase inhibitors may develop.
- Lactic acidosis and severe hepatomegaly with steatosis (which can be fatal) have occurred when using nucleoside analogues.

Pharmacokinetics

The pharmacokinetics of the biological response modifier interferon alfa-2b is largely unstudied. The main site of catabolism, the reduction of a drug to smaller usable units, is in the kidneys.

The absorption of entecavir is delayed by food intake. It is distributed almost entirely into systemic tissues. Approximately two thirds of the drug is excreted unchanged through the kidneys.

Sofosbuvir is administered and absorbed through the GI tract without regard to food intake. About two thirds of the drug binds to human plasma, which is its main route of distribution. Sofosbuvir is metabolized in the liver and almost entirely eliminated through urine and feces.

Virus proliferation inhibitors, peginterferon alfa-2a and peginterferon alfa-2b, like the interferons, have limited studies regarding pharmacokinetics. They are both administered subcutaneously, and at least 30% of peginterferon alfa-2b is thought to be cleared through the kidneys.

Pharmacodynamics

Biological response modifiers (interferon alfa-2b) bind to specific membrane receptors on the cell surface, initiating a complex sequence of events and inducing the antiviral immune response. These intracellular events are necessary to inhibit HBV replication.

Entecavir competes with natural substances to inhibit the essential activities necessary for HBV genetic strand transcription and viral cell reproduction.

Sofosbuvir is a nucleotide prodrug. It is inactive when administered, but following metabolism, it is incorporated into the HCV genetic strand where it terminates chain formation.

Pleiotropic peginterferons

Pleiotropic means having more than one effect. Peginterferon alfa-2a and peginterferon alfa-2b bind to interferon receptors activating multiple intracellular pathways. These include, but are not limited to, suppression of cell cycle progression and enhancement of phagocytic activity.

Pharmacotherapeutics

Interferon alfa-2b is indicated for use with chronic HBV. Interferon alfa-2b is also used in the treatment of various cancers to include AIDS-related Kaposi's sarcoma.

Entecavir and sofosbuvir are only indicated for the use in the treatment of HBV. Peginterferon alfa-2a and peginterferon alfa-2b are used in the combination therapeutic treatment of CHC. These drugs should not be administered alone.

Drug interactions

Biological response modifiers (interferon alfa-2b) should be administered cautiously with myelosuppressives, such as zidovudine. The patient should be monitored for toxicity. Interferon alfa-2b should not be given with theophylline because it blocks theophylline clearance, increasing serum concentrations to 100%.

Each of the interferons and peginterferons listed here are often administered as part of combination therapy with ribavirin. They should not be administered to anyone that has a known reaction to ribavirin.

Entecavir is eliminated by the kidneys. Kidney functions should be monitored closely if it is coadministered with any drug that decreases renal function.

Sofosbuvir should not be given with rifampin or St. John's wort because it significantly decreases plasma concentrations. Serious symptomatic bradycardia can develop with the use of amiodarone and other antiviral medications. Sofosbuvir metabolism involves P-glycoprotein inducers. A wide variety of drugs fall into this class, including anticonvulsants, antimycobacterials, herbal supplements, and HIV protease inhibitors. Drug-drug interactions should be considered whenever therapy with sofosbuvir is warranted.

Administration of peginterferon alfa-2a and peginterferon alfa-2b with nucleoside analogues requires close monitor for toxicities. Dose adjustments or termination of therapy may be required. Increased narcotic effects or methadone toxicity is possible with coadministration of methadone. Peginterferon alfa-2a must be monitored closely when given with drugs metabolized through the CYP1A2 pathway. Monitor for worsening neutropenia or anemia with coadministration of zidovudine. Peginterferon alfa-2b must be monitored closely when coadministered with drugs utilizing the CYP450, CYP2C8/9, or CYP2D6 pathways for metabolism. Coadministration is contraindicated with peginterferon alfa-2b when combined with ribavirin.

No babies allowed

Many of the drugs available for the treatment of liver disease must be given as part of a combination therapy. Interferon alfa-2b, sofosbuvir, peginterferon alfa-2a, and peginterferon alfa-2b may all routinely be administered with ribavirin.

These drugs may cause birth defects and fetal deaths. Natal sex women who may become pregnant and individuals with partners who may become pregnant must follow specific precautions. A negative pregnancy test must be obtained prior to treatment along with monthly retesting. Two forms of birth control must be used at all times including up to 6 months posttreatment.

Black Box Warning

Interferon Alfa-2B and Sofosbuvir

Carefully review black box warnings for any of these drugs. For example, interferon alfa-2b carries a warning about the possibility of development of fatal or life-threatening neuropsychiatric, autoimmune, ischemic, and infectious disorders (Epocrates, 2021b). As another example, sofosbuvir carries a warning about the possibility of fulminant hepatitis, hepatic failure, and/or death occurring in patients with HBV and HCV who completed HCV direct-acting antiviral treatment but were not on treatment for HBV (Epocrates, 2021c).

Check the boxes

Interferons and peginterferons, interferon alfa-2b, peginterferon alfa-2a, and peginterferon alfa-2b, carry additional serious warnings. They may cause or exacerbate fatal or life-threatening neuropsychiatric, autoimmune, ischemic, and infectious disorders. Patients must be clinically evaluated, including labs, regularly and with great detail. Severe, persistent, or exacerbated symptoms may warrant withdrawal from therapy.

Common adverse reactions related to HBV and HBC antivirals include:
- flulike symptoms (headache, fever, myalgia, fatigue, and nausea)
- chills
- abdominal pain
- neutropenia
- injection site reactions.

The Three-Step Approach

Nursing management for patients undergoing treatment with these drugs that treat HBV and HBCs is similar to that of management of patients receiving other drugs that are designed to treat HBV that have been discussed earlier. Key additional actions include:
- Monitor renal and hepatic function, CBC, and platelet count regularly.
- Monitor electrolyte levels (calcium, phosphate, magnesium, and potassium).
- Monitor creatinine clearance two to three times weekly during induction and at least once every 1 to 2 weeks during maintenance.

As with any drug administration, be certain to pay particular attention to the type of drug being given and personalize care.

Antitubercular drugs

Antitubercular drugs are used to treat tuberculosis (TB), which is caused by *M. tuberculosis*. These drugs also are effective against less common mycobacterial infections caused by *Mycobacterium kansasii*, *M. avium-intracellulare*, *Mycobacterium fortuitum*, and related organisms. Although not always curative, these drugs can halt the progression of a mycobacterial infection.

Compliance can get complicated

Unlike most antibacterials, antitubercular drugs may need to be administered over many months. This creates such problems as patient nonadherencce, the development of bacterial resistance, and drug toxicity.

Tag team therapy

Traditionally, isoniazid, rifampin, and ethambutol hydrochloride were the mainstays of multidrug TB therapy and successfully prevented the emergence of drug resistance.

Because of the current incidence of drug-resistant TB strains, however, a four-drug regimen is now recommended for initial treatment:

* isoniazid
* rifampin (Rifadin)
* pyrazinamide
* ethambutol (Myambutol).

Because of the necessity of combination therapy for best practices, these medications are rarely manufactured alone; more commonly, they are manufactured in combination drugs such as rifampin/isoniazid and pyrazinamide/rifampin/isoniazid. The actions, reactions, and interactions of these combination drugs are the same as those of the individual drugs from which they are made.

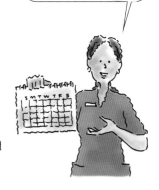

Antitubercular drugs may need to be administered over many months.

Times to modify

The antitubercular regimen should be modified if local testing shows resistance to one or more of these drugs. If local outbreaks of TB resistant to isoniazid and rifampin are occurring in institutions (for example, health care or correctional facilities), then other multidrug regimens are recommended as initial therapy.

Pharmacokinetics

Most antitubercular drugs are administered orally. When given orally, these drugs are well absorbed from the GI tract and widely distributed throughout the body. They're metabolized primarily in the liver and excreted by the kidneys.

Pharmacodynamics

Antitubercular drugs are specific for mycobacteria. At usual dosages, ethambutol and isoniazid are tuberculostatic, meaning that they inhibit the growth of *M. tuberculosis*. In contrast, rifampin is tuberculocidal, meaning that it destroys the mycobacteria. Because bacterial resistance to isoniazid and rifampin can develop rapidly, they should always be used with other antitubercular drugs.

Doubly inhibited

Ethambutol affects lipid synthesis, which results in the inhibition of mycolic acid incorporation into the cell wall, thereby inhibiting protein synthesis. Ethambutol acts only against replicating bacteria.

Tag team match

Isoniazid is taken up by mycobacterial cells and undergoes hydrolysis to isonicotinic acid, which reacts with cofactor nicotinamide adenine dinucleotide (NAD) to form a defective NAD that is no longer active as a coenzyme for certain life-sustaining reactions in the *M. tuberculosis* organism. Only replicating, not resting, bacteria appear to be inhibited. (See *Antitubercular drugs: Isoniazid*.)

RNA repressor

Rifampin inhibits RNA synthesis in susceptible organisms. The drug is effective primarily in replicating bacteria but may have some effect on resting bacteria as well.

Acid wash

The exact mechanism of action of pyrazinamide isn't known, but the antimycobacterial activity appears to be linked to the drug's conversion to the active metabolite pyrazinoic acid. Pyrazinoic acid, in turn, creates an acidic environment in which mycobacteria can't replicate.

Pharmacotherapeutics

Isoniazid is usually used with ethambutol, rifampin, or amikacin. This is because combination therapy for TB and other mycobacterial infections can prevent or delay the development of resistance.

For uncomplicated pulmonary TB

Ethambutol is used with isoniazid and rifampin to treat patients with uncomplicated pulmonary TB. It's also used to treat infections resulting from *Mycobacterium bovis* and most strains of *M. kansasii*.

Preventive power

Although isoniazid is the most important drug for treating TB, bacterial resistance develops rapidly if it's used alone. However, resistance doesn't pose a problem when isoniazid is used alone to

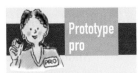

Prototype pro

Antitubercular drugs: Isoniazid

Actions
• Inhibits cell wall protein synthesis by interfering with mycolic acid incorporation

Indications
• TB

Nursing considerations
• Monitor the patient for adverse effects, such as peripheral neuropathy, seizures, hematologic disorders, hepatitis, and hypersensitivity reactions.
• Always give isoniazid with other antitubercular drugs to prevent the development of resistant organisms.

prevent TB in individuals who have been exposed to the disease, and no evidence exists of cross-resistance between isoniazid and other antitubercular drugs. Isoniazid is typically given orally but may be given IM or IV if necessary.

Rapid resistance

Rifampin is used to treat pulmonary TB with other antitubercular drugs. It combats many gram-positive and some gram-negative bacteria but is seldom used for nonmycobacterial infections because bacterial resistance develops rapidly. It's used to treat asymptomatic carriers of *Neisseria meningitidis* when the risk of meningitis is high, but it isn't used to treat infection due to this organism because of the potential for bacterial resistance.

First in line

Pyrazinamide is currently recommended as a first-line TB drug in combination with ethambutol, rifampin, and isoniazid. Pyrazinamide is a highly specific drug that's active only against *M. tuberculosis*. Resistance to pyrazinamide may develop rapidly when it's used alone.

Drug interactions

Antitubercular drugs may interact with a number of other drugs:
- Isoniazid may increase levels of phenytoin, carbamazepine, diazepam, ethosuximide, primidone, theophylline, and warfarin.
- Rifampin interferes with the action of oral contraceptives.
- When corticosteroids and isoniazid are taken together, the effectiveness of isoniazid is reduced, whereas the effects of corticosteroids are increased.
- Isoniazid may reduce the plasma concentration of ketoconazole, itraconazole, and oral antidiabetic drugs.
- When given together, the combination of rifampin, isoniazid, ethionamide, and pyrazinamide increases the risk of hepatotoxicity.
- Pyrazinamide combined with phenytoin may increase phenytoin levels.

Adverse reactions

Adverse reactions to antitubercular drugs vary:
- Ethambutol may cause itching, joint pain, GI distress, malaise, retrobulbar neuritis and blindness, leukopenia, headache, dizziness, numbness and tingling of the extremities, and confusion. Although rare, hypersensitivity reactions to ethambutol may produce rash and fever. Anaphylaxis may also occur.
- Peripheral neuropathy is the most common adverse reaction to isoniazid. Severe and occasionally fatal hepatitis associated with isoniazid may occur even many months after treatment has stopped. Patients must be monitored carefully.

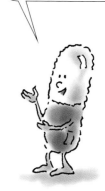

Isoniazid is the most important drug for treating TB. It's nice to get the recognition I deserve!

- The most common adverse reactions to rifampin include epigastric pain, nausea, vomiting, abdominal cramps, flatulence, anorexia, diarrhea and red-orange-brown discoloration of urine, tears, sweat, and sputum.
- Liver toxicity is the major limiting adverse reaction to pyrazinamide. GI disturbances include nausea, vomiting, and anorexia.

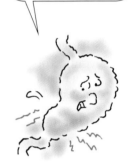

Common adverse reactions to rifampin include—ouch—epigastric pain and abdominal cramps.

The Three-Step Approach

Nursing management for patients undergoing treatment with antitubercular drugs, including newer ones rifapentine (Priftin) and bedaquiline fumarate (Sirturo) (see *Newer TB drugs: Rifapentine (Priftin) and bedaquiline fumarate (Sirturo)*), is similar to that of management of patients receiving other anti-infective therapies. Key additional actions include:

- Administer oral doses 1 hour before or 2 hours after meals to avoid decreased absorption.
- Follow the protocol for IM or IV dosage if prescribed via one of these routes. Collaborate with the health care provider to switch to the oral form as soon as possible.

Newer TB drugs: Rifapentine (Priftin) and bedaquiline fumarate (Sirturo)

Latent TB infection

Rifapentine (Priftin) is a cyclopentyl rifamycin that acts by inhibiting RN transcriptase, preventing chain formation and leading to cell death. It is indicated for the treatment of latent TB infection (LTBI) but also used as part of combination-drug therapy in the treatment of active TB.

Rifapentine is absorbed through the GI tract with food and distributed via plasma proteins. The majority of the drug is metabolized within 7 days and mainly excreted through feces.

Contraindications include known hypersensitivity to any rifamycin. Rifapentine is metabolized through the P450 pathway. Coadministered drugs that utilize the same pathway may increase or decrease serum levels; these include protease inhibitors, reverse transcriptase inhibitors, and hormonal contraceptives. Dose adjustments of drugs may be necessary, although a second form of contraception is indicated.

Multiple reported common adverse reactions include anemia, lymphopenia, neutropenia, arthralgia, conjunctivitis, headache, nausea, vomiting, diarrhea, pruritus, rash, anorexia, and lymphadenopathy.

Multidrug-resistant TB

Bedaquiline fumarate (Sirturo) is a diarylquinoline antimycobacterial drug that disrupts the intracellular process necessary for energy generation in *M. tuberculosis*. Bedaquiline is indicated for multidrug-resistant TB (MDR-TB) only when effective alternative treatments cannot be achieved. It must be used in combination with three to four other antitubercular drugs depending on known sensitivities.

Bedaquiline is well absorbed in the GI tract with food. It binds to plasma proteins for distribution, whereas metabolism is accomplished through the CYP3A4 pathway. Complete elimination of the drug can take up to 5.5 months; it is excreted through feces.

The most common adverse reactions are nausea, arthralgia, headache, hemoptysis, and chest pain.

Black Box Warning

Antitubercular drugs

Bedaquiline fumarate (Sirturo) carries a boxed warning for an increased risk of mortality and QT prolongation with therapy. For this reason, use with other drugs known to cause QT prolongation is contraindicated.

Education edge

Teaching about antitubercular drugs

If antitubercular drugs are prescribed, review these points with the patient and caregivers:
• Use a form of birth control while on antitubercular therapy.
• Take the drug with food if GI irritation occurs.
• Avoid alcohol use during drug therapy.

• Avoid certain foods, including fish (such as tuna) and products containing tyramine (such as aged cheese, beer, and chocolate), because the drug has some MAO inhibitor activity.
• Notify the health care provider immediately if signs and symptoms of liver impairment (loss of appetite, fatigue, malaise, jaundice, or dark urine) occur.

• Monitor for paresthesia of the hands and feet, which usually precedes peripheral neuropathy, especially in patients with malnourishment, diabetes, or alcohol use disorder.
• Monitor hepatic function closely for changes.
• Provider appropriate patient teaching. (See *Teaching about antitubercular drugs*.)

Antifungal drugs

Antifungal, or antimycotic, drugs are used to treat fungal infections. They include:
• polyenes
• flucytosine
• ketoconazole
• synthetic triazoles
• glucan synthesis inhibitors. (See *Other antifungal drugs*, page 632.)

Other antifungal drugs

Several other antifungal drugs offer alternative forms of treatment for topical fungal infections.

Clotrimazole

An imidazole derivative, clotrimazole is used:
- topically to treat dermatophyte and *Candida albicans* infections
- orally to treat mild oral candidiasis
- vaginally to treat vulvovaginal candidiasis.

Griseofulvin

Griseofulvin is used to treat fungal infections of the:
- skin (tinea corporis)
- feet (tinea pedis)
- groin (tinea cruris)
- beard area of the face and neck (tinea barbae)
- nails (onychomycosis)
- scalp (tinea capitis).

No relapse allowed

To prevent a relapse, griseofulvin therapy must continue until the fungus is eradicated and the infected skin or nails are replaced.

Miconazole

Available as miconazole or miconazole nitrate, this imidazole derivative is used to treat local fungal infections, such as vaginal and vulvar candidiasis, and topical fungal infections, such as chronic candidiasis of the skin and mucous membranes.

Delivery options

Miconazole may be administered:
- orally to treat oropharyngeal candidiasis
- locally to treat vaginal infections
- topically to treat topical infections.

Other topical antimycotic drugs

Ciclopirox, econazole nitrate, butoconazole nitrate (Gynazole-1), naftifine, tioconazole, terconazole, butenafine hydrochloride, sulconazole nitrate (Exelderm), and oxiconazole nitrate are available only as topical drugs.

Polyenes

The polyenes include amphotericin B, natamycin (Natacin), and nystatin. The potency of amphotericin B has made it the most widely used antifungal drug for severe systemic fungal infections. Nystatin is used only topically or orally to treat local fungal infections because it's extremely toxic when administered parenterally. Natamycin is used to treat fungal infections of the eye.

Pharmacokinetics

After IV administration, amphotericin B is distributed throughout the body and excreted by the kidneys. Its metabolism isn't well defined.

Not much circulation

Oral nystatin undergoes little or no absorption, distribution, or metabolism. It's excreted unchanged in feces. Topical nystatin isn't absorbed through intact skin or mucous membranes. Natamycin is not absorbed systemically.

Pharmacodynamics

Amphotericin B works by binding to sterol (a lipid) in the fungal cell membrane, altering cell permeability and allowing intracellular components to leak out.

Fungi town

Amphotericin B usually acts as a fungistatic drug (inhibiting fungal growth and multiplication) but can become fungicidal (destroying fungi) if it reaches high concentrations in the fungi.

Manipulating membranes

Nystatin and natamycin bind to sterols in fungal cell membranes and alters the permeability of the membranes, leading to loss of cell components. Nystatin can act as a fungicidal or fungistatic drug, depending on the organism present.

Pharmacotherapeutics

Amphotericin B is usually administered to treat severe systemic fungal infections and meningitis caused by fungi sensitive to the drug. It's never used for noninvasive forms of fungal disease because it's highly toxic. It's usually the drug of choice for severe infections caused by a wide variety of fungi, including *Candida*, *Aspergillus fumigatus*, *Scedosporium*, and some *Fusarium* species.

Amphotericin B comes along and thinks it can just send me and all my friends packing!

Know the limits

Because amphotericin B is highly toxic, its use is limited to patients who have a definitive diagnosis of life-threatening infection and are under close medical supervision.

Canning candidal infections

Different forms of nystatin are available for treating different types of candidal infections:
- Topical nystatin is used to treat candidal skin or mucous membrane infections, such as oral thrush, diaper rash, vaginal and vulvar candidiasis, and candidiasis between skin folds.
- Oral nystatin is used to treat GI infections.
- Natamycin is used to treat fungal forms of keratitis, blepharitis, and conjunctivitis.

Drug interactions

Amphotericin B may have significant interactions with many drugs:
- Because of the synergistic effects between flucytosine and amphotericin B, these two drugs are commonly combined in therapy for candidal or cryptococcal infections, especially for cryptococcal meningitis.
- The risk of kidney toxicity increases when amphotericin B is taken with aminoglycosides, cyclosporine, or acyclovir.
- Corticosteroids, extended-spectrum penicillins, and digoxin may worsen hypokalemia (low blood potassium levels) produced by amphotericin B, possibly leading to heart problems. Moreover, the risk of digoxin toxicity is increased.

- Amphotericin B increases muscle relaxation when given with nondepolarizing skeletal muscle relaxants (such as pancuronium).
- Amphotericin B may cause hypokalemia when given with thiazide diuretics.
- Electrolyte solutions may inactivate amphotericin B when diluted in the same solution. Amphotericin B preparations must be mixed with D_5W; they can't be mixed with saline solutions.

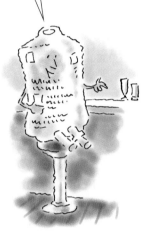

Don't mix amphotericin B preparations with saline solutions! They must be mixed with D5W.

Wallflowers

Nystatin and natamycin do not interact significantly with other drugs.

Adverse reactions

Almost all patients receiving IV amphotericin B, particularly at the beginning of low-dose therapy, experience:

- chills
- fever
- nausea and vomiting
- anorexia
- muscle and joint pain
- indigestion.

Watch those RBCs

Most patients also develop normochromic (adequate hemoglobin in each RBC) or normocytic anemia (too few RBCs) that significantly decreases hematocrit.

Altered electrolytes

Hypomagnesemia and hypokalemia may occur, causing ECG changes requiring replacement electrolyte therapy. Magnesium and potassium levels and renal function must be monitored frequently in patients receiving amphotericin B.

Losing concentration

Many patients may develop some degree of kidney toxicity, causing the kidneys to lose their ability to concentrate urine.

The higher the dosage, the harder they react

Reactions to nystatin may include hypotension, tachycardia, headache, and malaise, but high dosages may produce:

- diarrhea
- nausea and vomiting
- abdominal pain
- a bitter taste
- hypersensitivity reactions
- skin irritation (topical form).

The Three-Step Approach

Nursing management for patients undergoing treatment with polyenes is similar to that of management of patients receiving other anti-infective therapies. Key additional actions include:

- The lozenge form of the drug should be dissolved slowly.
- Parenteral IV use is for hospitalized patients *only* after diagnosis of potentially fatal fungal infection is confirmed. The initial dose is usually given as a test dose, administered over 20 to 30 minutes.
- Use an infusion pump and in-line filter with a mean pore diameter larger than 1 micron. Infuse over 2 to 6 hours; rapid infusion may cause cardiovascular collapse.
- Give antibacterials separately; don't mix them or give them piggyback with other drugs.
- Monitor pulse, respiratory rate, temperature, and blood pressure every 30 minutes for at least 4 hours after giving the drug IV; fever, shaking chills, anorexia, nausea, vomiting, headache, tachypnea, and hypotension may appear 1 to 3 hours after the start of an IV infusion. Signs and symptoms are usually more severe with initial doses.
- Monitor BUN, creatinine (or creatinine clearance), and electrolyte levels; CBC; and liver function test results at least weekly. If the BUN level exceeds 40 mg/dL or if the creatinine level exceeds 3 mg/dL, notify the health care provider who may reduce or stop the drug until renal function improves.
- If the patient has severe adverse infusion reactions to the initial dose, stop the infusion and notify the health care provider. The provider may prescribe antipyretics, antihistamines, antiemetics, or small doses of corticosteroids. To prevent reactions during subsequent infusions, collaborate with the health care provider regarding premedicating the patient with these drugs or give amphotericin B on an alternate-day schedule.

As with any drug administration, be certain to pay particular attention to the type of drug being given and personalize care.

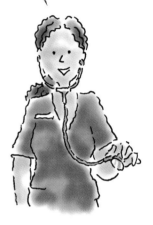

Take the patient's blood pressure every 30 minutes for at least 4 hours after giving polyenes IV.

Flucytosine

Flucytosine, a fluorinated pyrimidine analogue, is the only antimetabolite that acts as an antifungal. Flucytosine is a purine and pyrimidine inhibitor.

Pharmacokinetics

After oral administration, flucytosine is well absorbed from the GI tract and widely distributed. It undergoes little metabolism and is excreted primarily by the kidneys.

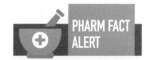

PHARM FACT ALERT

If a drug is fungicidal, it destroys the fungus—*cidus* is a Latin term for "killing." If it's fungistatic, it prevents fungal growth and multiplication—*stasis* is a Greek term for "halting."

Pharmacodynamics

Flucytosine penetrates fungal cells, where it's converted to its active metabolite, fluorouracil. Fluorouracil is then incorporated into the RNA of the fungal cells, altering their protein synthesis and causing cell death.

Pharmacotherapeutics

Flucytosine is used primarily with another antifungal drug such as amphotericin B to treat systemic fungal infections. For example, although amphotericin B is effective in treating candidal and cryptococcal meningitis alone, flucytosine is given with it to reduce the dosage of amphotericin B and the risk of toxicity. This combination therapy is the treatment of choice for cryptococcal meningitis.

Drug interactions

Cytarabine may antagonize the antifungal activity of flucytosine, possibly by competitive inhibition. Hematologic, kidney, and liver function must be closely monitored during flucytosine therapy because of the drug's serious risk of toxicity.

Adverse reactions

Flucytosine may produce unpredictable adverse reactions, including:
- confusion
- headache
- drowsiness
- vertigo
- hallucinations
- difficulty breathing
- respiratory arrest
- rash
- nausea and vomiting
- abdominal distention
- diarrhea
- anorexia.

The Three-Step Approach

Nursing management for patients undergoing treatment with flucytosine is similar to that of management of patients receiving other anti-infective therapies. Key additional actions include:
- Before therapy, obtain hematologic tests and renal and liver function studies. Make sure susceptibility tests showing that the organism is flucytosine sensitive are included on the patient's chart.
- Monitor blood and liver and renal function studies frequently; obtain susceptibility tests weekly to monitor drug resistance.

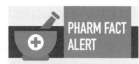

PHARM FACT ALERT

An antimetabolite is a substance that closely resembles one required for normal physiologic functioning and that exerts its effect by interfering with metabolism.

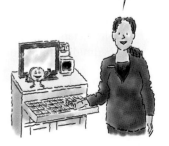

Flucytosine reduces the risk of amphotericin B toxicity when the drugs are given together.

- Collaborate with the health care provider to see if routine blood level assays of the drug to maintain flucytosine at therapeutic levels (25 to 120 mcg/mL) will be ordered. This is especially helpful when patients with renal impairment are prescribed this drug. Higher blood levels may be toxic.
    As with any drug administration, be certain to pay particular attention to the type of drug being given and personalize care.

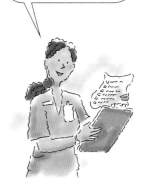

Before starting therapy, make sure susceptibility tests showing that the organism is flucytosine-sensitive are included on the patient's chart.

Ketoconazole

Ketoconazole, a synthetic imidazole derivative, is an effective oral antifungal drug with a broad spectrum of activity.

Pharmacokinetics

When given orally, ketoconazole is absorbed variably and distributed widely. It undergoes extensive liver metabolism and is excreted in bile and feces.

Pharmacodynamics

Within the fungal cells, ketoconazole interferes with sterol synthesis, damaging the cell membrane and increasing its permeability. This leads to a loss of essential intracellular elements and inhibition of cell growth.

Fungicidal tendencies

Ketoconazole usually produces fungistatic effects but can also produce fungicidal effects under certain conditions.

Pharmacotherapeutics

Ketoconazole is used to treat topical and systemic infections caused by susceptible fungi, which include dermatophytes and most other fungi.

Drug interactions

Ketoconazole may have significant interactions with other drugs:
- Ketoconazole use with drugs that decrease gastric acidity, such as cimetidine, ranitidine, famotidine, nizatidine, antacids, and anticholinergic drugs, may decrease absorption of ketoconazole and reduce its antimycotic effects. If the patient must take these drugs, delay administration of ketoconazole by at least 2 hours.
- Taking ketoconazole with phenytoin may alter metabolism and increase blood levels of both drugs.
- When taken with theophylline, ketoconazole may decrease the serum theophylline level.
- Use with other hepatotoxic drugs may increase the risk of liver disease.

- Combined with cyclosporine therapy, ketoconazole may increase cyclosporine and serum creatinine levels.
- Ketoconazole increases the effect of oral anticoagulants and can cause hemorrhage.

Feeling a bit inhibited

- Ketoconazole can inhibit metabolism (and possibly increase concentrations) of quinidine, sulfonylureas, carbamazepine, and protease inhibitors.
- Ketoconazole shouldn't be given with rifampin because serum ketoconazole concentrations may decrease.

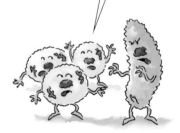

Help! We need antifungal activity!

Adverse reactions

The most common adverse reactions to ketoconazole are nausea and vomiting. Less frequent reactions include:

- anaphylaxis
- flulike symptoms
- tinnitus
- impotence
- photophobia
- hepatotoxicity (very rare; usually reversible when the drug is stopped).

The Three-Step Approach

Nursing management for patients undergoing treatment with a ketoconazole is similar to that of management of patients receiving other anti-infective therapies. Key additional actions include:

- Because of the risk of serious hepatotoxicity, the drug shouldn't be used for less serious conditions, such as fungal infections of the skin or nails.
- To minimize nausea, divide the daily amount into two doses and give the drug with meals.

As with any drug administration, be certain to pay particular attention to the type of drug being given and personalize care.

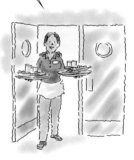

To minimize nausea, give the drug with meals. For breakfast, would you like some cereal, toast, and milk?

Synthetic triazoles

The synthetic triazoles include fluconazole (Diflucan), itraconazole (Sporanox), voriconazole (Vfend), and posaconazole (Noxafil).

Pharmacokinetics

After oral administration, fluconazole is almost completely absorbed. It's distributed into all body fluids, and most of the drug is excreted unchanged in urine.

With and without food

Oral bioavailability is greatest for itraconazole and posaconazole when they are taken with food; voriconazole is more effective if taken 1 hour before or after a meal. Both itraconazole and voriconazole are bound to plasma proteins and extensively metabolized in the liver into a large number of metabolites. They're minimally excreted in feces.

Pharmacodynamics

Fluconazole and posaconazole inhibit fungal cytochrome P450, an enzyme responsible for fungal sterol synthesis, causing fungal cell walls to weaken.

The wall comes tumbling down

Itraconazole and voriconazole interfere with fungal cell wall synthesis by inhibiting the formation of ergosterol and increasing cell wall permeability, making the fungus susceptible to osmotic instability.

Pharmacotherapeutics

The synthetic triazoles treat various infections:
- Fluconazole is used to treat mouth, throat, and esophageal candidiasis and serious systemic candidal infections, including UTIs, peritonitis, and pneumonia. It's also used to treat cryptococcal meningitis.
- Itraconazole is used to treat blastomycosis, nonmeningeal histoplasmosis, candidiasis, aspergillosis, and fungal nail disease.
- Voriconazole is used to treat invasive aspergillosis and serious fungal infections caused by *Scedosporium apiospermum* and *Fusarium* species.
- Posaconazole is used as prophylaxis against invasive *Aspergillus* and *Candida* in high-risk patients. It is also used for the treatment of oropharyngeal candidiasis.

Drug interactions

Fluconazole may have these drug interactions:
- Use with warfarin may increase the risk of bleeding.
- It may increase levels of phenytoin and cyclosporine.
- It may increase the plasma concentration of oral antidiabetic drugs, such as glyburide, tolbutamide, and glipizide, increasing the risk of hypoglycemia.
- Rifampin and cimetidine enhance the metabolism of fluconazole, reducing its plasma level.
- It may increase the activity of zidovudine.

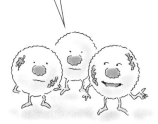

So here's how it works, people. Synthetic triazoles either cause fungal cell walls to weaken or interfere with cell wall synthesis. Got it?

And the interactions just keep coming...

Itraconazole and voriconazole have these drug interactions:

- Both may increase the risk of bleeding when combined with oral anticoagulants.
- Antacids, H_2-receptor antagonists, phenytoin, and rifampin lower plasma itraconazole levels.
- Voriconazole may inhibit the metabolism of phenytoin, benzodiazepines, calcium channel blockers, sulfonylureas, and tacrolimus.
- Voriconazole is contraindicated with sirolimus and ergot alkaloids because it may increase plasma concentrations of these drugs.
- Voriconazole is contraindicated with quinidine and pimozide because of the risk of prolonged QT intervals and, rarely, torsades de pointes.

Check your pathways

Metabolism of posaconazole takes place through the UDP-glucuronidation pathway and is a substrate of P-glycoprotein efflux. Drugs that inhibit or induce these pathways may significantly affect plasma concentrations of posaconazole. It is a strong inhibitor of CYP3A4, coadministration of drugs also using this pathway may increase their serum levels. Monitor for drug-drug interactions with all medications coadministered with posaconazole.

Adverse reactions

Adverse reactions to fluconazole, voriconazole, and posaconazole include:

- abdominal pain
- diarrhea
- dizziness
- headache
- increase in liver enzymes
- nausea and vomiting
- rash.

   Adverse reactions to itraconazole include:
- hypertension
- impaired liver function.

The Three-Step Approach

Nursing management for patients undergoing treatment with a synthetic triazole is similar to that of management of patients receiving other anti-infective therapies. Key additional actions include:

- Don't remove protective overwraps from IV bags of fluconazole until just before use to ensure product sterility.

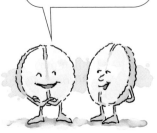

This list of adverse reactions makes me dizzy—just one of the possible side effects of synthetic triazoles.

- Give by continuous infusion with an infusion pump at a rate of no more than 200 mg/hour. To prevent air embolism, don't give the drug in a series with other infusions.
- Don't add other drugs to the solution.
- If the patient develops a mild rash, monitor closely. Stop the drug if lesions progress and notify the health care provider.
  As with any drug administration, be certain to pay particular attention to the type of drug being given and personalize care.

Glucan synthesis inhibitors

Caspofungin acetate (Cancidas), anidulafungin (Eraxis), and micafungin (Mycamine) are a group of drugs in a class known as *glucan synthesis inhibitors* (also known as *echinocandins*).

Pharmacokinetics

These drugs are given IV and are highly protein bound, with little distribution into RBCs. They are slowly metabolized and excreted in urine and feces.

Pharmacodynamics

Caspofungin, anidulafungin, and micafungin inhibit the synthesis of beta (1,3)-D-glucan, an enzyme present in fungal but not mammalian cells. This inhibition disrupts fungal cell wall development.

Pharmacotherapeutics

Caspofungin is used to treat invasive aspergillosis in patients who have failed to respond to, or can't tolerate, other antifungals, such as amphotericin B or itraconazole. It hasn't been studied as an initial treatment for invasive aspergillosis.

Anidulafungin is indicated in the treatment of candidemia, esophageal candidiasis, and other forms of *Candida* infection. Micafungin is also used to treat candidemia and esophageal candidiasis. It is also used as prophylaxis in patients undergoing stem cell transplants and with acute disseminated candidiasis.

Drug interactions

Glucan synthesis inhibitors are known to cause these drug interactions:

- Patients taking caspofungin and tacrolimus may need higher doses of tacrolimus because caspofungin decreases the blood tacrolimus level.
- These drugs should not be given to anyone with a known hypersensitivity to any glucan synthesis inhibitors, also known as *echinocandins*.

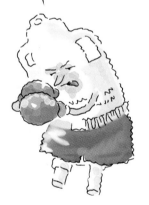

Caspofungin is called into the ring when other antifungal therapies have failed.

Clearance concerns

- Inducers of drug clearance, such as phenytoin, carbamazepine, efavirenz, nevirapine, and nelfinavir, may lower caspofungin clearance.
- Concurrent use of caspofungin and cyclosporine may result in elevated liver enzyme levels and decreased caspofungin clearance; their use together isn't recommended.

Adverse reactions

Adverse reactions common to the group include nausea, vomiting, diarrhea, and pyrexia. Anidulafungin may cause insomnia, anemia, headache, or dyspepsia. Micafungin carries a risk of thrombocytopenia and headache. Additional adverse reactions specific to caspofungin include:

- paresthesia
- tachycardia
- tachypnea
- rash
- facial swelling.

The Three–Step Approach

Nursing management for patients undergoing treatment with a glucose synthesis inhibitor is similar to that of management of patients receiving other anti-infective therapies. Key additional actions include:

- Assess the patient's hepatic function before starting drug therapy.
- Observe the patient for histamine-mediated reactions (rash, facial swelling, pruritus, sensation of warmth).

As with any drug administration, be certain to pay particular attention to the type of drug being given and personalize care.

Quick quiz

1. Which condition is an adverse reaction to fluoroquinolones?
    A. Increased appetite
    B. Hyponatremia
    C. Glaucoma
    D. Tendinitis/tendon rupture

Answer: D. Adverse reactions to fluoroquinolones include tendonitis/ tendon rupture, QT prolongation, aortic dissection, and *C. difficile*– associated diarrhea.

2. Which bacterial infection are the drugs isoniazid, rifampin, and ethambutol hydrochloride used to treat?
    A. *Escherichia coli*
    B. *Mycobacterium tuberculosis*
    C. *Pneumocystis carinii*
    D. *Haemophilus influenzae*

Answer: B. These drugs are used in combination as first-line therapy to treat tuberculosis caused by *Mycobacterium tuberculosis*.

3. Which condition is often treated with a tetracycline? (Select all that apply.)
    A. Lyme disease
    B. Q fever
    C. Brucellosis
    D. Urinary tract infection
    E. Chlamydiae

Answer: A, B, C, E. Tetracyclines are often used to treat Lyme disease, Q fever, brucellosis, and chlamydiae; they are not often used in the treatment of urinary tract infections.

4. Because of their chemical makeup, there is a small chance of cross-reactivity between cephalosporins and which other group of antibiotics?
    A. Aminoglycosides
    B. Tetracyclines
    C. Carbapenems
    D. Penicillins

Answer: D: Penicillins have a known cross-reactivity with cephalosporins. Aminoglycosides, tetracyclines, and carbapenems do not have this same cross-reactivity.

Scoring

★★★ If you answered all four questions correctly, impeccable! You're privy to the pills that pounce those pesky pathogens.

★★ If you answered three questions correctly, magnificent! Those malicious microorganisms are marked now that you're on the scene.

★ If you answered two or less questions correctly, don't get in a funk. You'll be fluent in antifungals and all the rest before you know it.

Suggested References

Byron May, D. (2020). Tetracyclines. In *UpToDate*. Retrieved from https://www.uptodate.com/contents/tetracyclines?search=tetracycline&source=search_result&selectedTitle=2~148&usage_type=default&display_rank=1

Cies, J. J., Moore, W. S. II, Enache, A., & Chopra, A. (2020). Ceftaroline cerebrospinal fluid penetration in the treatment of a ventriculopleural shunt infection: A case report. *The Journal of Pediatric Pharmacology and Therapeutics: JPPT: the Official Journal of PPAG, 25*(4), 336–339. https://doi.org/10.5863/1551-6776-25.4.336

Drew, R. (2020a). Aminoglycosides. In *UpToDate*. Retrieved from https://www.uptodate.com/contents/aminoglycosides?search=aminoglycosides&source=search_result&selectedTitle=1~150&usage_type=default&display_rank=1

Drew, R. (2020b). Linezolid and tedizolid (oxazolidinones): An overview. In *UpToDate*. Retrieved from https://www.uptodate.com/contents/linezolid-and-tedizolid-oxazolidinones-an-overview?search=tedizolid&source=search_result&selectedTitle=2~19&usage_type=default&display_rank=1

Epocrates. (2021a). *Entecavir: Black box warnings*. Retrieved from https://online.epocrates.com/drugs/409711/entecavir/Black-Box-Warnings

Epocrates. (2021b). *Interferon alfa-2b: Black box warnings*. Retrieved from https://online.epocrates.com/drugs/329111/Pegasys/Black-Box-Warnings

Epocrates. (2021c). *Sofosbuvir: Black box warnings*. Retrieved from https://online.epocrates.com/drugs/677711/Sovaldi/Black-Box-Warnings

Fletcher, C. (2021). Overview of antiretroviral agents used to treat HIV. In *UpToDate*. Retrieved from https://www.uptodate.com/contents/overview-of-antiretroviral-agents-used-to-treat-hiv?search=nnrti&sectionRank=2&usage_type=default&anchor=H3604592045&source=machineLearning&selectedTitle=2~150&display_rank=2#H3604592045

HIV.info.NIH.gov. (2021). *HIV and lactic acidosis*. Retrieved from https://hivinfo.nih.gov/understanding-hiv/fact-sheets/hiv-and-lactic-acidosis

Hooper, D. (2021). Fluoroquinolones. In *UpToDate*. Retrieved from https://www.uptodate.com/contents/fluoroquinolones?search=fluoroquinolones&source=search_result&selectedTitle=2~149&usage_type=default&display_rank=1

Letourneau, A. (2021). Cephalosporins. In *UpToDate*. Retrieved from https://www.uptodate.com/contents/cephalosporins?search=cephalosporins&source=search_result&selectedTitle=2~139&usage_type=default&display_rank=1

Martel, T., Jamil, R., & King, K. (2021). Vancomycin flushing syndrome. [Updated 2021 Sep 12]. In: *StatPearls* [Internet]. Treasure Island, FL: StatPearls Publishing. Retrieved from https://www.ncbi.nlm.nih.gov/books/NBK482506/

Werth, B. (2020a). Carbapenems. In *Merck manual professional version*. Retrieved from https://www.merckmanuals.com/professional/infectious-diseases/bacteria-and-antibacterial-drugs/carbapenems

Werth, B. (2020b). Fluoroquinolones. In *Merck manual professional version*. Retrieved from https://www.merckmanuals.com/professional/infectious-diseases/bacteria-and-antibacterial-drugs/fluoroquinolones

Werth, B. (2020c). Macrolides. In *Merck manual professional version*. Retrieved from https://www.merckmanuals.com/professional/infectious-diseases/bacteria-and-antibacterial-drugs/macrolides

Chapter 17

Anti-inflammatory, antiallergy, and immunosuppressant drugs

Just the facts

In this chapter, you'll learn:

♦ classes of drugs that modify immune or inflammatory responses

♦ uses and varying actions of these drugs

♦ absorption, distribution, metabolization, and excretion of these drugs

♦ drug interactions and adverse reactions to these drugs.

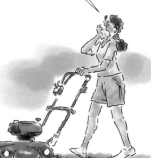

Antihistamines can be used to treat mild seasonal allergies.

Drugs and the immune system

Immune and inflammatory responses protect the body from invading foreign substances. Certain classes of drugs can modify these responses:

- *Antihistamines* block the effects of histamine on target tissues.
- *Corticosteroids* suppress immune responses and reduce inflammation.
- *Immunosuppressants (noncorticosteroids)* prevent rejection of transplanted organs and can be used to treat autoimmune diseases.
- *Uricosurics* control the occurrence of gout attacks.

Antihistamines

Antihistamines primarily act to block histamine effects that occur in an immediate (type I) hypersensitivity reaction, commonly called an *allergic reaction*. They are available by themselves or in combination products, and may be obtained by prescription or purchased over the counter.

Histamine-1 receptor antagonists

The term *antihistamine* refers to drugs that act as histamine-1 (H_1)-receptor antagonists; they compete with histamine for H_1-receptor sites throughout the body. However, they don't displace histamines already bound to receptors.

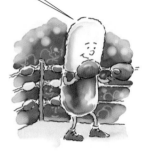

Come on, histamine! I can take you on.

It's all about chemistry

Antihistamines are categorized into major classes based on their chemical structures:

- *Ethanolamines* include clemastine fumarate (Dayhist), dimenhydrinate (Dramamine), and diphenhydramine hydrochloride (Benadryl).
- *Alkylamines* include brompheniramine (Dimetapp), chlorpheniramine (Aller-Chlor), and dexchlorpheniramine (no trade name at time of publication).
- *Phenothiazines* include promethazine hydrochloride (Phenergan).
- *Piperidines* include cetirizine (Zyrtec), cyproheptadine hydrochloride (no trade name at time of publication), desloratadine (no trade name at time of publication), fexofenadine (Allegra), loratadine (Claritin), and meclizine hydrochloride (Antivert).
- Miscellaneous drugs, such as hydroxyzine hydrochloride (Vistaril) and hydroxyzine pamoate (no trade name at time of publication), also act as antihistamines.

Pharmacokinetics

H_1-receptor antagonists are absorbed well after oral or parenteral administration. Some can also be given rectally. Except for loratadine and desloratadine, antihistamines are distributed widely throughout the body and central nervous system (CNS).

On the alert

Fexofenadine, desloratadine, and loratadine are nonsedating antihistamines. Because these drugs only minimally penetrate the blood-brain barrier, they aren't widely distributed throughout the CNS. As a result, they produce fewer sedative effects than other antihistamines.

Antihistamines are metabolized by liver enzymes and excreted in urine, with small amounts secreted in breast milk. Fexofenadine, mainly excreted in feces, is an exception. Cetirizine undergoes hepatic metabolism.

Pharmacodynamics

H_1-receptor antagonists compete with histamine for H_1 receptors on effector cells (the cells that cause allergic signs and symptoms), blocking histamine from producing its effects.

Antagonizing line of attack

H_1-receptor antagonists produce their effects by:
- blocking the action of histamine on small blood vessels
- decreasing arteriole dilation and tissue engorgement
- reducing leakage of plasma proteins and fluids out of the capillaries (capillary permeability), thereby lessening edema
- inhibiting most smooth muscle responses to histamine (in particular, blocking the constriction of bronchial, GI, and vascular smooth muscle)
- relieving symptoms by acting on the terminal nerve endings in the skin that flare and itch when stimulated by histamine
- suppressing adrenal medulla stimulation, autonomic ganglia stimulation, and exocrine gland secretion, such as lacrimal and salivary secretion.

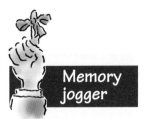

Memory jogger

Anti- is a familiar prefix that means *opposing*. And that's exactly what antihistamines do: They oppose histamine effects (or allergic reactions).

It's all in your head

Several antihistamines have a high affinity for H_1 receptors in the brain and are used for their CNS effects. These drugs include diphenhydramine, dimenhydrinate, promethazine, and various piperidine derivatives. (See *Antihistamines: Diphenhydramine (Benadryl)*, page 648.)

H_1-receptor antagonists don't affect parietal cell secretion in the stomach because the receptors of these cells are H_2 receptors, not H_1 receptors.

Pharmacotherapeutics

Antihistamines are used to treat signs and symptoms of type I hypersensitivity reactions, such as:
- allergic rhinitis (runny nose and itchy eyes caused by a local sensitivity reaction)
- vasomotor rhinitis (rhinitis not caused by allergy or infection)
- allergic conjunctivitis (inflammation of the eye membranes)
- urticaria (hives)
- angioedema (submucosal swelling in the hands, face, and feet).

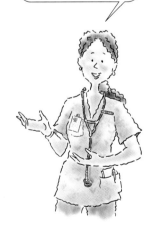

Antihistamines relieve the signs and symptoms of an allergic reaction. However, they don't give the body immunity to the allergy itself.

Prototype pro

Antihistamines: Diphenhydramine (Benadryl)

Actions
- Competes with histamine for H₁ receptor sites on the smooth muscle of the bronchi, GI tract, uterus, and large blood vessels, binding to the cellular receptors and preventing access and subsequent activity of histamine
- Antagonizes the action of histamine that causes increased capillary permeability and resultant edema and suppresses flare and pruritus associated with endogenous release of histamine (doesn't directly alter histamine or prevent its release)

Indications
- Rhinitis
- Allergy symptoms
- Motion sickness
- Parkinson's disease

Nursing considerations
- Monitor for common adverse effects, such as drowsiness, sedation, nausea, and dry mouth.
- Serious, although rare, adverse effects include thrombocytopenia, agranulocytosis, thickening of secretions, and anaphylactic shock.
- Monitor older adults carefully for confusion, delirium, and fall risk; monitor dosage calculations carefully in pediatric patients.
- Use with extreme caution in patients with prostatic hyperplasia, asthma, chronic obstructive pulmonary disease, hyperthyroidism, cardiovascular disease, or hypertension.

Beyond the obvious

Antihistamines have other therapeutic uses. Many are used primarily as antiemetics (to control nausea and vomiting). They can also be used as adjunctive therapy to treat an anaphylactic reaction after serious signs and symptoms are controlled. For example, diphenhydramine (Benadryl) can be used to help treat vertigo and drug-induced extrapyramidal reactions (abnormal involuntary movements).

Drug interactions

Antihistamines interact with many other drugs, sometimes with life-threatening consequences. Here are a few examples:
- Antihistamines may block or reverse the vasopressor effects of epinephrine (Emerphed), producing vasodilation, increased heart rate, and dangerously low blood pressure.
- Antihistamines may mask toxic signs and symptoms of ototoxicity (a detrimental effect on hearing) associated with aminoglycosides or large doses of salicylates.
- Antihistamines may increase the sedative and respiratory depressant effects of CNS depressants, such as tranquilizers and alcohol.

> Beware of the potentially dangerous drug interactions that may occur when giving antihistamines.

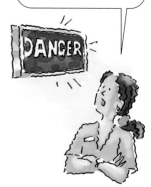

- Loratadine (Claritin) may cause serious cardiac effects when taken with macrolide antibiotics (such as erythromycin), fluconazole (Diflucan), ketoconazole (no trade name at time of publication), itraconazole (Sporanox), miconazole (Oravig), cimetidine (Tagamet HB), ciprofloxacin (Cipro), and clarithromycin (Biaxin XL).

Adverse reactions

The most common adverse reaction to antihistamines (with the exception of fexofenadine, loratadine, and desloratadine) is CNS depression. Other CNS reactions include:
- dizziness
- fatigue
- disturbed coordination
- muscle weakness.

Gut reactions

GI reactions may include:
- epigastric distress
- loss of appetite
- nausea and vomiting
- constipation
- diarrhea
- dryness of the mouth, nose, and throat.

Cardiac concerns

Cardiovascular reactions may include:
- hypotension
- hypertension
- rapid heart rate
- arrhythmias.

A sensitive issue

Sensitivity reactions can also occur.

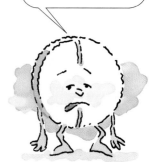

Sigh. I guess I'm just feeling a bit sensitive about the sensitivity reactions I can sometimes cause.

The Three-Step Approach

Nursing management for patients receiving antihistamine therapy includes these three steps. Be certain to pay particular attention to the type of antihistamine being given, and personalize care accordingly.

Preadministration

(Recognize and analyze cues)

- Conduct a baseline physical assessment before therapy begins and watch for significant changes.
- Assess severity of specific symptoms (for example, rhinitis, sneezing, immune response, etc.) prior to administration so that comparison can be done afterward to determine efficacy.

(Prioritize Hypothesis—Priority Patient Problems)

- Immunity alteration
- Potential for injury if CNS depression occurs (with certain antihistamines)

(Generate solutions)

- Specific symptoms related to immunity alteration will be alleviated.
- CNS depression will not occur.

Medication Administration

(Take action)

- Determine whether the patient is taking other medication that could depress the CNS; collaborate with the health care provider if needed.
- If hospitalized, make sure that the patient has a call light in hand. Remind not to get out of bed without calling for a nurse.
- Ensure that the room is free from clutter that may increase the risk for falls.
- Reduce GI distress by giving antihistamines with food.
- If administering the drug IM, alternate injection sites to prevent irritation. Give IM injections into large muscles such as the deltoid of the arm, vastus lateralis of the thigh, ventrogluteal of the hip, and dorsogluteal of the buttocks.
- Encourage fluid intake (if allowed) or humidify the air to decrease thickened secretions.
- Notify the health care provider if tolerance is observed because a substitute antihistamine may be indicated.

Postadministration

(Evaluate outcomes)

- Conduct a follow-up assessment to determine if specific symptoms are alleviated.
- Monitor for adverse reactions (especially CNS depression) and drug interactions.
- Monitor blood counts during long-term therapy; watch for signs of blood dyscrasia.
- For patients undergoing outpatient therapy, teach to use sugarless gum, hard candy, or ice chips to relieve dry mouth.
- Provide teaching as included in *Teaching about antihistamines*, page 651.

Teaching about antihistamines

If antihistamine therapy is prescribed, teach about these points:

- Avoid caffeine, nicotine, alcohol, tranquilizers, sedative, pain medication, and sleeping medication while taking an antihistamine, as these can also affect the central nervous system (in addition to the antihistamine).
- Use warm water rinses, artificial saliva, ice chips, or sugarless gum or candy to relieve dry mouth.

- If using to prevent motion sickness, take the drug 30 minutes before travel.
- If using for insomnia, administer 20 minutes before sleep.
- Avoid hazardous activities such as driving until the full CNS effects of the drug are known.
- If you are having diagnostic skin tests done, discuss if or when to discontinue antihistamine therapy prior to testing to preserve the accuracy of test results.

- Notify the health care provider if tolerance develops because a different antihistamine may need to be prescribed.
- Be aware that antihistamines may cause photosensitivity. Use sunblock or wear protective clothing.
- Avoid using other products containing diphenhydramine (including over-the-counter and topical forms) while breast-feeding because of the risk of adverse reactions.

Corticosteroids

Corticosteroids suppress immune responses and reduce inflammation. They're available in natural or synthetic forms.

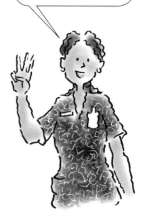

Glucocorticoids work in three ways, exerting anti-inflammatory, metabolic, and immunosuppressant effects.

Nature's bounty

Natural corticosteroids are hormones produced by the adrenal cortex; most corticosteroid drugs are synthetic forms of these hormones.

Natural and synthetic corticosteroids are classified according to their biological activities:

- *Glucocorticoids*, such as cortisone and dexamethasone, affect carbohydrate, fat, and protein metabolism.
- *Mineralocorticoids*, such as aldosterone and fludrocortisone acetate, regulate electrolyte and water balance.

Glucocorticoids

Most glucocorticoids are synthetic analogues of hormones secreted by the adrenal cortex. They exert anti-inflammatory, metabolic, and immunosuppressant effects. Drugs in this class include:

- beclomethasone (Beconase AQ)
- betamethasone (Celestone Soluspan)

- budesonide (Pulmicort Flexhaler, Pulmicort Respules)
- cortisone (no trade name at time of publication)
- dexamethasone (no trade name at time of publication)
- fluticasone (Flonase Allergy Relief, over-the-counter)
- hydrocortisone (Solu-cortef)
- methylprednisolone (Solu-medrol)
- prednisolone (Orapred ODT)
- prednisone (Rayos)
- triamcinolone (Nasacort Allergy 24-Hour, over-the-counter)

Pharmacokinetics

Glucocorticoids are well absorbed when administered orally. After IM administration, they're completely absorbed. Glucocorticoids can also be absorbed through inhalation through the lining of the lungs with the use of an inhaler.

Glucocorticoids are bound to plasma proteins and distributed through the blood. They're metabolized in the liver and excreted by the kidneys.

Pharmacodynamics

Glucocorticoids suppress hypersensitivity and immune responses through a process that isn't entirely understood.

The research suggests…

Researchers believe that glucocorticoids inhibit immune responses by:
- suppressing or preventing cell-mediated immune reactions
- reducing levels of leukocytes, monocytes, and eosinophils
- decreasing the binding of immunoglobulins to cell surface receptors
- inhibiting interleukin synthesis.

So soothing

Glucocorticoids suppress the redness, edema, heat, and tenderness associated with the inflammatory response. They start on the cellular level by stabilizing the lysosomal membrane (a structure within the cell that contains digestive enzymes) so that it doesn't release its store of hydrolytic enzymes into the cells. (See *Corticosteroids: Prednisone*.)

Prototype pro

Corticosteroids: Prednisone

Actions
- Decreases inflammation by stabilizing leukocyte lysosomal membranes, suppressing immune response, stimulating bone marrow, and influencing protein, fat, and carbohydrate metabolism

Indications
- Severe inflammation
- Immunosuppression

Nursing considerations
- Monitor for adverse effects, such as euphoria, insomnia, heart failure, thromboembolism, peptic ulcers, and acute adrenal insufficiency.
- Monitor for Cushing effects, such as moon face, buffalo hump, central obesity, thinning hair, and increased susceptibility to infection.
- Monitor and trend weight, blood pressure, and serum electrolytes.
- Teach that this drug may mask signs of infection.
- Recognize that dosage must be gradually reduced after long-term therapy.

A job well done

Glucocorticoids prevent leakage of plasma from capillaries, suppress the migration of polymorphonuclear leukocytes (cells that kill and digest microorganisms), and inhibit phagocytosis (cellular ingestion and destruction of solid substances).

To ensure a job well done, glucocorticoids decrease antibody formation in injured or infected tissues and disrupt histamine synthesis, fibroblast development, collagen deposition, capillary dilation, and capillary permeability. (See *How methylprednisolone works*, page 654.)

Pharmacotherapeutics

Glucocorticoids are used as replacement therapy for patients with adrenocortical insufficiency. They're also prescribed for immunosuppression (such as in allergic reactions, organ transplants, and autoimmune disorders) and disorders requiring treatment by reduction of inflammation (such as arthritis, asthma, and chronic obstructive pulmonary disease). They are also prescribed for their effects on the blood and lymphatic systems.

Drug interactions

There are numerous drug interactions with glucocorticoids. Some of the most common include the following:

- Efficacy of the COVID-19 vaccine and other immunizations may be diminished if glucocorticoids are taken at time of immunization
- The hypokalemic effect of loop diuretics may be increased when taken with systemic corticosteroids
- The effects of antidiabetic drugs may be reduced, resulting in increased blood glucose levels.
- Estrogen and hormonal contraceptives that contain estrogen increase the effects of glucocorticoids.
- Glucocorticoids reduce the serum concentration and effects of salicylates.
- The risk of GI bleeding, ulceration, and perforation associated with nonsteroidal anti-inflammatory drugs and salicylates is increased when these agents are taken with corticosteroids.

Pharm function

How methylprednisolone works

Tissue trauma normally leads to tissue irritation, edema, inflammation, and production of scar tissue. Methylprednisolone counteracts the initial effects of tissue trauma, promoting healing.

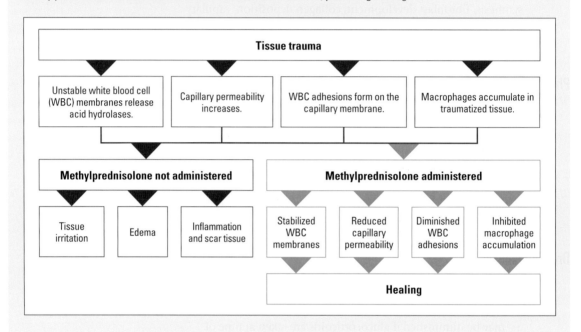

Adverse reactions

Glucocorticoids affect almost all body systems. Their widespread adverse effects are more common in long-term or high-dose use and include:

- insomnia
- increased sodium and water retention
- increased potassium excretion
- suppressed immune and inflammatory responses
- osteoporosis
- GI bleeding, ulceration, perforation
- impaired wound healing
- ocular hypertension and glaucoma
- hypertension
- personality changes
- increased susceptibility to infection.

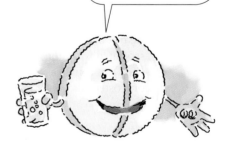

Glucocorticoids affect almost all body systems. You might say we're all inclusive.

Endocrine system

Endocrine system reactions may include:

- diabetes mellitus
- hyperlipidemia
- adrenal atrophy
- hypothalamic-pituitary axis suppression
- cushingoid signs and symptoms (such as buffalo hump, moon face, and elevated blood glucose levels).

The Three-Step Approach

Nursing management for patients receiving corticosteroid therapy includes these three steps. Be certain to pay particular attention to the type of corticosteroid being given, and personalize care accordingly.

Preadministration

(Recognize and analyze cues)

- Conduct a baseline physical assessment before therapy begins and watch for significant changes.
- Assess condition (for which the drug is being given) prior to administration so that comparison can be done afterward to determine efficacy.
- Establish baseline blood pressure, fluid and electrolyte status, and weight. For pediatric patients, establish height also.

(Prioritize hypothesis—priority patient problems)

- Need for immunosuppression (for example, due to allergic reaction, transplant, autoimmune disorder, asthma, etc.)
- Potential for infection due to immunosuppression
- Hyperglycemia related to drug-induced adverse reaction

(Generate solutions)

- Desired immunosuppression will be achieved
- Immunosuppression will not result in infection
- Hyperglycemia will not occur.

Medication administration

(Take action)

- Administer early in the day to mimic circadian rhythm.
- Give with food to prevent GI irritation.
- Unless contraindicated, offer a low-sodium diet that is high in potassium and protein. Administer potassium supplements as prescribed.
- If inhaled, teach to gargle and rinse mouth with water after each dose to reduce oral mucosal irritation and to prevent infections of the mouth.
- Take precautions to avoid exposure to infection.
- Expect to increase the drug dosage (as prescribed) during times of physiologic stress, such as surgery, trauma, or infection.

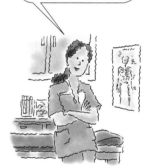

Glucocorticoids can reduce the effects of antidiabetic drugs. Monitor glucose levels of a patient with diabetes closely.

Postadministration

(Evaluate outcomes)

- Conduct ongoing follow-up assessments to determine if desired immunosuppression has occurred and to assure that no signs of infection are present.
- Monitor for adverse effects including depression, aggression, and adrenal insufficiency.
- Monitor closely for changes in weight and glycemic control (and height, for pediatric patients); report any concerning changes to the health care provider.
- Recognize that patients with diabetes may need dosage adjustments to insulin and that patients without diabetes may require insulin or antidiabetic drugs during therapy.
- Do not stop the drug abruptly. (See *Concerns regarding abrupt corticosteroid withdrawal.*)
- Work collaboratively with the health care provider to avoid prolonged use of corticosteroids, especially in children.

Mineralocorticoids

Mineralocorticoids affect electrolyte and water balance. One mineralocorticoid is fludrocortisone acetate (no trade name at time of publication), a synthetic analogue of hormones secreted by the adrenal cortex.

Pharmacokinetics

Fludrocortisone acetate is absorbed well and distributed to all parts of the body. It's metabolized in the liver to inactive metabolites and excreted by the kidneys.

Pharmacodynamics

Fludrocortisone acetate affects fluid and electrolyte balance by acting on the distal renal tubule to increase sodium reabsorption and potassium and hydrogen secretion.

Pharmacotherapeutics

Fludrocortisone acetate is used as replacement therapy for patients with adrenocortical insufficiency (reduced secretion of glucocorticoids, mineralocorticoids, and androgens).

Keeping things in balance

Fludrocortisone acetate may also be used to treat salt-losing congenital adrenogenital syndrome (characterized by a lack of cortisol and deficient aldosterone production) after the patient's electrolyte balance has been restored.

Concerns regarding abrupt corticosteroid withdrawal

If corticosteroids are rapidly withdrawn, adverse symptoms can occur. These include rebound inflammation, fatigue, weakness, arthralgia, fever, dizziness, lethargy, depression, fainting, orthostatic hypotension, dyspnea, anorexia, and hypoglycemia. After long-term therapy, increased stress or abrupt withdrawal may cause acute adrenal insufficiency. Sudden withdrawal after prolonged therapy can be fatal.

Teaching about corticosteroid therapy

If corticosteroid therapy is prescribed, review these points with the patient and caregivers:

• Take the drug exactly as prescribed and do not stop the drug suddenly. If you miss a dose, do not double the next dose. Continue with the next dose and follow up with the health care provider.

• Missed doses or suddenly stopping the drug may result in complications (especially if you're on long-term corticosteroid therapy). It's important to notify your prescriber of a change in your regular dosing schedule.

• Notify the health care provider if your stress level increases; the dosage may need to be temporarily adjusted.

• Take the oral form of the drug with food.

• Report sudden weight gain, swelling, slow healing, black tarry stools, bleeding, bruising, blurred vision, emotional changes, or other unusual effects.

• If receiving long-term therapy, eat a diet high in protein, calcium, and potassium and low in carbohydrates and sodium.

• Wear or carry medical identification at all times indicating the need for systemic glucocorticoids during stress.

• If receiving long-term therapy, watch for cushingoid signs and symptoms (weight gain, swelling of the face) and report them immediately.

• Be aware of early signs and symptoms of adrenal insufficiency, including fatigue, muscle weakness, joint pain, fever, anorexia, nausea, dyspnea, dizziness, and fainting.

• Keep regular medical checkups to help detect early adverse reactions, evaluate disease status, and assess drug response. Dosage adjustments may be needed.

• Don't take other medications, over-the-counter preparations, or herbal remedies without first consulting your health care provider.

• Discuss activity or exercise needed to help prevent or delay osteoporosis, a common adverse reaction, with your health care provider.

• Report signs and symptoms of infection.

• Avoid alcohol during therapy.

Drug interactions

The drug interactions associated with mineralocorticoids are similar to those associated with glucocorticoids.

Adverse reactions

The adverse reactions associated with mineralocorticoids are similar to those associated with glucocorticoids.

The Three-Step Approach

Nursing management for patients receiving mineralocorticoid therapy follows the same principles as the Three-Step Approach for patients receiving glucocorticoid therapy. A key concept to remember when administering a mineralocorticoid is to frequently evaluate fluid and electrolyte status and to be prepared to intervene if signs and symptoms of hypovolemia are present. Also, recognize that potassium supplementation may be needed depending on laboratory results or if the patient develops signs of hypokalemia including muscle cramps and/or electrocardiogram changes.

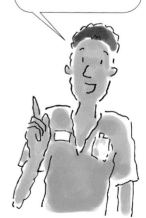

Mineralocorticoids and glucocorticoids have similar drug interactions.

Immunosuppressants

Several drugs used for their immunosuppressant effects in patients undergoing allograft transplantation (a transplant between two people who aren't identical twins) are also used experimentally to treat autoimmune diseases (diseases resulting from an inappropriate immune response directed against the self). They include:

- anakinra (Kineret)
- azathioprine (Imuran)
- basiliximab (Simulect)
- cyclosporine (Gengraf)
- daclizumab (Zinbryta)
- lymphocyte immune globulin (ATG [equine]) (Atgam)
- mycophenolate mofetil (CellCept)
- sirolimus (Rapamune)
- tacrolimus (Prograf)
- thymoglobulin (antithymocyte globulin [rabbit]) (Thymoglobulin)

ATG, anakinra, basiliximab, daclizumab, and thymoglobulin are administered only by IV injection.

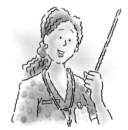

Pharmacokinetics

Immunosuppressants take different paths through the body:

- When administered orally, azathioprine is absorbed readily from the GI tract, whereas absorption of cyclosporine and sirolimus is varied and incomplete.
- The distributions of azathioprine, daclizumab, and basiliximab are not fully understood.
- Cyclosporine is distributed widely throughout the body.
- Azathioprine and cyclosporine cross the placental barrier.
- ATG is distributed by binding to circulating lymphocytes, granulocytes, platelets, bone and marrow cells.
- Distribution of tacrolimus depends on several factors, with the majority being protein bound. Sirolimus is almost completely protein-bound.

How it all adds up…

Azathioprine and cyclosporine are metabolized in the liver. The metabolism of ATG is unknown. Mycophenolate is metabolized in the liver to mycophenolate acid, an active metabolite, and then further metabolized to an inactive metabolite, which is excreted in urine and bile. The mycophenolate concentration may be increased in the presence of nephrotoxicity.

... and out

Azathioprine, anakinra, and ATG are excreted in urine; cyclosporine is excreted principally in bile. Tacrolimus is extensively metabolized and primarily excreted primarily in bile. Sirolimus is metabolized and excreted primarily in feces with a small amount excreted in urine. Metabolism and excretion of basiliximab and daclizumab aren't fully understood.

Pharmacodynamics

It is not fully understood how many immunosuppressants achieve their desired effects.

The jury's still out...

For example, the exact mechanisms of action of azathioprine, cyclosporine, and ATG are unknown; however, these drugs may undergo these processes:

- Azathioprine antagonizes the metabolism of the amino acid purine and, therefore, inhibits ribonucleic acid and deoxyribonucleic acid structure and synthesis. It may also inhibit coenzyme formation and function.
- Cyclosporine is thought to inhibit helper T cells and suppressor T cells.
- ATG may eliminate antigen-reactive T cells in the blood, alter T-cell function, or both.

... but this much is known

In a patient receiving a kidney allograft, azathioprine suppresses cell-mediated hypersensitivity reactions and produces various alterations in antibody production.

Anakinra, basiliximab, and daclizumab block the activity of interleukin. Mycophenolate inhibits responses of T and B lymphocytes, suppresses antibody formation by B lymphocytes, and may inhibit the recruitment of leukocytes into sites of inflammation and graft rejection. Sirolimus is an immunosuppressant that inhibits T-lymphocyte activation and proliferation that occurs in response to antigenic and cytokine stimulation; it also inhibits antibody formation.

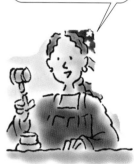

In my judgment, the jury's still out on the exact mechanism of action of several immunosuppressants. But let's hear from my colleagues below about their involvement...

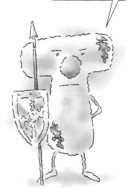

"I'd say we're definitely involved in the action..."

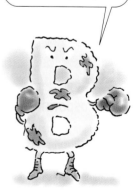

"Absolutely! Like that mycophenolate. It's always trying to inhibit our responses, no matter what kind of fight I put up!"

Pharmacotherapeutics

Immunosuppressants are mainly used to prevent rejection in patients undergoing organ transplantation. Cyclophosphamide is primarily used to treat cancer. Anakinra is indicated for adults with moderate to severely active rheumatoid arthritis who have taken at least one disease-modifying antirheumatic drug that has not worked.

Drug interactions

Drug interactions with this class commonly involve other immunosuppressant and anti-inflammatory drugs or various antibiotic and antimicrobial drugs:

- Allopurinol increases the blood levels of azathioprine.
- Verapamil increases the blood levels of sirolimus.
- Levels of cyclosporine may be increased by ketoconazole, calcium channel blockers, cimetidine, anabolic steroids, hormonal contraceptives, erythromycin, and metoclopramide.
- Coadministration of voriconazole and sirolimus is contraindicated because of the inhibition of cytochrome P450 3A4 enzymes by voriconazole, which increases sirolimus levels.
- The absorption of mycophenolate is decreased when taken with antacids or cholestyramine. Coadministration of mycophenolate with acyclovir may increase concentrations of both drugs, especially in a patient with renal impairment.

Kidney concerns

- The risk of toxicity to the kidneys increases when cyclosporine is taken with acyclovir, aminoglycosides, or amphotericin B.
- The risk of infection and lymphoma (neoplasm of the lymph tissue, most likely malignant) is increased when cyclosporine or sirolimus is taken with other immunosuppressants (except corticosteroids).
- Barbiturates, rifampin, phenytoin, sulfonamides, and trimethoprim decrease plasma cyclosporine and sirolimus levels.
- Serum digoxin levels may be increased when cyclosporine is taken with digoxin.

Black Box Warning

Cyclosporine

Cyclosporine carries a Black Box Warning stating that only providers experienced in immunosuppressant therapy (for example, treatment and management of organ transplants, located in a medical facility with adequate resources, etc.) should administer this medication. It also notes that there is skin malignancy risk when taken by people with psoriasis, and hypertension and nephrotoxicity risk even when given at recommended doses.

- Taking ATG, anakinra, basiliximab, daclizumab, or thymoglobulin with other immunosuppressant drugs increases the risk of infection and lymphoma. Anakinra therapy shouldn't be initiated in a patient with an active infection or neutropenia.

Adverse reactions

All immunosuppressants can cause hypersensitivity reactions. Other common adverse reactions include flu-like symptoms (nausea, vomiting, GI upset, fever, chills, and diarrhea). Some drugs can cause bone marrow suppression, liver toxicity, thrombosis, leukopenia, or thrombocytopenia. Be sure to carefully assess side effects of the individual drug given and be prepared to put proper interventions in place and monitor for specific side effects.

The Three–Step Approach

Nursing management for patients receiving immunosuppressant therapy includes these three steps. Be certain to pay particular attention to the type of immunosuppressant being given, and personalize care accordingly.

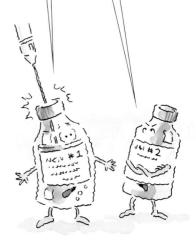

"Wait! What about all these adverse reactions we can cause?"

"Come on! You know we play a key role in helping prevent organ rejection in transplant patients."

Preadministration

(Recognize and analyze cues)

- Conduct a baseline physical assessment before therapy begins and watch for significant changes. Be sure to take a comprehensive history regarding the patient's immune status prior to the onset of therapy.
- Assure that baseline laboratory work including blood urea nitrogen (BUN), creatinine levels, glomerular filtration rate (GFR), potassium, alkaline phosphatase, and bilirubin are collected.

(Prioritize hypothesis—priority patient problems)

- Potential for injury due to organ rejection or drug-induced immunosuppression.

(Generate solutions)

- Organ will not be rejected.
- Drug-induced immunosuppression will not occur.

Medication administration

(Take action)

- Be prepared to reconstitute certain medications according to policy and procedure.
- Teach that the medication can take up to 12 weeks to be effective.
- Teach patients who may become pregnant to use protection while taking the medication and to avoid pregnancy for at least 4 months after stopping therapy.

Postadministration

(Evaluate outcomes)

- Conduct a follow-up assessment to determine how patient is tolerating drug therapy.
- Monitor the drug's effectiveness by observing for signs of organ rejection.
- Monitor for signs of infection and report fever, sore throat, and malaise to the health care provider.
- Monitor hemoglobin levels, hematocrit, and WBC and platelet counts at least once monthly (initially) or as prescribed by the health care provider.
- Recognize that drug therapy may need to be stopped if WBC is less than 3,000/μL.
- To prevent bleeding, avoid IM injections when the platelet count is below 100,000/μL.
- Monitor renal and liver function tests as prescribed by the health care provider.

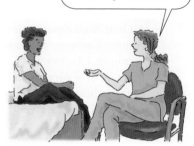

Remember, it may take up to 12 weeks for this medication to be fully effective.

Uricosurics

Uricosurics and other antigout drugs exert their anti-inflammatory actions through their effects on uric acid. Increased uric acid in the blood (hyperuricemia) results in gout, a specific form of inflammatory arthritis. Hyperuricemia occurs because of increased production of uric acid or because of decreased excretion of uric acid by the kidneys.

Uricosuric drug

A uricosuric drug acts by increasing uric acid excretion in urine. The primary goal in using this type of drug is to prevent or control the frequency of gout attacks. It is *not* used for acute gout attacks. One well-known uricosuric is probenecid (Probalan).

Pharmacokinetics

Probenecid (Probalan) is absorbed from the GI tract. Distribution is mostly protein-bound. Metabolism occurs in the liver, and excretion occurs primarily through the kidneys. Only small amounts of this drug are excreted in feces.

Pharmacodynamics

Probenecid (Probalan) reduces the reabsorption of uric acid at the proximal convoluted tubules of the kidneys. This results in excretion of uric acid in urine, reducing serum urate levels.

Pharmacotherapeutics

Probenecid (Probalan) is used to treat:

- symptoms of gout
- gout (one or more joints are inflamed due to the deposits inside the actual joints).

When acute, substitute

Probenecid (Probalan) should not be given during an acute attack of gout. If taken at that time, it will prolong inflammation. Because it may increase the chance of an acute gout attack when therapy begins and whenever the serum urate level changes rapidly, colchicine (Colcrys) is administered during the first 3 to 6 months of therapy.

Drug interactions

Many drug interactions, some potentially serious, can occur with this drug:

- It can significantly increase and prolong the effects of cephalosporins, penicillins, and sulfonamides.
- Serum urate levels may be increased when it is taken with antineoplastic drugs.
- Probenecid (Probalan) increases the serum concentration of methotrexate (Trexall), causing toxic reactions.

Adverse reactions

Adverse reactions to probenecid (Probalan) include uric acid stone formation (acute attack of gout), anemia, aplastic anemia, hemolytic anemia, leukopenia, headache, nausea, and vomiting.

During an acute attack of gout, I am "out of the game" because I can prolong inflammation and make the attack last longer.

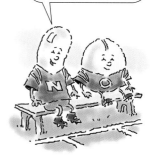

The Three-Step Approach

Nursing management for patients receiving uricosuric therapy follows the same principles as the Three-Step Approach for patients receiving other types of therapy. Be certain to pay particular attention to the uricosuric being given, and personalize care accordingly. Key concepts to remember include:

- monitoring BUN and renal function tests during long-term therapy
- giving with milk or food to minimize gastrointestinal distress
- encouraging fluids at a minimum of 2 L daily to prevent hematuria, renal colic, and uric acid stone formation
- teaching to avoid drugs containing aspirin, as these may precipitate gout, and to avoid alcohol as it increases the urate level
- teaching to avoid alcohol during drug therapy because it increases the urate level
- teaching to limit intake of foods high in purine, such as anchovies, liver, sardines, kidneys, sweetbreads, peas, and lentils.

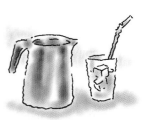

Other antigout drugs

Other antigout drugs include allopurinol (Zyloprim) and colchicine (Colcrys). Allopurinol (Zyloprim) is used to reduce uric acid production, preventing gout attacks. Colchicine (Colcrys) interferes with the WBC role in causing inflammation. Another antigout drug is febuxostat (Uloric), which is used for chronic management of hyperuricemia in patients with gout.

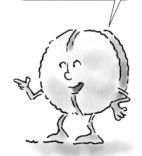

Other antigout drugs include allopurinol and colchicine.

Pharmacokinetics

All of these antigout drugs take somewhat different paths through the body.

All aboard allopurinol

When given orally, allopurinol (Zyloprim) is absorbed from the GI tract. Allopurinol (Zyloprim) and its metabolite oxypurinol are widely distributed throughout the body except in the brain, where drug concentrations are lower than those found in the rest of the body. It is metabolized by the liver and excreted in urine.

"Tracting" colchicine's course

Colchicine (Colcrys) is also absorbed from the GI tract. It is partially metabolized in the liver. This drug and its metabolites then reenter the intestinal tract through biliary secretions. After reabsorption from the intestines, it is distributed to various tissues before being excreted primarily in feces and to a lesser degree in urine.

Finding febuxostat

Absolute bioavailability of Febuxostat (Uloric) is unknown. It is heavily plasma protein-bound, heavily metabolized, and eliminated via the hepatic and renal pathways.

Pharmacodynamics

Allopurinol (Zyloprim) and its metabolite oxypurinol inhibit xanthine oxidase, the enzyme responsible to produce uric acid. By reducing uric acid formation, this drug eliminates the hazards of hyperuricosuria.

Colchicine (Colcrys) appears to reduce the inflammatory response to monosodium urate crystals deposited in joint tissues. This drug may produce its effects by inhibiting migration of WBCs to the inflamed joint. This reduces phagocytosis and lactic acid production by WBCs, decreasing urate crystal deposits and reducing inflammation.

Febuxostat (Uloric) decreases serum uric acid; it is not thought to inhibit other enzymes that take part in purine and pyrimidine synthesis and metabolism when given in therapeutic doses (Takeda Pharmaceuticals America, Inc., 2017).

Pharmacotherapeutics

Allopurinol (Zyloprim) helps to prevent acute gout attacks. It can be prescribed with a uricosuric when smaller dosages of each drug are ordered. It is used to:
- treat gout or hyperuricemia that may occur with blood abnormalities and during treatment of tumors or leukemia
- treat primary or secondary uric acid nephropathy (with or without the accompanying signs and symptoms of gout)
- treat and prevent recurrent uric acid stone formation
- treat patients who respond poorly to maximum dosages of uricosurics or who have allergic reactions or intolerance to uricosurics.

What a relief!

Colchicine (Colcrys) is used to decrease the inflammation associated with gout attacks. If given promptly, it's especially effective in relieving pain. Also, giving colchicine (Colcrys) during the first several months of allopurinol (Zyloprim) or probenecid (Probalan) therapy may prevent attacks that sometimes accompany the use of these drugs.

Febuxostat (Uloric) is indicated for treatment of chronic hyperuricemia.

Drug interactions

Colchicine (Colcrys) doesn't interact significantly with other drugs. Allopurinol (Zyloprim) and Febuxostat (Uloric) increase the serum concentrations of mercaptopurine (Purixan) and azathioprine (Azasan), increasing the risk of toxicity. When allopurinol (Zyloprim) is used with other drugs, the resulting interactions can be serious:
- It potentiates the effects of oral anticoagulants.
- Angiotensin-converting enzyme inhibitors increase the risk of hypersensitivity reactions to allopurinol (Zyloprim).
- It increases serum theophylline levels.
- The risk of bone marrow depression increases when cyclophosphamide (Cytoxan) is taken with allopurinol (Zyloprim).

Adverse reactions

Rash is a common adverse reaction to allopurinol (Zyloprim) and mercaptopurine (Purixan). Prolonged administration of colchicine (Colcrys) and mercaptopurine (Purixan) may cause bone marrow suppression.

All drugs commonly cause:
- nausea and vomiting
- diarrhea
- intermittent abdominal pain.

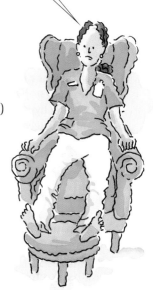

Colchicine decreases the inflammation associated with gout. Now, that feels better!

The Three-Step Approach

Nursing management for patients receiving antigout therapy follows the same principles as the Three-Step Approach for patients receiving other types of anti-inflammatory drugtherapy. Be certain to pay particular attention to the antigout medication being given, and personalize care accordingly. Key concepts to remember include the following:

- Assess the patient's uric acid level, joint stiffness, and pain before and during therapy. Optimal benefits may require 2 to 6 weeks of therapy.
- Monitor the complete blood count, and hepatic and renal function, at the start of therapy and periodically during therapy.
- Monitor the patient's fluid intake and output. Daily urine output of at least 2 L and maintenance of neutral or slightly alkaline urine are desirable.
- Give the medication with meals or immediately after to minimize GI distress.
- Encourage the patient to drink fluids while taking the drug unless contraindicated.
- Notify the prescriber if renal insufficiency occurs during treatment; this usually warrants a dosage reduction.
- Teach to refrain from driving or performing hazardous tasks requiring mental alertness until the CNS effects of the drug are known.
- Teach to reduce intake of animal protein, sodium, refined sugars, oxalate-rich foods, and calcium, and to avoid alcohol as this increases the serum urate level.
- Teach to stop the drug at the first sign of a rash, which may precede a severe hypersensitivity or another adverse reaction, and to immediately report this adverse reaction. A rash is more common in patients taking diuretics and in those with renal disorders.

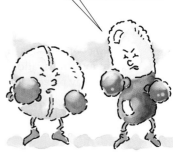

Colchicine and allopurinol together give a 1 to 2 punch against gout.

Quick quiz

1. A patient is taking digoxin (Lanoxin), furosemide (Lasix), diazepam (Valium), and amoxicillin (Amoxil). Which medication is most likely to cause a drug interaction with the antihistamine the health care provider prescribed?

    A. Digoxin (Lanoxin)
    B. Furosemide (Lasix)
    C. Diazepam (Valium)
    D. Amoxicillin (Amoxil)

Answer: C. Antihistamines can interact with many drugs, sometimes with life-threatening consequences. A drug interaction with diazepam (Valium) is most likely, due to the additive effect of depressing the central nervous system. Interactions with the other medications are less likely.

2. Which medication interacts with allopurinol?
A. Oral anticoagulants
B. Antihistamines
C. Cardiac glycosides
D. Antidiabetic agents

Answer: A. Allopurinol potentiates the effects of oral anticoagulants. It does not interact with antihistamines, cardiac glycosides, or antidiabetic agents.

3. A patient with chronic obstructive pulmonary disease (COPD) presents with shortness of breath and wheezing in all lung fields. Which drug does the nurse anticipate administering?
A. Fexofenadine (Allegra)
B. Methylprednisolone (Solu-medrol)
C. Allopurinol (Zyloprim)
D. Diphenhydramine (Benadryl)

Answer: B. Wheezing indicates inflammation of the airways within the lung. Methylprednisolone (Solu-medrol) will decrease lung tissue inflammation, so the nurse anticipates this will be the drug given. Fexofenadine (Allegra) is used for allergies. Allopurinol (Zyloprim) is used for gout. Diphenhydramine (Benadryl) is used for allergies and less severe reactions.

4. A patient is receiving fludrocortisone acetate for adrenal insufficiency. Which electrolyte must be closely monitored during drug therapy? **Select all that apply.**
A. Potassium
B. Sodium
C. Calcium
D. Phosphorus
E. Magnesium
F. Chloride

Answer: A, B. Fludrocortisone affects the reabsorption of sodium and excretion of potassium in the kidney, so these electrolytes must be closely monitored. The other electrolytes can be routinely monitored.

Scoring

☆☆☆ If you answered all four questions correctly, extraordinary! You certainly aren't allergic to smarts!

☆☆ If you answered three questions correctly, congratulations! You're taking the sting out of learning!

☆ If you answered fewer than three questions correctly, keep trying! With continued improvement, the next chapter should have you feeling better!

Suggested References

Burcham, J., & Rosenthal, L. (2019). *Lehne's pharmacology for nursing care* (10th ed.). St, Louis, MO: Elsevier.

Epocrates. (2021a). *Allopurinol.* Retrieved from https://online.epocrates.com/drugs/129/allopurinol

Epocrates. (2021b). *Fexofenadine.* Retrieved from https://online.epocrates.com/drugs/374/fexofenadine

Epocrates. (2021c). *Loratadine.* Retrieved from https://online.epocrates.com/drugs/503/loratadine

Ignatavicius, D. D., Workman, M. L., Rebar, C., & Heimgartner, N. (2021). *Medical-surgical nursing: Concepts for interprofessional collaborative care* (10th ed.). St. Louis, MO: Elsevier.

Lexicomp. (2021). *Drug information.* Retrieved from www.uptodate.com

Lilley, L. L., Collins, S. R., Harrington, S., & Snyder, J. S. (2020). *Pharmacology and the nursing process* (9th ed.). St. Louis, MO: Mosby.

Takeda Pharmaceuticals America, Inc. (2017). *Uloric (febuxostat) tablet for oral use.* Retrieved from https://www.accessdata.fda.gov/drugsatfda_docs/label/2017/021856s011lbl.pdf

Tucker, R. (2020). *2021 Lippincott pocket drug guide for nurses.* Philadelphia, PA: Wolters Kluwer.

U.S. National Library of Medicine. (2021). *Probenecid: Lannett company.* Retrieved from https://dailymed.nlm.nih.gov/dailymed/drugInfo.cfm?setid=ab497fd8-00c3-4364-b003-b39d21fbdf38

Whalen, K. (2018). *Lippincott illustrated reviews: Pharmacology* (7th ed.). Philadelphia, PA: Lippincott, Williams, and Wilkins.

Chapter 18

Antineoplastic drugs

Just the facts

In this chapter, you will learn:

◆ classes of drugs used to treat cancer

◆ uses and varying actions of these drugs

◆ absorption, distribution, metabolization, and excretion of these drugs

◆ drug interactions, safe administration, and adverse reactions to these drugs.

Drugs and cancer

In the 1940s, antineoplastic (chemotherapeutic) drugs were developed to treat cancer. However, these agents commonly cause serious adverse reactions.

A change for the better

With modern chemotherapy, childhood malignancies such as acute lymphoblastic leukemia and adult cancers such as testicular cancer are curable in most cases. Therapeutic strategies, such as monoclonal antibodies and targeting specific proteins, are prolonging patient's lives and increasing cures. In addition, immunotherapy is being used to treat patients with cancer.

Handle with care

Hazardous drugs require special protocols for storage, compounding, mixing, and administration. Nurses must take additional training to be safe and competent in providing antineoplastic chemotherapy.

Chemoprotective personal protective equipment (PPE) is required for all antineoplastic administration. Direct contact with these drugs or their vapors can cause severe reactions, especially to the skin, eyes, and respiratory tract. Use facility guidelines and established protocols for storing, mixing, administering, and disposing of all chemotherapy.

Antineoplastic agents are composed of intravenous (IV) and oral treatments and can be used as single agents or in combination. Common categories of antineoplastic agents include the following:

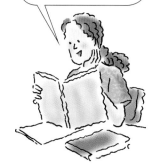

News flash! Antineoplastic drugs were developed to treat cancer in the 1940s.

- **Cytotoxic antineoplastics**
  - ○ Alkylating drugs
  - ○ Antimetabolite drugs
  - ○ Antibiotic antineoplastic drugs
  - ○ Natural antineoplastic drugs
  - ○ Topoisomerase I inhibitors
  - ○ Unclassified antineoplastic drugs
- **Monoclonal antibodies and immunotherapy**
  - ○ Monoclonal antibodies
  - ○ Immunotherapy
- **Targeted treatments**
  - ○ Targeted therapies
  - ○ Endocrine and hormone modulators

Cytotoxic antineoplastics

Alkylating drugs

Alkylating drugs, either given alone or with other drugs, effectively act against various malignant neoplasms. These drugs are categorized into one of five classes:
- nitrogen mustards
- alkyl sulfonates
- nitrosoureas
- triazines
- alkylating-like drugs.

Unfazed at any phase

Alkylating drugs produce their antineoplastic effects by damaging deoxyribonucleic acid (DNA). They halt DNA's replication process by cross-linking its strands so that amino acids do not pair up correctly. Alkylating drugs are cell cycle phase nonspecific. This means that their alkylating actions may take place at any phase of the cell cycle.

Nitrogen mustards

Nitrogen mustards represent the largest group of alkylating drugs. They include:
- bendamustine (Treanda, Bendeka)
- chlorambucil (Leukeran)
- cyclophosphamide (Cytoxan)
- estramustine (Emcyt)
- ifosfamide (Ifex)
- melphalan (Alkeran).

The opening act

Cyclophosphamide (Cytoxan) is a common nitrogen mustard and is commonly used for breast cancer and some leukemias.

Pharmacokinetics

As with most alkylating drugs, the absorption and distribution of nitrogen mustards vary widely. Nitrogen mustards are metabolized in the liver and excreted by the kidneys. Cyclophosphamide (Cytoxan) has a half-life of 3 to 12 hours when given IV and can be prolonged if renal impairment is present.

Pharmacodynamics

Nitrogen mustards form covalent bonds with DNA molecules in a chemical reaction known as *alkylation*. Alkylated DNA cannot replicate properly, thereby resulting in cell death. Unfortunately, cells may develop resistance to the cytotoxic effects of nitrogen mustards. (See *How alkylating drugs work*.)

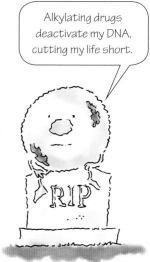

Alkylating drugs deactivate my DNA, cutting my life short.

 Pharm function

How alkylating drugs work

Alkylating drugs can attack DNA in two ways, as shown in the illustrations below.

Bifunctional alkylation
Some drugs become inserted between two base pairs in the DNA chain, forming an irreversible bond between them. This is called *bifunctional alkylation*, which causes cytotoxic effects capable of destroying or poisoning cells.

Monofunctional alkylation
Other drugs react with just one part of a pair, separating it from its partner and eventually causing it and its attached sugar to break away from the DNA molecule. This is called *monofunctional alkylation*, which eventually may cause permanent cell damage.

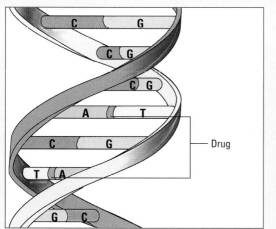

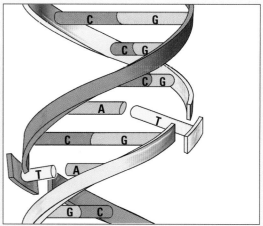

Pharmacotherapeutics

Because they produce leukopenia (a reduced number of white blood cells [WBCs]), nitrogen mustards are effective in treating malignant neoplasms, such as Hodgkin's lymphoma (cancer that causes painless enlargement of the lymph nodes, spleen, and lymphoid tissues) and leukemia (cancer of the blood-forming tissues) that can have an associated elevated WBC count.

Nitrogen bomb

Nitrogen mustards also have proven effective against lymphoma (cancer of the lymphoid tissue), multiple myeloma (cancer of the marrow plasma cells), and cancer of the breast, ovaries, uterus, lung, brain, testes, and prostate.

Drug interactions

Nitrogen mustards interact with several other drugs:
- Calcium-containing drugs and foods, such as antacids and dairy products, reduce absorption of estramustine (Emcyt).
- Taking cyclophosphamide (Cytoxan) with cardiotoxic drugs produces additive cardiac effects.
- Cyclophosphamide (Cytoxan) can reduce serum digoxin levels.
- An increased risk of ifosfamide (Ifex) toxicity exists when the drug is taken with allopurinol, barbiturates, or phenytoin (Dilantin).
- The lung toxicity threshold of carmustine (BiCNU) may be reduced when taken with melphalan.

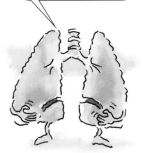

Direct contact with nitrogen mustards can cause severe skin, eye, and respiratory reactions. That's just so irritating!

Side effects/Adverse reactions

Many patients experience fatigue during nitrogen mustard therapy. Other adverse reactions include:
- bone marrow suppression, leading to severe neutropenia and thrombocytopenia
- nausea and vomiting from central nervous system (CNS) irritation
- stomatitis
- reversible hair loss.
  Cyclophosphamide (Cytoxan) can cause hemorrhagic cystitis if aggressive hydration is not maintained.

The three-step approach for ALL cytotoxic antineoplastic chemotherapy

All cytotoxic antineoplastic chemotherapy has standard assessment, administration, and postadministration monitoring that is required for safe care in the oncology setting. In this feature, the standard three-step approach to administration of ANY antineoplastic chemotherapy is presented. Refer to this box frequently. In addition, relevant specific information will be presented with each category throughout the chapter. Refer to this broader three-step approach when preparing or administering these drugs.

Preadministration

(Recognize and analyze cues)

- Perform a complete assessment before therapy begins, including medication reconciliation.
- Review provider's orders for clarity and appropriateness.
- Perform thorough education. (See *Teaching about chemotherapy,* page 674.)
- Refer to provider order and current resources to ensure that appropriate lab work has been drawn and resulted prior to administration.
- The dose should not be administered unless the platelet count is greater than 100,000/mcL and ANC is greater than 1,000/mcL. Doses may be adjusted based of abnormal kidney and liver functions.
- Ensure that the patient is not pregnant or nursing prior to administration. Teach women of childbearing age and men to use effective contraceptive methods during therapy and for at least 6 months following the completion of therapy.
- Ensure that the patient has knowledge of self-care and side effects after treatment.

Medication administration

(Take action)

- Monitor for adverse reactions and drug interactions throughout therapy.
- Set infusion rate at prescribed rate.
- Monitor the patient's vital signs and catheter or IV-line patency throughout drug administration. Monitor for redness, pain, swelling, or lack of blood return from IV site or central line. Local tissue injury and scarring may result from tissue infiltration at the infusion site.
- Stop infusion immediately if an infusion reaction is suspected. Keep diphenhydramine, hydrocortisone, epinephrine, and necessary emergency equipment available to establish an airway in case of anaphylaxis.

Postadministration

(Evaluate outcomes)

- Promote measures to relieve nausea, vomiting, and other signs and symptoms of treatment toxicity.
- Observe for signs of infection and fever.

- Monitor for decreased blood cells, including WBCs, granulocytes (ANC), and hemoglobin and platelets. Provide supportive care or transfusions if warranted.
- Continue to reinforce self-care and symptom management.
- The patient and family will demonstrate an understanding of drug therapy and diagnosis.

Education edge

Teaching about chemotherapy

If chemotherapy is prescribed, review these points with the patient and caregivers:

Avoid people with bacterial or viral infections because chemotherapy can increase susceptibility. Watch for signs and symptoms of infection (fever, sore throat, and fatigue) and bleeding (easy bruising, nosebleeds, bleeding gums, and melena). Take your temperature daily and report signs of infection or fever 100.4°F or greater promptly to health care team.

- Perform meticulous oral hygiene, including cautious use of a toothbrush, dental floss, and toothpicks. Chemotherapy can increase the risk of microbial infection, delayed healing, and bleeding gums.
- Complete dental work before therapy begins or delay it until your blood counts are normal.
- Be aware that you may bruise easily because of the drug's effect on your platelet count.
- Use an electric razor to help minimize bleeding.
- Do not take over-the-counter (OTC) products, medications, or herbal remedies without first consulting your prescriber.
- Avoid OTC products that contain aspirin or fever reducing properties.
- Take medications as directed, including antinausea medication. Report uncontrolled side effects such as

nausea or vomiting, diarrhea or constipation, rash, or other concerning side effects.

- Keep all appointments for chemotherapy, blood tests, and follow ups.
- Maintain an adequate hydration and intake of nutritious food; consult with a dietitian to help design a diet that meets your needs.
- Hair loss will occur; it usually starts 2 to 3 weeks after treatment and hair will regrow after completion of treatment. If you experience hair loss, use of wigs, scarves, or hats can help with body image and need for warmth.
- Report redness, pain, or swelling at the injection site. Local tissue injury and scarring may result from tissue infiltration at the infusion site.
- Inform any other physician, dentist, or health care provider before any treatment that you are receiving chemotherapy.
- Defer immunizations if possible until blood counts have returned to normal limits.
- If you are of childbearing age, you should use effective contraception during and for at least 6 months after chemotherapy.
- Stop breast-feeding during therapy because of the risk of toxicity to the infant.

The Three-Step Approach

Nursing management for patients needing nitrogen mustard therapy includes these three steps.

Reminder to review the broader *The three-step approach* that applies to ALL cytotoxic antineoplastic chemotherapy (see page 672).

Preadministration
(Recognize and analyze cues)
- Review lab work, including CBC, for platelet and total and differential white blood cell (WBC) counts as well as hemoglobin, hematocrit, alanine aminotransferase (ALT), aspartate aminotransferase (AST), lactate dehydrogenase (LDH), bilirubin, blood urea nitrogen (BUN), serum creatinine, uric acid, and other lab work as needed.
- Ensure that hydration is ordered for patients receiving cyclophosphamide (Cytoxan).
- Ensure that the patient is premedicated with antiemetics prior to administration.

(Prioritize hypothesis—priority patient problems)
- Infection risk
- Fluid imbalance risk

(Generate solutions)
- The patient will not develop infection from drug-induced neutropenia.
- The patient and family will demonstrate an understanding of side effect management.

Medication administration
(Take action)
- Administer adequate hydration and monitor intake and output.

Postadministration
(Evaluate outcomes)
- Ensure that the patient has appropriate intake and output.
- Ensure that the patient remains free from hemorrhagic cystitis or uncontrolled nausea.

Alkyl sulfonates

The alkyl sulfonate busulfan has historically been used to treat chronic myelogenous leukemia (CML), polycythemia vera (increased red blood cell [RBC] mass and an increased number of WBCs and platelets), and other myeloproliferative (pertaining to overactive bone marrow) disorders. Busulfan is used at high doses to treat leukemia during bone marrow transplantation.

Pharmacokinetics

Busulfan is absorbed rapidly and well from the GI tract. Little is known about its distribution. Busulfan is metabolized extensively in the liver before urinary excretion. Its half-life is 2 to 3 hours.

Pharmacodynamics

As an alkyl sulfonate, busulfan forms covalent bonds with the DNA molecules in alkylation.

Pharmacotherapeutics

Busulfan primarily affects granulocytes (a type of WBC) and, to a lesser degree, platelets. Because of its action on granulocytes, it has been used for treating chronic myelogenous leukemia and in conditioning regimens for bone marrow transplantation.

To a screeching halt

Busulfan is also effective in treating polycythemia vera. However, other drugs are usually used to treat polycythemia vera because busulfan can cause severe myelosuppression (halting of bone marrow function).

Drug interactions

There can be an increased risk of bleeding when busulfan is taken with anticoagulants or aspirin. Use with antifungals can result in increased busulfan serum concentration and an increased risk of busulfan toxicity.

Side effects/Adverse reactions

The major adverse reaction to busulfan is bone marrow suppression, producing severe neutropenia, anemia, and thrombocytopenia (reduced WBCs, RBCs, and platelets, respectively), which is usually dose-related and reversible.

A latecomer

Pulmonary fibrosis may occur 4 months to 10 years after treatment. (The average onset of symptoms is 4 years after therapy.) Seizures are also a concern. (See *Busulfan warning*.)

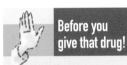

Before you give that drug!

Busulfan warning

Seizures can occur as an adverse reaction to IV infusion of busulfan. The patient may be started on a prophylactic anticonvulsant to decrease the risk of seizures.

The Three-Step Approach

These nursing steps are appropriate for patients undergoing treatment with alkyl sulfonates.

Reminder to review the broader *The three-step approach* that applies to ALL cytotoxic antineoplastic chemotherapy (see page 672).

Preadministration
(Recognize and analyze cues)
- Ensure that antiemetics are ordered and given prior to treatment.
- Ensure that the patient has been started on prophylactic anticonvulsants.

(Prioritize hypothesis—priority patient problems)
- Infection risk
- Seizure risk
- Nausea and vomiting risk
- Knowledge deficiency

(Generate solutions)
- The patient will remain free from infection.
- The patient will remain free of seizures.
- The patient will have controlled nausea and vomiting.
- The patient and family will demonstrate an understanding of drug therapy.

Medication administration

(Take action)
- Give the drug at the same time each day.
- Treat extravasation promptly.
- Administer adequate hydration and monitor intake and output.
- The dosage is adjusted based on the patient's weekly WBC count, and the prescriber may temporarily stop drug therapy if severe neutropenia develops. Therapeutic effects are commonly accompanied by toxicity.

Postadministration

(Evaluate outcomes)
- Promote measures to relieve nausea, vomiting, and other signs and symptoms of treatment toxicity.
- Observe for signs of infection.
- Observe for seizures, and protect from injury if seizures occur.
- Monitor the patient's WBC and platelet counts weekly during therapy. The WBC count falls about 10 days after the start of therapy and continues to fall for 2 weeks after stopping the drug.

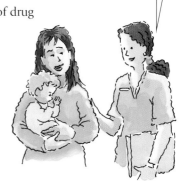

It's often best to stop breast-feeding during drug therapy because of the possible risk of infant toxicity.

Nitrosoureas

Nitrosoureas are alkylating agents that halt cancer cell reproduction. They include:
- carmustine (BiCNU)
- lomustine
- streptozocin.

Pharmacokinetics

When administered IV, carmustine (BiCNU) achieves a steady-state volume of distribution. With oral administration, lomustine is absorbed adequately, although incomplete.

Don't go PO

Streptozocin is administered IV because it is poorly absorbed orally.

The fat of the matter is...

Nitrosoureas are lipophilic (attracted to fat) drugs and are distributed to fatty tissues and cerebrospinal fluid (CSF). They are metabolized extensively before urine excretion.

Pharmacodynamics

During a process called *bifunctional alkylation*, nitrosoureas interfere with amino acids, purines, and DNA needed for cancer cells to divide, thus halting their reproduction.

Pharmacotherapeutics

The nitrosoureas are highly lipid soluble, which allows them or their metabolites to easily cross the blood-brain barrier. Because of this ability, nitrosoureas are used to treat brain tumors and meningeal leukemias.

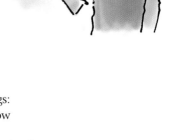

Cimetidine may increase carmustine's bone marrow toxicity.

Drug interactions

Each of the nitrosoureas has its own interactions with other drugs:

- Cimetidine (Tagamet) may increase carmustine's bone marrow toxicity.
- Lomustine used with anticoagulants or aspirin increases the risk of bleeding; avoid using these drugs together.

Side effects/Adverse reactions

All the nitrosoureas can produce severe nausea and vomiting.

Bad to the bone

Carmustine and lomustine produce bone marrow suppression that begins 4 to 6 weeks after treatment and lasts 1 to 2 weeks. These drugs should not be given more frequently than every 6 weeks.

Kidney concerns

Kidney toxicity and kidney failure may also occur in patients taking nitrosoureas. Streptozocin may produce reversible hepatotoxicity.

Pulmonary problems

Carmustine (BiCNU) may cause delayed lung toxicity characterized by lung infiltrates or fibrosis (scarring) that can occur years after treatment.

In patients who receive prolonged therapy with total dosages greater than 1,400 mg/m², pulmonary toxicity can occur anywhere from 9 days to 15 years after treatment. (See *Carmustine (BiCNU) warning.*)

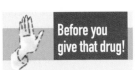

Before you give that drug!

Carmustine (BiCNU) warning

Obtain baseline pulmonary function tests before therapy with carmustine (BiCNU) because pulmonary toxicity appears to be related to the dosage and may occur from 9 days to 15 years after treatment. Be sure to evaluate results of the liver, renal, and pulmonary function tests periodically thereafter.

The Three-Step Approach

Nursing management for patients needing nitrosoureas therapy includes these three steps.

Reminder to review the broader *The three-step approach* that applies to ALL cytotoxic antineoplastic chemotherapy (see page 672).

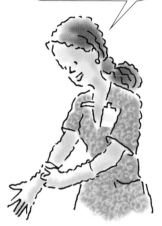

Use double gloves when handling carmustine wafer in the operating room.

Preadministration

(Recognize and analyze cues)
- Obtain baseline pulmonary function tests before therapy.

(Prioritize hypothesis—priority patient problems)
- Infection risk
- Nausea and vomiting
- Knowledge deficiency

(Generate solutions)
- The patient will not develop infection from drug-induced immunosuppression.
- The patient will have controlled nausea and vomiting.
- The patient and family will demonstrate an understanding of drug therapy and diagnosis.

Medication administration

(Take action)
- Give an antiemetic before giving the drug to reduce nausea.
- Use carmustine (BiCNU) only in glass containers. The solution is unstable in plastic IV bags. Avoid contact with skin because carmustine will cause a brown stain. If skin contact occurs, wash the drug off thoroughly.
- Repeat lomustine administration only when CBC results reveal safe hematologic parameters.

Postadministration

(Evaluate outcomes)
- Evaluate the liver, renal, and pulmonary function tests periodically.
- Monitor for and treat drug-induced adverse reactions (such as nausea and vomiting) proactively.

Triazines

Dacarbazine, a triazine, functions as an alkylating drug only after it has been activated by the liver.

Pharmacokinetics

After IV injection, dacarbazine is distributed throughout the body and metabolized in the liver. Within 6 hours, 30% to 46% of a dose is excreted by the kidneys (half is excreted unchanged; the other half is excreted as one of the metabolites).

Dysfunction junction

In a patient with kidney or liver dysfunction, the drug's half-life may increase to 7 hours.

Pharmacodynamics

Dacarbazine first must be metabolized in the liver to become an alkylating drug. It seems to inhibit ribonucleic acid (RNA) and protein synthesis. Like other alkylating drugs, dacarbazine is cell cycle nonspecific.

Pharmacotherapeutics

Dacarbazine is used primarily to treat patients with Hodgkin's lymphoma. It is also used with other drugs to treat patients with malignant melanoma.

Drug interactions

No significant drug interactions have been reported with dacarbazine.

Side effects/Adverse reactions

Dacarbazine use may cause the following adverse reactions:
- leukopenia
- thrombocytopenia
- nausea and vomiting (which begin within 1 to 3 hours after administration in most cases and may last up to 12 hours)
- photosensitivity
- flulike syndrome (which may begin 7 days after treatment and last from 7 to 21 days)
- hair loss.

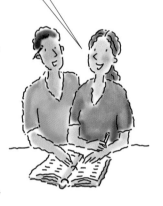

After IV injection, dacarbazine must be metabolized by the liver before it becomes an antineoplastic drug.

The Three-Step Approach

Nursing management for patients needing dacarbazine therapy includes these three steps.

Reminder to review the broader *The three-step approach* that applies to ALL cytotoxic antineoplastic chemotherapy (see page 672).

Preadministration

(Recognize and analyze cues)
- Anticipate dosage reduction if severe kidney or renal impairment.
- Ensure that the patient is premedicated with antiemetics prior to administration.

(Prioritize hypothesis—priority patient problems)
- Infection risk
- Nausea and vomiting risk
- Knowledge deficiency

(Generate solutions)
- The patient will not experience infection from drug-induced immunosuppression.
- The patient will have controlled nausea and vomiting.

Medication administration

(Take action)
- During infusion, protect the bag from direct sunlight to avoid drug breakdown. The solution may be diluted further or the infusion slowed to decrease pain at the infusion site.
- Advise the patient to avoid sunlight and sunlamps for the first 2 days after treatment.
- Reassure the patient that flulike syndrome may be treated with mild antipyretics such as acetaminophen (Tylenol). Avoid aspirin.

Not-so-pretty in pink

- Discard the drug if the solution turns pink; this is a sign of decomposition.
- Take care to avoid extravasation during infusion. If the IV site infiltrates, discontinue the infusion immediately, apply ice to the area for 24 to 48 hours, and notify the prescriber.

Postadministration

(Evaluate outcomes)
- Assess for signs of infection that could occur from drug-induced immunosuppression and report to the provider.

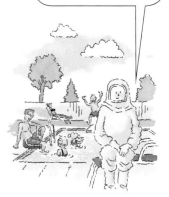

Advise the patient to avoid sunlight and sunlamps for the first 2 days after treatment. Although this might be taking it to a bit of an extreme...

Alkylating-like drugs

Carboplatin, oxaliplatin, and cisplatin are heavy metal complexes that contain platinum. Because their action resembles that of a bifunctional alkylating drug, these drugs are called *alkylating-like drugs*.

Pharmacokinetics

The distribution and metabolism of carboplatin are not clearly defined. After IV administration, carboplatin is eliminated primarily by the kidneys. Carboplatin is always dosed as area under the curve (AUC).

By and bi

The elimination of carboplatin is biphasic. It has an initial half-life of 1 to 2 hours and a terminal half-life of $2\frac{1}{2}$ to 6 hours. Oxaliplatin is 70% to 90% bound to plasma proteins and is eliminated primarily by the kidneys. When administered intrapleurally (into the pleural space around the lungs) or intraperitoneally (into the peritoneum), cisplatin may exhibit significant systemic absorption.

Reaching new heights

Highly protein-bound cisplatin reaches high concentrations in the kidneys, liver, intestines, and testes but has poor CNS penetration. The drug undergoes some liver metabolism, followed by excretion through the kidneys.

Pharmacodynamics

Like alkylating drugs, carboplatin, oxaliplatin, and cisplatin are cell cycle nonspecific. They act like bifunctional alkylating drugs by cross-linking strands of DNA and inhibiting DNA synthesis. (See *Alkylating-like drugs: Cisplatin.*)

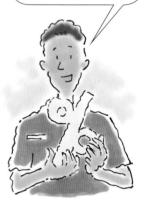

Talk about a good return on your investment. After IV administration, thiotepa is 100% bioavailable.

Pharmacotherapeutics

These alkylating-like drugs are used to treat several cancers:
- Carboplatin is used primarily to treat ovarian and lung cancer.
- Cisplatin is prescribed to treat bladder, metastatic, ovarian, and testicular cancers.
- Cisplatin may also be used to treat head, neck, and lung cancer. (Although these indications are clinically accepted, they are currently unlabeled uses.)
- Oxaliplatin is used in combination with other agents in pancreatic and colorectal cancer.

Drug interactions

These alkylating-like drugs interact with a few other drugs:
- When carboplatin, cisplatin, or oxaliplatin is administered with an aminoglycoside, the risk of toxicity to the kidney increases.

Prototype pro

Alkylating-like drugs: Cisplatin

Actions
- Probably cross-links strands of cellular DNA and interferes with RNA transcription, causing growth imbalance that leads to cell death
- Kills selected cancer cells

Indications
- Adjunct therapy in metastatic testicular and ovarian cancer
- Advanced bladder and esophageal cancer
- Head and neck cancer
- Cervical cancer
- Non–small cell lung cancer
- Brain tumor
- Osteosarcoma

Nursing considerations
- Monitor for adverse effects, such as peripheral neuropathy, seizures, tinnitus, hearing loss, nausea and vomiting, severe renal toxicity, myelosuppression, neutropenia, thrombocytopenia, anemia, and anaphylactic reaction.
- Assess the underlying neoplastic disease before therapy and reassess regularly throughout therapy.

What's that you say?

- Taking carboplatin or cisplatin with medications to treat edema such as bumetanide, ethacrynic acid, or furosemide (Lasix) increases the risk of ototoxicity (damage to the organs of hearing and balance).
- Cisplatin may reduce serum phenytoin (Dilantin) levels.

Side effects/Adverse reactions

Carboplatin and cisplatin produce many of the same adverse reactions as the alkylating drugs:

- Carboplatin can produce bone marrow suppression.
- Kidney toxicity can occur with cisplatin, usually after multiple courses of therapy. Carboplatin is less toxic to the kidneys.
- With long-term cisplatin therapy, neurotoxicity can occur. Neurotoxicity is less common with carboplatin.
- Tinnitus and hearing loss may occur with cisplatin; these effects are much less common with carboplatin.
- Cisplatin can also produce marked nausea and vomiting.

The Three-Step Approach

Nursing management for patients undergoing treatment with alkylating-like drugs includes this three-step approach.

Reminder to review the broader *The three-step approach* that applies to ALL cytotoxic antineoplastic chemotherapy (see page 672).

Preadministration

(Recognize and analyze cues)

- Review lab work including platelet and total and differential white blood cell (WBC) counts as well as hemoglobin, hematocrit, alanine aminotransferase (ALT), aspartate aminotransferase (AST), lactate dehydrogenase (LDH), bilirubin, blood urea nitrogen (BUN), serum creatinine, and electrolyte levels (especially potassium and magnesium). Anticipate possible dose reduction due to decreased renal function.
- The dose should not be given unless the patient's platelet count is greater than 100,000/mcL, ANC is greater than 1,000/mcL, creatinine level is under 1.5 mg/dL, or BUN level is under 25 mg/dL.
- Review orders for antiemetics as premedication.
- Ensure that hydration orders are in place for cisplatin. Rigorous hydration is required to help protect renal function. Occasionally, mannitol may be ordered to promote diuresis.
- Ensure that the patient has baseline hearing (audiology) test completed if required.

(Prioritize hypothesis—priority patient problems)

- Infection risk

- Nausea and vomiting
- Electrolyte imbalance risk
- Knowledge deficiency

(Generate solutions)
- The patient will not develop infection from drug-induced immunosuppression.
- The patient will have controlled nausea and vomiting.
- The patient will maintain electrolyte balance.
- The patient and family will demonstrate an understanding of drug therapy.

Medication administration
(Take action)
- Treat extravasation promptly.
- Administer adequate hydration and monitor intake and output.
- Monitor the patient's renal function because renal toxicity is cumulative. Renal function must return to normal before receiving the next dose.
- Administer an antiemetic, as ordered; nausea and vomiting may be severe and delayed (up to 24 hours). Ondansetron (Zofran) or granisetron (Kytril) has been used effectively to prevent and treat nausea and vomiting. Some clinicians may combine dexamethasone (Decadron) with ondansetron (Zofran) or granisetron (Kytril). Provide aggressive management of nausea.
- To prevent hypokalemia, potassium chloride (10 to 20 mEq/L) is commonly added to IV fluids before and after cisplatin therapy.
- Patients receiving oxaliplatin infusions will experience extreme cold sensitivity, including bronchospasms, cold triggered neuropathy, and paresthesia. These may affect ADLs. Ensure that the patient does not have any cold exposure, including food, drink, or cold air.
- Stop infusion immediately if an infusion reaction is suspected. Give epinephrine, corticosteroids, or antihistamines for anaphylactic reactions. Teach the patient to report tinnitus immediately as well as edema or a decrease in urine output (if recording intake and output at home).

Postadministration
(Evaluate outcomes
- The patient will not develop infection related to drug-induced immunosuppression.
- The patient will remain free of renal impairment and maintain electrolyte balance.
- Delayed vomiting (3 to 5 days after treatment) has been reported. The patient may need prolonged antiemetic treatment to control symptoms of nausea and vomiting.

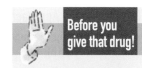
Before you give that drug!

Cisplatin warning

Follow facility policy to reduce risks. Reminder: Chemoprotective PPE is required for all antineoplastic administration.

Aggressive hydration is given before, during, and after cisplatin infusion to maintain diuresis of 100 to 400 mL/hour for up to 24 hours after therapy. Prehydration and diuresis may reduce renal toxicity and ototoxicity significantly. Patients are at significant risk of renal failure with cisplatin.

Antimetabolite drugs

Because antimetabolite drugs structurally resemble DNA base pairs, they can become involved in processes associated with DNA base pairs—that is, the synthesis of nucleic acids and proteins.

Getting specific

Antimetabolites differ significantly from the DNA base pairs in how they interfere with this synthesis. Because the antimetabolites are cell cycle specific and primarily affect cells that actively synthesize DNA, they are referred to as *S phase specific*. Normal cells that are reproducing actively as well as the cancer cells are affected by the antimetabolites.

Each according to its metabolite

These drugs are subclassified according to the metabolite affected and include:
- folic acid analogues
- pyrimidine analogues
- purine analogues.

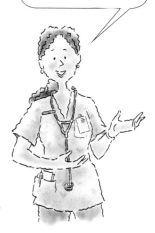

The antimetabolite drugs are cell cycle specific. They're referred to as *S phase specific* because they primarily affect cells that actively synthesize DNA.

Folic acid analogues

The early compound methotrexate remains the most commonly used of all the folic acid analogues.

Pharmacokinetics

Methotrexate is absorbed well and distributed throughout the body. It can accumulate in any fluid collection, such as ascites or pleural or pericardial effusion. This can result in prolonged elimination and higher-than-expected toxicity, especially myelosuppression.

Do not enter

At usual dosages, methotrexate does not enter the CNS readily. Although methotrexate is metabolized partially, it is excreted primarily unchanged in urine.

A disappearing act

Methotrexate exhibits a three-part disappearance from plasma; the rapid distributive phase is followed by a second phase, which reflects kidney clearance. The last phase, the terminal half-life, is 3 to 10 hours for a low dose and 8 to 15 hours for a high dose.

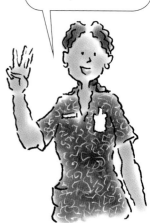

Methotrexate exhibits a three-part disappearance from plasma.

Antimetabolite drugs: Methotrexate

Actions
- Prevents the reduction of folic acid to tetrahydrofolate by binding to dihydrofolate reductase
- Kills certain cancer cells and reduces inflammation

Indications
- Trophoblastic tumors (choriocarcinoma, hydatidiform mole)
- Acute lymphoblastic and lymphocytic leukemia, meningeal leukemia
- Burkitt's lymphoma
- Osteosarcoma

Nursing considerations
- Monitor for adverse reactions, such as stomatitis, diarrhea, intestinal perforation, nausea, vomiting, renal failure, anemia, neutropenia, thrombocytopenia, acute hepatotoxicity, pulmonary fibrosis, urticaria, and sudden death.
- Assess the underlying neoplastic disease before therapy and reassess regularly throughout therapy.
- Follow facility policy for reconstitution and administration. Nurses of childbearing years can choose to opt out of patients receiving antineoplastic therapy.
- High-dose methotrexate requires leucovorin rescue.

Pharmacodynamics

Methotrexate reversibly inhibits the action of the enzyme dihydrofolate reductase. This blocks normal folic acid processing, which inhibits DNA and RNA synthesis. The result is cell death. (See *Antimetabolite drugs: Methotrexate.*)

Pharmacotherapeutics

Methotrexate is especially useful in treating:
- acute lymphoblastic leukemia (abnormal growth of lymphocyte precursors, the lymphoblasts), the most common leukemia in children
- acute lymphocytic leukemia (abnormal growth of lymphocytes); may be given as treatment and prophylaxis for meningeal leukemia
- CNS diseases (given intrathecally)
- choriocarcinoma (cancer that develops from the chorionic portions of the products of conception)
- osteogenic sarcoma (bone cancer)
- malignant lymphomas.

Unconventional treatment

The drug is also prescribed in low doses to treat severe psoriasis, autoimmune diseases, graft versus host disease, or rheumatoid arthritis that does not respond to conventional therapy. Methotrexate has also been used in treatment of ectopic pregnancy.

Drug interactions

Methotrexate interacts with several other drugs:

- Probenecid decreases methotrexate excretion, increasing the risk of methotrexate toxicity, including fatigue, bone marrow suppression, and stomatitis (mouth inflammation).
- Salicylates and nonsteroidal anti-inflammatory drugs (NSAIDs), especially diclofenac (Cambia), ketoprofen, indomethacin (Indocin), and naproxen (Aleve), also increase methotrexate toxicity and severe bone marrow suppression.
- Cholestyramine reduces the absorption of methotrexate from the GI tract.
- Concurrent use of alcohol and methotrexate increases the risk of liver toxicity.
- Taking trimethoprim and sulfamethoxazole (Bactrim) with methotrexate may produce blood cell abnormalities.
- Penicillin decreases renal tubular secretion of methotrexate, increasing the risk of methotrexate toxicity.

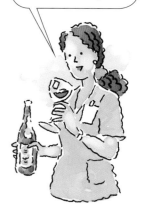

Consuming alcohol while taking methotrexate increases the risk of liver toxicity.

Side effects/Adverse reactions

Side effects/adverse reactions to methotrexate include:

- bone marrow suppression
- stomatitis
- pulmonary toxicity, exhibited as pneumonitis or pulmonary fibrosis
- skin reactions, such as photosensitivity and hair loss.

To the rescue

Kidney toxicity can also occur with high doses of methotrexate. During high-dose therapy, leucovorin (folinic acid) may be used to minimize adverse reactions. This process is known as *leucovorin rescue*.

Intrathecal threats

Adverse reactions to intrathecal administration (through the dura into the subarachnoid space) of methotrexate may include seizures, paralysis, and death. Other less severe adverse reactions may also occur, such as headache, fever, neck stiffness, confusion, and irritability.

The Three-Step Approach

Nursing management for patients needing methotrexate therapy includes these three steps.

Reminder to review the broader *The three-step approach* that applies to ALL cytotoxic antineoplastic chemotherapy (see page 672).

Preadministration
(Recognize and analyze cues
- Review lab work including platelet and total and differential white blood cell (WBC) counts as well as hemoglobin, hematocrit, alanine aminotransferase (ALT), aspartate aminotransferase (AST), lactate dehydrogenase (LDH), serum bilirubin, blood urea nitrogen (BUN), serum creatinine, urine pH, and other lab work as needed.
- The dose should not be given unless the patient's platelet count is greater than 100,000/mcL, ANC is greater than 1,000/mcL, creatinine level is under 1.5 mg/dL, or BUN level is under 25 mg/dL.
- Ensure that the patient remains hydrated. Monitor intake and output.
- Ensure that the patient does not drink alcohol during treatment.
- Review orders: higher doses may cause nausea and may require leucovorin rescue.
- If the patient is receiving intrathecal (IT) methotrexate, ensure that there are no other syringes near, and the methotrexate syringe has a label identifying it as "intrathecal" use only. Fatal events have occurred when mix ups occur.
- If the patient is receiving oral methotrexate, ensure that tablets are not touched.

(Prioritize hypothesis—priority patient problems)
- Infection risk
- Bleeding risk
- Knowledge deficiency

(Generate solutions)
- The patient will not develop infection from drug-induced immunosuppression.
- The patient will remain free of myelosuppressive complications such as bleeding.
- The patient and family will demonstrate an understanding of drug therapy.

Medication administration
(Take action)
- Give an antiemetic before giving the drug to lessen nausea, if ordered. This is usually prescribed for high doses.
- Provide diligent mouth care to prevent stomatitis with methotrexate therapy.
- Anticipate the need for leucovorin rescue with high-dose methotrexate therapy.
- Give methotrexate with correct route verified. It can be given PO, IV, IM, and IT. If given IM, be sure to use the ventrogluteal muscle.

Postadministration
(Evaluate outcomes)
- Monitor for signs of infection that can develop from drug-induced immunosuppression.

- Evaluate for bleeding, a complication of myelosuppression.
- Evaluate the patient's and family's understanding of drug therapy and diagnosis.

Pyrimidine analogues

Pyrimidine analogues are a diverse group of drugs that inhibit production of pyrimidine nucleotides necessary for DNA synthesis. They include:
- capecitabine (Xeloda)
- cytarabine
- floxuridine
- fluorouracil
- gemcitabine (Gemzar).

Pharmacokinetics

Because pyrimidine analogues are generally absorbed poorly when given orally, they are usually administered by other routes. Except for cytarabine, pyrimidine analogues are distributed well throughout the body, including the CSF. They are metabolized extensively in the liver and are excreted in urine. Intrathecal (IT) cytarabine may be given with or without cranial radiation to treat CNS leukemia.

Pharmacodynamics

Pyrimidine analogues kill cancer cells by interfering with the natural function of pyrimidine nucleotides. (See *How pyrimidine analogues work*.)

Pharm function

How pyrimidine analogues work

To understand how pyrimidine analogues work, it helps to consider the basic structure of DNA.

Climbing the ladder to understanding
DNA resembles a ladder that has been twisted. The rungs of the ladder consist of pairs of nitrogenous bases: adenine always pairs with thymine, and guanine always pairs with cytosine. Cytosine and thymine are pyrimidines; adenine and guanine are purines.

One part sugar...
The basic unit of DNA is the nucleotide. A nucleotide is the building block of nucleic acids. It consists of a sugar, a nitrogen-containing base, and a phosphate group. It is on these components that pyrimidine analogues do their work.

In the guise of a nucleotide
After pyrimidine analogues are converted into nucleotides, they are incorporated into DNA, where they may inhibit DNA and RNA synthesis as well as other metabolic reactions necessary for proper cell growth.

Pharmacotherapeutics

Pyrimidine analogues may be used to treat many types of tumors. However, they are primarily indicated in the treatment of:

- acute leukemias
- GI tract adenocarcinomas, such as colorectal, pancreatic, esophageal, and stomach cancers
- carcinomas of the breast
- malignant lymphomas.

Drug interactions

No significant drug interactions occur with most of the pyrimidine analogues; however, several are possible with capecitabine (Xeloda):

- Capecitabine (Xeloda) may have increased absorption when coadministered with antacids.
- Capecitabine (Xeloda) can increase the pharmacodynamic effects of warfarin, thereby increasing the risk of bleeding.
- Capecitabine (Xeloda) may increase serum phenytoin levels.

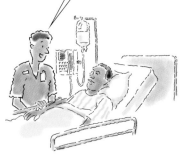

Like most antineoplastic drugs, pyrimidine analogues can cause such adverse effects as fatigue, nausea, and anorexia.

Side effects/Adverse reactions

Like most antineoplastic drugs, pyrimidine analogues can cause:

- fatigue
- inflammation of the mouth, esophagus, and throat, leading to painful ulcerations and tissue sloughing
- bone marrow suppression
- nausea and vomiting
- anorexia.

A range of reactions

High-dose cytarabine can cause severe cerebellar neurotoxicity, chemical conjunctivitis, diarrhea, fever, and hand-foot syndrome (numbness, paresthesia, tingling, painless or painful swelling, erythema, desquamation, blistering, and severe pain of the hands or feet). Other adverse reactions with fluorouracil include diarrhea and hair loss. Gemcitabine (Gemzar) can cause flulike reactions, including fever, within the first 12 hours of the infusion. Inform the provider as patient may need infectious workup with fever.

The Three-Step Approach

Nursing management for patients needing treatment with pyrimidine analogues are listed below.

Reminder to review the broader *The three-step approach* that applies to ALL cytotoxic antineoplastic chemotherapy (see page 672).

Preadministration

(Recognize and analyze cues)
- Review lab work including platelet and total and differential white blood cell (WBC) counts as well as hemoglobin, hematocrit, alanine aminotransferase (ALT), aspartate aminotransferase (AST), lactate dehydrogenase (LDH), serum bilirubin, blood urea nitrogen (BUN), serum creatinine, uric acid, and other lab work as needed.
- The dose should not be given unless the patient's platelet count is greater than 100,000/mcL, ANC is greater than 1,000/mcL, creatinine level is under 1.5 mg/dL, or BUN level is under 25 mg/dL.

(Prioritize hypothesis—priority patient problems)
- Infection risk
- Electrolyte imbalance risk
- Altered skin integrity risk
- Knowledge deficiency

(Generate solutions)
- The patient will not develop infection from drug-induced immunosuppression.
- The patient will maintain electrolyte balance with controlled diarrhea and vomiting and adequate hydration.
- The patient and family will demonstrate an understanding of drug therapy and side effect management.

Medication administration

(Take action)
- If the patient is receiving intrathecal (IT) cytarabine, ensure that there are no other syringes near, and the cytarabine syringe has a label identifying it as "intrathecal" use only. Fatal events have occurred when mix ups occur.
- If the patient is receiving oral capecitabine (Xeloda), ensure that tablets are not touched. The tablets need to be taken within 30 minutes after a meal.
- If the patient is receiving oral capecitabine (Xeloda), monitor the patient for hand-foot syndrome and hyperbilirubinemia. Drug therapy will need to be adjusted.

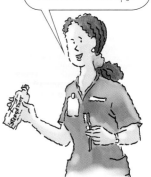

Provide diligent mouth care to prevent stomatitis with cytarabine and fluorouracil therapy.

Postadministration

(Evaluate outcomes)
- Monitor for signs of infection that can develop from drug-induced immunosuppression.
- Evaluate for and proactively address nausea and vomiting.

Purine analogues

Purine analogues are incorporated into DNA and RNA, interfering with nucleic acid synthesis and replication. They include:

- cladribine
- fludarabine
- mercaptopurine (Purixan)
- pentostatin
- thioguanine.

Pharmacokinetics

The pharmacokinetics of purine analogues are not defined clearly. They are largely metabolized in the liver and excreted in urine.

Pharmacodynamics

As with the other antimetabolites, fludarabine, mercaptopurine, and thioguanine first must undergo conversion via phosphorylation to the nucleotide level to be active. The resulting nucleotides are then incorporated into DNA, where they may inhibit DNA and RNA synthesis as well as other metabolic reactions necessary for proper cell growth. Cladribine responds in a similar fashion. Pentostatin inhibits adenosine deaminase (ADA), causing an increase in intracellular levels of deoxyadenosine triphosphate. This leads to cell damage and death. The greatest activity of ADA is in cells of the lymphoid system, especially malignant T cells.

Analogous to pyrimidine analogues

This conversion to nucleotides is the same process that pyrimidine analogues experience but, in this case, it is purine nucleotides that are affected. Purine analogues are cell cycle specific as well, exerting their effect during that same S phase.

Pharmacotherapeutics

Purine analogues are used to treat acute and chronic leukemias and may be useful in the treatment of lymphomas.

Drug interactions

No significant interactions occur with cladribine or thioguanine.

A serious flub with fludarabine

Taking fludarabine and pentostatin together may cause severe pulmonary toxicity, which can be fatal. Taking pentostatin with allopurinol may increase the risk of rash.

No bones about it

Concomitant administration of mercaptopurine (Purixan) and allopurinol may increase bone marrow suppression by decreasing mercaptopurine (Purixan) metabolism. Dose of mercaptopurine (Purixan) may need to be reduced as much as one third if used with allopurinol.

Side effects/Adverse reactions

Purine analogues can produce:
- bone marrow suppression
- nausea and vomiting
- anorexia
- mild diarrhea
- stomatitis
- rise in uric acid levels (a result of the breakdown of purine).

High-dose horrors

Fludarabine, when used at high doses, may cause severe neurologic effects, including blindness, coma, and death.

The Three-Step Approach

Nursing management for patients needing purine analog therapy includes these three steps.

Reminder to review the broader *The three-step approach* **that applies to ALL cytotoxic antineoplastic chemotherapy (see page 672).**

Preadministration

(Recognize and analyze cues)
- Review lab work including platelet and total and differential white blood cell (WBC) counts as well as hemoglobin, hematocrit, alanine aminotransferase (ALT), aspartate aminotransferase (AST), lactate dehydrogenase (LDH), serum bilirubin, blood urea nitrogen (BUN), serum creatinine, uric acid, and other lab work as needed.
- Monitor the patient's fluid intake and output daily. Anticipate hydration or allopurinol orders if risk of tumor lysis syndrome (TLS) is a possibility.

(Prioritize hypothesis—priority patient problems)
- Infection risk
- Electrolyte imbalance risk
- Knowledge deficiency

(Generate solutions)
- The patient will not develop infection from drug-induced immunosuppression.

- The patient will not develop evidence of tumor lysis syndrome (TLS), which can cause electrolyte imbalance.
- The patient and family will demonstrate an understanding of drug therapy.

Medication administration

(Take action)

- For oral preparations, ensure administration at the same time every day. Avoid milk products with administration.
- For oral preparations, ensure that you do not touch the tablets.
- Provide careful hematologic monitoring, especially of neutrophil and platelet counts. Bone marrow suppression can be significant.
- Hepatotoxicity can occur approximately 1 to 2 months into treatment.

Postadministration

(Evaluate outcomes)

- Monitor for signs of infection that can develop from drug-induced immunosuppression.
- Evaluate for signs of tumor lysis syndrome that can cause electrolyte imbalance. The patient will need frequent lab work to continue to evaluate CBC, liver, and kidney function.

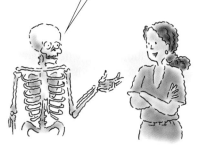

Now, you promise to monitor my neutrophil and platelet counts closely? I don't want my marrow suppressed!

Antibiotic antineoplastic drugs

Antibiotic antineoplastic drugs are antimicrobial products that produce tumoricidal (tumor-destroying) effects by binding with DNA. These drugs inhibit the cellular processes of normal and malignant cells. They include:

- anthracyclines (daunorubicin, doxorubicin [Adriamycin], epirubicin, and idarubicin)
- bleomycin
- dactinomycin
- mitomycin
- mitoxantrone.

Pharmacokinetics

Because antibiotic antineoplastic drugs are usually administered IV, no absorption occurs. They are considered 100% bioavailable.

Direct delivery

Some of the drugs are also directly administered into the body cavity being treated. Mitomycin can be sometimes given as

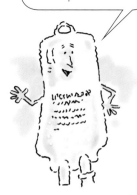

Because antibiotic antineoplastic drugs are usually administered IV, no absorption occurs.

Prototype pro

Antibiotic antineoplastic drugs: Doxorubicin hydrochloride (Adriamycin)

Actions
- Thought to interfere with DNA-dependent RNA synthesis by intercalation (chemical effect unknown)
- Hinders or kills certain cancer cells

Indications
- Bladder, breast, ovarian (liposomal formulation), gastric, testicular, and thyroid carcinomas
- Hodgkin's and non-Hodgkin's lymphoma
- Acute lymphoblastic and myeloblastic leukemia
- Wilms' tumor
- Neuroblastoma
- Soft tissue sarcoma and osteosarcoma

Nursing considerations
- Doxorubicin (Adriamycin) has a high emetic potential. Ensure that the patient is premedicated to prevent nausea and vomiting.

- Monitor for adverse reactions, such as arrhythmias, significant myelosuppression, alopecia, cardiotoxicity (acute and delayed).
- Severe mucositis can occur. Ensure meticulous oral hygiene to prevent infection and decreased intake.
- Heart failure can occur. Perform ECHO prior to treatment and in regular intervals after treatment. Drug therapy may need to change if decrease in ejection fraction (EF) occurs.
- Doxorubicin (Adriamycin) is potent vesicant and can cause extreme tissue damage if the IV extravasates. Central line is usually required for administration.
- Drug is red-orange and will cause urine discoloration.
- Doxorubicin can be in the form of drug-eluting beads and used for chemoembolization in hepatic lesions.
- Follow facility policy for reconstitution and administration.

postsurgical bladder instillation. When bleomycin is injected into the pleural space for malignant effusions, up to one half of the dose is absorbed.

Distribution of antibiotic antineoplastic drugs throughout the body varies as does their metabolism and elimination. (See *Antibiotic antineoplastic drugs: Doxorubicin hydrochloride (Adriamycin)*.)

Pharmacodynamics

Except for mitomycin, antibiotic antineoplastic drugs intercalate, or insert themselves, between adjacent base pairs of a DNA molecule, physically separating them.

Worming their way in

Remember, DNA looks like a twisted ladder with the rungs made up of pairs of nitrogenous bases. Antibiotic antineoplastic drugs insert themselves between these nitrogenous bases. Then, when the DNA chain replicates, an extra base is inserted opposite the intercalated antibiotic, resulting in a mutant DNA molecule. The overall effect is cell death.

Breaking the chain

Mitomycin is activated inside the cell to a bifunctional or trifunctional alkylating drug. It produces single-strand breakage of DNA, cross-links DNA, and inhibits DNA synthesis.

Pharmacotherapeutics

Antibiotic antineoplastic drugs act against many cancers, including:
- Hodgkin's lymphoma and other malignant lymphomas
- testicular carcinoma
- squamous cell carcinoma of the head, neck, and cervix
- Wilms' tumor (a malignant neoplasm of the kidney, occurring in young children)
- osteogenic sarcoma and rhabdomyosarcoma (a malignant neoplasm composed of striated muscle cells)
- Ewing's sarcoma (a malignant tumor that originates in bone marrow, typically in long bones or the pelvis) and other soft tissue sarcomas
- breast, ovarian, and bladder cancer
- carcinomas of the upper GI tract
- choriocarcinoma
- acute leukemia
- neuroblastoma.

Drug interactions

Antibiotic antineoplastic drugs interact with many other drugs:
- Concurrent therapy with fludarabine and idarubicin is not recommended because of the risk of fatal lung toxicity.
- Bleomycin may decrease serum digoxin and serum phenytoin (Dilantin) levels.
- Doxorubicin (Adriamycin) may reduce serum digoxin levels.
- Combination chemotherapies increase risk of leukopenia and thrombocytopenia.
- Mitomycin and vinca alkaloids may cause acute respiratory distress.
- Black cohosh and St. John's wort should be avoided during antineoplastic therapy.

Side effects/Adverse reactions

The primary adverse reaction to antibiotic antineoplastic drugs is bone marrow suppression. Irreversible cardiomyopathy and acute electrocardiogram (ECG) changes can also occur as well as nausea and vomiting. The patient's ejection fraction may drop. As such, routine

ECHO is required prior to and regularly during therapy. There is also a risk of secondary malignancies for patients receiving antibiotic antineoplastic drugs.

Running hot and cold

An antihistamine and antipyretic should be given before bleomycin to prevent fever and chills. An anaphylactic reaction can occur in patients receiving bleomycin, so test doses are recommended. Bleomycin can also cause pulmonary fibrosis. This can be acute or delayed.

Seeing red . . . or blue-green

Doxorubicin (Adriamycin), daunorubicin, epirubicin, and idarubicin may color urine red; mitoxantrone may color it blue-green.

The Three-Step Approach

Nursing management for patients needing antitumor antibiotic includes these three steps.

Reminder to review the broader *The three-step approach* **that applies to ALL cytotoxic antineoplastic chemotherapy (see page 672).**

Preadministration

(Recognize and analyze cues)

- Review lab work including platelet and total and differential white blood cell (WBC) counts as well as hemoglobin, hematocrit, alanine aminotransferase (ALT), aspartate aminotransferase (AST), lactate dehydrogenase (LDH), serum bilirubin, blood urea nitrogen (BUN), serum creatinine, uric acid, and other lab work as needed.
- The dose should not be given unless the patient's platelet count is greater than 100,000/mcL, ANC is greater than 1,500/mcL, creatinine level is under 1.5 mg/dL, or BUN level is under 25 mg/dL.
- Ensure that the patient is premedicated with antiemetics prior to administration.
- Ensure that the patient has a patent IV; central line may be required. Follow facility guidelines.
- Perform ECHO prior to anthracycline therapy. Perform pulmonary function test (PFT) prior to bleomycin administration. Ensure that these are repeated at frequent intervals.
- Stop infusion immediately upon suspecting an infusion reaction. Keep epinephrine, corticosteroids, and antihistamines available

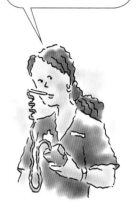

An antihistamine and antipyretic should be given before bleomycin to prevent fever and chills.

during therapy. Anaphylactic reactions may occur, especially with bleomycin. Test dose of bleomycin is required.

- Ensure knowledge on how to manage extravasation, should it occur.

(Prioritize hypothesis—priority patient problems)
- Infection risk
- Nausea and vomiting
- Safety risk
- Knowledge deficiency

(Generate solutions)
- The patient will not develop infection associated with drug-induced immunosuppression.
- The patient will have controlled nausea and vomiting.
- Promptly recognize and address any respiratory or cardiac side effects to ensure patient safety.
- The patient and family will demonstrate an understanding of drug therapy.

Medication administration

(Take action)
- Vesicants are usually given in a free-flowing compatible solution via push. Check for blood return at defined intervals, usually every 2 to 5 mL or per facility policy.
- Treat extravasation promptly. If extravasation occurs, stop the infusion immediately and disconnect (leave cannula/needle in place), gently aspirate extravasated solution (do **NOT** flush the line), remove needle/cannula, and elevate extremity. Initiate antidote (dexrazoxane or dimethyl sulfate [DMSO]) (Lexicomp, 2020).
- Provide careful hematologic monitoring, especially of neutrophil and platelet counts. Bone marrow suppression can be severe. The patient will need frequent lab work to continue to evaluate CBC, liver, and kidney function.
- Anticipate the need for growth factor support.

Postadministration

(Evaluate outcomes)
- The patient will not develop infection associated with drug-induced immunosuppression.
- Evaluate for and proactively address nausea and vomiting.
- Protect patient safety with identification and prompt treatment of acute cardiac or respiratory side effects.

Teaching about antibiotic antineoplastic drugs

If antibiotic antineoplastic therapy is prescribed, review these additional points with the patient and caregivers:

• Report redness, pain, or swelling at the injection site immediately. Local tissue injury and scarring may result if IV infiltration occurs.

• If you are taking daunorubicin, doxorubicin (Adriamycin), epirubicin, or idarubicin, your urine may turn orange or red for 1 to 2 days after therapy begins. Mitoxantrone may turn your urine a blue-green color.

• Educate the patient that cardiac and respiratory issues may arise. This may be acute or delayed. Patients reporting symptoms of cardiac or respiratory failure should report their chemotherapy history to their provider.

Natural antineoplastic drugs

A subclass of antineoplastic drugs known as *natural products* includes:
• vinca alkaloids
• podophyllotoxins.

Vinca alkaloids

Vinca alkaloids are nitrogenous bases derived from the periwinkle plant. These drugs are cell cycle specific for the *M and S* phase and include:
• vinblastine
• vincristine
• vinorelbine (Navelbine).

Pharmacokinetics

After IV administration, the vinca alkaloids are distributed well throughout the body. They undergo moderate liver metabolism before being eliminated through different phases, primarily in feces, with a small percentage eliminated in urine.

Pharmacodynamics

Vinca alkaloids may disrupt the normal function of the microtubules (structures within cells that are associated with the movement of DNA) by binding to the protein tubulin in the microtubules.

Separation anxiety

With the microtubules unable to separate chromosomes properly, the chromosomes are dispersed throughout the cytoplasm or arranged in unusual groupings. As a result, formation of the mitotic spindle is prevented, and the cells cannot complete mitosis (cell division).

Under arrest

Cell division is arrested in metaphase, causing cell death. Therefore, vinca alkaloids are cell cycle M and S phase specific. Interruption of the microtubule function may also impair some types of cellular movement, phagocytosis (engulfing and destroying microorganisms and cellular debris), and CNS functions.

Pharmacotherapeutics

Vinca alkaloids are used in several therapeutic situations:
- Vinblastine is used to treat metastatic testicular carcinoma, lymphomas, Kaposi's sarcoma (the most common acquired immunodeficiency syndrome [AIDS]-related cancer), and neuroblastoma (a highly malignant tumor originating in the sympathetic nervous system).
- Vincristine is used in combination therapy to treat Hodgkin's lymphoma, non-Hodgkin's lymphoma, Wilms' tumor, rhabdomyosarcoma, choriocarcinoma, and acute lymphocytic leukemia.
- Vinorelbine (Navelbine) is used to treat non–small cell lung cancer. It may also be used in the treatment of metastatic breast carcinoma, rhabdomyosarcoma, cisplatin-resistant ovarian carcinoma, and Hodgkin's lymphoma.

Drug interactions

Vinca alkaloids interact in many ways with other drugs:
- Erythromycin may increase the toxicity of vinblastine.
- Vinblastine decreases the plasma levels of phenytoin (Dilantin).
- Aprepitant (Emend) may increase serum concentration of vincristine.
- Fluconazole (Diflucan) may increase serum concentration of vincristine and cause worsening neuropathy.
- Calcium channel blockers enhance vincristine accumulation, increasing the tendency for toxicity.

Side effects/Adverse reactions

Vinca alkaloids may cause the following adverse reactions:
- nausea and vomiting
- constipation or paralytic ileus
- peripheral neuropathy

- jaw pain
- stomatitis (mouth inflammation).
- Vinblastine and vinorelbine (Navelbine) toxicities occur primarily as bone marrow suppression. Neurotoxicity may frequently occur with vincristine and vinorelbine (Navelbine) and occasionally with vinblastine therapy.

Hair scare

Reversible alopecia occurs in up to one half of patients receiving vinca alkaloids; it is more likely to occur with vinblastine than with vincristine.

The Three-Step Approach

Nursing management for patients needing vinca alkaloid therapy includes these three steps.

Reminder to review the broader *The three-step approach* that applies to ALL cytotoxic antineoplastic chemotherapy (see page 672).

Preadministration
(Recognize and analyze cues)
- Review lab work including platelet and total and differential white blood cell (WBC) counts as well as hemoglobin, hematocrit, alanine aminotransferase (ALT), aspartate aminotransferase (AST), lactate dehydrogenase (LDH), serum bilirubin, blood urea nitrogen (BUN), serum creatinine, uric acid, and other lab work as needed.
- The dose should not be given unless the patient's platelet count is greater than 100,000/mcL and ANC is greater than 1,000/mcL.
- Ensure that the patient is premedicated with antiemetics prior to administration.
- Use caution to avoid confusion with vinBLAStine, vinCRIStine, and vinorelBINE. Use of TALL lettering helps decrease confusion.

(Prioritize hypothesis—priority patient problems)
- Infection risk
- Nausea and vomiting
- Constipation
- Knowledge deficiency

(Generate solutions)
- The patient will not develop infection associated with drug-induced immunosuppression.
- The patient will have controlled nausea and vomiting.
- The patient will not experience adverse effects such as constipation.
- The patient and family will demonstrate an understanding of drug therapy.

More on vinblastine and vincristine

Vinblastine and vincristine are fatal if given intrathecally; they are for IV use only.

If extravasation occurs, stop infusion immediately. If IV line is still in place, instill hyaluronidase into existing line. If IV not in place, inject hyaluronidase SQ in clockwise manner. Apply dry warm compresses for 20 minutes 4 times a day.

Medication administration

(Take action)

- Vinca alkaloids are vesicants, use precautions and follow facility policy for administration. Central line is preferred. (See *More on vinblastine and vincristine*.) Monitor IV site before, during, and after infusion for blood return.
- Vinca alkaloids are fatal if given via intrathecally. They should always be prepared in a mini bag, not syringe, and never stored in a location where intrathecal (IT) treatment is given.
- They should be given via free-flowing compatible solution or via pump over a short duration.

Postadministration

(Evaluate outcomes)

- Assess for neurotoxicity and neuropathy (numbness and tingling in the patient's hands and feet). Vinblastine is less neurotoxic than vincristine.
- Ensure patient safety if neurotoxicity or neuropathy develops.
- The patient will remain free from infection. Check CBC at regular intervals. Monitor for decreased blood cells, including WBCs, granulocytes (ANC), and hemoglobin and platelets. Provide supportive care or transfusions if warranted.
- The patient will have controlled nausea and vomiting.
- The patient will start a prophylactic bowel regimen. Monitor for severe constipation or ileus.
- The patient will need frequent lab work to continue to evaluate CBC, liver, and kidney function.

> If extravasation occurs, stop the infusion at once and notify the prescriber.

Podophyllotoxins

Podophyllotoxin is a semisynthetic glycoside that is cell cycle specific and act during the early G2 and late S phases of the cell cycle. They include:

- etoposide (Toposar, VePesid).

Pharmacokinetics

When taken orally, etoposide is only moderately absorbed. Although the drugs are distributed widely throughout the body, they achieve poor CSF levels. Etoposide undergoes liver metabolism and is excreted primarily in urine.

Pharmacodynamics

Etoposide (Toposar, VePesid) may inhibit mitochondrial transport. It appears to cause DNA strand breaks.

Pharmacotherapeutics

Etoposide (Toposar, VePesid) is used to treat testicular cancer and small cell lung cancer.

Drug interactions

Etoposide (Toposar, VePesid) has a few significant interactions with other drugs:

- Etoposide (Toposar, VePesid) may increase the risk of bleeding in a patient taking warfarin (Coumadin).
- St. John's wort decreases etoposide (Toposar, VePesid) levels.

Side effects/Adverse reactions

Most patients receiving podophyllotoxins experience hair loss. Other adverse reactions include:

- nausea and vomiting; this is to a lesser extent with oral etoposide
- anorexia
- stomatitis
- bone marrow suppression, causing leukopenia and, less commonly, thrombocytopenia
- acute hypotension (if infused too rapidly by the IV route).

The Three-Step Approach

Nursing management for patients needing etoposide therapy includes these three steps.

Reminder to review the broader *The three-step approach* **that applies to ALL cytotoxic antineoplastic chemotherapy (see page 672).**

Preadministration

(Recognize and analyze cues)

- Review lab work including platelet and total and differential white blood cell (WBC) counts as well as hemoglobin, hematocrit, alanine aminotransferase (ALT), aspartate aminotransferase (AST), lactate dehydrogenase (LDH), serum bilirubin, blood urea nitrogen (BUN), serum creatinine, uric acid, and other lab work as needed.
- The dose should not be given unless the patient's platelet count is greater than 100,000/mcL, ANC is greater than 1,000/mcL, creatinine level is under 1.5 mg/dL, or BUN level is under 25 mg/dL.

- Ensure that the patient is premedicated with antiemetics prior to administration.

(Prioritize hypothesis—priority patient problems)
- Infection risk related to drug-induced immunosuppression
- Nausea and vomiting risk
- Hypotension risk, due to too rapid IV infusion
- Knowledge deficiency related to drug therapy and diagnosis

(Generate solutions)
- The patient will remain free from infection.
- The patient will have controlled nausea and vomiting.
- The patient will have no adverse effects from infusion.
- The patient and family will demonstrate an understanding of drug therapy.

Medication administration

(Take action)
- Stop infusion immediately upon suspecting an infusion reaction. Keep diphenhydramine, hydrocortisone, epinephrine, and necessary emergency equipment available to establish an airway in case of anaphylaxis.
- If oral etoposide is ordered, do not touch tablets. Wear gloves when administering. Doses less than 200 mg/day are a single daily dose. Greater than 200 mg/day should be given in two divided doses.
- Ensure that pump is programmed to infuse at least 30 to 60 minutes to prevent hypotension. If the patient's blood pressure drops, stop infusion immediately and notify the provider.
- Etoposide is an irritant; use caution to prevent extravasation. Monitor IV site before, during, and after infusion for blood return.

Postadministration

(Evaluate outcomes)
- Monitor the patient's CBC. Observe the patient for signs of bone marrow suppression.
- The risk of injury to the patient will be minimized, including hypotension.
- The patient will remain free from infection.
- The patient will have controlled nausea and vomiting.

Topoisomerase I inhibitors

As the name implies, topoisomerase I inhibitors inhibit the enzyme topoisomerase I. These agents are derived from a naturally occurring alkaloid from the Chinese tree *Camptotheca acuminata*. Currently available drugs include:
- irinotecan (Camptosar)
- topotecan (Hycamtin).

Pharmacokinetics

Irinotecan (Camptosar) and topotecan (Hycamtin) are minimally absorbed and must be given IV. Irinotecan (Camptosar) undergoes metabolic changes to become the active metabolite SN-38. The half-life of SN-38 is approximately 10 hours, and it is eliminated through biliary excretion. Topotecan (Hycamtin) is metabolized hepatically, although renal excretion is a significant elimination pathway.

Pharmacodynamics

These agents exert their cytotoxic effect by inhibiting the topoisomerase I enzyme, an essential enzyme that mediates the relaxation of supercoiled DNA. Topoisomerase inhibitors bind to the DNA topoisomerase I complex and prevent resealing, thereby causing DNA strand breaks, resulting in impaired DNA synthesis.

Pharmacotherapeutics

Topoisomerase I inhibitors are active against solid tumors and hematologic malignancies. Topotecan (Hycamtin) is administered for ovarian cancer and small cell lung cancer. Irinotecan (Camptosar) is administered to patients with colorectal cancer or small cell lung cancer.

Drug interactions

Irinotecan (Camptosar) is associated with the following drug interactions:
- Ketoconazole can significantly increase SN-38 serum concentrations when given with irinotecan (Camptosar), increasing the risk of associated toxicities.
- Concurrent administration of diuretics may exacerbate dehydration caused by irinotecan-induced diarrhea.
- Concurrent administration of laxatives with irinotecan (Camptosar) can induce diarrhea.

Side effects/Adverse reactions

Diarrhea is the most common adverse reaction to topoisomerase I inhibitors, especially irinotecan (Camptosar), which is cholinergically mediated; this can be reversed with atropine.

Delayed reaction

Late-onset diarrhea, which may persist for up to 1 week, can occur several days after chemotherapy has been administered. Treatment consists of loperamide (Imodium) given every 2 hours until stools become formed.

Common conditions, part two

Besides diarrhea, the more common adverse reactions to topoisomerase I inhibitors, particularly irinotecan (Camptosar), include:
- increased sweating and saliva production

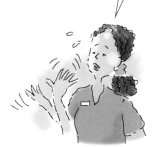

Irinotecan can cause an increase in sweating and saliva production. It can also cause watery eyes.

- watery eyes
- abdominal cramps
- nausea and vomiting
- loss of appetite
- fatigue
- hair loss or thinning.

Serious situation

These reactions rarely occur but are more serious:
- Both drugs are associated with significant myelosuppression, especially topotecan (Hycamtin).
- Irinotecan (Camptosar) has been associated with thromboembolic events.

The Three-Step Approach

Nursing management for patients needing topoisomerase I inhibitor therapy includes these three steps.

Reminder to review the broader *The three-step approach* that applies to ALL cytotoxic antineoplastic chemotherapy (see page 672).

Preadministration

(Recognize and analyze cues)
- Review lab work including platelet and total and differential white blood cell (WBC) counts as well as hemoglobin, hematocrit, alanine aminotransferase (ALT), aspartate aminotransferase (AST), lactate dehydrogenase (LDH), serum bilirubin, blood urea nitrogen (BUN), serum creatinine, uric acid, electrolytes, and other lab work as needed.
- The dose should not be given unless the patient's platelet count is greater than 100,000/mcL, ANC is greater than 1,000/mcL, creatinine level is under 1.5 mg/dL, or BUN level is under 25 mg/dL.
- Ensure that the patient is premedicated with antiemetics prior to administration.
- Ensure that orders for atropine and loperamide (Imodium) are received. IV atropine is given prior to irinotecan (Camptosar) to reduce acute onset diarrhea.

(Prioritize hypothesis—priority patient problems)
- Diarrhea (associated with irinotecan [Camptosar])
- Hypovolemia risk
- Infection risk
- Nausea and vomiting
- Knowledge deficiency

(Generate solutions)
- The patient will not develop infection associated with drug-induced immunosuppression.

- The patient will have controlled nausea, vomiting, and diarrhea.
- The patient will maintain hydration and fluid volume status.
- The patient and family will demonstrate an understanding of drug therapy.

Medication administration
(Take action)
- Give a topotecan IV infusion over 30 minutes; give an irinotecan IV infusion over at least 90 minutes.
- Ensure that atropine was given as premedication.
- Topotecan (Hycamtin) is an irritant.

Postadministration
(Evaluate outcomes)
- Management of late onset diarrhea is loperamide (Imodium) at onset of diarrhea,
- Evaluate for and promptly address signs of infection associated with drug-induced immunosuppression.
- Evaluate for and proactively address nausea and vomiting.

Unclassified antineoplastic drugs

Many other antineoplastic drugs cannot be included in existing classifications. These drugs include:
- asparaginases
- procarbazine
- taxanes.

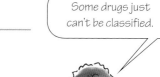

Some drugs just can't be classified.

Asparaginases

Asparaginases are cell cycle specific and act during the G_1 phase. They include:
- asparaginase (Elspar)
- pegaspargase.

Pharmacokinetics

Asparaginase (Elspar) is administered parenterally. It is considered 100% bioavailable when administered IV and about 50% bioavailable when administered IM.

After administration, asparaginase (Elspar) remains inside the blood vessels, with minimal distribution elsewhere. The metabolism of asparaginase (Elspar) is unknown; only trace amounts appear in urine.

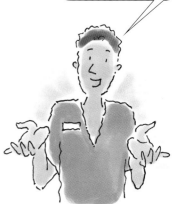

Pharmacodynamics

Asparaginase (Elspar) and pegaspargase capitalize on the biochemical differences between normal and tumor cells.

Eat your asparagines, or else

Most normal cells can synthesize asparagine (Elspar), but some tumor cells depend on other sources of asparagine for survival. Asparaginase (Elspar) and pegaspargase help to degrade asparagine to aspartic acid and ammonia. Deprived of their supply of asparagine, the tumor cells die.

Pharmacotherapeutics

Asparaginase (Elspar) is used primarily to induce remission in patients with acute lymphocytic leukemia in combination with standard chemotherapy.

If allergic to the natives

Pegaspargase is used to treat acute lymphocytic leukemia in patients who are allergic to the native form of asparaginase (Elspar).

Drug interactions

Asparaginase (Elspar) and pegaspargase can reduce the effectiveness of methotrexate. Concurrent use of asparaginase (Elspar) with dexamethasone (Decadron) or vincristine (Oncovin) increases the risk of adverse reactions.

Side effects/Adverse reactions

Many patients receiving asparaginase (Elspar) and pegaspargase develop nausea and vomiting. Fever, headache, abdominal pain, pancreatitis, coagulopathy, and liver toxicity can also occur. Hyperglycemia and hypersensitivity reactions can occur during and after administration.

Raising the risk

Asparaginase (Elspar) and pegaspargase can cause anaphylaxis, which is more likely to occur with intermittent IV dosing than with daily IV dosing or IM injections. The risk of a reaction rises with each successive treatment. Hypersensitivity reactions may also occur.

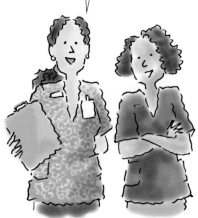

Asparaginases can cause anaphylaxis, especially with intermittent IV dosing rather than daily dosing.

The Three–Step Approach

Nursing management for patients needing asparaginase therapy includes these three steps.

Reminder to review the broader *The three-step approach* **that applies to ALL cytotoxic antineoplastic chemotherapy (see page 672).**

Preadministration

(Recognize and analyze cues)
- Review lab work including platelet and total and differential white blood cell (WBC) counts as well as hemoglobin, hematocrit, alanine aminotransferase (ALT), aspartate aminotransferase (AST), lactate dehydrogenase (LDH), serum bilirubin, blood urea nitrogen (BUN), serum creatinine, uric acid, blood glucose, and other lab work as needed.
- Withhold treatment if bilirubin is greater than 3 to 10 times upper limit of normal.
- Ensure that the patient is premedicated with antiemetics prior to administration.
- Hormonal contraceptives may not be effective, and alternative methods should be considered.

(Prioritize hypothesis—priority patient problems)
- Infection risk
- Nausea and vomiting risk
- Hyperglycemia risk
- Knowledge deficiency

(Generate solutions)
- The patient will not develop infection associated with drug-induced immunosuppression.
- The patient will have controlled nausea and vomiting.
- The patient will demonstrate controlled blood sugar.
- Evaluate the patient's and family's understanding of drug therapy.

Medication administration

(Take action)
- Stop infusion immediately upon suspecting an infusion reaction. Keep diphenhydramine, hydrocortisone, epinephrine, and necessary emergency equipment available to establish an airway in case of hypersensitivity or anaphylaxis. Risk of anaphylaxis can occur with each dose.
- Pegaspargase can be given IM or IV. For IM injections, give no more than 2 mL per injection. Administer deep IM into a large muscle. For IV infusions, give over 1 to 2 hours through a running IV infusion line with compatible solution.
- Treat hyperglycemia according to facility protocol.

Postadministration

(Evaluate outcomes)
- Monitor the patient for 1 hour post administration for hypersensitivity reaction.
- The patient will remain free from infection, bleeding, or anaphylaxis.
- The patient will have controlled nausea and vomiting.

- The patient will need frequent lab work to continue to evaluate CBC, liver, and kidney function. The patient is at risk for pancreatitis. Monitor for signs and symptoms.
- Prolonged bone marrow suppression can occur, and the patient should report bleeding, bruising, or signs and symptoms of infection or bleeding. Transfusion support may be required.

Procarbazine

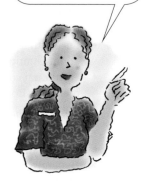

Procarbazine is used to treat Hodgkin's disease, lymphoma, and primary and metastatic brain tumors.

Procarbazine hydrochloride, a methylhydrazine derivative with monoamine oxidase (MAO)-inhibiting properties, is cell cycle specific and acts on the S phase.

Pharmacokinetics

After oral administration, procarbazine is absorbed well. It readily crosses the blood-brain barrier and is well distributed into CSF.

To activate, just add enzymes

Procarbazine is metabolized rapidly in the liver and must be activated metabolically by microsomal enzymes. It is excreted in urine, primarily as metabolites.

Pharmacodynamics

An inert drug, procarbazine must be activated metabolically in the liver before it can produce various cell changes. It can cause chromosomal damage, suppress mitosis, and inhibit DNA, RNA, and protein synthesis.

Pharmacotherapeutics

Procarbazine is used to treat Hodgkin's lymphoma, primary and metastatic brain tumors, and relapsed or refractory non-Hodgkin's lymphoma.

Drug interactions

Interactions with procarbazine can be significant:
- Procarbazine produces an additive effect when administered with CNS depressants.
- Taken with meperidine (Demerol), procarbazine may result in severe hypotension and death.

Mirroring MAO

- Because of procarbazine's MAO-inhibiting properties, hypertensive reactions may occur when it is administered concurrently with sympathomimetics, antidepressants, and tyramine-rich foods (for example, smoked or cured meats, aged cheeses, beer, sauerkraut, and soybean-based condiments).
- Procarbazine taken with caffeine may result in arrhythmias and severe hypertension.

Side effects/Adverse reactions

Delayed-onset bone marrow suppression is the most common dose-limiting toxicity associated with procarbazine. Interstitial pneumonitis and pulmonary fibrosis may also occur.

A gut feeling

GI reactions include nausea, vomiting, stomatitis, and diarrhea.

The Three-Step Approach

Nursing management for patients needing procarbazine therapy includes these three steps.

Reminder to review the broader *The three-step approach* **that applies to ALL cytotoxic antineoplastic chemotherapy (see page 672).**

Preadministration

(Recognize and analyze cues)

• Instruct the patient on avoiding foods that interact with monoamine oxidase inhibitor (MAOI).
• Review lab work including platelet and total and differential white blood cell (WBC) counts as well as hemoglobin, hematocrit, alanine aminotransferase (ALT), aspartate aminotransferase (AST), lactate dehydrogenase (LDH), serum bilirubin, blood urea nitrogen (BUN), serum creatinine, uric acid, and other lab work as needed.
• Ensure that the patient is premedicated with antiemetics prior to administration.

(Prioritize hypothesis—priority patient problems)

• Infection risk
• Nausea and vomiting
• Nonadherence
• Knowledge deficiency

(Generate solutions)

• The patient will not develop infection associated with drug-induced immunosuppression.
• The patient will have controlled nausea and vomiting.
• The patient will adhere to dietary needs to prevent adverse effects.
• The patient and family will demonstrate an understanding of drug therapy, including dosing schedule and importance of taking their medication.

Medication administration

(Take action)

• Procarbazine can be given daily or in divided doses.
• Monitor vital signs at ordered intervals.
• Monitor for CNS toxicity. Stop the drug and notify the prescriber if a disulfiram-like reaction occurs (chest pain, rapid or irregular heartbeat, severe headache, and stiff neck).

Postadministration

(Evaluate outcomes)
- The patient will remain free from infection.
- The patient will have controlled nausea and vomiting.
- Monitor for CNS toxicity.
- The patient will need frequent lab work to continue to evaluate CBC, liver, and kidney function.
- The patient will remain free of myelosuppression complications.

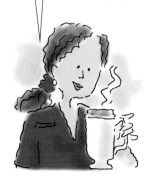

Advise the patient taking procarbazine to avoid caffeine. I suppose decaf will have to do…

Taxanes

Taxanes have many uses and are usually in combination with other chemotherapy or immunotherapy. Taxanes include:
- albumin-bound paclitaxel (Abraxane)
- cabazitaxel (Jevtana)
- docetaxel (Taxotere)
- paclitaxel (Taxol).

Pharmacokinetics

After IV administration, paclitaxel (Taxol) is highly bound to plasma proteins. Docetaxel (Taxotere) is administered IV with a rapid onset of action. Paclitaxel (Taxol) and nab-paclitaxel (Abraxane) are metabolized primarily in the liver, with a small amount excreted unchanged in urine. Docetaxel (Taxotere) and cabazitaxel (Jevtana) are excreted primarily in feces.

Pharmacodynamics

Taxanes exert their chemotherapeutic effect by disrupting the microtubule network that is essential for mitosis and other vital cellular functions.

Pharmacotherapeutics

Paclitaxel (Taxol) is used as first-line chemotherapy for ovarian cancer, breast cancer, and non–small cell lung cancer. The taxanes may also be used to treat head and neck cancer, prostate cancer, and unknown primary adenocarcinomas. Paclitaxel (Taxol) is also a treatment for AIDS-related Kaposi's sarcoma.

Drug interactions

Taxanes have few interactions with other drugs:
- Concomitant use of paclitaxel (Taxol) and cisplatin may cause additive myelosuppressive effects.
- Cyclosporine, ketoconazole, and erythromycin may modify docetaxel (Taxotere) metabolism.
- Phenytoin (Dilantin) may decrease paclitaxel (Taxol) serum concentrations, leading to a loss of efficacy.

- Drugs that inhibit cytochrome P-450, such as cyclosporine, dexamethasone (Decadron), diazepam (Valium), etoposide (Toposar, VePesid), ketoconazole, quinidine, retinoic acid, teniposide, testosterone, verapamil, and vincristine (Oncovin), may increase paclitaxel (Taxol) levels. Monitor the patient for toxicity.

Side effects/Adverse reactions

Side effects/adverse reactions to taxanes include:
- bone marrow suppression
- hypersensitivity reactions
- abnormal electrocardiogram (EKG)
- peripheral neuropathy
- muscle and joint pain
- fluid retention and peripheral edema—docetaxel (Taxotere) and cabazitaxel (Jevtana)
- nausea and vomiting
- diarrhea
- constipation—albumin bound paclitaxel (Abraxane)
- mucous membrane inflammation/stomatitis
- hair loss.

The Three-Step Approach

Nursing management for patients needing taxane therapy includes these three steps.

Reminder to review the broader *The three-step approach* **that applies to ALL cytotoxic antineoplastic chemotherapy (see page 672).**

Preadministration

(Recognize and analyze cues)
- Review lab work including platelet and total and differential white blood cell (WBC) counts as well as hemoglobin, hematocrit, alanine aminotransferase (ALT), aspartate aminotransferase (AST), lactate dehydrogenase (LDH), serum bilirubin, blood urea nitrogen (BUN), serum creatinine, uric acid, and other lab work as needed.
- Doses may need to be reduced in hepatic impairment.
- Ensure that the patient is premedicated with antiemetics prior to administration.
- Ensure that the patient is premedicated with an antihistamine, corticosteroid, and an H2 antagonist at least 30 minutes prior to infusion. Albumin-bound paclitaxel (Abraxane) does not need premedicating for hypersensitivity reactions.
- To prevent fluid retention and peripheral edema with docetaxel (Taxotere) and cabazitaxel (Jevtana), corticosteroids can be given 3 days starting the day prior to infusion.

(Prioritize hypothesis—priority patient problems)
- Infection risk
- Nausea and vomiting risk
- Knowledge deficiency

(Generate solutions)
- The patient will remain free from infection.
- The patient will have controlled nausea and vomiting.
- The patient and family will demonstrate an understanding of drug therapy.

Medication administration

(Take action)
- Central line is not required, but taxanes are irritants with vesicant-like properties. Monitor IV site before, during, and after infusion for blood return.
- Stop infusion immediately upon suspecting an infusion reaction. Keep diphenhydramine, hydrocortisone, epinephrine, and necessary emergency equipment available to establish an airway in case of anaphylaxis.
- Use polyethylene-lined (non-PVC) administration set and a 0.22-micrometer inline filter with cabazitaxel (Jevtana) and paclitaxel (Taxol).
- Use polyethylene-lined (non-DEHP) tubing for administration of docetaxel (Taxotere).
- When taxanes are given with other antineoplastics, refer to facility protocol for sequencing.
- Albumin-bound paclitaxel (Abraxane) is given over 30 minutes.

Postadministration

(Evaluate outcomes)
- Evaluate for and promptly address signs of infection associated with drug-induced immunosuppression.
- Evaluate for and proactively address nausea and vomiting.
- The patient will need frequent lab work to continue to evaluate CBC, liver, and kidney function.

Monoclonal antibodies and immunotherapy

With the development of monoclonal antibodies and immunotherapy, there has been a new way to treat cancer that is not cytotoxic in nature. While these medications are not without side effects, the toxicity typically associated with traditional chemotherapy regimens is not as pronounced. These agents can be single agents or in combination with each other or with chemotherapy.

Monoclonal antibodies

Recombinant DNA technology has allowed for the development of monoclonal antibodies directed at targets that are on the surface of some tumor cells. Having these antigens allows these directed agents to work directly on the tumor. They include:

- blinatumomab (Blincyto)
- brentuximab vedotin (Adcetris)
- daratumumab (Darzalex)
- dinutuximab (Unituxin)
- ibritumomab tiuxetan (Zevalin)
- nivolumab (Opdivo)
- obinutuzumab (Gazyva)
- pertuzumab (Perjeta)
- rituximab (Rituxan)
- trastuzumab (Herceptin).

Monoclonal antibodies are further characterized by being chimeric or humanized. Chimeric formulated monoclonal antibodies have higher risk of infusion-related hypersensitivity reactions.

Pharmacokinetics

The monoclonal antibodies, by virtue of their large protein molecule structure, are not given orally. They are mostly given IV; however, some subcutaneous administrations are approved.

Here's to a long (half) life

These drugs may have a limited volume of distribution as well as a long half-life, sometimes measured in weeks.

The monoclonal antibodies bind to target receptor or cancer cells and can cause tumor death via several mechanisms. They can induce programmed cell death and recruit other elements of the immune system to attack the cancer cell.

Targeting in

Ibritumomab tiuxetan (Zevalin) can deliver a radiation dose to the site of the tumor.

Pharmacotherapeutics

Monoclonal antibodies have demonstrated activity in solid tumors and hematologic malignancies. The cells must have these receptors on the surface to be effective.

- Acute lymphoblastic leukemia—blinatumomab (Blincyto) targets CD19 and CD22 B cells.

Biosimilar— What's so similar?

Biosimilar drugs are biologic therapies that are highly like the reference product in clinical potency and toxicity but may have slight differences in components that do not appear to affect their clinical efficacy or toxicity. Biosimilar monoclonal antibodies are named as the reference drug plus a four-letter suffix that consists of four unique and meaningless lowercase letters (Manis, 2020).

An example is trastuzumab-pkrb.

- Hodgkin's lymphoma—brentuximab vedotin (Adcetris) targets CD30.
- Non-Hodgkin's lymphoma—rituximab (Rituxan), obinutuzumab (Gazyva), and ibritumomab tiuxetan (Zevalin) target CD20 or malignant B lymphocytes.
- Breast cancer—trastuzumab (Herceptin) and pertuzumab (Perjeta)—patient must have HER2 protein receptors (HER2 +) overexpression.
- Pediatric neuroblastoma—dinutuximab (Unituxin) targets GD2 glycolipid cells.
- Daratumumab (Darzalex) targets CD38 on multiple myeloma cells.

Drug interactions

- There are no known drug interactions with pertuzumab (Perjeta) or dinutuximab (Unituxin).
- Ibritumomab tiuxetan (Zevalin) may cause cytopenias (decreased cell count) and may interfere with such drugs as warfarin (Coumadin), aspirin, clopidogrel, ticlopidine, NSAIDs, azathioprine, cyclosporine, and corticosteroids.
- Trastuzumab (Herceptin) increases the cardiac toxicity associated with anthracycline administration.
- Rituximab (Rituxan) used with cisplatin may cause renal toxicity.

Side effects/Adverse reactions

All monoclonal antibodies are associated with infusion-related toxicities, such as fever, chills, shortness of breath, low blood pressure, and anaphylaxis. Fatalities have been reported.

Inviting infection in

- Monoclonal antibodies are frequently given with cytotoxic chemotherapy. Myelosuppression may be enhanced with combination therapy.
- Ibritumomab tiuxetan (Zevalin) is associated with increased myelosuppression.
- Pertuzumab (Perjeta) can cause life-threatening diarrhea.

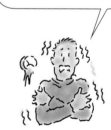

Chills are one of the infusion-related toxicities associated with monoclonal antibodies

The Three-Step Approach

Nursing management for patients needing monoclonal antibody therapy includes these three steps.

Preadministration

(Recognize and analyze cues)

- Review lab work including platelet and total and differential white blood cell (WBC) counts as well as hemoglobin, hematocrit, alanine aminotransferase (ALT), aspartate aminotransferase

(AST), lactate dehydrogenase (LDH), serum bilirubin, blood urea nitrogen (BUN), serum creatinine, potassium, uric acid, electrolytes, and other lab work as needed.

- Ensure that the patient is premedicated with antiemetics prior to administration.
- Ensure premedications to prevent or reduce hypersensitivity. Corticosteroids, antihistamines, and an antipyretic are usually ordered.
- Allopurinol may be started if the patient is at high risk for tumor lysis syndrome.
- Ensure that hydration orders are ordered, especially if cytokine release syndrome (CRS) or tumor lysis syndrome (TLS) is expected.
  - ○ CRS—blinatumomab (Blincyto)
  - ○ TLS—rituximab (Rituxan); obinutuzumab (Gazyva)
- Complete ECHO prior to trastuzumab (Herceptin) and pertuzumab (Perjeta) therapy as it can reduce ejection fraction (EF).
- Perform thorough education on monoclonal antibodies. Include cytotoxic chemotherapy teaching, if applicable. (See *Teaching about chemotherapy*, page 674.)
- Monoclonal antibodies may cause reactivation of latent infections. The patient may need antibiotic, antiviral, and antifungal prophylaxis.
- Ensure that the patient is not pregnant or nursing prior to administration. Teach women of childbearing age and men to use effective contraceptive methods during therapy and for at least 6 months following the completion of therapy.
- Ensure that the patient has knowledge of self-care and side effects after treatment.

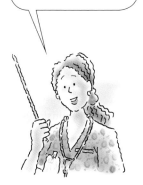

Teach women of childbearing age and men to use effective contraceptive methods during therapy and for at least 6 months following the completion of therapy

(Prioritize hypothesis—priority patient problems)
- Altered breathing pattern
- Infection risk
- Nausea and vomiting
- Diarrhea
- Knowledge deficiency

(Generate solutions)
- The patient will remain safe from adverse reactions (such as altered breathing patterns that can occur with hypersensitivity) during infusion.
- The patient will not develop infection associated with drug-induced immunosuppression.
- Manage diarrhea to prevent life-threatening complications, such as hypokalemia and fluid imbalance.
- The patient and family will demonstrate an understanding of drug therapy.

Medication administration

(Take action)

- Follow the established procedures for safe and proper handling, administration, and disposal of drugs. Chemoprotective PPE is required for all monoclonal antibody administration.
- Monitor IV site before, during, and after infusion to ensure extravasation does not occur.
- Set infusion rate at prescribed rate. Monoclonal antibodies are usually titrated at set intervals.
- All infusions should have a dedicated IV line. Verify compatible solution as some are not compatible with normal saline. Follow drug-specific protocols.
- Monitor for adverse reactions. Stop infusion immediately if an infusion reaction is suspected. Keep diphenhydramine, hydrocortisone, epinephrine, and necessary emergency equipment available to establish an airway in case of anaphylaxis. Provide supportive care such as oxygen and positioning. Notify the provider to receive orders to resume or follow preestablished protocols.
- Never administer monoclonal antibodies via IV push.
- Monitor the patient's vital signs and catheter or IV line patency throughout drug administration. Monitor for redness, pain, or swelling or lack of blood return from IV site or central line. Local tissue injury and scarring may result from tissue infiltration at the infusion site.
- Blinatumomab (Blincyto), daratumumab (Darzalex), and ibritumomab tiuxetan (Zevalin) require use of a 0.22-micrometer filter.
- Ibritumomab tiuxetan (Zevalin) is radiopharmaceutical. Use appropriate shielding when preparing, administering, and disposing drugs.

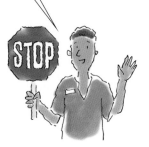

Stop infusion immediately if an infusion reaction is suspected.

Postadministration

(Evaluate outcomes)

- The patient and family will demonstrate an understanding of drug therapy and diagnosis.
- Monitor the patient for delayed hypersensitivity. Trastuzumab (Herceptin) and pertuzumab (Perjeta) require a monitoring period after each dose.
- Patients may experience myelosuppression and renal or hepatic changes after dose. Monitor CBC, liver, and kidney function at regular intervals.
- The patient will not develop infection associated with drug-induced immunosuppression.
- Evaluate for and proactively address nausea and vomiting.
- Patients receiving pertuzumab (Perjeta) will have controlled diarrhea and normal potassium levels.

Immunotherapy

Newer antitumor agents activates the person's own immune response to target and kill the cancer. Immunotherapy drugs, also referred to as checkpoint inhibitors, block certain signaling pathways on the cell, allowing one's own immune system to recognize and destroy the cancer cell. There has been great survival data for those who are able to receive immunotherapy; however, these drugs are not without significant complications.

Anti-CTLA4—cytotoxic T lymphocyte antigen-4 blocking antibody
- Ipilimumab (Yervoy)

Anti-PD-1—programmed cell death protein 1
- Cemiplimab (Libtayo)
- Nivolumab (Opdivo)
- Pembrolizumab (Keytruda)

Anti-PD-L1—programmed cell death-ligand 1
- Atezolizumab (Tecentriq)
- Avelumab (Bavencio)
- Durvalumab (Imfinzi)

Pharmacokinetics

Immunotherapy drugs have a long half-life and are steadily excreted.

Pharmacodynamics

Immunotherapy allows for enhanced T-cell activation and proliferation. This activates the body's natural immune system to target and destroy cancer cells. Each category binds to their specific receptor: cytotoxic T lymphocyte antigen-4 (CTLA-4), programmed death-1 (PD-1), and the programmed death-ligand 1 (PD-L1), blocking these receptors allows for the antitumor immune response. Cancer cells escape normal immune surveillance; however, with the addition of immunotherapy, the body's immune system is reactivated, and cancer cells are marked for destruction.

Pharmacotherapeutics

Immunotherapy has shown great improvement in survival for colorectal cancer, non–small cell lung cancer, head and neck cancer, melanoma, hepatocellular carcinoma, triple negative breast cancer, gastric cancer bladder or renal cell, Hodgkin's lymphoma, and cutaneous squamous cell carcinoma. Historically, antineoplastic drugs with a high side effect profile and limited survival are being retired as more indications for immunotherapy are discovered. Immunotherapy can be given in combination with antineoplastic chemotherapies, combination immunotherapy regimens, or as single agents.

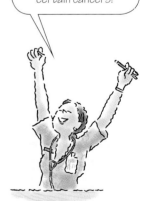

Good news!! Immunotherapy has shown great improvement in survival rates for certain cancers!

Drug interactions

Systemic corticosteroids may significantly diminish therapeutic effect of immunotherapy. Consider different treatment or avoid all together. However, if a patient is experiencing an adverse reaction, corticosteroids are used to help reverse immune-mediated reactions.

Vemurafenib in combination with ipilimumab (Yervoy) may enhance hepatotoxic effect.

Side effects/Adverse reactions

Immune-mediated adverse reactions include dermatologic toxicity, endocrinopathies, including type 1 diabetes, thyroid disorders, and adrenal insufficiency. Colitis, hepatitis, nephritis, ocular toxicity, pneumonitis, neurologic, and other toxicities of any organ system or tissue can occur and be life threatening if not treated.

The Three-Step Approach

Nursing management for patients needing immunotherapy includes these three steps. If the patient is receiving cytotoxic antineoplastic chemotherapy in combination with immunotherapy, refer to chemotherapy education and safe management and administration of cytotoxic antineoplastics.

Preadministration

(Recognize and analyze cues)

- Perform a complete assessment before therapy begins, including medication reconciliation. If the patient is on steroids, notify the prescriber.
- Review lab work including platelet and total and differential white blood cell (WBC) counts as well as hemoglobin, hematocrit, alanine aminotransferase (ALT), aspartate aminotransferase (AST), serum bilirubin, blood urea nitrogen (BUN), serum creatinine, glucose, TSH, T3 and T4, ACTH, and other lab work as needed.
- Ensure stability of electrolytes on blood work. Provide replacements as needed.
- Ensure that the patient is not pregnant or nursing prior to administration. Teach women of childbearing age and men to use effective contraceptive methods during therapy and for at least 6 months following the completion of therapy.
- Obtain a baseline weight before therapy, and weigh the patient daily throughout therapy. Evaluate and treat unexpected and rapid weight gain.
- Monitor vital signs at ordered intervals.

(Prioritize hypothesis—priority patient problems)

- Infection risk
- Safety risk
- Knowledge deficiency

(Generate solutions)

- The patient will remain free from infection from drug-induced immunosuppression.
- The patient will report signs and symptoms of immune-mediated adverse reactions.
- The patient and family will demonstrate an understanding of drug therapy, including dosing schedule and importance of taking their medication.

Medication administration

(Take action)

- Follow the established procedures for safe and proper handling, administration, and disposal of drugs. Chemoprotective PPE is required for immunotherapy administration.
- Monitor the patient's vital signs and catheter or IV line patency throughout drug administration. Central line is usually not required.
- Monitor for signs and symptoms of infusion reactions. Premedicate prior to infusion. Interrupt or slow the infusion for grade 1 or 2 infusion reactions. Discontinue if the patient experiences grade 3 or 4 infusion-related reaction after premedications.
- Give immunotherapy through a dedicated IV line using a 0.22-micrometer filter.
- Infusion is usually 30 to 60 minutes and does not require titration.

Postadministration

(Evaluate outcomes)

- The patient will remain free from infection.
- Monitor the patient for adverse reactions and drug interactions on an ongoing basis. Monitor closely for clinical signs/symptoms of immune-mediated adverse reactions, including adrenal insufficiency, colitis/diarrhea, dermatologic toxicity, diabetes/hyperglycemia, hepatitis/hepatotoxicity, hypophysitis or hypopituitarism, pneumonitis, ocular toxicity, and thyroid disorders.
- The patient and family will demonstrate an understanding of drug therapy, including dosing schedule.
- The patient will need frequent lab work to continue to evaluate CBC, thyroid, endocrine function, liver, and kidney function.

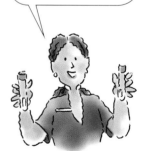

The patient will need frequent lab work to continue to evaluate levels.

Targeted treatments

A groundbreaking approach to anticancer therapies is to target proteins associated with the growth patterns for a specific type of cancer. This allows a specific protein to be targeted, rather than damaging all cells as with traditional cytotoxic chemotherapy.

Targeted therapies

These targeted therapies include:
- epidermal growth factor receptor (EGFR) inhibitors
- tyrosine kinase inhibitors (TKIs)
- vascular endothelial growth factor (VEGF) inhibitors
- proteasome inhibitors.

Targeted therapies

Targeted therapies can be intravenous (IV), subcutaneous, or oral, depending on the drug. Side effects can be less pronounced than with traditional cytotoxic antineoplastic agents but still require monitoring and assessment to prevent untoward adverse effects. These can be given in combination with cytotoxic antineoplastic agents or as single agent treatment.

Preadministration

(Recognize and analyze cues)
- Perform a complete assessment before therapy begins, including medication reconciliation.
- Review lab work.
- Ensure stability of electrolytes on blood work. Provide replacements as needed.
- Ensure that medication for prevention of skin rash is ordered. Instruct the patient to report skin changes promptly.
- Ensure that the patient is not pregnant or nursing prior to administration. Teach women of childbearing age and men to use effective contraceptive methods during therapy and for at least 6 months following the completion of therapy.
- Obtain a baseline weight before therapy, and weigh the patient daily throughout therapy. Evaluate and treat unexpected and rapid weight gain.
- Monitor vital signs at ordered intervals.

Medication administration

(Take action)
- Follow the established procedures for safe and proper handling, administration, and disposal of drugs. Chemoprotective PPE is required for all antineoplastic administration. Do not cut, crush, or touch oral medications. Wear gloves when administering oral medications.

The three-step approach for ALL targeted therapies

The following three-step process is standard for ALL targeted therapy agents regardless of administration route. Refer to this broader three-step approach when preparing or administering these drugs.

Postadministration

(Evaluate outcomes)

- The patient will remain free from infection, including skin infections.
- The patient will establish a rigorous skin care regimen to prevent complications with EGFR rash.
- Monitor the patient closely for fluid retention, which can be severe.
- Monitor the patient for adverse reactions and drug interactions on an ongoing basis. Patients will need to be monitored for 1 hour post cetuximab (Erbitux) and panitumumab (Vectibix) infusion for reaction.
- Evaluate the patient's and family's understanding of drug therapy, including dosing schedule and importance of taking their medication.
- The patient will need frequent lab work to continue to evaluate CBC, liver, and kidney function and electrolytes.

Epidermal growth factor receptor (EGFR) inhibitors

Epidermal growth factor proteins promote cell proliferation and differentiation. Their antitumor effects are mediated in part by inhibition of tumor angiogenesis as well as a reduced production of proangiogenic factors by tumor cells.

- Cetuximab (Erbitux)
- Erlotinib (Tarceva)
- Panitumumab (Vectibix)

Pharmacokinetics

The half-life of cetuximab (Erbitux) is 112 hours, and for erlotinib (Tarceva), it is 36 hours. Dosing adjustments need to occur for severe renal or hepatic impairment. Erlotinib (Tarceva) is 100% bioavailable when taken with food; however, it needs to be taken on an empty stomach.

Pharmacodynamics

EGFR inhibitors bind specifically to the epidermal growth factor receptor and competitively inhibits the binding of epidermal growth factor and other ligands. This results in inhibition of cell growth, induction of apoptosis, and decreased vascular endothelial growth factor production.

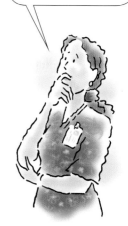

Dosing adjustments need to occur for severe renal or hepatic impairment.

Pharmacotherapeutics

Cancers that have an overexpression of EGFR are certain lung cancers, colorectal cancers, and head and neck cancers. The tumor cell must have the overexpression of EGFR to respond to this treatment. Cetuximab (Erbitux) is used for KRAS wild-type colorectal and squamous cell head and neck cancers. Erlotinib (Tarceva) is used for non–small cell lung cancer with exon 19 deletion or exon 21 substitution mutation and unresectable or metastatic pancreatic cancer.

Drug interactions

There are no known significant drug interactions with cetuximab (Erbitux). The following drug interactions are associated with erlotinib (Tarceva).

- Avoid tobacco if possible. If not able, dose increases need to occur at 2-week intervals in 50 mg increments.
- Avoid grapefruit and grapefruit juice.
- Avoid concomitant use with proton pump inhibitors or antacids.

Side effects/Adverse reactions

- Skin changes (acneiform, erythema, erythematous rash, desquamation, nail bed changes). The rash usually starts within the first 2 weeks of therapy.
- Fatigue.
- Electrolyte imbalances—can be life threatening.
- Peripheral edema.
- GI perforation.
- Diarrhea.
- Cough.
- Hyperbilirubinemia.
- Thrombocytopenia.
- Ocular toxicities.

The Three-Step Nursing Approach

Nursing management for patients needing EGFR therapy includes these three steps.

Reminder to review the broader *The three-step approach* that applies to ALL targeted therapies on page 672.

Preadministration

(Recognize and analyze cues)
- Review lab work including platelet and total and differential white blood cell (WBC) counts as well as hemoglobin, hematocrit, alanine aminotransferase (ALT), aspartate aminotransferase (AST), lactate dehydrogenase (LDH), serum bilirubin, blood urea nitrogen (BUN), serum creatinine, uric acid, electrolytes, magnesium, and other lab work as needed.

- Ensure that replacement electrolytes are ordered prior to infusion of cetuximab (Erbitux). Severe imbalances can occur.
- Obtain a baseline weight before therapy and weigh the patient daily throughout therapy. Evaluate and treat unexpected and rapid weight gain.
- Ensure that medication for prevention of skin rash is ordered. Instruct the patient to report skin changes promptly.

(Prioritize hypothesis—priority patient problems)
- Infection risk
- Electrolyte imbalance risk
- Nonadherence to oral drug regimen
- Knowledge deficiency

(Generate solutions)
- The patient will remain free from infection.
- The patient's electrolytes will remain within normal limits or be corrected in a timely manner.
- The patient and family will demonstrate an understanding of drug therapy, including dosing schedule and importance of taking their medication.

Medication administration
(Take action)
- Premedicate with antihistamine prior to cetuximab (Erbitux) and panitumumab (Vectibix) infusion. Stop infusion immediately upon infusion reaction. Keep diphenhydramine, hydrocortisone, and epinephrine, in case of infusion reaction. Keep necessary emergency equipment available to establish an airway in case of anaphylaxis.
- Use a 0.22-micrometer filter with cetuximab (Erbitux) and panitumumab (Vectibix).
- Give erlotinib (Tarceva) greater than 1 hour before meals or 2 hours after.
- Give erlotinib (Tarceva) at the same time every day.

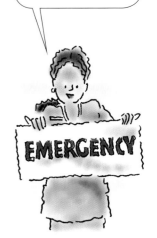

Keep diphenhydramine, hydrocortisone, and epinephrine, in case of infusion reaction. Keep necessary emergency equipment available to establish an airway in case of anaphylaxis.

Postadministration
(Evaluate outcomes)
- The patient will remain free from infection, including skin infections.
- The patient will establish a rigorous skin care regimen to prevent complications with EGFR rash.
- Monitor the patient closely for fluid retention, which can be severe.
- Monitor the patient for adverse reactions and drug interactions on an ongoing basis. Patients will need to be monitored for 1 hour post cetuximab (Erbitux) and panitumumab (Vectibix) infusion for reaction.

- Evaluate the patient's and family's understanding of drug therapy, including dosing schedule and importance of taking their medication.
- The patient will need frequent lab work to continue to evaluate CBC, liver, and kidney function and electrolytes.

Tyrosine kinase inhibitors (TKIs)

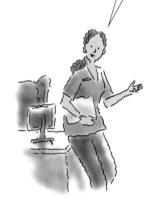

Tyrosine kinase inhibitors (TKIs) have demonstrated promising antitumor activities in a variety of malignancies.

Tyrosine kinase inhibitors (TKIs) have demonstrated promising antitumor activities in a variety of malignancies. Unlike monoclonal antibodies, these drugs have the bioavailability to be dosed orally (Kuo, 2020). There are similarities in the EGFR and TKI receptor categories; the drugs can fit into several categories based off mechanism of action. There is some crossover to EGFR and TKI receptors and drug categorization.

- Dasatinib (Sprycel)
- Gefitinib (Iressa)
- Ibrutinib (Imbruvica)
- Imatinib (Gleevec)
- Nilotinib (Tasigna)

Pharmacokinetics

Gefitinib (Iressa) is available in an oral form of which approximately half the dose is absorbed. The drug is widely distributed in tissues. It undergoes hepatic metabolism with minimal urinary excretion.

Imatinib (Gleevec) is available in an oral form, which is almost completely absorbed. It is 95% bound to plasma proteins and extensively metabolized by the liver. The half-life is approximately 15 hours.

Pharmacodynamics

Gefitinib (Iressa) inhibits the epidermal growth factor receptor-1 tyrosine kinase, which is overexpressed with certain cancers, such as non–small cell lung cancer. This blocks signaling pathways for the growth, survival, and metastasis of cancer.

In a bind

Imatinib (Gleevec) binds to the adenosine triphosphate–binding domain of the BCR-ABL protein, which stimulates other tyrosine kinase proteins to result in abnormally high production of WBCs in chronic myeloid leukemia. This binding of imatinib (Gleevec) effectively shuts down the abnormal WBC production.

Pharmacotherapeutics

Gefitinib (Iressa) is used for patients with non–small cell lung cancer. Imatinib (Gleevec) is used to treat chronic myeloid leukemia, acute lymphoid leukemia, and GI stromal tumors.

Drug interactions

- Administration of gefitinib (Iressa) or imatinib with warfarin (Coumadin) causes elevations in the international normalized ratio (INR), increasing the risk of bleeding.
- Drugs that inhibit the CYP3A4 family (such as clarithromycin, erythromycin, itraconazole, and ketoconazole) when taken with gefitinib (Iressa) and imatinib (Gleevec) may increase gefitinib (Iressa) and imatinib (Gleevec) plasma levels.
- Imatinib (Gleevec) administered with CYP3A4 inducers (carbamazepine [Tegretol], dexamethasone [Decadron], phenobarbital, phenytoin [Dilantin], and rifampin) may increase the metabolism of imatinib (Gleevec) and decrease imatinib (Gleevec) levels.
- Imatinib (Gleevec) given with simvastatin (Zocor) increases simvastatin (Zocor) levels about threefold.
- Imatinib (Gleevec) increases plasma levels of other CYP3A4-metabolized drugs, such as triazolobenzodiazepines, dihydropyridine, calcium channel blockers, and certain HMG-CoA reductase inhibitors.
- Avoid grapefruit and grapefruit juice with imatinib (Gleevec). Gefitinib (Iressa) may have increased serum concentrations with grapefruit; monitor closely.

Side effects/Adverse reactions

Gefitinib (Iressa)

- Skin rash
- Diarrhea
- Abnormal eyelash growth, ocular toxicity
- GI perforation
- Lung and liver damage

Imatinib (Gleevec)

- Skin rash
- Edema (periorbital and lower limb), which may result in pulmonary edema, effusions, and heart or renal failure; management includes treatment with diuretics and supportive measures such as decreasing the dosage
- Nausea, vomiting, liver function abnormalities, and myelosuppression (especially neutropenia and thrombocytopenia)

The Three-Step Approach

Nursing management for patients needing targeted TKI therapy includes these three steps.

Reminder to review the broader *The three-step approach* **that applies to ALL targeted therapies on page 672.**

Preadministration

(Recognize and analyze cues)

- Review lab work including platelet and total and differential white blood cell (WBC) counts as well as hemoglobin, hematocrit, alanine aminotransferase (ALT), aspartate aminotransferase (AST), lactate dehydrogenase (LDH), serum bilirubin, blood urea nitrogen (BUN), serum creatinine, uric acid, electrolytes, and other lab work as needed.

(Prioritize hypothesis—priority patient problems)

- Infection risk
- Nonadherence risk
- Knowledge deficiency

(Generate solutions)

- The patient will not develop infection associated with drug-induced immunosuppression.
- The patient and family will demonstrate an understanding of drug therapy, including dosing schedule and importance of taking their medication.

Medication administration

(Take action)

- Gefitinib (Iressa) can be given without regard to food.
- Imatinib (Gleevec) should be given with a meal and a large glass of water. Antiemetics may need to be administered.
- Give gefitinib (Iressa) and imatinib (Gleevec) at the same time every day.

Postadministration

(Evaluate outcomes)

- The patient will remain free from infection.
- Monitor the patient closely for fluid retention, which can be severe.
- Monitor the patient for adverse reactions and drug interactions on an ongoing basis.
- Evaluate the patient's and family's understanding of drug therapy, including dosing schedule and importance of taking their medication.
- The patient will need frequent lab work to continue to evaluate CBC, liver, and kidney function.
- Instruct the patient to report skin changes, vision changes, severe abdominal pain, or signs of hepatic impairment.

Vascular endothelial growth factor (VEGF) inhibitors

Vascular growth factors work selectively on vascular endothelial cells and are capable of stimulating angiogenesis. These inhibitors work to stop this from occurring. Drugs included in this category:

- axitinib (Inlyta)
- bevacizumab (Avastin)
- lenvatinib (Lenvima)
- ramucirumab (Cyramza)
- sunitinib (Sutent)
- sorafenib (NexAVAR)
- pazopanib (Votrient).

Pharmacokinetics

Bevacizumab (Avastin) and ramucirumab (Cyramza) are given as infusion.

Sunitinib (Sutent) is metabolized hepatically by CYP3A4 with a half-life of 40 to 60 hours. It is primarily excreted through feces.

Pharmacodynamics

This category of VEGF inhibitors also has activity on the tyrosine kinase inhibitor of vascular endothelial growth factor (VEGF) receptors. Inhibition of these receptor tyrosine kinases leads to decreased tumor growth and slowing of cancer progression.

Pharmacotherapeutics

Bevacizumab (Avastin) is used in metastatic colorectal cancer and glioblastoma.

Lenvatinib (Lenvima) is used to treat metastatic or locally advanced thyroid malignancy. It can also be used in hepatocellular or renal cell carcinoma.

Sunitinib (Sutent) is used in GI stromal tumor, pancreatic neuroendocrine tumors, and renal cell carcinoma.

Drug interactions

Prolongation of the QT interval can occur with these drugs. Use caution with other drugs that may prolong the QT interval. Avoid concomitant use of bevacizumab (Avastin), sunitinib (Sutent), and sorafenib (Nexavar).

Side effects/Adverse reactions

- Dose adjustments or discontinuation is likely based on severity of side effects. Delayed wound healing and thrombotic events can occur with these drugs. Gastrointestinal perforation can also occur.

Bevacizumab (Avastin)
Side effects/adverse reactions to bevacizumab include:
- hemorrhage
- hypertension
- proteinuria.

Lenvatinib (Lenvima)

Side effects/adverse reactions to lenvatinib include:

- hypertension
- abdominal pain, nausea, vomiting, diarrhea, stomatitis
- arthralgia.

The Three-Step Approach

Nursing management for patients needing targeted VEGF inhibitor therapy includes these three steps.

Reminder to review *The three-step approach* that applies to ALL targeted therapies on page 672.

Preadministration

(Recognize and analyze cues)

- Review lab work including platelet and total and differential white blood cell (WBC) counts as well as hemoglobin, hematocrit, alanine aminotransferase (ALT), aspartate aminotransferase (AST), lactate dehydrogenase (LDH), serum bilirubin, blood urea nitrogen (BUN), serum creatinine, uric acid, electrolytes, urinalysis (UA), and other lab work as needed.
- Ensure that the patient has not had surgery within 28 days of bevacizumab (Avastin) infusion. Delayed wound healing and increased bleeding risk can occur.

(Prioritize hypothesis—priority patient problems)

- Infection risk
- Bleeding risk
- Nonadherence risk
- Knowledge deficiency

(Generate solutions)

- The patient will not develop infection associated with drug-induced immunosuppression.
- The patient will remain free from bleeding or clotting events.
- The patient and family will demonstrate an understanding of drug therapy, including dosing schedule and importance of taking their medication.

Medication administration

(Take action)

- Because GI irritation is common, antiemetics may need to be given.
- Bevacizumab (Avastin) and ramucirumab (Cyramza) have risk of infusion-related reaction. Ramucirumab (Cyramza) requires premedication and use of a 0.22-micron inline filter.
- Stop infusion immediately if an infusion reaction is suspected. Keep diphenhydramine, hydrocortisone, epinephrine, and necessary emergency equipment available to establish an airway in case of anaphylaxis.

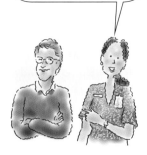

Ensure that the patient has not had surgery within 28 days of bevacizumab (Avastin) infusion.

- Check urine for protein prior to each bevacizumab (Avastin) infusion or as ordered.
- Lenvatinib (Lenvima) and sunitinib (Sutent) may be given with or without regard to food. Sorafenib (NexAVAR) must be administered without food.
- Lenvatinib (Lenvima) and sorafenib (NexAVAR) capsules may be dissolved in a small amount of water. Ensure dosing at least 1 hour before or 2 hours after a meal.
- Give oral preparations at the same time every day.

Postadministration
(Evaluate outcomes)
- Monitor for and promptly address signs of infection.
- Evaluate for and proactively address nausea and vomiting.
- Monitor the patient closely for hypertension and bleeding, which can be severe.
- Monitor the patient for adverse reactions and drug interactions on an ongoing basis.
- Evaluate the patient's and family's understanding of drug therapy, including dosing schedule and importance of taking their medication.
- The patient will need frequent lab work to continue to evaluate CBC, liver, and kidney function.
- The patient should be instructed to report bleeding or abnormal bruising.

Proteasome inhibitors

Cancer cells produce proteins that promote both cell survival and proliferation, and/or inhibit apoptosis. Proteasome inhibitors effectively block this pathway providing a very valuable treatment option. Discovery of the proteasome pathway led to significantly improved outcomes for multiple myeloma.

These drugs include:
- bortezomib (Velcade)
- carfilzomib (Kyprolis)
- ixazomib (Ninlaro).

Pharmacokinetics

Bortezomib (Velcade) is not absorbed orally and usually given subcutaneously. It can also be given intravenously. It is extensively distributed into body tissues and hepatically metabolized. Ixazomib (Ninlaro) has a terminal half-life of 9.5 days. Dosing may need to be adjusted with renal and hepatic impairments.

Pharmacodynamics

Feeling a bit inhibited...

Proteasome inhibitors inhibit proteasomes, which are integral to cell cycle function and promote tumor growth. Proteolysis by these drugs results in the disruption of normal homeostatic mechanisms and leads to cell death.

Drug interactions

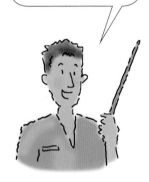

Bortezomib (Velcade) when taken with drugs that are inhibitors or inducers of CYP3A4 may cause either toxicities or reduced efficacy of these drugs.

- Bortezomib (Velcade) when taken with drugs that are inhibitors or inducers of CYP3A4 may cause either toxicities or reduced efficacy of these drugs. Inhibitors of CYP3A4 include amiodarone, cimetidine, erythromycin, diltiazem, disulfiram, fluoxetine, grapefruit juice, verapamil, zafirlukast, and zileuton. Inducers of CYP3A4 include amiodarone, carbamazepine, nevirapine, phenobarbital, phenytoin, and rifampin.
- Bortezomib, when taken with oral antidiabetic agents, may cause hypoglycemia or hyperglycemia in patients with diabetes.
- Ixazomib (Ninlaro) may decrease serum concentrations of estrogen and progestins. Patients should use a nonhormonal barrier contraception while undergoing treatment.
- Carfilzomib (Kyprolis) may increase thrombogenic effect of estrogen and progestins. Consider alternative nonhormonal contraceptive methods.

Side effects/Adverse reactions

Bortezomib (Velcade)

The most common adverse reactions to bortezomib (Velcade) include asthenic conditions (fatigue, malaise, and weakness), nausea, diarrhea, appetite loss (anorexia), constipation, pyrexia, and vomiting. Other reactions include:

- peripheral neuropathy (usually reversible), headache, hypotension, liver toxicity, thrombocytopenia, and renal toxicity
- cardiac toxicity (arrhythmias, such as bradycardia, ventricular tachycardia, atrial fibrillation, and atrial flutter; heart failure; myocardial ischemia and infarction; pulmonary edema; and pericardial effusion).

Depending on the severity of the reactions, the dosage may need to be reduced or the drug withheld until toxicity resolves. Severe reactions may require discontinuing the medication.

The Three-Step Approach

Nursing management for patients receiving proteasome inhibitor therapy includes these three steps.

Reminder to review *The three-step approach* that applies to ALL targeted therapies on page 672.

Preadministration

(Recognize and analyze cues)

- Review lab work including platelet and total and differential white blood cell (WBC) counts as well as hemoglobin, hematocrit, alanine aminotransferase (ALT), aspartate aminotransferase (AST), lactate dehydrogenase (LDH), serum bilirubin, blood urea nitrogen (BUN), serum creatinine, uric acid, and other lab work as needed.
- The dose of bortezomib (Velcade) should not be given unless the patient's platelet count is greater than 70,000/mcL, ANC is greater than 1,000/mcL.
- Hormonal contraceptives may have decreased efficacy; additional considerations should be taken.
- Bortezomib (Velcade) can cause hypotension.

(Prioritize hypothesis—priority patient problems)

- Infection risk
- Nonadherence
- Knowledge deficiency

(Generate solutions)

- The patient will not develop infection associated with drug-induced immunosuppression.
- The patient will have normal blood pressure measurements. Dose adjustments of antihypertensives may be warranted.
- The patient and family will demonstrate an understanding of drug therapy, including dosing schedule and importance of taking their medication.

Medication administration

(Take action)

- Because GI irritation is common, antiemetics may need to be given.
- Bortezomib (Velcade) is given subcutaneously. Ensure that skin is intact and avoid scarred areas. Rotate injection sites. If IV administration is ordered, monitor IV site before, during, and after infusion for blood return. It is given as a rapid IV push over 3 to 5 seconds.

Postadministration

(Evaluate outcomes)

- The patient will not develop infection associated with drug-induced immunosuppression.
- Evaluate for signs of and promptly address hypotension associated with bortezomib (Velcade).
- Monitor the patient closely for fluid retention, which can be severe.

- Monitor the patient for adverse reactions and drug interactions on an ongoing basis.
- Evaluate the patient's and family's understanding of drug therapy, including dosing schedule and importance of taking their medication.
- The patient will need frequent lab work to continue to evaluate CBC, liver, and kidney function.

Endocrine and hormone modulators

Endocrine and hormone modulators are prescribed to alter the growth of malignant neoplasms. These drugs fall into four classes:
- aromatase inhibitors
- antiestrogens
- antiandrogens
- gonadotropin-releasing hormone analogues.

Hitting them where it hurts

Hormonal therapies and hormone modulators prove effective against hormone-dependent tumors, such as cancers of the prostate, breast, and endometrium. Lymphomas and leukemias are usually treated with therapies that include corticosteroids because of their potential for affecting lymphocytes.

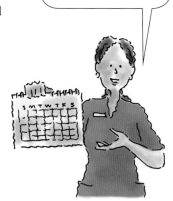

Steady-state plasma levels after daily doses of aromatase inhibitors are reached in 2 to 6 weeks.

Aromatase inhibitors

Aromatase inhibitors (AI) prevent androgen from being converted into estrogen in postmenopausal women. This blocks estrogen's ability to activate cancer cells by limiting the amount of estrogen reaching the cancer cells to promote growth. Aromatase inhibitors may be type 1 steroidal inhibitors, such as the drug exemestane (Aromasin), or type 2 nonsteroidal inhibitors, such as anastrozole (Arimidex) and letrozole (Femara).

Pharmacokinetics

Aromatase inhibitors are taken orally in pill form and are generally well tolerated by most women. Steady-state plasma levels after daily doses are reached in 2 to 6 weeks. Inactive metabolites are excreted in urine.

Pharmacodynamics

In postmenopausal women, estrogen is produced through aromatase, an enzyme that converts hormone precursors into estrogen. Aromatase inhibitors work by lowering the body's production of the female hormone estrogen. In approximately 75% of patients with breast cancer, the tumor growth is dependent on estrogen (Pritchard, 2020).

After the pause

Aromatase inhibitors are used in postmenopausal women because they lower the amount of circulating estrogen that is produced outside the ovaries in muscle and fat tissue. Because they induce estrogen deprivation, bone thinning and osteoporosis may develop in time.

What's your type?

Type 1 inhibitors irreversibly inhibit the aromatase enzyme, whereas type 2 inhibitors reversibly inhibit the aromatase enzyme. It has also been suggested that type 1 aromatase inhibitors might have some effect after the failure of a type 2 aromatase inhibitor.

Exemestane (Aromasin) selectively inhibits estrogen synthesis and does not affect synthesis of adrenocorticosteroid, aldosterone, or thyroid hormones. Anastrozole (Arimidex) and letrozole (Femara) act by inhibiting aromatase, and the conversion of androstenedione to estrone and testosterones to estradiol is prevented. They do not affect synthesis of adrenocorticosteroid, aldosterone, or thyroid hormones.

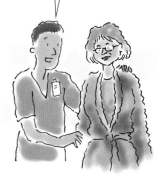

Aromatase inhibitors lower the amount of estrogen that's produced outside the ovaries in muscle and fat tissue. They're primarily used for postmenopausal women with metastatic breast cancer.

Pharmacotherapeutics

Aromatase inhibitors are indicated primarily for postmenopausal women with breast cancer. These are usually started after adjuvant treatment is complete.

Drug interactions

- Certain drugs may decrease the effectiveness of anastrozole (Arimidex), including tamoxifen and estrogen-containing drugs.
- Exemestane (Aromasin) given in combination with cytochrome P-450 isoenzyme 3A4 (CYP3A4) inducers may result in decreased serum exemestane (Aromasin) concentrations.
- St. John's wort decreases serum concentration of exemestane (Aromasin).

Side effects/Adverse reactions

Side effects/adverse reactions to aromatase inhibitors are rare but may include dizziness, fever, pharyngitis, mild nausea, anorexia, urinary tract infections, mild muscle and joint aches, hot flashes, alopecia, and increased sweating. They can also affect cholesterol levels; anastrozole (Arimidex) may elevate high-density lipoprotein and low-density lipoprotein levels. Bone mineral density loss and osteoporosis may occur. Patients have experienced swelling of the face, lips, and throat after administration.

Preadministration
(Recognize and analyze cues)
- Perform a complete assessment before therapy begins, including medication reconciliation. Ensure that there are no estrogen-containing medications, including vaginal or topical preparations. Ensure that no testosterone-containing supplements are being taken.
- Ensure that patients have had a baseline bone mineral density test.
- Ensure that the patient is not pregnant or nursing prior to administration. Teach women of childbearing age and men to use effective contraceptive methods during therapy and for at least 6 months following the completion of therapy.
- Monitor vital signs for hypertension.

Medication administration
(Take action)
- Follow the established procedures for safe and proper handling, administration, and disposal of drugs. Chemoprotective PPE is required for all hormonal treatment administration. Wear gloves when administering medication.
- Oral drug dosing should be the same time every day.

Postadministration
(Evaluate outcomes)
- The patient will not experience activity intolerance associated with acute bone and joint pain during drug initiation.
- Evaluate for and promptly address pain associated with drug side effects. Use supportive treatments to help manage side effects from the treatment.
- Encourage the patient to incorporate routine exercise and stretching to help prevent musculoskeletal side effects. Weight-bearing activities can help prevent bone density loss.
- The patient should also be on vitamin D and calcium supplementation.
- Evaluate the patient's and family's understanding of drug therapy.
- Monitor lipid levels during long-term therapy in patients with hyperlipidemia.
- Arrange for consult to dietitian if the patient has persistently elevated glucose levels.
- Ensure that the patient understands that frequent lab work to continue to evaluate CBC, liver, and kidney function.
- Evaluate the patient's and family's understanding of drug therapy.

The three-step approach for ALL endocrine and hormone modulators

General nursing management for endocrine and hormonal treatments are listed below. Drug specifics will still be listed under each header. Refer to this broader three-step approach when preparing or administering these drugs.

The Three-Step Approach

Nursing management for patients needing aromatase inhibitor (AI) therapy includes these three steps.

Remember to refer to the broader *The three-step approach* for ALL endocrine and hormone modulators listed on page 672.

Preadministration

(Recognize and analyze cues)

- Review lab work including platelet and total and differential white blood cell (WBC) counts as well as hemoglobin, hematocrit, alanine aminotransferase (ALT), aspartate aminotransferase (AST), lactate dehydrogenase (LDH), serum bilirubin, blood urea nitrogen (BUN), serum creatinine, uric acid, cholesterol, LDL, vitamin D, and other lab work as needed.
- Ensure that the patient is postmenopausal prior to administration. Do not use AIs in premenopausal women unless ovarian function is suppressed.

(Prioritize hypothesis—priority patient problems)

- Activity intolerance
- Knowledge deficiency

(Generate solutions)

- The patient will not experience activity intolerance associated with acute bone and joint pain during drug initiation.
- The patient and family will demonstrate an understanding of drug therapy.

Medication administration

(Take action)

- Dose can be given with or without food. Exemestane (Aromasin) should be given after a meal.

Postadministration

(Evaluate outcomes)

- Monitor for and promptly address any adverse effects such as bone and joint pain that would affect activity.

Antiestrogens

Antiestrogens bind to estrogen receptors and block estrogen action. The antiestrogens include tamoxifen citrate, toremifene citrate, and fulvestrant (Faslodex).

Feeling antagonistic?

Tamoxifen and toremifene are nonsteroidal estrogen agonist-antagonists. Fulvestrant (Faslodex) is a pure estrogen antagonist.

Pharmacokinetics

After oral administration, tamoxifen is absorbed well and undergoes extensive metabolism in the liver before being excreted in feces. IM injection of fulvestrant (Faslodex) yields peak serum levels in 7 to 9 days; fulvestrant (Faslodex) has a half-life of 40 days. Toremifene is well absorbed and is not influenced by food.

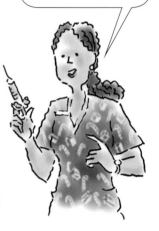

IM injection of fulvestrant results in peak serum levels in 7 to 9 days.

Pharmacodynamics

The exact action of these agents is unknown. However, it is known that they act as estrogen antagonists. Estrogen receptors, found in the cancer cells of half of premenopausal and three fourths of postmenopausal women with breast cancer, respond to estrogen to induce tumor growth.

It's bound to inhibit growth

Tamoxifen, toremifene, and fulvestrant (Faslodex) bind to estrogen receptors and inhibit estrogen-mediated tumor growth in breast tissue. Tamoxifen can retain estrogen antagonist activity in other tissue such as bone. Ultimately, DNA synthesis and cell growth are inhibited.

Pharmacotherapeutics

The antiestrogen tamoxifen citrate is used alone in high-risk or premenopausal women diagnosed with estrogen receptor–positive cancer.

Further tales of tamoxifen

It is also used for breast cancer in postmenopausal women who have estrogen receptor–positive tumors. Tumors in postmenopausal women are more responsive to tamoxifen than those in premenopausal women. Tamoxifen may also be used to reduce the incidence of breast cancer in healthy women at high risk for breast cancer. (See *Who benefits from tamoxifen?*, page 739.)

Toremifene is used to treat metastatic breast cancer in postmenopausal women with estrogen receptor–positive tumors. Fulvestrant (Faslodex) is used in postmenopausal women with receptor-positive metastatic breast cancer with disease progression after treatment with tamoxifen.

Drug interactions

- Fulvestrant (Faslodex) has no known drug interactions.
- Tamoxifen and toremifene may increase the effects of warfarin sodium (Coumadin), increasing prothrombin time (PT), and the risk of bleeding.
- Tamoxifen should not be taken with aromatase inhibitors.
- Bromocriptine (Cycloset; Parlodel) increases the effects of tamoxifen.
- QT prolongation—use caution if concurrent medications have this risk.

Who benefits from tamoxifen?

The current indication for the use of tamoxifen is based on the 1998 results of the Breast Cancer Prevention Trial (BCPT) sponsored by the National Cancer Institute. Results indicated that tamoxifen reduced the rate of breast cancer in healthy high-risk women by one half. However, tamoxifen can cause serious adverse reactions, including potentially fatal blood clots and uterine cancer. The question is whether these risks are worth the benefits in healthy women.

The National Cancer Institute's report

To help answer this question, the National Cancer Institute published a report in November 1999. It concluded that most women over age 60 would receive more harm than benefit from tamoxifen. Even though women under age 60 could benefit from taking tamoxifen, they were still at risk unless they had undergone a hysterectomy, which eliminated the risk of uterine cancer, or were in the very high-risk group for developing breast cancer.

Breaking it down further

The report also concluded that the risks of tamoxifen were greater than the benefits for black women over age 60 and for almost all other women over age 60 who still had a uterus. But for older women without a uterus and with a 3.5% chance of developing breast cancer over the next 5 years, the benefits may outweigh the risks.

NSABP studies update

A report from the 2000 annual meeting of the American Society of Clinical Oncology presented an analysis of data gathered from the National Surgical Adjuvant Breast and Bowel Project, which carried out nine studies of adjuvant tamoxifen therapy for breast cancer. The analysis indicated that tamoxifen is as effective in black women as in white women in reducing the occurrence of contralateral breast cancer (breast cancer that develops in the healthy breast after treatment in the opposite breast).

New findings

The Study of Tamoxifen and Raloxifene (STAR) is a clinical trial being conducted to determine whether raloxifene can prevent breast cancer better and with fewer adverse effects than tamoxifen.

The study, which began in 1999 and continued to enroll women until 2004, produced initial results in 2006. These results indicated that raloxifene is as effective as tamoxifen in reducing the risk of breast cancer. It also showed that the women who took raloxifene had fewer incidences of uterine cancer and fewer blood clots than the women who took tamoxifen. For more information on this study, go to http://www.cancer.gov/types/breast/research/star-trial-results-qa.

In 2007, follow-up studies of individuals from the BCPT revealed a reduction in risks of the serious adverse effects (blood clots, endometrial cancer) and a continuation of the beneficial effects even years after the drug was stopped.

Side effects/Adverse reactions

Side effects/adverse reactions to antiestrogens vary by drug. In general, antiestrogens are relatively nontoxic drugs.

Tamoxifen

The most common adverse reactions to tamoxifen include:

- hot flashes
- nausea and vomiting
- diarrhea
- fluid retention
- leukopenia or thrombocytopenia.

Toremifene

Side effects/adverse reactions to toremifene include:

- hot flashes
- sweating
- nausea and vomiting
- vaginal discharge or bleeding
- edema.

Fulvestrant (Faslodex)

Side effects/adverse reactions to fulvestrant (Faslodex) include:

- hot flashes
- nausea and vomiting
- diarrhea or constipation
- abdominal pain
- headache
- back pain
- pharyngitis.

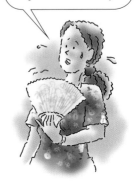

Whew! All of the antiestrogen drugs seem to cause hot flashes. I'd better keep my fan at the ready!

The Three-Step Approach

Nursing management for patients needing antiestrogen therapy includes these three steps.

Reminder to refer to the broader *The three-step approach* for ALL endocrine and hormone modulators approach listed on page 672.

Reminder to refer to the broader *The three-step approach* for ALL endocrine and hormone modulators approach listed on page 672.

Preadministration

(Recognize and analyze cues)

- Review lab work including platelet and total and differential white blood cell (WBC) counts as well as hemoglobin, hematocrit, alanine aminotransferase (ALT), aspartate aminotransferase (AST), lactate dehydrogenase (LDH), serum bilirubin, blood urea nitrogen (BUN), serum creatinine, and other lab work as needed.
- Educate the patient on increased risk of uterine cancer and blood clots with tamoxifen.

(Prioritize hypothesis—priority patient problems)

- Activity intolerance
- Knowledge deficiency

(Generate solutions)

- The patient will not experience activity intolerance associated with acute bone and joint pain during drug initiation.
- The patient and family will demonstrate an understanding of drug therapy.

Teaching about tamoxifen

If tamoxifen therapy is prescribed, review these points with the patient and caregivers:

• Report signs and symptoms of a pulmonary embolism (chest pain, difficulty breathing, rapid breathing, sweating, and fainting).

• Report signs and symptoms of a stroke, including headache, vision changes, confusion, difficulty speaking or walking, and weakness in the face, arm, or leg, especially on one side of the body.

• Encourage the patient to incorporate routine exercise and stretching to help prevent musculoskeletal side effects.

• Have regular gynecologic examinations because of an increased risk of uterine cancer.

• If you are taking the drug to reduce the risk of breast cancer, use the proper technique for breast self-examination. Review this with your health care provider.

• It is important to keep appointments for clinical breast examinations, annual mammograms, and gynecologic examinations.

• If you are premenopausal, use a barrier form of contraception because short-term therapy induces ovulation.

• If you are of childbearing age, avoid becoming pregnant during therapy and consult with your prescriber before becoming pregnant.

• Do not take any estrogen-containing formulations, including vaginal creams.

Medication administration

(Take action)

• Dose can be given with or without food.

Postadministration

(Evaluate outcomes)

• The patient will not experience activity intolerance associated with acute bone and joint pain during drug initiation.

• Encourage the patient to incorporate routine exercise and stretching to help prevent musculoskeletal side effects. Weight-bearing activities can help prevent bone density loss.

• Monitor lipid levels during long-term therapy in patients with hyperlipidemia.

• Evaluate the patient's and family's understanding of drug therapy. (See *Teaching about tamoxifen*.)

Antiandrogens

Antiandrogens are used as an adjunct therapy with gonadotropin-releasing hormone analogues in treating advanced prostate cancer. These drugs include:

• abiraterone (Zytiga)

• bicalutamide (Casodex)

- enzalutamide (Xtandi)
- flutamide
- nilutamide.

> Antiandrogens are used with a gonadotropin-releasing hormone analogue to treat metastatic prostate cancer.

Pharmacokinetics

After oral administration, antiandrogens are absorbed rapidly and completely. They are metabolized rapidly and extensively and excreted primarily in urine.

Pharmacodynamics

They exert their antiandrogenic action by inhibiting androgen uptake or preventing androgen binding in cell nuclei in target tissues.

Pharmacotherapeutics

Antiandrogens are used with a gonadotropin-releasing hormone analogue, such as leuprolide acetate (Lupron), to treat metastatic prostate cancer.

Drug interactions

Antiandrogens do not interact significantly with other drugs. However, flutamide and bicalutamide (Casodex) may affect clotting times (PT) in a patient receiving warfarin. Bicalutamide (Casodex) inhibits CYP3A4. Many interactions can occur.

Side effects/Adverse reactions

When an antiandrogen is used with a gonadotropin-releasing hormone analogue, the most common adverse reactions are:
- hot flashes
- decreased libido
- impotence
- blue-green or orange urine (flutamide)
- diarrhea
- nausea and vomiting
- breast enlargement.

The Three-Step Approach

Nursing management for patients needing antiandrogen therapy includes these three steps.

Reminder to refer to the broader *The three-step approach* for ALL endocrine and hormone modulators on page 672.

Preadministration
(Recognize and analyze cues)
- Review lab work including platelet and total and differential white blood cell (WBC) counts as well as hemoglobin, hematocrit,

alanine aminotransferase (ALT), aspartate aminotransferase (AST), lactate dehydrogenase (LDH), serum bilirubin, blood urea nitrogen (BUN), serum creatinine, potassium, PT/INR, testosterone, and other lab work as needed.

- Monitor liver function every 2 weeks for the first 3 months of therapy and then monthly thereafter.
- Ensure that the patient is receiving leuprolide acetate (Lupron) while on antiandrogen therapy.

(Prioritize hypothesis—priority patient problems)
Knowledge deficiency related to drug therapy and diagnosis.

(Generate solutions)
- The patient and family will demonstrate an understanding of drug therapy.
- The patient will respond well to drug therapy.

Medication administration

(Take action)
- Enzalutamide can be given with or without food. Abiraterone must be taken on an empty stomach.
- Swallow capsules whole. Do not crush, break, dissolve, or open them.
- Monitor for signs and symptoms of adrenocorticoid insufficiency.

Postadministration

(Evaluate outcomes)
- The patient will need to keep follow-up schedule for leuprolide acetate (Lupron) injections.
- The patient will need frequent follow-up lab work.
- The patient must prevent childbearing while on therapy.

Don't stop those drugs!

Teach the patient that they must take flutamide continuously with a drug used for medical castration, such as leuprolide acetate (Lupron), to allow for the full benefit of therapy. Leuprolide (Lupron) suppresses testosterone production, whereas flutamide inhibits testosterone action at the cellular level. Together, they can impair the growth of androgen-responsive tumors. Advise the patient not to discontinue either drug.

- Monitor the patient for adverse reactions and drug interactions.

Gonadotropin-releasing hormone analogues

Gonadotropin-releasing hormone analogues are used to treat advanced prostate cancer. Goserelin can help down regulate estrogen in estrogen receptor–positive breast cancer. They include:

- goserelin acetate (Zoladex)
- leuprolide acetate (Lupron, IM; Eligard, SQ)
- triptorelin pamoate (Trelstar).

Pharmacokinetics

Subcutaneous goserelin (Zoladex) is absorbed slowly for the first 8 days of therapy and rapidly and continuously thereafter. After subQ injection, leuprolide (Eligard) is absorbed well. The distribution, metabolism, and excretion of these drugs is not clearly defined. Triptorelin (Trelstar) reaches peak serum levels within 1 week of IM injection, with serum levels remaining detectable for 4 weeks.

Pharmacodynamics

Initially, leuprolide (Lupron, Eligard) acts on the pituitary gland of a male patient to increase luteinizing hormone (LH) secretion, which in turn stimulates testosterone production. Goserelin (Zoladex) decreases the testosterone or estradiol level.

The rise . . .

The peak testosterone level is reached 5 to 12 days after administration. Triptorelin is a potent inhibitor of gonadotropin secretion. After the first dose, levels of LH, follicle-stimulating hormone (FSH), testosterone, and estradiol surge transiently. It takes 2 to 4 weeks to achieve a sustained decrease of these hormones.

. . . and fall

After long-term, continuous administration, LH and FSH secretion steadily declines and testicular steroidogenesis decreases. In men, testosterone declines to a level typically seen in surgically castrated men. As a result, tissues and functions that depend on these hormones become inactive.

Reversing course

The drop in LH secretion occurs because, with long-term administration, goserelin (Zoladex) and leuprolide (Lupron, Eligard) inhibit LH release from the pituitary gland, which subsequently inhibits testicular release of testosterone. Because prostate tumor cells are stimulated by testosterone, the reduced testosterone level inhibits tumor growth.

Pharmacotherapeutics

Goserelin (Zoladex), leuprolide (Lupron, Eligard), and triptorelin (Trelstar) are used for the palliative treatment of metastatic prostate cancer. These drugs lower the testosterone level without the adverse psychological effects of surgical castration. These drugs can also be used as adjuvant therapy with oral antiestrogens to help premenopausal breast cancer patients achieve ovarian suppression.

Drug interactions

No direct drug interactions have been identified; however, they have a risk of prolonging the QT interval. Use with caution with other drugs that may prolong the QT interval.

Side effects/Adverse reactions

Hot flashes, impotence, and decreased sexual desire are commonly reported reactions to goserelin (Zoladex), leuprolide (Faslodex), and triptorelin (Trelstar). Other adverse reactions include:

- peripheral edema
- nausea and vomiting
- constipation
- local reactions at injection site.

On the rise

Oncology disease symptoms and pain may worsen or flare during the first 2 weeks of goserelin (Zoladex) or leuprolide (Lupron, Eligard) therapy. The flare can be fatal in patients with bony vertebral metastasis. Androgen deprivation therapy (ADT) can lead to an increased risk for cardiovascular disease and hyperglycemia.

The Three-Step Approach

Nursing management for patients needing gonadotropin-releasing hormone analogue therapy includes these three steps.

Reminder to refer to the broader *The three-step approach* for ALL endocrine and hormone modulators on page 672.

Preadministration

(Recognize and analyze cues)

- Review lab work including platelet and total and differential white blood cell (WBC) counts as well as hemoglobin, hematocrit, alanine aminotransferase (ALT), aspartate aminotransferase (AST), lactate dehydrogenase (LDH), serum bilirubin, blood urea nitrogen (BUN), serum creatinine, uric acid, cholesterol and LDL, glucose, HbA1c, and other lab work as needed.
- The dose should not be given unless the patient's platelet count is greater than 100,000/mcL.

(Prioritize hypothesis—priority patient problems)

- Acute pain
- Hyperglycemia risk
- Knowledge deficiency

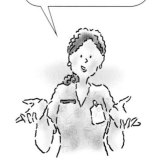

Oncology disease symptoms and pain may worsen during the first 2 weeks of goserelin (Zoladex) or leuprolide (Lupron, Eligard) therapy.

(Generate solutions)
- The patient's pain level will be controlled.
- The patient will not demonstrate hyperglycemia.
- The patient and family will demonstrate an understanding of drug therapy; including routine follow-up.

Medication administration

(Take action)
- Leuprolide (Lupron) is given deep IM on a monthly, every 3- or 6-month schedule. Reconstitute with provided diluent. Administer the milky suspension deep IM.
- Leuprolide (Eligard) is given subcutaneously. Bring to room temperature prior reconstitution. Administer within 30 minutes. If self-administered, teach the patient or caregiver proper storage, injection technique, and syringe/needle disposal. Wash hands before and after injection.
- The implant form of goserelin (Zoladex) comes in a preloaded syringe. If the package is damaged, do not use the syringe. Make sure that the drug pellet is visible in the translucent chamber. Repeat every 28 days.
- After implantation, withdraw the needle and apply a bandage to the area.
- Implant may be detected by ultrasound if removal is required.
- Monitor the patient for adverse reactions.

Postadministration

(Evaluate outcomes)
- Evaluate for and promptly address pain associated with drug side effects. Use supportive treatments to help manage side effects from the treatment.
- Ensure that the patient understands that they must continue to receive injections at predefined intervals.
- Arrange for consult to dietitian if the patient has persistently elevated glucose levels.

The inhibitors

As more genetic and cellular pathways are discovered, more targeted treatments become available to treat cancers. This category of drugs focuses solely specific pathways to inhibit cancer growth.

Histone deacetylase (HDAC) inhibitors

- Panobinostat (Farydak)
- Romidepsin (Istodax)
- Vorinostat (Zolinza)

Pharmacokinetics

Administered orally, panobinostat (Farydak) is highly bound to plasma proteins. It is metabolized extensively in the liver and excreted in the stool and urine. Half-life is 37 hours.

Belinostat (Beleodaq), romidepsin (Istodax), and vorinostat (Zolinza) are protein bound and largely excreted in urine. Hepatic impairment can slow metabolism.

Pharmacodynamics

HDAC inhibitors work to inhibit the removal of acetyl groups from the lysine residues of histones and some nonhistone proteins. This induces cell cycle arrest and apoptosis occurs.

Pharmacotherapeutics

Belinostat (Beleodaq) is used in relapsed or refractory peripheral T-cell lymphoma. Panobinostat (Farydak) is used to treat multiple myeloma, after first-line therapy. It is used in conjunction with bortezomib (Velcade) or carfilzomib (Kyprolis) and dexamethasone (Decadron). Romidepsin (Istodax) and vorinostat (Zolinza) are used for primary cutaneous lymphomas.

Drug interactions

- Use with strong CYP3A inhibitors can result in increased panobinostat (Farydak) exposure.
- Phenytoin (Dilantin) may increase QT prolongation.
- Warfarin (Coumadin) may have enhanced anticoagulant effect with romidepsin (Istodax) and vorinostat (Zolinza).
- Avoid star fruit, pomegranate or pomegranate juice, and grapefruit or grapefruit juice.

Side effects/Adverse reactions

- Abnormal T waves on EKG
- Bone marrow suppression
- Electrolyte imbalances
- Nausea, vomiting, diarrhea, or constipation
- Fatigue

The Three-Step Approach

Nursing management for patients needing HDAC inhibitor therapy includes these three steps. If the patient is receiving cytotoxic antineoplastic chemotherapy in combination with HDAC inhibitors, refer to chemotherapy education (see *Teaching about chemotherapy*) and safe management and administration of cytotoxic antineoplastics.

Preadministration
(Recognize and analyze cues)
- Perform a complete assessment before therapy begins, including medication reconciliation.
- Review lab work including CBC, for platelet and total and differential white blood cell (WBC) counts, as well as hemoglobin, hematocrit, alanine aminotransferase (ALT), aspartate aminotransferase (AST), lactate dehydrogenase (LDH), serum bilirubin, blood urea nitrogen (BUN), serum creatinine, uric acid, electrolytes, magnesium, and other lab work as needed.
- The dose should not be given unless the patient's platelet count is greater than 50,000/mcL (100,000/mcL for Panobinostat) and ANC is greater than 1,000/mcL.
- Ensure that the patient is not pregnant or nursing prior to administration. Teach women of childbearing age and men to use effective contraceptive methods during therapy and for at least 6 months following the completion of therapy.
- Monitor vital signs at ordered intervals.
- Premedicate with antiemetic prior.
- Perform EKG as baseline if drugs that prolong QT interval are ordered.
- Correct electrolyte imbalances prior to administering medications.

(Prioritize hypothesis—priority patient problems)
- Infection risk
- Electrolyte imbalance risk
- Nonadherence to oral drug regimen
- Knowledge deficiency related to drug therapy and diagnosis

(Generate solutions)
- The patient will remain free from infection related to drug-induced immunosuppression.
- The patient will have normal or corrected electrolyte imbalances without any untoward effect.
- The patient and family will demonstrate an understanding of drug therapy, including dosing schedule and importance of taking their medication.

Medication administration
(Take action)
- Infuse belinostat (Beleodaq) over 30 minutes with a 0.22-micron inline filter. Monitor IV site during infusion.

> Teach women of childbearing age and men to use effective contraceptive methods during therapy and for at least 6 months following the completion of therapy.

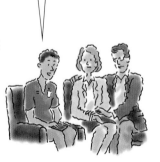

- Administer panobinostat (Farydak) orally at the same time every day. It may be administered with or without food. It is given every other day for three doses during the first 2 weeks in 21-day cycle.
- Infuse romidepsin (Istodax) over 4 hours. Monitor IV site during infusion.
- Administer vorinostat (Zolinza) daily with food. Maintain adequate hydration (greater than 2 L/day of fluids).

Postadministration

(Evaluate outcomes)

- The patient will remain free from infection.
- Monitor the patient closely for electrolyte imbalances and correct, as necessary.
- Monitor the patient for adverse reactions and drug interactions on an ongoing basis.
- Evaluate the patient's and family's understanding of drug therapy, including dosing schedule and importance of taking their medication.
- The patient will need frequent lab work to continue to evaluate CBC, liver, and kidney function and electrolytes.

CDK 4 and CDK 6 inhibitors (cyclin-dependent kinases)

This newer category of drug has provided improved survival for those diagnosed with metastatic breast cancer.

- Abemaciclib (Verzenio)
- Palbociclib (Ibrance)
- Ribociclib (Kisqali)

Pharmacokinetics

Administered orally, CDK 4 and CDK 6 inhibitors bind well with plasma proteins. They are metabolized primarily in the liver and are mainly excreted in the stool, while a small amount is excreted in urine.

Pharmacodynamics

CDK 4 and CDK 6 inhibitors reduce the cellular proliferation of estrogen receptor–positive breast cancer cells. It does so by blocking the progression of the cell from the G_1 to the S phase (Teh & Aplin, 2019). It is combined with letrozole (Femara) to increase the inhibition of retinoblastoma protein phosphorylation.

Pharmacotherapeutics

CDK 4 and CDK 6 inhibitors are used to treat metastatic breast cancer, which is HER2 negative and estrogen receptor positive in postmenopausal women. It is used in combination with letrozole (Femara).

Drug interactions

- Use with carbamazepine (Tegretol) suppresses the effects of palbociclib (Ibrance) and increased exposure to carbamazepine (Tegretol).
- Use with CYP3A substrates with a narrow therapeutic index may result in increased exposure to CYP3A substrates. Conversely, use with selected strong CYP3A inhibitors can increase palbociclib (Ibrance).
- Avoid grapefruit and grapefruit juice with CDK 4/6 inhibitors.

Side effects/Adverse reactions

During clinical trials, 25% or more of patients experienced these adverse reactions:

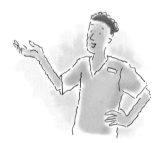

- alopecia
- decreased appetite, diarrhea, nausea, vomiting, stomatitis
- cytopenias
- increased serum creatinine and liver enzymes
- fatigue.

The Three-Step Approach

Nursing management for patients needing CDK 4 or CDK 6 inhibitor therapy includes these three steps. Many times, these are in combination with antiestrogen or hormonal treatment. Refer to the specifics for those drugs when giving.

Preadministration

(Recognize and analyze cues)

- Perform a complete assessment before therapy begins, including medication reconciliation.
- Review lab work including platelet and total and differential white blood cell (WBC) counts as well as hemoglobin, hematocrit, alanine aminotransferase (ALT), aspartate aminotransferase (AST), lactate dehydrogenase (LDH), serum bilirubin, blood urea nitrogen (BUN), serum creatinine, uric acid, and other lab work as needed.
- Monitor lab work every 2 weeks for the first two cycles, then prior to each cycle for six cycles then as clinically indicated.
- Ensure that the patient is not pregnant or nursing prior to administration. Teach women of childbearing age and men to use effective contraceptive methods during therapy and for at least 6 months following the completion of therapy.
- Monitor vital signs at ordered intervals.
- Ensure that antiemetics are ordered as abemaciclib (Verzenio) and ribociclib (Kisqali) can cause nausea and vomiting.

(Prioritize hypothesis—priority patient problems)
- Infection risk
- Nonadherence
- Knowledge deficiency

(Generate solutions)
- The patient will remain free from infection.
- The patient and family will demonstrate an understanding of drug therapy, including dosing schedule and importance of taking their medication.

Medication administration

(Take action)
- Follow the established procedures for safe and proper handling, administration, and disposal of drugs. Chemoprotective PPE is required for all antineoplastic administration. Do not cut, crush, or touch oral medications. Wear gloves when administering oral medications.
- Abemaciclib (Verzenio) should be taken at same time of the day, without regard to food.
- Palbociclib (Ibrance) should be taken at same time of the day. Administer tablets with or without food and capsules with food.
- Ribociclib (Kisqali) should be taken at same time of the day, preferably AM, without regard to food.
- Palbociclib (Ibrance) and ribociclib (Kisqali) are dosed 21 days on with 7-day rest period per cycle. Abemaciclib (Verzenio) is dosed BID continuously with no rest period.

Postadministration

(Evaluate outcomes)
- The patient will not develop infection associated with drug-induced immunosuppression.
- Monitor the patient for adverse reactions and drug interactions on an ongoing basis.
- Evaluate the patient's and family's understanding of drug therapy, including dosing schedule and importance of taking their medication.
- The patient will need frequent lab work to continue to evaluate CBC, liver, and kidney function. The patient is at risk for severe neutropenia and increased liver enzymes.

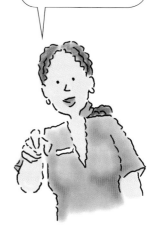

Follow the established procedures for safe and proper handling, administration, and disposal of drugs.

PARP inhibitors

PARP inhibitors (poly (ADP-ribose) polymerase) are a newer class of drug. Patients who have BRCA 1 or 2 mutations have a higher risk of breast and ovarian cancer. Options after chemotherapy to prevent recurrence have been very limited. PARP inhibitors are one of the few categories that have efficacy against BRCA mutations to reduce recurrence risk.

These drugs include:
- olaparib (Lynparza)
- niraparib (Zejula)
- rucaparib (Rubraca).

Pharmacokinetics

PARP inhibitors are highly protein bound, metabolized primarily by the liver, and excreted by urine and feces.

Pharmacodynamics

Inhibiting PARP enzymatic activity results in DNA damage, apoptosis, and cell death.

Pharmacotherapeutics

PARP inhibitors have shown efficacy in maintenance therapy for ovarian cancer. BRCA mutations and HER2-negative breast cancer can be more challenging to treat. PARP inhibitors have shown improvement in survival after first-line therapy.

Drug interactions

Rucaparib (Rubraca) inhibits CYP1A2 and may increase serum concentrations of caffeine, duloxetine (Cymbalta), phenytoin. It also can react with warfarin (Coumadin).

Side effects/Adverse reactions

- Significant cytopenias
- Increased liver enzymes
- Increased creatinine and serum cholesterol
- Hypertension
- GI distress
- Skin rash (higher with rucaparib [Rubraca])
- Secondary malignancies or myelodysplastic syndrome (MDS)

The Three–Step Approach

Nursing management for patients needing PARP inhibitors includes these three steps.

Preadministration
(Recognize and analyze cues)
- Perform a complete assessment before therapy begins, including medication reconciliation.
- Review lab work including platelet and total and differential white blood cell (WBC) counts as well as hemoglobin, hematocrit, alanine aminotransferase (ALT), aspartate aminotransferase (AST),

serum bilirubin, blood urea nitrogen (BUN), serum creatinine, cholesterol, and other lab work as needed.

- Ensure that the patient is not pregnant or nursing prior to administration. Teach women of childbearing age and men to use effective contraceptive methods during therapy and for at least 6 months following the completion of therapy.
- Monitor vital signs at ordered intervals.
- Ensure that the patient has BRCA status results and the patient has the genetic mutation BCRA 1 or 2.

(Prioritize hypothesis—priority patient problems)
- Infection risk
- Nonadherence
- Knowledge deficiency

(Generate solutions)
- The patient will remain free from infection.
- The patient and family will demonstrate an understanding of drug therapy, including dosing schedule and importance of taking their medication.

Medication administration

(Take action)
- Follow the established procedures for safe and proper handling, administration, and disposal of drugs. Chemoprotective PPE is required for all antineoplastic administration. Do not cut, crush, or touch oral medications. Wear gloves when administering oral medications.
- Do not substitute capsules for tablets. They are not interchangeable.
- Olaparib (Lynparza) administer capsules every 12 hours with or without food. However, patients may experience higher rates of nausea and vomiting when fasting.
- Niraparib (Zejula) administer capsules at the same time every day, with or without food. Provide antiemetics prior to dose as needed. Consider administering at bedtime to diminish the potential of nausea and vomiting.
- Rucaparib (Rubraca) administer orally twice daily (about 12 hours) with or without food. Provide antiemetics prior to dose as needed.
- There is no dose adjustment for renal or hepatic impairment.

Postadministration

(Evaluate outcomes)
- The patient will remain free from infection.
- Monitor the patient closely for peripheral edema and rash.
- Monitor the patient for adverse reactions and drug interactions on an ongoing basis.

- The patient and family will demonstrate an understanding of drug therapy, including dosing schedule and importance of taking their medication.
- The patient will need frequent lab work to continue to evaluate CBC, liver, and kidney function. The patient should get weekly lab work until blood counts recover. Dose reductions may be needed for prolonged hematologic toxicity.
- The patient will need to have regular blood pressure checks to monitor hypertension risk.

Quick quiz

1. Which of these adverse effects would be considered life threatening and dose limiting?
   A. Hair loss
   B. Stomatitis
   C. Neutropenia
   D. Skin rash

Answer: C. While stomatitis and skin rash can be dose limiting and risk of infection is present, neutropenia is the only life-threatening adverse effect. Monitor the patient for infection. Hair loss is cosmetic, although difficult emotionally.

2. The nurse is reviewing the patient's medical history and notices a history of a paralytic ileus. Which medication will the nurse anticipate holding or monitoring closely after administration?
   A. Irinotecan (Camptosar)
   B. Paclitaxel (Taxol)
   C. Doxorubicin (Adriamycin)
   D. Vincristine (Vincasar)

Answer: D. Vincristine (Vincasar) has an adverse effect of constipation and paralytic ileus. Irinotecan (Camptosar) can cause extreme diarrhea. Paclitaxel (Taxol) and doxorubicin (Adriamycin) can cause either diarrhea or constipation but are usually not severe.

3. Which action would the nurse perform before treatment with rituximab (Rituxan)?
   A. Monitor blood glucose.
   B. Perform ECG.
   C. Ensure skin regimen is ordered.
   D. Premedicate with antihistamine and corticosteroid.

Answer: D. Hypersensitivity infusion reactions can occur. Premedicating can reduce the incidence of hypersensitivity reaction. Rituximab (Rituxan) does not raise blood glucose levels, and cardiac rhythm changes or rash is not anticipated as a side effect.

Scoring

  If you answered all three questions correctly, extraordinary! You really mowed down the malignant neoplasms!

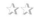 If you answered two questions correctly, congratulations! You are competent to combat cancer.

  If you answered fewer than two questions correctly, give it another shot. Remember, practice makes perfect!

Suggested References

Kuo, C. J. (2020). Overview of angiogenesis inhibitors. In *UptoDate*. Retrieved from https://www.uptodate.com/contents/overview-of-angiogenesis-inhibitors

Lexicomp. (2020). *Management of drug extravasations.* Lexicomp. Retrieved from http://online.lexi.com/lco/action/doc/retrieve/docid/patch_f/4111?cesid=2hQrbe4Y2WG&searchUrl=%2Flco%2Faction%2Fsearch%3Fq%3Dextravasation%26t%3Dname%26va%3Dextravasation#

Manis, J. P. (2020). Overview of therapeutic monoclonal antibodies. In *UptoDate*. Retrieved from https://www.uptodate.com/contents/overview-of-therapeutic-monoclonal-antibodies

Oncology Nursing Society. (2019). *Chemotherapy and Immunotherapy guidelines and recommendation for practice.*

Pritchard, K. I. (2020). Adjuvant endocrine therapy for postmenopausal women with hormone receptor-positive breast cancer. In *UptoDate*. Retrieved from https://www.uptodate.com/contents/adjuvant-endocrine-therapy-for-postmenopausal-women-with-hormone-receptor-positive-breast-cancer

Teh, J., & Aplin, A. E. (2019). Arrested developments: CDK4/6 inhibitor resistance and alterations in the tumor immune microenvironment. *Clinical cancer research, 25*(3), 921–927. https://doi.org/10.1158/1078-0432.CCR-18-1967

Chapter 19

Drugs for fluid and electrolyte balance

Just the facts

In this chapter, you'll learn:

◆ classes of drugs used to treat fluid and electrolyte disorders

◆ uses and varying actions of these drugs

◆ absorption, distribution, metabolization, and excretion of these drugs

◆ drug interactions, side effects, and adverse reactions to these drugs.

Drugs and homeostasis

Many factors can easily disrupt the delicate homeostatic mechanisms that help maintain normal fluid and electrolyte balance. Often, during illness, this balance is altered. Additionally, occurrences such as loss of appetite, medication administration, vomiting, surgery, and diagnostic tests can also alter this delicate balance.

Fortunately, several drugs can help correct imbalances and bring the body back to homeostasis (the stability of body fluid composition and volume).

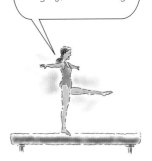

Many factors can disrupt normal fluid and electrolyte balance, including illness, loss of appetite, medication administration, surgery, and vomiting.

Electrolyte replacement drugs

An electrolyte is a compound or element that carries an electric charge when dissolved in water. Electrolyte replacement drugs are inorganic or organic salts that increase depleted or deficient electrolyte levels, helping to maintain homeostasis. These drugs include:

- potassium, the primary intracellular fluid (ICF) electrolyte
- calcium, a major extracellular fluid (ECF) electrolyte
- magnesium, an electrolyte essential for homeostasis found in ICF
- sodium, the principal electrolyte in ECF necessary for homeostasis.

Potassium

Potassium is the major positively charged ion (cation) in ICF. Because the body can't store potassium, adequate amounts must be ingested daily. If this isn't possible, potassium can be replaced orally or IV with potassium replacements, such as:

- potassium acetate
- potassium chloride
- potassium gluconate
- potassium citrate
- potassium bicarbonate
- potassium phosphate.

Pharmacokinetics

Oral potassium is absorbed readily from the GI tract. After absorption into the ECF, almost all potassium passes into the ICF. There, the enzyme adenosine triphosphatase maintains the concentration of potassium by pumping sodium out of the cell in exchange for potassium.

Normal serum levels of potassium are maintained by the kidneys, which excrete most excess potassium in urine. The rest is excreted in feces and sweat. A majority of potassium in the intestine is reabsorbed.

Pharmacodynamics

Potassium moves quickly into ICF through active transport to restore depleted potassium levels and reestablish balance. It's an essential element in determining cell membrane potential and excitability.

Nervous about potassium?

Potassium is necessary for proper functioning of all nerve and muscle cells and for nerve impulse transmission. It's also essential for tissue growth and repair and for maintenance of acid-base balance.

Pharmacotherapeutics

Potassium replacement therapy corrects hypokalemia (low levels of potassium in the blood). Hypokalemia is a common occurrence in conditions that increase potassium excretion or depletion, such as:

- vomiting, diarrhea, or nasogastric suction
- excessive urination
- some kidney diseases
- cystic fibrosis
- increased insulin
- burns
- excessive antidiuretic hormone levels
- therapy with a potassium-depleting diuretic
- beta adrenergic agonists medications (albuterol, terbutaline, and dobutamine)
- laxative abuse

- antipsychotics such as risperidone
- sympathomimetic medications (OTC decongestants with pseudoephedrine, OTC diet medications with ephedrine)
- alkalosis
- hypothermia
- insufficient potassium intake from starvation, anorexia nervosa, alcoholism, or clay ingestion
- administration of a glucocorticoid, IV amphotericin B, vitamin B_{12}, folic acid, granulocyte-macrophage colony–stimulating factor, or IV solutions that contain insufficient potassium (Mount, 2021).

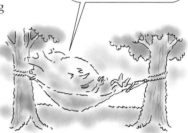

Because potassium inhibits my excitability, it decreases the toxic effects of digoxin— which leaves me feeling quite relaxed.

Be still my heart

Potassium can balance the toxic effects of digoxin. Potassium can inhibit the excitability of the heart. Because they share the same mechanism of binding for transport through the cells (Na/K channel), only one can bind. In normal potassium levels, the channels are fully bound by potassium; thus, it moderates the action of digoxin, reducing the chance of toxicity.

Drug interactions

Potassium should be used cautiously in patients receiving potassium-sparing diuretics (such as amiloride, spironolactone, and triamterene) or angiotensin-converting enzyme (ACE) inhibitors (such as captopril, enalapril, and lisinopril) to avoid hyperkalemia.

Side effects/adverse reactions

Most side effects and adverse reactions to potassium are related to the method of administration. Oral potassium sometimes causes nausea, vomiting, abdominal pain, and diarrhea. Enteric-coated tablets may cause small bowel ulcerations, stenosis, hemorrhage, and obstruction. An IV infusion can cause pain at the IV site, phlebitis (vein inflammation), and even cardiac arrest if administered too rapidly. It is never given faster intravenously than over one hour, and NEVER by IV push. Infusion of potassium in patients with decreased urine production and/or impaired renal function also increases the risk of hyperkalemia.

The Three-Step Approach

Nursing management for the patient receiving treatment with potassium replacement therapy includes these three steps.

Preadministration

(Recognize and analyze cues)
- Monitor the patient's potassium level. Be particularly alert for hyperkalemia if the patient's urine output decreases during therapy.

Before you give that drug!

Signs and symptoms of hyperkalemia

Potassium replacement therapy can lead to overcorrection and hyperkalemia. To prevent this, closely monitor the patient for signs and symptoms of hyperkalemia, including:

- abdominal cramping
- confusion
- diarrhea
- electrocardiogram changes (tall, tented T wave)
- hypotension
- irregular pulse rate
- irritability
- muscle weakness
- nausea
- paresthesia.

- Monitor the patient for signs and symptoms of hyperkalemia. (See *Signs and symptoms of hyperkalemia.*)
- Assess for conditions that may impact potassium levels.
- Watch for adverse reactions and drug interactions.
- Monitor the patient's electrocardiogram (ECG) for changes that suggest hyperkalemia, such as prolonged PR intervals; widened QRS complexes; depressed ST segments; and tall, tented T waves.
- Monitor infusion site for any signs of phlebitis.
- Monitor the patient's intake and output if nausea, vomiting, or diarrhea occurs.

(Priority hypothesis—priority patient problems)
- Dehydration
- Hypovolemia
- Electrolyte imbalance
- Knowledge deficiency

(Generate solutions)
- The patient's fluid intake and output will remain at an appropriate level for age and condition.
- The patient's electrolyte status will be maintained for homeostasis without complications associated with hypokalemia/hyperkalemia.
- The patient and family members will understand drug therapy.

Medication administration
(Take action)
- Use potassium cautiously if the patient is also receiving a potassium-sparing diuretic or an ACE inhibitor.
- When administering potassium IV, dilute the preparation before infusion.
- Give diluted IV potassium slowly to prevent life-threatening hyperkalemia.
- NEVER give potassium as an IV bolus or IM injection.
- For severe cases of hypokalemia requiring aggressive IV repletion, a central venous catheter may be required.

Teaching about potassium therapy

See Education edge: Teaching template in Chapter 3, page 38 for general teaching for all medications. Specific points to review with patients and family for potassium replacement therapy:

• Take oral potassium with or after meals to minimize GI distress.

• Dissolve all powders and tablets in at least 4 oz (120 mL) of water or fruit juice, and sip the solution slowly over 5 to 10 minutes. Also, take capsules or tablets with plenty of liquid.

• Make sure not to crush or chew extended-release tablets, which will defeat the purpose of the special coating. Also understand that although the remnants of the wax matrix may appear in your stools, the drug has been absorbed.

• Make sure you keep appointments for periodic blood tests to measure potassium level.

• If you experience GI distress or signs and symptoms of hyperkalemia, such as diarrhea, muscle weakness, or confusion, notify your primary care provider.

Nix that mix

- Don't mix IV potassium phosphate with or in a solution that contains calcium or magnesium because precipitates will form.
- Monitor the patient's IV site regularly for pain, discomfort, and signs of phlebitis. If minor discomfort occurs with infusion, a reduced infusion time may be ordered. It may also be administered as a piggyback infusion. If phlebitis or worsening pain occurs, stop the infusion and change the site.
- Give oral potassium with or after meals to minimize GI distress.
- Give antiemetics or antidiarrheals as needed if the patient develops vomiting or diarrhea.
- Teach the patient and family members about potassium therapy. (See *Teaching about potassium therapy*.)

Postadministration

(Evaluate outcomes)

- The patient maintains adequate hydration.
- The patient maintains normal potassium levels.
- The patient and family members demonstrate an understanding of drug therapy.

Give oral potassium with or after meals to minimize GI distress.

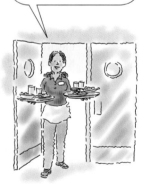

Calcium

Calcium is a major cation in ECF. Almost all of the calcium in the body (99%) is stored in bone, where it can be mobilized if necessary.

When dietary intake isn't enough to meet metabolic needs, calcium stores in bone are reduced.

Bound, complexed, ionized

Extracellular calcium exists in three forms—bound to plasma protein (mainly albumin); complexed with substances such as phosphate, citrate, or sulfate; and ionized. About 47% of the ionized calcium is physiologically active and plays a role in cellular functions (Hogan & Goldfarb, 2021).

Salting the body

Chronic insufficient calcium intake can result in bone demineralization. Calcium is replaced orally or IV most commonly with the calcium salts, calcium carbonate, and calcium citrate. Other calcium salts include:
- calcium acetate
- calcium chloride
- calcium glubionate
- calcium gluconate
- calcium lactate.

Pharmacokinetics

Oral calcium is absorbed readily from the duodenum and proximal jejunum. A pH of 5 to 7, parathyroid hormone (PTH), calcitriol, and vitamin D all aid calcium absorption (Hogan & Goldfarb, 2021).

A soapy situation

Absorption also depends on dietary factors, such as calcium binding to fiber, phytates, and oxalates, and on fatty acids, with which calcium salts form insoluble soaps.

Calcium is distributed primarily in bone. Calcium salts are eliminated primarily in feces, with the remainder excreted in urine.

Pharmacodynamics

Calcium moves quickly into ECF to restore calcium levels and reestablish balance. It has several vital functions:
- Extracellular ionized calcium plays an essential role in normal nerve and muscle excitability.
- Calcium is integral to normal functioning of the heart, kidneys, and lungs, and it affects the blood coagulation rate as well as cell membrane and capillary permeability.
- Calcium is a factor in neurotransmitter and hormone activity, amino acid metabolism, vitamin B_{12} absorption, and gastrin secretion.
- Calcium plays a major role in normal bone and tooth formation. (See *Calcium in balance*, page 762.)

Pharm function

Calcium in balance

Extracellular calcium levels are normally kept constant by several interrelated processes that move calcium ions into and out of ECF. Calcium enters the extracellular space through resorption of calcium ions from bone, through the absorption of dietary calcium in the GI tract, and through reabsorption of calcium from the kidneys. Calcium leaves ECF as it's excreted in feces and urine and deposited in bone tissues. This illustration shows how calcium moves throughout the body.

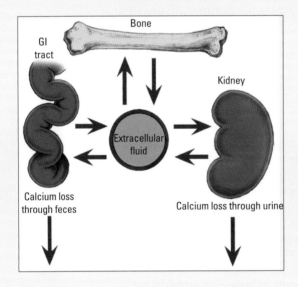

Pharmacotherapeutics

Calcium is helpful in treating magnesium intoxication. It also helps strengthen myocardial tissue after defibrillation or a poor response to epinephrine during resuscitation. Pregnancy and breast-feeding increase calcium requirements, as do periods of bone growth during childhood and adolescence.

In the IV league

The major clinical indication for IV calcium is acute hypocalcemia (low serum calcium levels), which necessitates a rapid increase in serum calcium levels. Acute hypocalcemia can occur in tetany, cardiac arrest, vitamin D deficiency, parathyroid surgery, and alkalosis. IV calcium is also used to prevent a hypocalcemic reaction during exchange transfusions.

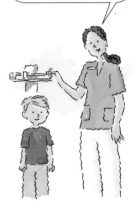

When a child is going through a period of bone growth, he needs extra calcium. I think he has grown another inch!

Mouth medicine

Oral calcium is commonly used to supplement a calcium-deficient diet and prevent osteoporosis. Chronic hypocalcemia from such conditions as chronic hypoparathyroidism (a deficiency of PTH), osteomalacia (softening of bones), long-term glucocorticoid therapy, and vitamin D deficiency is also treated with oral calcium.

Drug interactions

Calcium has significant interactions with other drugs:
- Preparations administered with digoxin may cause cardiac arrhythmias.
- Calcium replacement drugs may reduce the response to calcium channel blockers.
- Calcium replacements may inactivate tetracyclines.
- Calcium supplements may decrease the amount of atenolol available to the tissues, resulting in decreased effectiveness of the drug.
- Ceftriaxone with IV calcium can precipitate and should not be infused together. In neonates, the two medicines should not be infused simultaneously due to fatal pulmonary and renal injuries.

An insoluble problem

- When given in total parenteral nutrition, calcium may react with phosphorus present in the solution to form insoluble calcium phosphate granules, which may find their way into pulmonary arterioles, causing emboli and possibly death.

Side effects/adverse reactions

Calcium preparations may produce hypercalcemia if calcium levels aren't monitored closely. Early signs include drowsiness, lethargy, muscle weakness, headache, constipation, and a metallic taste in the mouth. ECG changes that occur with elevated serum calcium levels include a shortened QT interval and heart block. Severe hypercalcemia can cause cardiac arrhythmias, cardiac arrest, and coma.

A burning issue

With IV administration, calcium may cause venous irritation and even necrosis if infiltration occurs. Subcutaneous or IM injection of calcium may cause severe local reactions, such as burning, necrosis, and tissue sloughing. Because of this reaction, calcium is only given PO and IV. In some cases, central venous access may be needed. The severe reaction of necrosis and skin sloughing that can occur is called calcinosis cutis. In rare cases, it can be severe.

The Three-Step Approach

Nursing management for the patient receiving treatment with calcium replacement therapy includes these three steps.

Preadministration

(Recognize and analyze cues)
- Monitor the patient's calcium level.
- Assess for conditions that may impact calcium levels.
- Monitor the patient for signs of hypocalcemia and hypercalcemia including ECG changes.
- Monitor administration site with IV administration for signs of infiltration.

(Priority hypothesis—priority patient problems)
- Electrolyte imbalance
- Injury risk
- Knowledge deficiency

(Generate solutions)
- The patient will maintain normal calcium levels.
- The patient won't develop an increased risk of fractures or complications associated with hypocalcemia/hypercalcemia.
- The patient will demonstrate understanding of drug therapy.

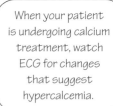

When your patient is undergoing calcium treatment, watch ECG for changes that suggest hypercalcemia.

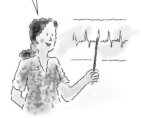

Medication administration

- Only give PO or IV.
- Give an IV infusion slowly to prevent hypercalcemia which may result in arrhythmias and cardiac arrest.
- Keep the patient recumbent for 15 minutes after injecting calcium.
- If extravasation occurs, stop the IV infusion and apply warm, moist compresses to the area.
- During emergency may give calcium via intraosseous catheter, but this is not preferred.
- Give oral calcium supplements 1 to 2 hours after meals.
- Give calcium and digoxin slowly and in small amounts to avoid precipitating arrhythmias during therapy with both drugs.
- Teach the patient about calcium. (See *Teaching about oral calcium.*)

Education edge

Teaching about oral calcium

See Education edge: Teaching template in Chapter 3, page 38 for general teaching for all medications. Specific points to review with patients and family for oral calcium replacement therapy:

- Don't take calcium with foods that interfere with calcium absorption, such as spinach, rhubarb, bran, whole grain cereals and breads, and fresh fruits and vegetables; take calcium tablets 1 to 2 hours after eating.
- Eat foods containing vitamin D to enhance calcium absorption.

- Don't skip follow-up blood tests to monitor calcium levels.
- Report signs and symptoms of hypercalcemia, including nausea and vomiting, constipation, muscle weakness, lethargy, and fatigue, to your primary care provider.

Postadministration

(Evaluate outcomes)

- The patient maintains normal calcium levels as evidenced by normal vital signs and ECG.
- The patient avoided injuries or complications associated with hypercalcemia or hypocalcemia.
- The patient and family members demonstrate an understanding of drug therapy.

Magnesium

Magnesium is the most abundant cation in ICF after potassium. It's essential in transmitting nerve impulses to muscle and activating enzymes necessary for carbohydrate and protein metabolism. About 65% of all magnesium is in bone and 20% is in muscle.

Officiating in the ICF

Magnesium stimulates PTH secretion, thus regulating ICF calcium levels.

Traffic control

Magnesium also aids in cell metabolism and the movement of sodium and potassium across cell membranes.

A run on magnesium

Magnesium stores may be depleted by:

- malabsorption
- chronic diarrhea
- prolonged treatment with diuretics
- nasogastric suctioning
- prolonged therapy with parenteral fluids not containing magnesium
- prolonged therapy with proton pump inhibitors
- hyperaldosteronism
- hypoparathyroidism or hyperparathyroidism
- excessive release of adrenocortical hormones
- acute and chronic alcohol consumption
- uncontrolled diabetes mellitus
- drugs, such as cisplatin, aminoglycosides, cyclosporine, and amphotericin B (Yu, 2021).

Low magnesium… low calcium…low potassium

Hypomagnesemia interferes with calcium metabolism and results in hypocalcemia (Yu et al., 2021). Other symptoms of hypomagnesemia include:

- neuromuscular: tremors, tetany, seizures
- cardiovascular: QRS widening, PR widening, atrial and ventricular arrhythmias
- electrolytes: hypokalemia and hypocalcemia.

Restocking the mineral stores

Magnesium is typically replaced in the form of magnesium sulfate when administered IV (preferred) or in the form of magnesium oxide if given orally. Other forms of magnesium include magnesium carbonate, magnesium chloride, magnesium citrate, magnesium glucoheptonate, and magnesium gluconate.

Pharmacokinetics

Magnesium sulfate is distributed widely throughout the body. IV magnesium sulfate acts immediately, whereas it acts within 30 minutes after IM administration. However, IM injections can be painful, induce sclerosis, and need to be repeated frequently. Therefore, IM dosing is not routinely utilized and is dose adjusted down when administered. Magnesium sulfate isn't metabolized and is excreted unchanged in urine; some appears in breast milk.

Pharmacodynamics

Magnesium sulfate replenishes and prevents magnesium deficiencies. As an oral medication, it increases the flow in the colon and promotes bowel movements by increasing osmotic retention of fluid. It also prevents or controls seizures by blocking neuromuscular transmission. Magnesium sulfate stabilizes excitable membranes of the uterus and pericardium. Additionally, IV magnesium can help stabilize pulmonary smooth muscle during an asthma exacerbation.

Pharmacotherapeutics

IV magnesium sulfate is the drug of choice for replacement therapy in symptomatic magnesium deficiency (hypomagnesemia). It's widely used to treat or prevent preeclampsia and eclamptic seizure activity. It's also used to treat ventricular arrhythmias such as torsades de pointes, seizures, severe toxemia, and acute nephritis in children.

Drug interactions

Magnesium has significant interactions with other drugs:
- Magnesium used with digoxin may lead to heart block.
- Magnesium taken with gabapentin can increase CNS depression.
- Magnesium taken orally with certain oral antibiotics like quinolones and tetracyclines can decrease their effectiveness if taken together. To reduce this, they should be taken separately.
- Magnesium taken orally together with levothyroxine can reduce the absorption and blood levels of levothyroxine. They should be taken at least four hours apart.

So depressing…
- Combining magnesium sulfate with alcohol, opioids, antianxiety drugs, barbiturates, antidepressants, hypnotics, antipsychotic drugs, or general anesthetics may increase central nervous system depressant effects.

- Using magnesium sulfate with succinylcholine potentiates and prolongs the neuromuscular blocking action of the drug.

Side effects/adverse reactions

Side effects and adverse reactions to magnesium sulfate can be life-threatening. They include:
- hypotension
- circulatory collapse
- flushing
- depressed reflexes
- respiratory paralysis.
- IM injections of magnesium can cause pain and induce sclerosis.

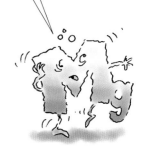

Adverse reactions to magnesium sulfate can be life-threatening! Just the thought of it makes me feel faint.

The Three–Step Approach

Nursing management for the patient receiving treatment with magnesium replacement therapy includes these three steps.

Preadministration

(Recognize and analyze cues)
- Monitor the patient's serum electrolyte levels before, during, and after treatment.
- Assess for conditions that may impact magnesium levels.
- Monitor the patient's intake and output. Magnesium may not be administered if the patient's urine output is less than 100 mL in 4 hours.
- Monitor the patient's vital signs and ECG tracings, looking for signs of hypotension, arrhythmias, and respiratory distress.

(Priority hypothesis—priority patient problems)
- Electrolyte imbalance
- Altered breathing pattern risk
- Knowledge deficiency

(Generate solutions)
- The patient will maintain normal electrolyte levels without complications.
- The patient will have regular breathing patterns.
- The patient and family members will demonstrate an understanding of drug therapy.

Medication administration

(Take action)
- Keep IV calcium gluconate available to reverse the respiratory depression that an infusion of magnesium sulfate can cause.

A knee-jerk reaction

- It is of critical importance to test the patient's knee-jerk and patellar reflexes before giving each dose. If a reflex is absent, notify the primary care provider right away and withhold the dose until the patient's reflexes return. Otherwise, the patient may develop temporary respiratory failure and need cardiopulmonary resuscitation or IV administration of calcium.

- Patients with neuromuscular disorders such as Myasthenia Gravis should avoid an infusion of IV magnesium and should take caution with oral magnesium due to the relaxation effect of magnesium on the muscle from its effect on acetylcholine release.
- Use parenteral magnesium cautiously in a patient with renal impairment because renal impairment increases the risk of hypermagnesemia.
- Administer magnesium sulfate slowly! Injecting a bolus dose too rapidly can trigger cardiac arrest.
- Monitor the patient's vital signs and deep tendon reflexes during an infusion of magnesium. Watch for signs and symptoms of overdose, including hypotension and respiratory distress.
- Check the patient's serum magnesium level after each bolus dose; if the patient is receiving a continuous IV drip, check the serum magnesium level at least every 6 hours.
- Place the patient on continuous cardiac monitoring during replacement therapy.
- Monitor the patient's urine output before, during, and after magnesium sulfate infusion. Notify the primary care provider if the output is less than 100 mL over 4 hours.

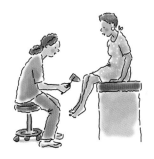

Postadministration

(Evaluate outcomes)

- The patient maintains normal electrolyte and fluid balance without complications associated with hypomagnesemia and hypermagnesemia.
- The patient maintains regular breathing patterns and cardiac output as evidenced by normal vital signs and ECG.
- The patient and family members demonstrate an understanding of drug therapy.

> Conditions that deplete sodium include anorexia, excessive GI fluid loss, and excessive perspiration. Speaking of excessive perspiration, I think it's time to get out of this heat!

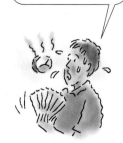

Sodium

Sodium is the major cation in ECF. Sodium performs many functions:

- It maintains the osmotic pressure and concentration of ECF, acid-base balance, and water balance.
- It contributes to nerve conduction and neuromuscular function.
- It plays a role in glandular secretion.

The truth about sodium and water balance

Sodium and water balance are intertwined. Plasma sodium levels are regulated by water intake and excretion. Low sodium levels (hyponatremia) are generally associated with water that cannot be excreted, and high sodium levels (hypernatremia) are usually associated with loss of water (Sterns, 2021).

Sweating it out

Sodium replacement is necessary in conditions that rapidly deplete sodium, such as anorexia, excessive loss of GI fluids, and excessive perspiration. Diuretics and tap water enemas can also deplete sodium, particularly when fluids are replaced by plain water.

Sodium also can be lost in trauma or wound drainage, adrenal gland insufficiency, cirrhosis of the liver with ascites, syndrome of inappropriate antidiuretic hormone, and prolonged IV infusion of dextrose in water without other solutes. Sodium is typically replaced in the form of sodium chloride.

Pharmacokinetics

Oral and parenteral sodium chloride are quickly absorbed and distributed widely throughout the body. Sodium chloride isn't significantly metabolized. It's eliminated primarily in urine but also in sweat, tears, and saliva.

Pharmacodynamics

Sodium chloride solution replaces deficiencies of sodium and chloride ions in blood plasma.

Pharmacotherapeutics

Sodium chloride is used for water and electrolyte replacement in patients with hyponatremia from electrolyte loss or severe sodium chloride depletion.

In cases of cerebral edema, the osmotic effect of sodium can help to shift the intracerebral fluid balance and temporarily stabilize intracranial pressure. In these cases, hypertonic infusions of saline are utilized.

A welcome infusion

Severe symptomatic sodium deficiency may be treated by IV infusion of a solution containing sodium chloride. If hypertonic solutions are used, they must be infused through a central venous catheter.

Drug interactions

No significant drug interactions have been reported with sodium chloride.

Side effects/adverse reactions

Side effects and adverse reactions to sodium include pulmonary edema if it's given too rapidly or in excess, hypernatremia, and potassium loss.

The Three-Step Approach

Nursing management for the patient receiving treatment with sodium replacement therapy includes these three steps.

Preadministration

(Recognize and analyze cues)
- Monitor the patient's intake and output.
- Monitor the patient's serum electrolyte levels before, during, and after treatment.
- Assess for conditions that may impact sodium and water balance.
- Monitor for complications of hyponatremia including brain herniation.
- Assess the patient and family members' knowledge about drug therapy.

(Priority hypothesis—priority patient problems)
- Electrolyte imbalance
- Hypovolemia
- Fluid overload risk
- Knowledge deficiency

(Generate solutions)
- The patient will maintain normal sodium (electrolytes) and fluid levels for age and condition.
- The patient and family members will demonstrate an understanding of drug therapy.

Medication administration

(Take action)
- Use cautiously in older adults and postoperative patients as well as in patients with heart failure, circulatory insufficiency, renal impairment, or hypoproteinemia.
- Use a central venous catheter to infuse prescribed hypertonic saline solutions.

Every breath you take

- Teach the patient to recognize signs and symptoms of pulmonary edema, including shortness of breath, coughing, anxiety, wheezing, and pallor; tell the patient to notify the primary care provider if these symptoms are experienced.

Postadministration

(Evaluate outcomes)
- The patient maintains normal electrolyte and fluid balance.
- The patient and family members demonstrate understanding of drug therapy.

Alkalinizing and acidifying drugs

Alkalinizing and acidifying drugs act to correct acid-base imbalances in the blood. A shift too far in either direction in the body's pH can mean death. Alkalinizing drugs are used to treat metabolic acidosis, a condition in which excess hydrogen ions in the ECF result in a decreased serum pH. Acidifying drugs are used for metabolic alkalosis, in which excess bicarbonate in the ECF increases serum pH.

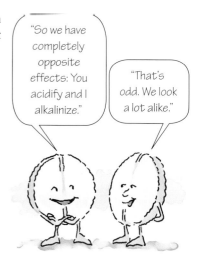

"So we have completely opposite effects: You acidify and I alkalinize."

"That's odd. We look a lot alike."

Odd couple

Alkalinizing and acidifying drugs have opposite effects:
- An alkalinizing drug increases the pH of the blood and decreases the concentration of hydrogen ions.
- An acidifying drug decreases the pH of the blood and increases the concentration of hydrogen ions.

Rx for overdose?

Some of these drugs also alter urine pH, making them useful in treating some urinary tract infections and drug overdoses.

Alkalinizing drugs

Alkalinizing drugs used to treat metabolic acidosis and increase blood pH include sodium bicarbonate (also used to increase urine pH) and tromethamine.

Pharmacokinetics

The alkalinizing drugs are absorbed well when given orally. Sodium bicarbonate isn't metabolized. Tromethamine undergoes little or no metabolization and is excreted unchanged in urine.

Pharmacodynamics

Sodium bicarbonate separates in the blood, providing bicarbonate ions that are used in the blood's buffer system to decrease the hydrogen ion concentration and raise blood pH. (Buffers prevent extreme changes in pH by taking or giving up hydrogen ions to neutralize acids or bases.) As the bicarbonate ions are excreted in urine, urine pH rises. (See *Alkalinizing drugs: Sodium bicarbonate*, page 772.)

While these drugs work to help life-threatening acidosis, it is important to remember that they only work temporarily. The underlying problem must be resolved to prevent further episodes of acidosis.

Hitching up with hydrogen

Tromethamine acts by combining with hydrogen ions to alkalinize the blood; the resulting tromethamine-hydrogen ion complex is excreted in urine.

Pharmacotherapeutics

Alkalinizing drugs are commonly used to treat metabolic acidosis. Additional benefits include raising urine pH. This can be beneficial to help remove certain substances such as phenobarbital, tricyclic antidepressants, and salicylates after an overdose.

Drug interactions

The alkalinizing drug sodium bicarbonate can interact with a wide range of drugs to increase or decrease their pharmacologic effects:
- The drugs may increase the excretion and reduce the effects of ketoconazole, lithium, and salicylates.
- It may reduce the excretion and increase the effects of amphetamines, quinidine, and pseudoephedrine.
- The antibacterial effects of methenamine are reduced when taken with alkalinizing drugs.
- Tromethamine doesn't have any significant drug interactions.

Side effects/adverse reactions

Side effects and adverse reactions to alkalinizing drugs vary with the drug.

Sodium bicarbonate

An overdose of sodium bicarbonate or any alkalinizing drugs can lead to metabolic alkalosis, the most severe adverse reaction. If the drug is administered too rapidly to a patient with diabetic ketoacidosis, the patient may experience cerebral dysfunction, tissue hypoxia, and lactic acidosis. The drug's high sodium content can cause water retention and edema. Oral sodium bicarbonate may cause gastric distention and flatulence.

Tromethamine

Mild reactions to tromethamine include phlebitis or irritation at the injection site. Severe reactions include hypoglycemia, respiratory depression, and hyperkalemia.

Toxic time bomb

If tromethamine is given for more than 24 hours, toxic drug levels can occur.

The Three-Step Approach

Nursing management for the patient receiving treatment with alkalinizing drugs includes these three steps.

Preadministration

(Recognize and analyze cues)
- Monitor the patient's pH and bicarbonate levels before, during, and after treatment.

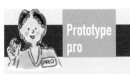

Alkalinizing drugs: Sodium bicarbonate

Actions
- Neutralizes excess acid in the body
- Restores the blood's buffer system

Indications
- Respiratory acidosis (in some cases)
- Metabolic, systemic, or urinary acidosis
- Gastric acidity (works as an antacid)

Nursing considerations
- If the patient has diabetic ketoacidosis, give the drug slowly to prevent cerebral dysfunction, tissue hypoxia, and lactic acidosis.
- Monitor the patient for signs and symptoms of fluid retention, such as crackles, peripheral edema, and jugular vein distention.
- Watch for respiratory depression.
- Inspect the IV site for signs of extravasation.
- If the drug is used to treat urinary alkalinization, monitor the patient's urine pH.

- Monitor respiratory status for an acute change during and after treatment.
- Monitor for signs and symptoms of overdose, including hyperirritability and tetany.
- Monitor the patient's intake and output.
- Assess for conditions that impact acid/base balance.
- Watch for adverse reactions and drug interactions.
- Assess the patient and family members' knowledge of drug therapy.

(Priority hypothesis—priority patient problems)
- Electrolyte imbalance
- Safety
- Injury risk
- Fluid overload risk
- Knowledge deficiency
- Impaired gas exchange risk
- Hypoglycemia risk

(Generate solutions)
- The patient will have fluid/electrolyte and acid/base balance.
- The patient will be free of injuries and complications associated with acid/base and electrolyte imbalances.
- The patient and family members will demonstrate an understanding of drug therapy.

Medication administration
(Take action)
- If the patient is receiving sodium bicarbonate or tromethamine, watch the IV site for extravasation. If extravasation occurs, elevate the affected limb, apply warm compresses, and administer lidocaine.
- For a patient receiving tromethamine, check the IV site for phlebitis or irritation and don't give the drug for more than 24 hours.
- Teach the patient and caregivers about the prescribed drug. (See *Teaching about alkalinizing drugs,* page 774.)

Postadministration
- The patient maintains normal fluid/electrolyte and acid/base balance.
- The patient is free from injuries and complications associated with fluid/electrolyte and acid/base imbalances.
- The patient and family members demonstrate an understanding of drug therapy.

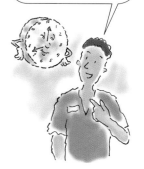

Keep in mind that giving tromethamine for more than 24 hours can result in toxic levels.

Teaching about alkalinizing drugs

See Education edge: Teaching template in Chapter 3, page 38 for general teaching for all medications. Specific points to review with patients and family for alkalinizing therapy:
- Prolonged therapy with sodium bicarbonate tablets can cause GI distress and flatulence. Report these symptoms to your primary care provider.
- Watch for signs and symptoms of fluid retention, such as ankle swelling and tightness of rings on your fingers and report them to your primary care provider.
- If you're taking tromethamine (THAM), monitor your glucose level carefully because THAM can cause hypoglycemia.
- Avoid milk while taking sodium bicarbonate to avoid milk-alkali syndrome, hypercalcemia, and renal calculi production.

Acidifying drugs

Acidifying drugs used to correct metabolic alkalosis include acetazolamide (used to treat acute mountain sickness and wide-angle glaucoma) and ammonium chloride. Ascorbic acid, along with ammonium chloride, serves as a urinary acidifier.

Pharmacokinetics

The action of most acidifying drugs is immediate. Acetazolamide inhibits the enzyme carbonic anhydrase, which blocks hydrogen ion secretion in the renal tubule, resulting in increased excretion of bicarbonate and a lower pH. Acetazolamide also acidifies urine but may produce metabolic acidosis in normal patients. Orally administered ammonium chloride is absorbed completely in 3 to 6 hours. It's metabolized in the liver to form urea, which is excreted by the kidneys.

Ascorbic acid is best absorbed after oral administration. It's metabolized in the liver and excreted by the kidneys.

Pharmacodynamics

Acidifying drugs have several actions:
- Acetazolamide increases the excretion of bicarbonate, lowering blood pH (Mehta & Emmett, 2021).
- Ammonium chloride lowers the blood pH after being metabolized to urea and hydrochloric acid, which provides hydrogen ions to acidify the blood or urine.
- Ascorbic acid directly acidifies urine, providing hydrogen ions and lowering urine pH.

Pharmacotherapeutics

A patient with metabolic alkalosis requires therapy with an acidifying drug that provides hydrogen ions; such a patient may need chloride ion therapy as well.

Safe and easy

Most patients receive both types of ions in oral or parenteral doses of ammonium chloride, a safer drug that's easy to prepare.

Kidney concerns

In patients with renal dysfunction, acetazolamide may be ineffective and cause the loss of potassium in urine.

Drug interactions

Acidifying drugs don't cause clinically significant drug interactions. However, concurrent use of ammonium chloride and spironolactone may cause increased systemic acidosis.

Side effects/adverse reactions

Side effects and adverse reactions are drug-related.

Acetazolamide

Acetazolamide can cause nausea and vomiting, hypokalemia, anorexia, paresthesia, diarrhea, altered taste, drowsiness, and aplastic anemia.

Ammonium chloride

Metabolic acidosis can result from ammonium chloride. Large doses can cause loss of electrolytes, especially potassium.

Ascorbic acid

Large doses of ascorbic acid can cause GI distress. Patients with glucose-6-phosphate dehydrogenase (G6PD) deficiency may experience hemolytic anemia. Individuals with an alteration in renal function may experience an increased risk and incidence of renal calculi.

The Three-Step Approach

Nursing management for the patient receiving treatment with acidifying drugs includes these three steps.

Preadministration

(Recognize and analyze cues)
- Monitor the patient's blood pH and bicarbonate and potassium levels before, during, and after treatment.
- Watch for signs of metabolic acidosis during and after treatment.
- Assess the patient for hypokalemia during therapy with large amounts of ammonium chloride.
- Assess periodically for signs of anemia.
- Assess conditions that may impact acid/base balance.

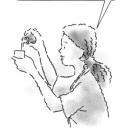

Most patients receive both hydrogen and chloride ions in oral or parenteral doses of ammonium chloride, a safer drug that's easy to prepare.

Keep a complete count

- If the patient has G6PD deficiency and is receiving high doses of ascorbic acid, monitor the complete blood count. Note changes that suggest hemolytic anemia.
- Assess the patient for adverse reactions and drug interactions.
- Assess the patient and family members' knowledge of drug therapy.
- Monitor urine output and consider adjustments if acute changes occur such as a drop to less than 100 mL in 4 hours.

(Priority hypothesis—priority patient problems)
- Electrolyte imbalance/risk
- Fluid overload risk
- Injury risk
- Knowledge deficiency

(Generate solutions)
- The patient will have electrolyte/fluid and acid/base balance.
- The risk of injury to the patient will be minimized.
- The patient and family members will demonstrate understanding of drug therapy.

Medication administration

(Take action)
- Administer an IV acidifying drug slowly to prevent pain or irritation at the infusion site as well as other adverse reactions.
- If hypokalemia occurs during therapy, notify the prescriber, check electrolyte levels, and start therapy to correct the imbalance.
- Teach the patient and family members about the prescribed drug and tell them to report adverse reactions to the primary care provider.
- Report severe GI reactions and monitor urine pH in the patient taking ascorbic acid or oral ammonium chloride.

Telltale twitch

- If twitching occurs with ammonium chloride therapy, withhold the next dose and notify the primary care provider. Twitching may indicate ammonium toxicity.
- Give a mild analgesic if a headache results from high-dose ascorbic acid therapy.
- If insomnia occurs, suggest relaxation techniques before bedtime. If insomnia persists, recommend further evaluation for underlying causes. Vitamin C has beneficial effects for sleep and should not cause insomnia.

Postadministration

(Evaluate outcomes)
- The patient maintains fluid/electrolyte and acid/base balance.
- The patient sustains no injury from adverse reactions.
- The patient and family members demonstrate an understanding of drug therapy.

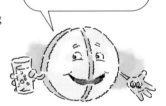

A mild analgesic can help relieve a headache that results from high-dose ascorbic acid therapy.

Quick quiz

1. A nurse is caring for a patient taking multiple medications. Which drug would the nurse monitor the client for hypomagnesemia?

    A. Atenolol—beta-blockers
    B. Omeprazole—proton pump inhibitors
    C. Spironolactone—potassium sparing diuretics
    D. Mylanta—antacids

Answer: B. Hypomagnesemia can often occur after prolonged administration of proton pump inhibitors due to altered absorption in the intestines. In contrast, potassium sparring diuretics and antacids have the potential to cause hypermagnesemia.

2. A nurse is caring for a patient taking spironolactone. Which electrolyte would the nurse monitor closely?

    A. Sodium
    B. Calcium
    C. Potassium
    D. Phosphates

Answer: C. Potassium should be monitored closely in patients receiving potassium-sparing diuretics such as spironolactone to avoid hyperkalemia.

3. A nurse is caring for a patient with an electrolyte imbalance who has calcium gluconate ordered for treatment. Which electrolyte would the nurse monitor to determine effectiveness of treatment?

    A. Sodium
    B. Calcium
    C. Potassium
    D. Magnesium

Answer: C. Calcium gluconate is given to reverse hyperkalemia by increasing the membrane potential and permeability for movement of electrolytes.

4. A nurse is caring for a patient with hyponatremia and has 3% saline ordered. Which route would the nurse anticipate administering the saline?

    A. Oral
    B. Central line
    C. IM injection
    D. Peripheral IV

Answer: B. 3% saline is a hypertonic solution. Hypertonic solutions, such as 3% saline, must be infused through a central venous catheter. Oral, IM injection, and peripheral IV routes are not appropriate for 3% saline administration.

5.   A nurse is caring for a patient with hypocalcemia who is receiving calcium therapy. Which nursing action will the nurse take? Select all that apply.
   A.   Give an IV infusion slowly to prevent arrhythmias and cardiac arrest.
   B.   Keep the patient recumbent for 15 minutes after injecting calcium.
   C.   If extravasation occurs, stop the IV infusion and apply warm, moist compresses to the area.
   D.   Give oral calcium supplements 1 to 2 hours after meals.
   E.   Eat foods such as spinach, rhubarb, bran, and whole grain cereals.

Answer: A, B, C, D. When giving calcium IV, infuse slowly. If extravasation occurs, stop the IV, and apply warm, moist compresses to the area. Keep the patient recumbent for 15 minutes after injecting calcium; and give oral calcium supplements 1 to 2 hours after meals for absorption. Avoid eating foods that interfere with calcium absorption such as spinach, rhubarb, bran, and whole grain cereals.

Scoring

☆☆☆   If you answered all five questions correctly, extraordinary! You're one well-balanced individual!

☆☆   If you answered three or four questions correctly, congratulations! You're moving closer to complete harmony!

☆   If you answered fewer than three questions correctly, try again! You can do it!

Suggested References

Burcham, J. R., & Rosenthal, L. D. (2015). *Lehne's pharmacology for nursing care* (9th ed.). St. Louis, MO: Elsevier Saunders.

Crees, Z. (2020). *The Washington manual of medical therapeutics* (36th ed.). Philadelphia, PA: Lippincott Williams & Wilkins.

Hogan, J., & Goldfarb, S. (2021). Regulation of calcium and phosphate. In R. H. Sterns (Ed.), *UpToDate.*

Mehta, A., & Emmett, M. (2021). Treatment of metabolic alkalosis. In R. H. Sterns (Ed.), *UpToDate.*

Mount, D. (2021). Causes of hypokalemia in adults. In R. S. Sterns & J. P. Forman (Eds.), *UpToDate.*

Sterns, R. (2021). General principles of disorders of water balance (hyponatremia and hypernatremia) and sodium balance (hypovolemia and edema). In M. Emmett (Ed.), *UpToDate.*

Wecker, L., et al. (2019). *Brody's human pharmacology: Mechanism-based therapeutics* (6th ed.). Philadelphia, PA: Elsevier, Inc.

Yu, A. (2021). Hypomagnesemia: Causes of hypomagnesemia. In S. Goldfarb (Ed.), *UpToDate*.

Yu, A., BChir, M., & Yarlagadda, S. (2021). Hypomagnesemia: Clinical manifestations of magnesium depletion. In S. Goldfarb (Ed.), *UpToDate*.

Chapter 20

Practice makes perfect

1. The nurse is caring for a client who wishes to prevent pregnancy. Which type of drug does the nurse anticipate will be prescribed?
   A. Estrogen and progestin combination
   B. 5a-reductase inhibitor
   C. Alpha blocker
   D. Potassium sparing diuretic

2. The nurse is caring for a client with fluid volume excess. Which drug does the nurse anticipate will be prescribed?
   A. Doxazosin
   B. Trospium
   C. Tamsulosin
   D. Hydrochlorothiazide

3. The nurse is caring for a client who has been prescribed trospium. Which teaching will the nurse provide?
   A. Exercise vigorously several days weekly.
   B. Take with meals to avoid gastrointestinal distress.
   C. Increase fluid intake to prevent constipation.
   D. Temporary blurred vision is an expected side effect.

4. The nurse is teaching a male client and his female partner about finasteride. Which education will the nurse provide? **Select all that apply.**
   A. This drug can treat benign prostatic hyperplasia.
   B. Erectile dysfunction is a possible side effect.
   C. Report any increase in breast tissue to the health care provider.
   D. Women of childbearing age should not handle this drug at any time.
   E. Go to the nearest emergency department if priapism occurs.

5. The nurse is teaching a client about signs and symptoms of bleeding while on coumadin. Which client statement indicates the need for further teaching?
   A. "I will avoid eating excess green leafy vegetables since I am on coumadin and it could reverse the effects of the medication."
   B. "Dark tarry stool is not uncommon when taking coumadin and I do not need to seek medical attention.
   C. "If I forget to take my medication for a week, I will notify my provider in case testing is needed prior to restarting my medication."
   D. "Drinking too much water can alter how coumadin affects my body."

6. The nurse is caring for a client who has been taking a benzodiazepine for years. Which client statement requires the nurse to intervene?
   A. "This kind of drug can become addictive over time."
   B. "I need to stop taking this medication immediately."
   C. "Benzodiazepines can cause respiratory depression."
   D. "I will not drink alcohol while I am taking this drug."

7. The nurse is caring for a client who has been prescribed diazepam for a short term. Which teaching will the nurse provide?
   A. "You will need to increase your intake of calcium."
   B. "It takes 2 to 3 weeks for the full effect to be noted."
   C. "Do not drive until you know how this drug affects you."
   D. "Limit alcohol to 1 to 2 drinks per day when taking diazepam."

8. A client with schizophrenia has been given haloperidol. Which reaction does the nurse document when the client's head is noted to be rotated to one side in a fixed position?
   A. Dystonia
   B. Akathisia
   C. Tardive dyskinesia
   D. Waxy flexibility

9. Which laboratory assessment will the nurse prioritize when caring for a client taking aripiprazole?
   A. Luteinizing hormone
   B. Potassium
   C. Hemoglobin
   D. Glucose

10. Which teaching will the nurse provide for a client who has just been prescribed lithium for bipolar disorder? **Select all that apply.**
   A. "Therapeutic blood levels will require ongoing monitoring."
   B. "Be careful to avoid development of dehydration."
   C. "Take your pulse and hold the dose if your pulse is less than 60 beats/minute."
   D. "Take this medication on an empty stomach."
   E. "Decrease sodium intake in your diet."

11. A history of which condition requires the nurse to collaborate with the health care provider for a client who has been prescribed bupropion?
   A. Penicillin allergy
   B. Closed head injury
   C. Thyroid dysfunction
   D. Excess weight gain

12. The nurse is preparing a client for an epidural injection. In which position would the nurse place the client?
  A. Prone
  B. Supine
  C. Sitting
  D. Standing

13. The nurse is reviewing a client's medical history before administering medications. Which client factors would affect absorption of medications? **Select all that apply.**
  A. Blood flow
  B. High fat diet
  C. Form of drug
  D. Route of administration
  E. Taking other medications

14. A nurse manager is listening to a new nurse discuss the therapeutic index of a medication. Which statement by the new nurse indicates understanding of therapeutic index?
  A. "How the drug binds with a protein."
  B. "It is the window between effective drug dosage and toxic drug dosage."
  C. "The drug goes to the liver and is metabolized before the drug enters the circulation."
  D. "Ability to change the drug from its dosage form to a water soluble form for excretion."

15. The nurse is caring for a client with pneumonia who has a temperature of 102°F and a moderate headache. Which type of drug does the nurse anticipate will be prescribed?
  A. Codeine
  B. Morphine
  C. Naloxone
  D. Acetaminophen

16. The nurse is caring for a client who has a sunburn and is using topical anesthetic benzocaine for pain relief. The client asks, "How does that work?" Which response would the nurse provide?
  A. "It numbs the skin surface, decreasing the perception of pain."
  B. "It freezes the skin surface, which prevents nerve impulse transmission."
  C. "It blocks nerve impulse transmission by preventing nerve cell depolarization."
  D. "It occupies sites on specialized receptors, modifying the release of neurotransmitters."

17. The nurse is caring for a client who has been prescribed oxycodone. Which teaching will the nurse provide?
 A. Avoid alcohol while taking the medication.
 B. Prevent diarrhea by increasing fiber in your diet.
 C. Report episodes of tachypnea caused by this medication.
 D. Hold the medication if your systolic blood pressure is elevated.

18. The nurse in the surgery clinic prepares to use acetylcholine eye drops during a client's ocular surgery. Which desired effects would the nurse anticipate from this drug?
 A. Eyelid paralysis
 B. Pupil constriction
 C. Increased intraocular pressure
 D. Decreased ocular musculature movement

19. The nurse instructs a family member of a client with Alzheimer's disease about taking donepezil, an anticholinesterase agent. Which teaching will the nurse provide?
 A. Report constipation.
 B. St. John's wort will increase absorption.
 C. Rise slowly from a lying or sitting position.
 D. This drug should be taken for less than 2 weeks.

20. A 72-year-old client is being treated for urinary incontinence with tolterodine, an anticholinergic agent. Which potential side effect would the nurse anticipate?
 A. Vomiting
 B. Confusion
 C. Increased sweating
 D. Decreased heart rate

21. The nurse is caring for a client with asthma who reports using their albuterol inhaler, a $beta_2$-adrenergic agonists, more often now, at least 6 times a day for the past 3 weeks to manage their asthma symptoms. Which action would the nurse take?
 A. Only documentation is needed as this is a normal finding.
 B. Assess the client's current respiratory status for drug effectiveness.
 C. Report finding to the health care provider as this may indicate poor asthma control.
 D. Teach the client to increase the use of the inhaler to 4 puffs every 4 hours day and night.

22. The nurse is educating the client to always close their eyes when using ipratropium, an anticholinergic. Which response would the nurse make when the client asks, "Why should I close my eyes?"
 A. "It can cause yellowing of the sclera."
 B. "The drug could result in acute narrow-angle glaucoma."
 C. "Proper administration can cause irreversible vision changes."
 D. "Macular degeneration can occur if the drug is absorbed systemically."

23. The nurse is caring for a 10-year-old boy who has exercise-induced asthma. Which type of medication would the nurse anticipate administering to the client?
- A. Corticosteroids
- B. Anticholinergics
- C. Mast cell stabilizers
- D. Beta$_2$-adrenergic agonists

24. A client who is taking an H$_2$-receptor antagonist reports side effects to the nurse. Which side effect is the priority when notifying the health care provider?
- A. Nausea
- B. Headache
- C. Muscle pain
- D. Black tarry stools

25. A client is taking lactulose. Which finding would require the nurse to intervene immediately?
- A. Nausea
- B. Serum glucose 138 mg/dL
- C. Serum potassium 2.9 mEq/L
- D. Four diarrheal stools in the past 24 hours

26. A nurse is caring for a client who has had a myocardial infarction. Which medication type would the nurse anticipate being ordered to prevent straining for a bowel movement?
- A. Antiflatulents
- B. Antidiarrheals
- C. Emollient laxatives
- D. Proton pump inhibitors

27. Which teaching will the nurse provide for a client who has just been prescribed insulin for type I diabetes mellitus? **Select all that apply.**
- A. Avoid skipping meals.
- B. Report symptoms of hypoglycemia.
- C. Carry carbohydrates with you in case of emergency.
- D. Once glucose returns to normal, insulin will not be needed.
- E. Maintain a routine diet, exercise, and medication administration schedule.

28. The nurse is teaching a client about medication safety for thyroid replacement hormones. Which side effect/adverse reaction would the nurse include in the teaching?
- A. Bradycardia
- B. Somnolence
- C. Muscle weakness
- D. Menstrual irregularities

29. The nurse is caring for a client who has been taking sulfonylureas. Which client statement requires the nurse to intervene? **Select all that apply.**
   A. "I wear long sleeves and a hat when I go outside."
   B. "Checking my blood sugar everyday is important."
   C. "At dinner last night, I had three glasses of white wine."
   D. "There is a pouch of tuna in my backpack in case I have a hypoglycemia reaction."
   E. "If I experience symptoms of hyperglycemia, I should call my health care provider."

30. A client who is taking a potassium supplement and reports side effects to the nurse. Which side effect is the priority when notifying the health care provider?
   A. Vomiting
   B. Diarrhea
   C. Confusion
   D. Abdominal pain

31. The nurse is preparing to administer medications. Which medication order would the nurse need to clarify with the health care provider? **Select all that apply.**
   A. Give potassium chloride as an IV bolus.
   B. Administer potassium chloride via IM injection.
   C. Oral potassium chloride to be administered with or after meals.
   D. IV normal saline with potassium phosphate and calcium chloride.
   E. Dissolve potassium chloride powder in at least 4 oz of water or juice.

32. The nurse is caring for a client with hyperaldosteronism. Which medication would the nurse anticipate administering?
   A. Ascorbic acid
   B. Sodium citrate
   C. Calcium chloride
   D. Magnesium oxide

33. A client with narcolepsy is seeing the health care provider today reporting sneezing, itchy eyes, and a mild sore throat. When the provider diagnoses the client with seasonal allergies, which medication does the nurse anticipate will be recommended?
   A. Fexofenadine
   B. Diphenhydramine
   C. Hydroxyzine hydrochloride
   D. Promethazine hydrochloride

34. The nurse is preparing to teach a client about medication for gout prevention. Which information will the nurse include?
    A.   Conduct home blood pressure checks.
    B.   Take medication on an empty stomach.
    C.   Consume at least 2 L of water per day.
    D.   Expect weekly monitoring of blood glucose levels.

35. The nurse will **prioritize** monitoring for which side effect after administering a client's first dose of azathioprine (Imuran)?
    A.   Liver toxicity
    B.   Nausea and vomiting
    C.   Bone marrow suppression
    D.   Hypersensitivity reaction

36. A client has been taking prednisone for several months. The nurse anticipates which laboratory draw will be ordered by the health care provider?
    A.   Calcium
    B.   Glucose
    C.   Potassium
    D.   Vitamin D

37. Which symptom is associated with Cushing's syndrome? **Select all that apply.**
    A.   Moon face
    B.   Hair growth
    C.   Hypertension
    D.   Buffalo hump
    E.   Thinning hair
    F.   Central obesity
    G.   Weight loss

38. A client has been diagnosed with trichomoniasis. Which drug does the nurse anticipate will be prescribed by the health care provider?
    A.   Mupirocin
    B.   Metronidazole
    C.   Sulfacetamide
    D.   Silver sulfadiazine

39. Prednisone has been prescribed for a client with rheumatoid arthritis who is already using mupirocin for impetigo. Which teaching will the nurse provide?
    A.   Mupirocin decreases the effect of prednisone.
    B.   Stop mupirocin for 1 week while taking prednisone.
    C.   Report any signs of infection to the health care provider.
    D.   Taking these drugs in combination decreases the effects of vaccines.

40. The nurse is caring for a client who was just prescribed ketoconazole. Which assessment finding does the nurse anticipate?
    A. White flakes on scalp
    B. Shallow puncture wound
    C. Burns with mild blistering
    D. Unilateral lesions on the back

41. The nurse is caring for a client who is 8 weeks pregnant with a folic acid deficiency. For which condition is the fetus at risk?
    A. Sickle cell anemia
    B. Iron deficiency anemia
    C. Spina bifida
    D. Congenital heart disease

42. Which medication will the nurse anticipate for a client on heparin who develops life-threatening bleeding?
    A. Vitamin K
    B. Protamine sulfate
    C. Enoxaparin
    D. Plavix

43. Which antiplatelet drug is used frequently to reduce the risk of death in clients with a previous myocardial infarction?
    A. Enoxaparin
    B. Warfarin
    C. Heparin
    D. Aspirin

44. A client presents to the emergency department and is diagnosed with an acute ischemic stroke. Which medication will the nurse anticipate for this client?
    A. Warfarin
    B. Aspirin
    C. Alteplase
    D. Lovenox

45. When caring for a client on intravenous heparin therapy which lab values will the nurse review as a priority? **Select all that apply.**
    A. Hemoglobin
    B. Hematocrit
    C. Platelet count
    D. Partial thromboplastin time (PTT)
    E. Potassium

46. The charge nurse is teaching a critical care course on the use of sodium nitroprusside for hypertensive crisis. Which teaching will the nurse include? **Select all that apply.**
    A. This drug must be shielded from light.
    B. Titration is unnecessary with this medication.
    C. Tachycardia is a common side effect of this medication.
    D. This drug is both an arterial and venous vasodilator.
    E. Cyanide toxicity can occur with this medication.

47. Which statement will the nurse use to explain the pharmacodynamics of ACE inhibitors?
    A. "ACE inhibitors are absorbed in the GI tract."
    B. "ACE inhibitors work by helping the body retain sodium."
    C. "ACE inhibitors prevent the conversion of angiotensin I to angiotensin II."
    D. "ACE inhibitors are commonly used in heart failure."

48. Which client statement indicates that additional teaching about metoprolol is needed?
    A. "I will hold the dose and call the provider if my heart rate is less than 60 bpm."
    B. "If I develop dizziness, I will stop the medication."
    C. "I will not crush the medication."
    D. "The metoprolol is for my blood pressure."

49. The nurse is caring for a client admitted with digoxin toxicity. What assessment data will the nurse anticipate?
    A. Atrial fibrillation
    B. Diarrhea
    C. Blurry vision
    D. Headache

50. The nurse is reviewing a client's chart who is on a chemotherapy regimen. The nurse notes the client's ejection fraction (EF) is 45%. Which medication will the nurse anticipate being removed from the chemotherapy regimen?
    A. Cyclophosphamide (Cytoxan)
    B. Trastuzumab (Herceptin)
    C. Gemcitabine (Gemzar)
    D. Fludarabine

51. Which client statement regarding capecitabine (Xeloda) indicates the need for further teaching?
    A. "I will take this medication within 30 minutes of a meal."
    B. "I will not share my medication with anyone else."
    C. "It is important to take this medication at the same time I take my warfarin."
    D. "I need to assess my skin and report changes to my provider."

52. The nurse is caring for a client who has had severe diarrhea for 2 days from irinotecan (Camptosar). What is the priority nursing concern and intervention?
    A. Hypomagnesemia; provide client with oral magnesium as ordered
    B. Bowel rest; place client on clear liquid diet
    C. Hypokalemia; monitor for arrhythmias
    D. Volume depletion; assess skin turgor regularly

53. Which side effect will the nurse teach the client who is taking dacarbazine?
- A. Photosensitivity
- B. Constipation
- C. Urinary retention
- D. Hand-foot syndrome

54. The nurse is caring for a client who is 2 weeks from the last dose of chemotherapy. The client's current absolute neutrophil count (ANC) is 700 mcL. What will the nurse anticipate for this client?
- A. Proceeding with the scheduled chemotherapy regimen
- B. Halting the client's chemotherapy regimen indefinitely
- C. Rescheduling the client for a repeat CBC in 1 week
- D. Providing education to the client to address the ANC level

55. The nurse is reviewing the home medication list for a client who is being started on the aromatase inhibitor, anastrozole (Arimidex). Which medication would prompt clarification?
- A. Metformin (Glucophage)
- B. Vaginal estrogen cream
- C. Azithromycin (Z-pack)
- D. Lisinopril (Prinivil)

56. Which drug requires leucovorin rescue when administered at high doses?
- A. Methotrexate (Rasuvo)
- B. Doxorubicin (Adriamycin)
- C. Palbociclib (Ibrance)
- D. Capecitabine (Xeloda)

57. The nurse is caring for a client recently admitted with a diagnosis of Guillain-Barré syndrome. Which assessment data would the nurse anticipate?
- A. Recent seizures or traumatic brain injury
- B. Meningitis within the last 5 years
- C. Back injury or trauma to the spinal cord
- D. Respiratory or gastrointestinal infection within the past month

58. The nurse is teaching a client with myasthenia gravis about the prevention of myasthenic and cholinergic crisis. Which teaching will the nurse include?
- A. Eat large, well-balanced meals.
- B. Do muscle strengthening exercises.
- C. Do chores early in the day while less fatigued.
- D. Take medications at the same time each day.

59. A client is admitted to the hospital for evaluation of balance and coordination problems, including possible Ménière's disease. What assessment data will the nurse anticipate?
    A.   Vertigo, tinnitus, and hearing loss
    B.   Vertigo, vomiting, and nystagmus
    C.   Vertigo, pain, and hearing impairment
    D.   Vertigo, blurred vision, and fever

60. A client with newly diagnosed multiple sclerosis (MS) is prescribed baclofen for spasticity. What teaching will the nurse include? **Select all that apply.**
    A.   If you experience dizziness, stop the medication and notify the provider.
    B.   Avoid the use of alcohol while taking this medication.
    C.   The drowsiness associated with the medication decreases over time.
    D.   You may not drive while taking this medication.
    E.   Urinary hesitancy can occur with this medication.

61. The nurse is teaching a client and the family about administration of a neuromuscular blocking drug. What teaching will the nurse provide?
    A.   "You will not be aware of your surroundings and will be asleep."
    B.   "You will be unable to move, but you may be able to speak."
    C.   "A ventilator will be used to support your breathing."
    D.   "If you are uncomfortable, you will be able to press the pain pump button."

62. A client with Parkinson's disease is experiencing brownish-orange urine. What would the nurse anticipate?
    A.   The client most likely has a urinary tract infection.
    B.   The client is most likely saw palmetto for dysuria.
    C.   The client is most likely taking COMT inhibiting medication.
    D.   The client is most likely dehydrated causing the change in urine.

63. The nurse is caring for a client who takes phenytoin for seizures. Which client statement requires further teaching?
    A.   "I know I have to take the same brand with each refill."
    B.   "I have a medical alert bracelet."
    C.   "I take melatonin for sleep and some herbal meds for anxiety."
    D.   "I know the medication may cause my urine to change colors."

64. Which nursing action is appropriate when administering ear drops to a child?
- A. Pull the ear up and slightly away from the body.
- B. Pull the ear down and slightly away from the body.
- C. Place the client in a prone position.
- D. Wait at least 3 to 5 minutes between each ear drop.

65. For which condition or procedure will the nurse anticipate the use of mydriatics and cycloplegics? **Select all that apply.**
- A. To perform an eye examination
- B. To conduct a procedure on the eye
- C. To treat a condition involving the iris
- D. To treat open-angle glaucoma
- E. To treat bacterial eye infections

66. The nurse is teaching a client about eye drop administration. Which teaching will the nurse include?
- A. Wait at least 3 to 5 minutes between instilling a different type of eye drop.
- B. Contact lenses do not affect the absorption of eye drops.
- C. Place the dropper on the eye if possible to make sure the full drop is administered.
- D. Wipe off excess medication on the eyelid and eye area immediately after administration.

67. Which side effect will the nurse include when teaching a client who is taking neomycin/polymyxin B/hydrocortisone otic?
- A. Ototoxicity
- B. Nephrotoxicity
- C. Hepatotoxicity
- D. Cataracts

68. Which medication will the nurse anticipate for a client with a significant build up of ear wax?
- A. Pilocarpine
- B. Mannitol
- C. Carbamide peroxide
- D. Tafluprost

69. Which action will the nurse take when administering ear drops to an adult?
- A. Pull the ear up and away from the body.
- B. Pull the ear down and away from the body.
- C. Pull the ear up and toward the body.
- D. Pull the ear down and toward the body.

70. How do osmotic agents reduce the volume of vitreous humor and decrease intraocular pressure?
    A. Elevating the osmolality of the blood
    B. Elevating the glomerular filtrate osmolarity
    C. Decreasing the glomerular filtrate osmolarity
    D. Decreasing the osmolality of the blood

71. How long should live attenuated influenza vaccines be avoided before and after administration of antivirals used for influenza A?
    A. Two weeks before and at least 48 hours after administration
    B. Two weeks before and at least 1 week after administration
    C. 48 hours before and at least 2 weeks after administration
    D. 48 hours before and at least 1 week after administration

72. Which condition will the nurse teach a client taking sulfonamides that may occur?
    A. Hypotension
    B. Hypoglycemia
    C. Hyperglycemia
    D. Hypertension

73. Which medication will the nurse question when it is prescribed for a client who is also taking levofloxacin?
    A. Tamsulosin
    B. Levothyroxine
    C. Amiodarone
    D. Allopurinol

74. Which medication does the nurse anticipate will be prescribed for a client newly diagnosed with *Clostridium difficile*?
    A. Vancomycin
    B. Metronidazole
    C. Doxycycline
    D. Cefuroxime

75. Which teaching point will the nurse provide to a 23-year-old female with otalgia taking amoxicillin?
    A. Monitor for an increase in acne since penicillins can alter hormone production.
    B. Avoid exposure to direct sunlight while taking this medication due to its photosensitizing effects.
    C. If symptoms resolve before therapy is completed, it is okay to discontinue the antibiotic.
    D. Use a second form of birth control to prevent pregnancy while taking this drug.

Answers

CN—Client Needs Category
CNS—Client Needs Subcategory
CL—Cognitive Level

1. Correct Answer: A. Estrogen and progestin combination therapy is used as a hormonal contraceptive, as these hormones taken together inhibit ovulation. 5a-reductase inhibitors, alpha blockers, and potassium-sparing diuretics do not prevent pregnancy.
CN: Health Promotion and Maintenance
CNS: Health Promotion/Disease Prevention
CL: Understanding

2. Correct Answer: D. Hydrochlorothiazide is a diuretic, used to treat fluid volume excess. Doxazosin and tamsulosin are alpha blockers which relax muscles and thus facilitate the flow of urine. Trospium is a urinary tract antispasmodic used to decrease muscle spasms.
CN: Pharmacological and Parenteral Therapies
CNS: Expected Actions/Outcomes
CL: Understanding

3. Correct Answer: C. Side effects of trospium can include dry mouth and constipation so the nurse will encourage increasing the intake of fluids to prevent these conditions. Increased or vigorous exercise should be discouraged, as urinary tract antispasmodic drugs can decrease the client's ability to sweat; thus, overheating is a concern. This drug should be taken at least 1 hour before meals or on an empty stomach to increase absorption, not with food. Blurred vision should be reported, as this is a concerning side effect of urinary tract antispasmodic drugs.
CN: Pharmacological and Parenteral Therapies
CNS: Expected Actions/Outcomes
CL: Applying

4. Correct Answer: A, B, C, D, E. The nurse will teach that finasteride is a drug prescribed to treat benign prostatic hyperplasia. Side effects include erectile dysfunction and gynecomastia (which should be reported to the provider). Pregnant women and women of childbearing age should not handle finasteride because it is a teratogenic drug. Priapism, another possible side effect, is a medical emergency that requires immediate treatment.
CN: Pharmacological and Parenteral Therapies
CNS: Adverse Effects/Contraindications/Side Effects/Interactions
CL: Applying

5. Correct Answer: B. Dark tarry stool is a sign of gastrointestinal bleeding which is a risk with warfarin. The client requires additional education regarding the need to seek medical direction if signs of bleeding, such as tarry stool, are observed.

    CN: Pharmacological and Parenteral Therapies
    CNS: Expected Actions/Outcomes
    CL: Applying

6. Correct Answer: B. The nurse will intervene when the client says they will stop taking the medication immediately. Benzodiazepine use must be tapered to avoid seizures. The nurse will remind the client to work with their health care provider on a weaning schedule. It is accurate that benzodiazepines are addictive, can cause respiratory depression, and should not be taken with alcohol, so the nurse does not need to intervene when the client makes these statements.

    CN: Pharmacological and Parenteral Therapies
    CNS: Adverse Effects/Contraindications/Side Effects/Interactions
    CL: Applying

7. Correct Answer: C. The nurse will teach that the client should not drive, make important decisions, or operate machinery until they know how the drug affects them, as diazepam can cause central nervous system depression. Taking diazepam does not require an additional intake of calcium. Therapeutic effects begin shortly after taking this drug. The client must be taught to completely avoid alcohol while taking diazepam, as this can cause further CNS depression.

    CN: Pharmacological and Parenteral Therapies
    CNS: Adverse Effects/Contraindications/Side Effects/Interactions
    CL: Applying

8. Correct Answer: A. Dystonia is an extrapyramidal (EP) adverse reaction to antipsychotic medications. It is characterized by a state of abnormal muscle tone resulting in muscular spasm. Akathisia is a movement disorder characterized by the feeling of restlessness. Tardive dyskinesia is characterized by abnormal and uncontrollable motor movements of the body and face. Waxy flexibility is characterized by the state of a client's limbs remaining in a fixed position after someone else manipulates them.

    CN: Pharmacological and Parenteral Therapies
    CNS: Adverse Effects/Contraindications/Side Effects/Interactions
    CL: Applying

9. Correct Answer: D. Atypical antipsychotics are associated with metabolic changes that include hyperglycemia, dyslipidemia, and

weight gain. Therefore, the nurse will prioritize checking the glucose result. All other laboratory values should be followed, yet glucose should be prioritized due to the risk for development of metabolic changes that can lead to other systemic problems.

CN: Pharmacological and Parenteral Therapies
CNS: Adverse Effects/Contraindications/Side Effects/Interactions
CL: Applying

10. Correct Answer: A, B. The nurse will teach the client that ongoing monitoring of blood levels is required while taking lithium, as it has a narrow therapeutic index. The nurse will also teach the client to avoid dehydration, as this can lead to lithium toxicity. There is no need to take the pulse before taking the medication. Lithium should be taken with food to avoid gastrointestinal distress. Regular sodium intake should be taught, as a reduced sodium diet can lead to lithium toxicity.

CN: Pharmacological and Parenteral Therapies
CNS: Adverse Effects/Contraindications/Side Effects/Interactions
CL: Analyzing

11. Correct Answer: B. Bupropion lowers the seizure threshold so it should be used with great caution in clients with seizures or head injuries that increase the risk for seizures. Penicillin allergy, thyroid dysfunction, and excess weight gain are not contraindications for the use of bupropion.

CN: Pharmacological and Parenteral Therapies
CNS: Adverse Effects/Contraindications/Side Effects/Interactions
CL: Analyzing

12. Correct Answer: C. Placing a client in the sitting or side lying position allows for straight entry of the needed into the epidural space. In other positions, it is more difficult to insert the needle straight into the epidural space.

CN: Reduction of Risk Potential
CNS: Therapeutic Procedures
CL: Understanding

13. Correct Answer: A, B, C, D, E. Factors that affect absorption of a drug includes blood flow, a high fat diet, form of the drug (capsule, tablet), route of administration, taking other medications, pain and stress, and first pass effect.

CN: Pharmacological and Parenteral Therapies
CNS: Medication Administration
CL: Analyzing

14. Correct Answer: B. The therapeutic index is a statistical number that indicates the safety margin of a drug; the window between drug effectiveness and toxicity. Protein binding describes how much a particular drug binds with a protein. First pass effect is when the drug goes to the liver and is metabolized before the drug enters the circulation. Biotransformation or metabolism is the body's ability to change the drug from its dosage form to a water-soluble form for excretion.

> CN: Pharmacological and Parenteral Therapies
> CNS: Medication Administration
> CL: Understanding

15. Correct Answer: D. Acetaminophen is used to reduce fever and relieve headache, muscle ache, and general pain. The pain control effects of acetaminophen works by inhibiting prostaglandin synthesis and reduces fever by acting directly on the heat-regulating center in the hypothalamus. While codeine and morphine, opioid agonists, are used for moderate to severe pain, these drugs do not reduce fever. Naloxone, an opioid antagonist, is prescribed for opioid overdose.

> CN: Pharmacological and Parenteral Therapies
> CNS: Expected Actions/Outcomes
> CL: Understanding

16. Correct Answer: C. Benzocaine prevents nerve cell depolarization, thus blocking nerve impulse transmission and relieving pain.

> CN: Pharmacological and Parenteral Therapies
> CNS: Expected Actions/Outcomes
> CL: Applying

17. Correct Answer: A. Teaching for a client who is prescribed oxycodone, an opioid agonist, includes avoiding alcohol, avoiding the operation of heavy machinery until effects of drug are known, preventing constipation as oxycodone decreases peristalsis, reporting bradypnea and bradycardia and taking the medication as prescribed.

> CN: Pharmacological and Parenteral Therapies
> CNS: Adverse Effects/Contraindications/Side Effects/Interactions
> CL: Applying

18. Correct Answer: B. Acetylcholine is a cholinergic agonist that acts directly on the cholinergic receptors to stimulate the release of acetylcholine. One of the desired effects in ocular surgery is to constrict the client's pupils, for example, after cataract lens extraction or iridectomy. It has a rapid onset and may begin to work almost immediately.

> CN: Pharmacological and Parenteral Therapies
> CNS: Expected Actions/Outcomes
> CL: Understanding

19. Correct Answer: C. A potential side effect of anticholinesterase agent, such as donepezil, is dizziness or syncope and diarrhea. Getting up slowly can help reduce fall risks. The client may need to take

this medication lifelong. The nurse would also teach to avoid herbal remedies while taking anticholinesterase agents as St. John's wort alters the absorption of donepezil.

CN: Pharmacological and Parenteral Therapies
CNS: Adverse Effects/Contraindications/Side Effects/Interactions
CL: Applying

20. Correct Answer: B. Adverse reactions to anticholinergic drugs like tolterodine include dry mouth, reduced bronchial secretion, increased heart rate, blurred vision, decreased sweating, confusion, delirium, and cognitive decline. Confusion, cognitive decline, and delirium are a potential concern for older adults taking anticholinergic drugs.

CN: Pharmacological and Parenteral Therapies
CNS: Adverse Effects/Contraindications/Side Effects/Interactions
CL: Understanding

21. Correct Answer: C. Some clients with COPD use short-acting inhaled beta$_2$-adrenergic agonists around the clock on a specified schedule. However, excessive use of these agents may indicate poor asthma control, requiring reassessment of the therapeutic regimen by the provider. The nurse would assess the client's current respiratory status, but this may not be indicative of overall asthma control. The nurse would not teach the client to increase medication frequency and dosage without a provider's prescription.

CN: Pharmacological and Parenteral Therapies
CNS: Expected Actions/Outcomes
CL: Applying

22. Correct Answer: B. The client should be instructed to keep eyes closed when using ipratropium because it can cause acute narrow-angle glaucoma if it gets in the eyes. Instruct the client to call the prescriber immediately if the drug gets in the eyes. Ipratropium does not cause yellowing of the sclera, irreversible vision changes, or macular degeneration.

CN: Pharmacological and Parenteral Therapies
CNS: Adverse Effects/Contraindications/Side Effects/Interactions
CL: Applying

23. Correct Answer: C. Mast cell stabilizers control the inflammatory process and are used for the prevention and long-term control of asthma symptoms. They are the agents of choice for children and clients with exercise-induced asthma.

CN: Pharmacological and Parenteral Therapies
CNS: Expected Actions/Outcomes
CL: Understanding

24. Correct Answer: D. The priority for the nurse would be to immediately notify the health care provider of reports of black tarry stools as this is indicative of a GI bleed. While nausea, headache, and muscle pain should be addressed, the priority is reporting black tarry stools.

    CN: Pharmacological and Parenteral Therapies
    CNS: Adverse Effects/Contraindications/Side Effects/Interactions
    CL: Analyzing

25. Correct Answer: C. Lactulose, an osmolar diuretic, can cause side effects including fluid and electrolyte imbalances (hypokalemia and hypernatremia), diarrhea, abdominal cramps, nausea and vomiting, and flatulence. Although the client is nauseated, has diarrhea, and has a above normal serum glucose, the potassium level is at a critical value and must be addressed immediately.

    CN: Pharmacological and Parenteral Therapies
    CNS: Adverse Effects/Contraindications/Side Effects/Interactions
    CL: Analyzing

26. Correct Answer: C. Emollient laxatives are frequently prescribed for clients after MI to reduce straining during bowel movements. Antiflatulent drugs help remove excess gas in the gastrointestinal tract. Antidiarrheal drugs are used to treat diarrhea. Proton pump inhibitors are used to treat peptic ulcers and GERD.

    CN: Pharmacological and Parenteral Therapies
    CNS: Expected Actions/Outcomes
    CL: Understanding

27. Correct Answer: A, B, C, E. A nurse would teach a client prescribed insulin to avoid skipping meals; report symptoms of hypoglycemia and hyperglycemia; carry carbohydrates in case of emergency; and maintain a routine diet, exercise, and medication administration schedule, and insulin is a lifelong hormone replacement.

    CN: Pharmacological and Parenteral Therapies
    CNS: Expected Actions/Outcomes
    CL: Analyzing

28. Correct Answer: D. The nurse would teach a client taking a thyroid hormone replacement drug side effects/adverse reactions including tachycardia, insomnia, heat intolerance, fever, nervousness, tremors, and menstrual irregularities.

    CN: Pharmacological and Parenteral Therapies
    CNS: Adverse Effects/Contraindications/Side Effects/Interactions
    CL: Understanding

29. Correct Answer: C, D. The nurse would intervene if a client stated they had alcohol at dinner and had a pouch of tuna in case of a hypoglycemic reaction. Alcohol with sulfonylureas can cause hypoglycemia. In cases of hypoglycemic reactions, the client requires a rapid-acting glucose (carbohydrate) to elevate glucose, not a protein. Sulfonylureas can cause photosensitivity and clients would need to protect their skin by wearing long sleeves and a hat to prevent sunburnlike skin reactions. A client stating that checking blood sugar regularly and reporting symptoms of hyperglycemia does not require nursing intervention.

    CN: Pharmacological and Parenteral Therapies
    CNS: Expected Actions/Outcomes
    CL: Analyzing

30. Correct Answer: C. For the client taking a potassium supplement, the nurse would teach the client to report symptoms of hyperkalemia which includes diarrhea, muscle weakness, cardiac dysrhythmias, vomiting, abdominal pain, and confusion. The priority for the nurse is to report confusion as this indicates the potassium level is affecting brain function.

    CN: Pharmacological and Parenteral Therapies
    CNS: Adverse Effects/Contraindications/Side Effects/Interactions
    CL: Analyzing

31. Correct Answer: A, B, D. The nurse would clarify the orders of administering potassium via the IM route or as an IV bolus as this could cause cardiac arrest. The nurse would also clarify the order to mix potassium with calcium in an IV solution together as this would cause precipitates to form. Oral potassium should be taken with or after meals to prevent GI distress and if the supplement is in powder form, the powder should be mixed in a minimum of 4 oz of water or juice and sipped slowly over 5 minutes.

    CN: Pharmacological and Parenteral Therapies
    CNS: Adverse Effects/Contraindications/Side Effects/Interactions
    CL: Analyzing

32. Correct Answer: C. Hyperaldosteronism depletes magnesium and may require a magnesium supplement. Ascorbic acid is an acidifying drug and sodium citrate is an alkalizing drug; neither of which would help with hyperaldosteronism. Calcium chloride is not generally used as a supplement to help manage electrolyte imbalances in hyperaldosteronism.

    CN: Pharmacological and Parenteral Therapies
    CNS: Expected Actions/Outcomes
    CL: Understanding

33. Correct Answer: A. Narcolepsy is a condition in which people fall asleep at unpredictable and unusual times, often quite suddenly. The nurse anticipates that the health care provider will recommend a nonsedating antihistamine like fexofenadine (Allegra). All other choices are sedating and should be avoided due to the preexisting condition of narcolepsy.

CN: Pharmacological and Parenteral Therapies
CNS: Adverse Effects/Contraindications/Side Effects/Interactions
CL: Understanding.

34. Correct Answer: C. Adequate fluid intake is necessary when taking medication to prevent gout. This helps to alkalize the urine which helps promote excretion of uric acid. The client will not need to conduct home blood pressure checks, take the medication on an empty stomach, or have blood glucose levels monitored.

CN: Pharmacological and Parenteral Therapies
CNS: Expected Actions/Outcomes
CL: Applying.

35. Correct Answer: D. All immunosuppressants like azathioprine (Imuran) can cause hypersensitivity reactions; therefore, the nurse will prioritize monitoring for this condition, as it may occur very quickly after the first dose(s). Side effects such as nausea and vomiting are not immediately critical and do not require prioritization. Adverse effects including bone marrow suppression and liver toxicity take a degree of time to develop, so these are not the priority immediately after initial dosing.

CN: Pharmacological and Parenteral Therapies
CNS: Adverse Effects/Contraindications/Side Effects/Interactions
CL: Applying.

36. Correct Answer: B. Corticosteroids affect almost all body systems. Endocrine system reactions may include decreased glucose tolerance, resulting in hyperglycemia and possibly precipitating diabetes mellitus. Therefore, the nurse will anticipate that a serum blood glucose laboratory order will be placed by the health care provider.

CN: Pharmacological and Parenteral Therapies
CNS: Adverse Effects/Contraindications/Side Effects/Interactions
CL: Applying.

37. Correct Answer: A, D, E, F. Cushing's syndrome is characterized by moon face, buffalo hump, thinning hair, and central obesity. It is not characterized by hair growth, hypertension, or weight loss.

CN: Pharmacological and Parenteral Therapies
CNS: Adverse Effects/Contraindications/Side Effects/Interactions
CL: Remembering

38. Correct Answer: B. Trichomoniasis is a sexually transmitted infection caused by a parasite. Metronidazole is a nitroimidazole antibiotic that is used to treat this type of infection. Mupirocin is used to treat methicillin-resistant staphylococcus aureus (MRSA). Sulfacetamide is used to treat seborrheic dermatitis. Silver sulfadiazine is used to treat burns.

    CN: Physiological Adaptation

    CNS: Alteration in Body Systems

    CL: Understanding

39. Correct Answer: C. Topical antibiotics like mupirocin, used in combination with a corticosteroid, may mask signs of infection or allergic reaction or increase risk for superimposed infection; the nurse will teach the client to report any signs of infection to the health care provider right away. Mupirocin and prednisone can be used together; mupirocin does not decrease the efficacy of prednisone. The nurse will never teach a client to stop another medication unless that is prescribed by the health care provider. Mafenide may reduce the efficacy of vaccinations; however, these drugs are not known to do so.

    CN: Physiological Adaptation

    CNS: Alteration in Body Systems

    CL: Applying

40. Correct Answer: A. Ketoconazole is regularly used for dandruff, a condition in which there are white flakes on the scalp and hair. This drug is not used to treat puncture wounds, burns, or shingles, which are unilateral lesions that arise on one side of the body.

    CN: Physiological Adaptation

    CNS: Alteration in Body Systems

    CL: Applying

41. Correct Answer: C. Lack of folic acid in pregnancy increases the risk for birth defects such as anencephaly and spina bifida.

    CN: Health Promotion and Maintenance

    CNS: Health Promotion/Disease Prevention

    CL: Understanding

42. Correct Answer: B. Protamine sulfate is the reversal agent for heparin and is used when life-threatening bleeding occurs in clients on heparin therapy.

    CN: Pharmacological and Parenteral Therapies

    CNS: Adverse Effects/Contraindications/Side Effects/Interactions

    CL: Applying

43. Correct Answer: D. Aspirin is an antiplatelet drug that is commonly used to reduce the risk of death in clients following a myocardial infarction.

    CN: Pharmacological and Parenteral Therapies

    CNS: Adverse Effects/Contraindications/Side Effects/Interactions

    CL: Understanding

44. Correct Answer: C. Alteplase is used to treat emboli, such as emboli associated with ischemic strokes, pulmonary embolism, myocardial infarction, and peripheral artery occlusion.

>   CN: Pharmacological and Parenteral Therapies
>   CNS: Adverse Effects/Contraindications/Side Effects/Interactions
>   CL: Applying

45. Correct Answer: A, B, C, D. Hemoglobin and hematocrit would be assessed as a priority for potential indication of hemorrhage. The PTT is used to evaluate the clotting time and the effectiveness of heparin. Platelet counts should be monitored for thrombocytopenia, which can be indicative of heparin-induced thrombocytopenia (HIT).

>   CN: Pharmacological and Parenteral Therapies
>   CNS: Adverse Effects/Contraindications/Side Effects/Interactions
>   CL: Applying

46. Correct Answer: A, C, D, E. Nitroprusside is a direct vasodilator affecting the arterial and venous system. The drug is light sensitive and must be shielded from light. Sodium nitroprusside is a very potent vasodilator that requires close monitoring and frequent titration. Tachycardia is a common side effect and cyanide toxicity can occur with this medication.

>   CN: Pharmacological and Parenteral Therapies
>   CNS: Adverse Effects/Contraindications/Side Effects/Interactions
>   CL: Applying

47. Correct Answer: C. Pharmacodynamics is how the drug acts on the body. ACE inhibitors prevent the conversion of angiotensin I to angiotensin II. ACE inhibitors promote the excretion of sodium and water (not retention of sodium). ACE inhibitors are absorbed in the GI tract. However, this process describes pharmacokinetics, not pharmacodynamics. ACE inhibitors are commonly used in heart failure; however, this process describes pharmacotherapeutics, not pharmacodynamics.

>   CN: Pharmacological and Parenteral Therapies
>   CNS: Adverse Effects/Contraindications/Side Effects/Interactions
>   CL: Applying

48. Correct Answer: B. Metoprolol has a black box warning regarding sudden cessation of the drug. Do not stop taking the drug suddenly. Rather, notify the provider regarding the dizziness and decrease the dose gradually over 1 to 2 weeks. The other client statements are accurate regarding the use of metoprolol.

>   CN: Pharmacological and Parenteral Therapies
>   CNS: Adverse Effects/Contraindications/Side Effects/Interactions
>   CL: Applying

49. Correct Answer: C. Digoxin has a narrow therapeutic index, so a dose adequate to produce therapeutic effects may produce signs of toxicity. Signs of digoxin toxicity include slow to rapid ventricular rhythms, nausea and vomiting, blurred vision, anorexia, abdominal discomfort, and mental changes.

    CN: Pharmacological and Parenteral Therapies
    CNS: Adverse Effects/Contraindications/Side Effects/Interactions
    CL: Applying

50. Correct Answer: B. Trastuzumab (Herceptin) is known to reduce the ejection fraction and must be held if the baseline EF drops. None of the other drugs reduce the ejection fraction.

    CN: Pharmacological and Parenteral Therapies
    CNS: Adverse Effects/Contraindications/Side Effects/Interactions
    CL: Applying

51. Correct Answer: C. Capecitabine (Xeloda) and warfarin (Coumadin) have been associated with substantial elevations in INR. This can lead to severe bleeding and death. Anticoagulant parameters (such as the INR) must be monitored closely and if these two drugs are combined, reduction in the warfarin dose will likely be required.

    CN: Pharmacological and Parenteral Therapies
    CNS: Adverse Effects/Contraindications/Side Effects/Interactions
    CL: Applying

52. Correct Answer: C. Significant electrolyte imbalance can occur from uncontrolled diarrhea. Hypokalemia is the most significant and life-threatening concern from those listed. Monitoring for arrhythmias is a priority intervention as arrhythmias can occur with hypokalemia. While hypomagnesemia could occur, oral magnesium can cause diarrhea so this would be avoided. Resting the bowel does not address the priority which is electrolyte imbalance. Volume depletion is a concern, however, assessing skin turgor is not the priority intervention.

    CN: Pharmacological and Parenteral Therapies
    CNS: Adverse Effects/Contraindications/Side Effects/Interactions
    CL: Applying

53. Correct Answer A. Photosensitivity is a side effect of dacarbazine. Constipation, urinary retention, and hand-foot syndrome are not side effects.

    CN: Pharmacological and Parenteral Therapies
    CNS: Adverse Effects/Contraindications/Side Effects/Interactions
    CL: Understanding

54. Correct Answer: C. Neutropenia is an expected side effect of chemotherapy. Absolute neutrophil counts usually recover prior to the next chemotherapy cycle. However, sometimes the bone marrow becomes slower in recovery. Assessing the client's blood counts in a week will allow the body additional time to recover without intervention. The client could experience life-threatening infections if the ANC remains low or if chemotherapy is continued with this lab value. Chemotherapy is not administered if the ANC is less than 1,000. Stopping the regimen indefinitely is not the first line of caution as a week for the body to recover would occur first, followed by a potential dose reduction. While the client can maintain hydration and nutrition, there are no self-directed interventions that will keep the white blood cells within normal limits.

> CN: Pharmacological and Parenteral Therapies
> CNS: Adverse Effects/Contraindications/Side Effects/Interactions;
> CL: Applying

55. Correct Answer: B. Aromatase inhibitors are intended to lower the body's production of estrogen to treat hormone-positive breast cancer. Anastrozole works by diminishing the biosynthesis of estrogens in peripheral tissues and cancer cells. A combination of this drug with vaginal estrogen cream could lead to decreased effectiveness of the aromatase inhibitors. The other medications have no known drug interactions with anastrozole.

> CN: Pharmacological and Parenteral Therapies
> CNS: Adverse Effects/Contraindications/Side Effects/Interactions
> CL: Applying

56. Correct Answer: A. Methotrexate is a folic acid analogue. This drug blocks normal folic acid processing and results in cell death. Leucovorin rescue helps reverse cell death and renal dysfunction from delayed methotrexate elimination. Leucovorin rescue usually starts about 24 hours after high-dose methotrexate. Leucovorin rescue is not used for standard methotrexate dosing.

> CN: Pharmacological and Parenteral Therapies
> CNS: Adverse Effects/Contraindications/Side Effects/Interactions
> CL: Understanding

57. Correct Answer: D. Guillain-Barré syndrome is a clinical syndrome of unknown origin that involves the cranial and peripheral nerves. Many clients report a history of respiratory or gastrointestinal illness 1 to 4 weeks prior to the onset of neurological deficit. Occasionally, the syndrome can be triggered by vaccinations or surgery.

> CN: Health Promotion and Maintenance
> CNS: Health Promotion/Disease Prevention
> CL: Understanding

58. Correct Answer: D. Clients with myasthenia gravis must be taught to take medications at the same time each day to maintain consistent levels versus levels of medication that are too high or too low. The client should be taught to space out activities over the course of the day to conserve energy. Muscle strengthening exercises are not helpful and can add additional fatigue.

CN: Pharmacological and Parenteral Therapies
CNS: Adverse Effects/Contraindications/Side Effects/Interactions
CL: Understanding

59. Correct Answer: A. Ménière's disease, an inner ear disease, is characterized by the triad of symptoms including vertigo, tinnitus, and hearing loss. The combination of vertigo, vomiting, and nystagmus would be anticipated with labyrinthitis. Ménière's disease rarely causes pain, blurred vision, or fever.

CN: Physiological Adaptation
CNS: Alterations in Body Systems
CL: Applying

60. Correct Answer: B, C, E. Skeletal muscle relaxants such as baclofen should not be stopped abruptly. Dizziness is a known side effect that may decrease over time or may require the provider to decrease the dose. However, abrupt cessation should be avoided. The use of alcohol with this medication should be avoided as it can intensify the effects. Drowsiness is a known side effect of baclofen that generally decreases with use. Clients can drive after a period of time with baclofen therapy. The key is to understand how the drug will affect the body, and the client should avoid driving or any hazardous activities until the CNS effects of the drug are known. Urinary hesitancy does occur with skeletal muscle relaxants.

CN: Pharmacological and Parenteral Therapies
CNS: Adverse Effects/Contraindications/Side Effects/Interactions
CL: Applying

61. Correct Answer: C. If neuromuscular blocking drugs are prescribed, the client is fully paralyzed, unable to move, speak, or breathe on their own. Ventilatory assistance is provided. These drugs do not cause sleep, and the client will be aware of their surroundings. Antianxiety medications are usually administered in conjunction with these medications. The client will not be able to push a button for pain control as this medication causes complete paralysis.

CN: Pharmacological and Parenteral Therapies
CNS: Adverse Effects/Contraindications/Side Effects/Interactions
CL: Applying

62. Correct Answer: C. One type of Parkinsonian medication is a COMT (catechol-O-methyltransferase) inhibitor. This class of medication is commonly used in the treatment of Parkinson disease and is known to change the urine color to a brownish-orange. This is the most likely cause of the urine color.

    CN: Pharmacological and Parenteral Therapies

    CNS: Adverse Effects/Contraindications/Side Effects/Interactions

    CL: Applying

63. Correct Answer C. Many over-the-counter and herbal preparations interfere with phenytoin. The client needs additional education to discuss this with the provider to evaluate for safety. Some herbal supplements can decrease the effectiveness of phenytoin, which could lead to seizure activity. All other statements are accurate.

    CN: Pharmacological and Parenteral Therapies

    CNS: Adverse Effects/Contraindications/Side Effects/Interactions

    CL: Applying

64. Correct Answer: B. When administering ear drops to a child, pull the bottom of the ear down and back, away from the body. It is not necessary to wait 3 to 5 minutes between each ear drop. However, it is important to keep the head tilted for 2 to 5 minutes to help with absorption.

    CN: Pharmacological and Parenteral Therapies

    CNS: Medication Administration

    CL: Applying

65. Correct Answer: A, B, C. Mydriatics and cycloplegics are used to perform diagnostic eye examinations, for procedures on the eye, and are also used to treat conditions involving the iris. Mydriatics dilate the eye and cycloplegics temporarily paralyze the eye muscles. Mydriatics and cycloplegics are not used to treat open-angle glaucoma or bacterial eye infections.

    CN: Pharmacological and Parenteral Therapies

    CNS: Adverse Effects/Contraindications/Side Effects/Interactions

    CL: Applying

66. Correct Answer: A. If more than one eye medication is prescribed, wait 3 to 5 minutes before instilling the next type of medication to allow for proper dosing and absorption. Contact lenses should be removed prior to administration of eye drops. The dropper should never touch the eye. While medication can be blotted near the eye to remove excess, avoid wiping the eyelid or on the eye to all as much medication to absorb into the eye as possible.

    CN: Pharmacological and Parenteral Therapies

    CNS: Medication Administration

    CL: Understanding

67. Correct Answer. A. Neomycin/polymyxin B/hydrocortisone otic may cause ototoxicity. It does not cause nephrotoxicity, hepatotoxicity, or cataracts.

    CN: Pharmacological and Parenteral Therapies
    CNS: Adverse Effects/Contraindications/Side Effects/Interactions
    CL: Understanding

68. Correct Answer: C. Carbamide peroxide (Debrox) is a ceruminolytic that releases oxygen to soften and help remove ear wax. Pilocarpine, mannitol, and tafluprost are not used for ear wax removal.

    CN: Pharmacological and Parenteral Therapies
    CNS: Adverse Effects/Contraindications/Side Effects/Interactions
    CL: Understanding

69. Correct Answer: A. When administering ear drops to an adult, pull the ear up and back, away from the body.

    CN: Pharmacological and Parenteral Therapies
    CNS: Medication Administration
    CL: Understanding

70. Correct Answer: B. Osmotic agents reduce the volume of vitreous humor and decrease IOP by elevating the glomerular filtrate osmolarity.

    CN: Pharmacological and Parenteral Therapies
    CNS: Adverse Effects/Contraindications/Side Effects/Interactions
    CL: Understanding

71. Correct Answer: A. Live attenuated influenza vaccines (LAIV) should be avoided for 2 weeks before and at least 48 hours after administration of peramivir, oseltamivir, or zanamivir due to their antiviral properties. All other time frames are incorrect.

    CN: Pharmacological and Parenteral Therapies
    CNS: Adverse Effects/Contraindications/Side Effects/Interactions
    CL: Remembering

72. Correct Answer: B. Hypoglycemia is a common side effect of sulfonamides. Hypotension, hyperglycemia, and hypertension are not expected side effects.

    CN: Pharmacological and Parenteral Therapies
    CNS: Adverse Effects/Contraindications/Side Effects/Interactions
    CL: Understanding

73. Correct Answer: C. The combination of levofloxacin and amiodarone increases the risk for QT prolongation, which can lead to dangerous cardiac arrhythmias. The same reaction is not expected when taking levofloxacin with tamsulosin, levothyroxine, or allopurinol.

    CN: Pharmacological and Parenteral Therapies
    CNS: Adverse Effects/Contraindications/Side Effects/Interactions
    CL: Applying

74. Correct Answer: A. Vancomycin is considered the gold standard treatment for clients newly diagnosed with *C. difficile*. Metronidazole, doxycycline, and cefuroxime are not used for this purpose.

    CN: Pharmacological and Parenteral Therapies
    CNS: Medication Administration
    CL: Understanding

75. Correct Answer: D. The effectiveness of hormonal contraceptives is reduced when taking penicillin so a back-up form of birth control should be used. An increase in acne and photosensitivity are not expected. The entire course of antibiotics must be taken to ensure eradication of the bacteria; the drug should not be stopped when feeling better.

    CN: Pharmacological and Parenteral Therapies
    CNS: Adverse Effects/Contraindications/Side Effects/Interactions
    CL: Applying

Appendices and index

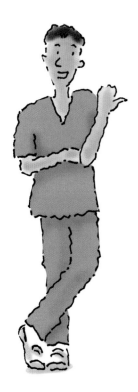

Emergency drugs, herbs/supplements, and vaccines

Emergency drugs

There are numerous drugs that are used emergently to treat a multitude of conditions. Often these drugs are kept in a "crash cart," a moveable collection of drugs and equipment that can be used in case of an emergency. Carts are often designed in keeping with the population they are meant to serve (for example, adult or pediatric) and contain many of the same medications, despite there not being a universal requirement regarding how a crash cart is stocked. The Joint Commission (2017) recommends that crash carts have the following contents related to medication:

- Drugs that are clearly labeled by name and arranged so they are easy to locate.
- Segregated pediatric medications (if a crash cart is shared for treating adults and children); these drugs can be placed in a plastic bag or in a completely different drawer than adult medications. Regardless of placement, clear labeling must be present to identify these drugs as pediatric.
- References for medication and proper medication doses for adult and pediatric emergencies. Again, all references must be clearly labeled.

Common drugs included in a crash cart include:

- adenosine
- albuterol
- amiodarone
- atropine
- calcium chloride
- dexamethasone
- diphenhydramine
- dobutamine
- epinephrine
- etomidate
- furosemide
- glucagon
- glucose
- hydralazine
- hydrocortisone
- ipratropium
- isoproterenol

- labetalol
- levetiracetam
- magnesium
- metoprolol
- naloxone
- nicardipine
- norepinephrine
- oxytocin
- phenylephrine
- phenytoin
- procainamide
- pyridoxine
- racemic epinephrine
- sodium bicarbonate
- thiamine
- thyroxine
- valproate
- verapamil
- vecuronium.

References

Jacquet, G., Hamade, B., Diab, K., Sawaya, R., Dagher, G., Hitti, E., & Bayram, J. (2018). The emergency department crash cart: A systematic review and suggested contents. *World Journal of Emergency Medicine, 9*(2), 93–98.

The Joint Commission. (2021). What are the Joint Commission's requirements and recommendations regarding crash carts? *Environment of Care News (EC News), 24*(7), 19–22. Retrieved from https://store.jcrinc.com/assets/1/7/ECN_24_2021_07.pdf

The Joint Commission. (2017). Crash cart preparedness. *Quick Safety, 32*, 1–3. Retrieved from https://www.jointcommission.org/-/media/tjc/documents/newsletters/quick_safety_issue_32_20171pdf.pdf

Herbal supplements

Encourage the client to discuss herbal supplements with their health care provider before using, especially if the individual has an acute or chronic health condition. Many common herbal supplements should be avoided when the individual is pregnant or lactating. The National Institute of Complementary and Integrative Health (2021) provides current research on efficacy on selected herbal supplements. The nurse needs to be well informed about herbal supplements before recommending their use to clients as common uses may not be supported by evidence. Information about specific herbs can be located at https://www.nccih.nih.gov/health/herbsataglance. This resource provides basic information about major herbal supplements commonly taken orally.

Vaccines

You can view the CDC Vaccine Schedules for "Recommended Child and Adolescent Immunization Schedule for ages 18 years or younger (2021) https://www.cdc.gov/vaccines/schedules/hcp/imz/child-adolescent.html" and "Recommended Adult Immunization Schedule for ages 19 years or older (2021) https://www.cdc.gov/vaccines/schedules/hcp/imz/adult.html"

Abbreviations to avoid

The Joint Commission has created an official "Do Not Use" list of abbreviations. In addition, the Institute for Safe Medicine Practices (ISMP) offers suggestions for other abbreviations and symbols to avoid.

The Joint Commission's Official "Do Not Use" List*

Do Not Use	Potential Problem	Use Instead
U, u (unit)	Mistaken for "0" (zero), the number "4" (four) or "cc"	Write "unit"
IU (International Unit)	Mistaken for "IV" (intravenous) or the number "10" (ten)	Write "International Unit"
Q.D., QD, q.d., qd (daily)	Mistaken for each other	Write "daily"
Q.O.D., QOD, q.o.d., qod (every other day)	Period after the Q mistaken for "I" and the "O" mistaken for "I"	Write "every other day"
Trailing zero (X.0 mg)† Lack of leading zero (.X mg)	Decimal point is missed	Write X mg Write 0.X mg
MS	Can mean morphine sulfate or magnesium sulfate	Write "morphine sulfate"
MSO₄ and MgSO₄	Confused for one another	Write "magnesium sulfate"

*Applies to all orders and all medication-related documentation that is handwritten (including free-text computer entry) or on preprinted forms.

†**Exception:** A "trailing zero" may be used only where required to demonstrate the level of precision of the value being reported, such as for laboratory results, imaging studies that report size of lesions, or catheter/tube sizes. It may not be used in medication orders or other medication-related documents.

ISMP list of error–prone abbreviations, symbols and dose designations

Error-prone abbreviations, symbols, and dose designations	Intended meaning	Misinterpretation	Best practice
Abbreviations for doses/measurement units			
cc	Cubic centimeters	Mistaken as u (units)	Use mL
IU*	International unit(s)	Mistaken as IV (intravenous) or the number 10	Use unit(s) (International units can be expressed as units alone)
l	Liter	Lowercase letter l mistaken as the number 1	Use L (UPPERCASE) for liter
ml	Milliliter		Use mL (lowercase m, UPPERCASE L) for milliliter
MM or M	Million	Mistaken as thousand	Use million
M or K	Thousand	Mistaken as million	Use thousand
		M has been used to abbreviate both million and thousand (M is the Roman numeral for thousand)	

(*continued*)

ISMP list of error-prone abbreviations, symbols and dose designations *(continued)*

Error-prone abbreviations, symbols, and dose designations	Intended meaning	Misinterpretation	Best practice
Ng or ng	Nanogram	Mistaken as mg Mistaken as nasogastric	Use nanogram or nanog
U or u*	Unit(s)	Mistaken as zero or the number 4, causing a 10-fold overdose or greater (e.g., 4U seen as 40 or 4u seen as 44) Mistaken as cc, leading to administering volume instead of units (e.g., 4u seen as 4cc)	Use unit(s)
μg	Microgram	Mistaken as mg	Use mcg
Abbreviations for Route of Administration			
AD, AS, AU	Right ear, left ear, each ear	Mistaken as OD, OS, OU (right eye, left eye, each eye)	Use right ear, left ear, or each ear
IN	Intranasal	Mistaken as IM or IV	Use NAS (all UPPERCASE letters) or intranasal
IT	Intrathecal	Mistaken as intratracheal, intratumor, intratympanic, or inhalation therapy	Use intrathecal
OD, OS, OU	Right eye, left eye, each eye	Mistaken as AD, AS, AU (right ear, left ear, each ear)	Use right eye, left eye, or each eye
Per os	By mouth, orally	The os was mistaken as left eye (OS, oculus sinister)	Use PO, by mouth, or orally
SC, SQ, sq, or sub q	Subcutaneous(ly)	SC and sc mistaken as SL or sl (sublingual) SQ mistaken as "5 every" The q in sub q has been mistaken as "every"	Use SUBQ (all UPPERCASE letters, without spaces or periods between letters) or subcutaneous(ly)
Abbreviations for frequency/instructions for use			
HS hs	Half-strength At bedtime, hours of sleep	Mistaken as bedtime Mistaken as half-strength	Use half-strength Use HS (all UPPERCASE letters) for bedtime
o.d. or OD	Once daily	Mistaken as right eye (OD, oculus dexter), leading to oral liquid medications administered in the eye	Use daily
Q.D., QD, q.d., or qd*	Every day	Mistaken as q.i.d., especially if the period after the q or the tail of a handwritten q is misunderstood as the letter i	Use daily

ISMP list of error-prone abbreviations, symbols and dose designations *(continued)*

Error-prone abbreviations, symbols, and dose designations	Intended meaning	Misinterpretation	Best practice
Qhs	Nightly at bedtime	Mistaken as qhr (every hour)	Use nightly or HS for bedtime
Qn	Nightly or at bedtime	Mistaken as qh (every hour)	Use nightly or HS for bedtime
Q.O.D., QOD, q.o.d., or qod*	Every other day	Mistaken as qd (daily) or qid (four times daily), especially if the "o" is poorly written	Use every other day
q1d	Daily	Mistaken as qid (four times daily)	Use daily
q6PM, etc.	Every evening at 6 PM	Mistaken as every 6 hours	Use daily at 6 PM or 6 PM daily
SSRI	Sliding scale regular insulin	Mistaken as selective serotonin reuptake inhibitor	Use sliding scale (insulin)
SSI	Sliding scale insulin	Mistaken as Strong Solution of Iodine (Lugol's)	
TIW or tiw	3 times a week	Mistaken as 3 times a day or twice in a week	Use 3 times weekly
BIW or biw	2 times a week	Mistaken as 2 times a day	Use 2 times weekly
UD	As directed (ut dictum)	Mistaken as unit dose (for example, an order for "dil**TIAZ**em infusion UD" was mistakenly administered as a unit [bolus] dose)	Use as directed
Miscellaneous abbreviations associated with medication use			
BBA	Baby boy A (twin)	B in BBA mistaken as twin B rather than gender (boy)	When assigning identifiers to newborns, use the mother's last name, the baby's gender (boy or girl), and a distinguishing identifier for all multiples (for example, Smith girl A, Smith girl B)
BGB	Baby girl B (twin)	B at end of BGB mistaken as gender (boy) not twin B	
D/C	Discharge or discontinue	Premature discontinuation of medications when D/C (intended to mean discharge) on a medication list was misinterpreted as discontinued	Use discharge and discontinue or stop
IJ	Injection	Mistaken as IV or intrajugular	Use injection
OJ	Orange juice	Mistaken as OD or OS (right or left eye); drugs meant to be diluted in orange juice may be given in the eye	Use orange juice
Period following abbreviations (for example, mg., mL.)†	mg or mL	Unnecessary period mistaken as the number 1, especially if written poorly	Use mg, mL, etc., without a terminal period

(continued)

ISMP list of error-prone abbreviations, symbols and dose designations *(continued)*

Error-prone abbreviations, symbols, and dose designations	Intended meaning	Misinterpretation	Best practice
		Drug name abbreviations	
To prevent confusion, avoid abbreviating drug names entirely. Exceptions may be made for multi-ingredient drug formulations, including vitamins, when there are electronic drug name field space constraints; however, drug name abbreviations should NEVER be used for any medications on the *ISMP List of High-Alert Medications* (in Acute Care Settings, Community/Ambulatory Settings, and Long-Term Care Settings). Examples of drug name abbreviations involved in serious medication errors include:			
Antiretroviral medications (for example, DOR, TAF, TDF)	DOR: doravirine	DOR: Dovato (dolutegravir and lami**VUD**ine)	Use complete drug names
	TAF: tenofovir alafenamide	TAF: tenofovir disoproxil fumarate	
	TDF: tenofovir disoproxil fumarate	TDF: tenofovir alafenamide	
APAP	Acetaminophen	Not recognized as acetaminophen	Use complete drug name
ARA A	Vidarabine	Mistaken as cytarabine ("ARA C")	Use complete drug name
AT II and AT III	AT II: angiotensin II (Giapreza)	AT II (angiotensin II) mistaken as AT III (antithrombin III)	Use complete drug names
	AT III: antithrombin III (Thrombate III)	AT III (antithrombin III) mistaken as AT II (angiotensin II)	
AZT	Zidovudine (Retrovir)	Mistaken as azithromycin, aza**THIO**prine, or aztreonam	Use complete drug name
CPZ	Compazine (prochlorperazine)	Mistaken as chlorpro**MAZINE**	Use complete drug name
DTO	Diluted tincture of opium or deodorized tincture of opium (Paregoric)	Mistaken as tincture of opium	Use complete drug name
HCT	Hydrocortisone	Mistaken as hydro**CHLORO**thiazide	Use complete drug name
HCTZ	Hydro**CHLORO**thiazide	Mistaken as hydrocortisone (for example, seen as HCT250 mg)	Use complete drug name
$MgSO_4$*	magnesium sulfate	Mistaken as morphine sulfate	Use complete drug name
MS, MSO4*	morphine sulfate	Mistaken as magnesium sulfate	Use complete drug name
MTX	Methotrexate	Mistaken as mito**XANTRONE**	Use complete drug name
Na at the beginning of a drug name (for example, Na bicarbonate)	Sodium bicarbonate	Mistaken as no bicarbonate	Use complete drug name
NoAC	Novel/new oral anticoagulant	Mistaken as no anticoagulant	Use complete drug name

ISMP list of error-prone abbreviations, symbols and dose designations *(continued)*

Error-prone abbreviations, symbols, and dose designations	Intended meaning	Misinterpretation	Best practice
OXY	Oxytocin	Mistaken as oxy**CODONE**, Oxy**CONTIN**	Use complete drug name
PCA	Procainamide	Mistaken as patient-controlled analgesia	Use complete drug name
PIT	Pitocin (oxytocin)	Mistaken as Pitressin, a discontinued brand of vasopressin still referred to as PIT	Use complete drug name
PNV	Prenatal vitamins	Mistaken as penicillin VK	Use complete drug name
PTU	Propylthiouracil	Mistaken as Purinethol (mercaptopurine)	Use complete drug name
T3	Tylenol with codeine No. 3	Mistaken as liothyronine, which is sometimes referred to as T3	Use complete drug name
TAC or tac	Triamcinolone or tacrolimus	Mistaken as tetracaine, Adrenaline, and cocaine; or as Taxotere, Adriamycin, and Cyclophosphamide	Use complete drug names Avoid drug regimen or protocol acronyms that may have a dual meaning or may be confused with other common acronyms, even if defined in an order set
TNK	TNKase	Mistaken as TPA	Use complete drug name
TPA or tPA	Tissue plasminogen activator, Activase (alteplase)	Mistaken as TNK (TNKase, tenecteplase), TXA (tranexamic acid), or less often as another tissue plasminogen activator, Retavase (reteplase)	Use complete drug name
TXA	Tranexamic acid	Mistaken as TPA (tissue plasminogen activator)	Use complete drug name
ZnSO4	Zinc sulfate	Mistaken as morphine sulfate	Use complete drug name
Stemmed/coined drug names			
Nitro drip	Nitroglycerin infusion	Mistaken as nitroprusside infusion	Use complete drug name
IV vanc	Intravenous vancomycin	Mistaken as Invanz	Use complete drug name
Levo	levofloxacin	Mistaken as Levophed (norepinephrine)	Use complete drug name
Neo	Neo-Synephrine, a well known but discontinued brand of phenylephrine	Mistaken as neostigmine	Use complete drug name

(continued)

ISMP list of error-prone abbreviations, symbols and dose designations *(continued)*

Error-prone abbreviations, symbols, and dose designations	Intended meaning	Misinterpretation	Best practice
Coined names for compounded products (for example, magic mouthwash, banana bag, GI cocktail, half and half, pink lady)	Specific ingredients compounded together	Mistaken ingredients	Use complete drug/product names for all ingredients Coined names for compounded products should only be used if the contents are standardized and readily available for reference to prescribers, pharmacists, and nurses
Number embedded in drug name (not part of the official name) (for example, 5-fluorouracil, 6-mercaptopurine)	fluorouracil mercaptopurine	Embedded number mistaken as the dose or number of tablets/capsules to be administered	Use complete drug names, without an embedded number if the number is not part of the official drug name
Dose designations and other information			
1/2 tablet	Half tablet	1 or 2 tablets	Use text (half tablet) or reduced font-size fractions (½ tablet)
Doses expressed as Roman numerals (for example, V)	5	Mistaken as the designated letter (for example, the letter V) or the wrong numeral (for example, 10 instead of 5)	Use only Arabic numerals (for example, 1, 2, 3) to express doses
Lack of a leading zero before a decimal point (e.g., .5 mg)*	0.5 mg	Mistaken as 5 mg if the decimal point is not seen	Use a leading zero before a decimal point when the dose is less than one measurement unit
Trailing zero after a decimal point (e.g., 1.0 mg)*	1 mg	Mistaken as 10 mg if the decimal point is not seen	Do not use trailing zeros for doses expressed in whole numbers
Ratio expression of a strength of a single-entity injectable drug product (for example, **EPINEPH**rine 1:1,000; 1:10,000; 1:100,000)	1:1,000: contains 1 mg/mL 1:10,000: contains 0.1 mg/mL 1:100,000: contains 0.01 mg/mL	Mistaken as the wrong strength	Express the strength in terms of quantity per total volume (for example, **EPINEPH**rine 1 mg per 10 mL) **Exception:** combination local anesthetics (for example, lidocaine 1% and **EPINEPH**rine 1:100,000)
Drug name and dose run together (problematic for drug names that end in the letter l [for example, propranolol20 mg; **TEG**retol300 mg])	Propranolol 20 mg **TEG**retol 300 mg	Mistaken as propranolol 120 mg Mistaken as **TEG**retol 1300 mg	Place adequate space between the drug name, dose, and unit of measure

ISMP list of error-prone abbreviations, symbols and dose designations *(continued)*

Error-prone abbreviations, symbols, and dose designations	Intended meaning	Misinterpretation	Best practice
Numerical dose and unit of measure run together (for example, 10mg, 10Units)	10 mg 10 mL	The m in mg, or U in Units, has been mistaken as one or two zeros when flush against the dose (for example, 10mg, 10Units), risking a 10- to 100-fold overdose	Place adequate space between the dose and unit of measure
Large doses without properly placed commas (for example, 100000 units; 1000000 units)	100,000 units	100000 has been mistaken as 10,000 or 1,000,000	Use commas for dosing units at or above 1,000 or use words such as 100 thousand or 1 million to improve readability
	1,000,000 units	1000000 has been mistaken as 100,000	**Note**: Use commas to separate digits only in the United States; commas are used in place of decimal points in some other countries
Symbols			
ʒ or	Dram	Symbol for dram mistaken as the number 3	Use the metric system
♏︎†	Minim	Symbol for minim mistaken as mL	
x1	Administer once	Administer for 1 day	Use explicit words (for example, for 1 dose)
> and <	More than and less than	Mistaken as opposite of intended	Use more than or less than
		Mistakenly have used the incorrect symbol	
		< mistaken as the number 4 when handwritten (for example, <10 misread as 40)	
↑ and ↓†	Increase and decrease	Mistaken as opposite of intended	Use increase and decrease
		Mistakenly have used the incorrect symbol	
		↑ mistaken as the letter T, leading to misinterpretation as the start of a drug name, or mistaken as the numbers 4 or 7	
/ (slash mark)†	Separates two doses or indicates per	Mistaken as the number 1 (for example, 25 units/10 units misread as 25 units and 110 units)	Use per rather than a slash mark to separate doses

(continued)

ISMP list of error-prone abbreviations, symbols and dose designations *(continued)*

Error-prone abbreviations, symbols, and dose designations	Intended meaning	Misinterpretation	Best practice
@†	At	Mistaken as the number 2	Use at
&†	And	Mistaken as the number 2	Use and
+†	Plus or and	Mistaken as the number 4	Use plus, and, or in addition to
°	Hour	Mistaken as a zero (for example, q2° seen as q20)	Use hr, h, or hour
Φ or ⊘†	Zero, null sign	Mistaken as the numbers 4, 6, 8, and 9	Use 0 or zero, or describe intent using whole words
#	Pound(s)	Mistaken as a number sign	Use the metric system (kg or g) rather than pounds
			Use lb if referring to pounds

Apothecary or household abbreviations			
*Explicit apothecary or household measurements may **ONLY** be safely used to express the directions for mixing dry ingredients to prepare topical products (for example, dissolve 2 capfuls of granules per gallon of warm water to prepare a magnesium sulfate soaking aid). Otherwise, metric system measurements should be used.*			
gr	Grain(s)	Mistaken as gram	Use the metric system (for example, mcg, g)
dr	Dram(s)	Mistaken as doctor	Use the metric system (for example, mL)
min	Minim(s)	Mistaken as minutes	Use the metric system (for example, mL)
oz	Ounce(s)	Mistaken as zero or 02	Use the metric system (for example, mL)
tsp	Teaspoon(s)	Mistaken as tablespoon(s)	Use the metric system (for example, mL)
tbsp or Tbsp	Tablespoon(s)	Mistaken as teaspoon(s)	Use the metric system (for example, mL)

Common Abbreviations with Contradictory Meanings	Contradictory Meanings		Correction
For additional information and tables from Neil Davis (MedAbbrev.com) containing additional examples of abbreviations with contradictory or ambiguous meanings, please visit: www.ismp.org/ext/6 8.			
B	Breast, brain, or bladder		Use breast, brain, or bladder
C	Cerebral, coronary, or carotid		Use cerebral, coronary, or carotid
D or d	Day or dose (for example, parameter-based dosing formulas using D or d [mg/kg/day] could be interpreted as either day or dose [mg/kg/day or mg/kg/dose]; or ×3 day could be interpreted as either 3 days or 3 doses)		Use day or dose

ISMP list of error-prone abbreviations, symbols and dose designations *(continued)*

Common Abbreviations with Contradictory Meanings	Contradictory Meanings	Correction
H	Hand or hip	Use hand or hip
I	Impaired or improvement	Use impaired or improvement
L	Liver or lung	Use liver or lung
N	No or normal	Use no or normal
P	Pancreas, prostate, preeclampsia, or psychosis	Use pancreas, prostate, preeclampsia, or psychosis
S	Special or standard	Use special or standard
SS or ss	Single strength, sliding scale (insulin), signs and symptoms, or ½ (apothecary) SS has also been mistaken as the number 55	Use single strength, sliding scale, signs and symptoms, or one-half or ½

* On The Joint Commission's "Do Not Use" list.

†Relevant mostly in handwritten medication information.

Institute for Safe Medication Practices. (2021). *List of error-prone abbreviations.* Retrieved from https://www.ismp.org/recommendations/error-prone-abbreviations-list

Glossary

acetylcholinesterase inhibitor: drug that increases parasympathetic activity and blocks the action of acetylcholinesterase, an enzyme that inhibits the action of acetylcholine

action potential: electrical impulse across nerve or muscle fibers that have been stimulated

adrenergic agonist: drug that mimics the effects of the sympathetic nervous system

adrenergic blocking drug: drug that interferes with transmission of nerve impulses to adrenergic receptors, allowing a parasympathetic response

agonist: drug that produces an effect similar to those produced by naturally occurring hormones, neurotransmitters, and other substances

agranulocytosis: severe and acute decrease in granulocytes (basophils, eosinophils, and neutrophils) as an adverse reaction to a drug or radiation therapy; results in high fever, exhaustion, and bleeding ulcers of the throat, mucous membranes, and GI tract

allergen: substance that induces an allergy or a hypersensitivity reaction

analgesia: loss of pain sensation

anaphylaxis: severe allergic reaction to a foreign substance

androgens: male sex hormones, primarily testosterone, secreted by the testes in men, the ovaries in women, and the adrenal cortex in both sexes

angioedema: life-threatening reaction causing sudden swelling of tissues around the face, neck, lips, tongue, throat, hands, feet, genitals, or intestines

antibody: immunoglobulin molecule that reacts only with the specific antigen that induced its formation in the lymph system

anticoagulant drug: drug that prevents clot formation or extension but doesn't speed dissolution of existing clots

antigen: foreign substance (such as bacteria or toxins) that induces antibody formation

antilipemic drug: drug used to prevent or treat increased accumulation of fatty substances (lipids) in the blood

antipyretic: pertaining to a substance that reduces fever

ataxia: incoordination of voluntary muscle action, particularly in activities as walking and reaching for objects

automaticity: ability of a cardiac cell to initiate an impulse on its own

bactericidal: causing death of bacteria

bioavailability: rate and extent to which a drug enters the circulation, thereby gaining access to target tissue

blood-brain barrier: barrier separating the parenchyma of the central nervous system from the circulating blood, preventing certain substances from reaching the brain or cerebrospinal fluid

body surface area (BSA): area covered by a person's external skin that's calculated in square meters (m^2) according to height and weight; used to calculate safe pediatric dosages for all drugs and safe dosages for adult patients receiving extremely potent drugs or drugs requiring great precision, such as antineoplastic and chemotherapeutic agents

bradykinesia: abnormally slow body movement

bronchospasm: narrowing of the bronchioles resulting from an increase in smooth muscle tone that causes wheezing

cerebral edema: increased fluid content in the brain; may result from correcting hypernatremia too rapidly

chemoreceptor trigger zone: center in the medulla of the brain that controls vomiting

conduction: transmission of electrical impulses through the myocardium

conductivity: ability of one cardiac cell to transmit an electrical impulse to another cell

contractility: ability of a cardiac cell to contract after receiving an impulse

cross-sensitivity: hypersensitivity or allergy to a drug in a particular class (e.g., penicillin) that may cause an allergic reaction to another drug in the same class

cytotoxic: destructive to cells

debriding drug: drug used to remove foreign material and dead or damaged tissue from a wound or burn

depolarization: response of a myocardial cell to an electrical impulse that causes movement of ions across the cell membrane, triggering myocardial contraction

diastole: phase of the cardiac cycle when both atria (atrial diastole) or both ventricles (ventricular diastole) are at rest and filling with blood

diplopia: double vision

directly observed therapy (DOT): a method of ensuring compliance with antitubercular therapy; a health care provider (or other responsible adult) directly observes the patient taking each dose of an antitubercular drug; recommended for all antitubercular drug regimens, it is considered mandatory in intermittent schedules and regimens for multidrug-resistant tuberculosis

dosage: the amount, frequency, and number of doses of a drug

dose: the amount of a drug to be given at one time

drip factor: number of drops to be delivered per milliliter of solution in an IV administration set; measured in drops per milliliter (gtt/mL); listed on the package containing the IV tubing administration set

drip rate: number of drops of IV solution to be infused per minute; based on the drip factor and calibrated for the selected IV tubing

emesis: act or instance of vomiting

excitability: ability of a cardiac cell to respond to an electrical stimulus

extrapyramidal symptoms: symptoms caused by an imbalance in the extrapyramidal portion of the nervous system; typically include pill-rolling motions, drooling, tremors, rigidity, and shuffling gait

extravasation: leakage of intravascular fluid into surrounding tissue; can be caused by such medications as chemotherapeutic drugs, dopamine, and calcium solutions that produce blistering and, eventually, tissue necrosis

flow rate: the number of milliliters of IV fluid to administer over 1 hour; based on the total volume to be infused in milliliters and the amount of time for the infusion

hepatotoxicity: quality of being toxic to or capable of destroying liver cells

hirsutism: excessive growth of dark, coarse body hair in a masculine distribution

histamine-2 (H-2) receptor: cells in the gastric mucosa that respond to histamine release by increasing gastric acid secretion

inhalation drug: drug that affects the respiratory tract locally; may be administered by handheld nebulizer, intermittent positive pressure breathing apparatus, nasal spray, or nose drops

insomnia: inability to sleep, sleep interrupted by periods of wakefulness, or sleep that ends prematurely

intradermal route (ID): drug administration into the dermis of the skin

intramuscular route (IM): drug administration into a muscle

intravenous route (IV): drug administration into a vein

ischemia: decreased blood supply to a body organ or tissue

leukocytosis: abnormal increase in circulating white blood cells

leukopenia: decrease in the number of white blood cell count

lipodystrophy: abnormal amount or distribution of adipose (fat) tissue

milliequivalent (mEq): one thousandth of an equivalent of a chemical element, radical, or compound

mydriasis: dilation of the pupil of the eye

necrotic: adjective describing premature cell death

nephrotoxicity: quality of being toxic to or capable of destroying kidney cells

neutropenia: abnormal decrease in circulating neutrophils

nonparenteral drug: drug administered by the oral, topical, or rectal route

nystagmus: involuntary eye movement

oral route (PO): drug administration through the mouth

ototoxicity: potentially irreversible damage to the auditory and vestibular branches of the eighth cranial nerve; may cause hearing or balance loss

pancytopenia: abnormal decrease in erythrocytes, white blood cells, and platelets

parasympatholytic drug: drug that blocks the effects of the parasympathetic nervous system, allowing a sympathetic response

parasympathomimetic drug: drug that mimics the effects of the parasympathetic nervous system

parenteral route: drug administration through a route other than the digestive tract, such as intravenous, intramuscular, and subcutaneous

paresthesia: abnormal sensations (including numbness, prickling, and tingling) with no known cause

paroxysmal: episode of something that starts and stops; recurrent

peak and trough drug concentration levels: serum drug concentration levels measured to determine whether the dosing regimen is therapeutic or toxic. Blood for peak concentration level is drawn at least 1 hour after the dose is completely administered; blood for trough concentration level is drawn just before the next dose is administered.

phlebitis: inflammation of a vein

photosensitivity reaction: increased reaction of the skin to sunlight; may result in edema, papules, urticaria, or acute burns

potentiate: to increase the action of another drug so that the combined effect of both drugs is greater than the sum of the effect of either drug alone

pruritus: itching

rectal route: drug administration (usually by suppository) through the rectum

refractory period: period of relaxation after muscle excitement

renin: enzyme secreted by the kidneys in response to an actual or perceived decline in extracellular fluid volume or decreased sodium level; important part of blood pressure regulation

repolarization: recovery of the myocardial cells after depolarization during which the cell membrane returns to its resting potential

rhabdomyolysis: acute and potentially fatal skeletal muscle disease

sedative-hypnotic drug: drug that exerts a tranquilizing effect while dulling the senses or inducing sleep

serotonin: neurotransmitter that affects functions such as mood and sleep

serum drug level: amount of a drug present in the blood at a given moment

status epilepticus: rapid succession of seizures without intervals of consciousness; constitutes a medical emergency

stomatitis: inflammation and ulceration of the mucous membranes of the mouth

subcutaneous route (subcut): drug administration into the subcutaneous tissue

sulfonamides: bacteriostatic agents that are used against a wide range of gram-positive and gram-negative bacteria

superinfection: new infection that develops in addition to one that's already present

sympatholytic drug: drug that inhibits sympathetic activity; may block receptors or prevent release of norepinephrine

sympathomimetic drug: drug that mimics the effects of the sympathetic nervous system

systole: phase of the cardiac cycle during which both of the atria (atrial systole) or the ventricles (ventricular systole) are contracting

tardive dyskinesia: disorder characterized by involuntary repetitious movements of the muscles of the face, limbs, and trunk; most commonly results from treatment with antipsychotic drugs

teratogenic: pertaining to the production of physical defects in an embryo or a fetus

thrombocytopenia: abnormal decrease in platelets, predisposing the patient to bleeding

thrombolytic drug: drug that dissolves a thrombus by activating plasminogen and converting it to plasmin

tophi: deposits of uric acid crystals in the joints, kidneys, and soft tissues

topical route: drug administration that works on the skin's surface usually in cream, ointment, or transdermal patch form

transdermal route: drug administration through the skin by which the drug is absorbed continuously and enter systemic circulation

United States Pharmacopeia (USP): compendium of drugs and their preparations that's issued annually by a national committee of experts

urticaria: itchy skin inflammation characterized by pale wheals with well-defined red edges; usually an allergic response to insect bites, food, or certain drugs; also called *hives*

vasopressor: drug that stimulates contraction of the muscle tissue of the capillaries and arteries

viral load: a measure of the amount of virus that can be detected in the blood of a person who is infected.

viscosity: state of being sticky

withdrawal symptoms: unpleasant and sometimes life-threatening physiologic changes occurring when certain drugs are withdrawn after prolonged, regular use

Index